GASTROINTESTINAL AND LIVER PATHOLOGY

Other books in this series:

 Busam: *Dermatopathology,*
978-0-443-06654-2

 Folpe & Inwards: *Bone and Soft Tissue Pathology,*
978-0-443-06688-7

 Hsi: *Hematopathology,*
978-0-443-06830-0

 Nucci & Oliva: *Gynecologic Pathology,*
978-0-443-06920-8

 O'Malley & Pinder: *Breast Pathology, 2e,*
978-1-4377-1750-0

 Prayson: *Neuropathology,*
978-0-443-06658-0

 Sidawy & Ali: *Fine Needle Aspiration Cytology,*
978-0-443-06731-0

 Thompson: *Endocrine Pathology,*
978-0-443-06685-6

 Thompson: *Head and Neck Pathology,*
978-0-443-06960-4

 Tubbs & Stoler: *Cell and Tissue Based Molecular Pathology,*
978-0-443-06901-7

 Zander & Farver: *Pulmonary Pathology,*
978-0-443-06741-9

 Zhou & Magi-Galluzzi: *Genitourinary Pathology,*
978-0-443-06677-1

GASTROINTESTINAL AND LIVER PATHOLOGY

A Volume in the Series
FOUNDATIONS IN DIAGNOSTIC PATHOLOGY
SECOND EDITION

EDITED BY

Christine A. Iacobuzio-Donahue, MD, PhD
Associate Professor of Pathology, Oncology, and Surgery
Johns Hopkins Medical Institutions
Department of Pathology
Division of Gastrointestinal and Liver Pathology
Baltimore, Maryland

Elizabeth Montgomery, MD
Professor of Pathology, Oncology, and Orthopedic Surgery
Johns Hopkins Medical Institutions
Department of Pathology
Division of Gastrointestinal and Liver Pathology
Baltimore, Maryland

SERIES EDITOR

John R. Goldblum, MD, FCAP, FASCP, FACG
Chairman, Department of Anatomic Pathology
The Cleveland Clinic Foundation
Cleveland Clinic Lerner College of Medicine
Case Western Reserve University
Cleveland, Ohio

ELSEVIER
SAUNDERS

SAUNDERS

1600 John F. Kennedy Blvd.
Ste 1800
Philadelphia, PA 19103-2899

GASTROINTESTINAL AND LIVER PATHOLOGY, SECOND EDITION   ISBN: 978-1-4377-0925-4
(A Volume in the Series Foundations in Diagnostic Pathology
Series edited by John R. Goldblum, MD)

ISBN: 978-1-4377-0925-4

Executive Publisher: William Schmitt
Senior Developmental Editor: Andrew Hall
Publishing Services Manager: Anne Altepeter
Senior Project Manager: Beth Hayes
Project Manager: Cindy Thoms
Senior Book Designer: Lou Forgione

Printed in China

Last digit is the print number: 9 8 7 6 5 4 3 2 1

To Tim—my husband, my best friend, my constant supporter,
and the most decent person I have ever known
—CID

To Sasha, Peter Alex, Sean, and Jonathan
—EM

Contributors

Carol Adair, MD
Pathology Residency Program Director
Baylor University Medical Center
Dallas, Texas
Pathology of the Anus

Syed Z. Ali, MD
Professor, Departments of Pathology and Radiology
Johns Hopkins University School of Medicine
Attending, Department of Pathology
Johns Hopkins Hospital
Baltimore, Maryland
*Non-Neoplastic and Neoplastic Pathology of the
Pancreas*

Pedram Argani, MD
Department of Pathology
Johns Hopkins University School of Medicine
Staff Pathologist
Johns Hopkins Hospital
Baltimore, Maryland
*Pathology of the Gallbladder and Extrahepatic Bile
Ducts*

David Baewer, MD, PhD
Department of Pathology
Johns Hopkins Medical Institutions
Baltimore, Maryland
Pathology of the Anus

Baishali Bhattacharya, MD, MPH
Surgical and Gastroenterology Pathologist
Caris Life Sciences
Phoenix, Arizona
Non-Neoplastic Disorders of the Stomach

Toby C. Cornish, MD, PhD
Johns Hopkins Hospital
Department of Surgical Pathology
Baltimore, Maryland
Neoplasms of the Small Intestine

H. Parry Dilworth, MD
Abbott Northwestern Laboratories
Minneapolis, Minnesota
*Epithelial Neoplasms of the Stomach, Neoplasms of
the Small Intestine, Gastrointestinal Lymphoma*

Theresa S. Emory, MD
Clinical Associate Professor
Department of Pathology
East Tennessee State University
Quillen College of Medicine
Johnson City, Tennessee
Highlands Pathology Consultants
Bristol, Tennessee
Idiopathic Inflammatory Bowel Disease

James R. Eshleman, MD, PhD
Department of Pathology
Department of Oncology
Associate Director
Molecular Diagnostics Laboratory
Johns Hopkins Medical Institutions
Baltimore, Maryland
Molecular Diagnostics in Gastrointestinal Pathology

Hubert H. Fenton, MD
Mercy Hospital
Baltimore, Maryland
*Epithelial Neoplasms of the Stomach, Gastrointestinal
Lymphoma*

Cyril Fisher, MD, DSc, FRCPath
Professor of Tumor Pathology
Department of Histopathology
Consultant Pathologist
Institute of Cancer Research
Royal Marsden Hospital
London, United Kingdom
Gastrointestinal Mesenchymal Tumors

Baojin Fu, MD
Department of Pathology
Johns Hopkins Medical Institutions
Baltimore, Maryland
Non-Neoplastic Disorders of the Esophagus

Christopher D. Gocke, MD
Associate Professor of Pathology and Oncology
Director of Hematology Molecular Diagnostics
Johns Hopkins University School of Medicine
Baltimore, Maryland
Gastrointestinal Lymphoma

Joel K. Greenson, MD
Professor, Department of Pathology
University of Michigan Medical School
Director, Surgical Pathology Fellowship Program
Department of Pathology
University of Michigan Health System
Ann Arbor, Michigan
Inflammatory/Descriptive/Iatrogenic Colitides

Ralph H. Hruban, MD
Professor, Departments of Pathology and Oncology
Johns Hopkins University School of Medicine
Pathologist, Department of Pathology
Johns Hopkins Hospital
Baltimore, Maryland
*Non-Neoplastic and Neoplastic Pathology of the
Pancreas*

Christine A. Iacobuzio-Donahue, MD, PhD
Associate Professor of Pathology, Oncology,
and Surgery
Johns Hopkins Medical Institutions
Department of Pathology
Division of Gastrointestinal and Liver Pathology
Baltimore, Maryland
*Non-Neoplastic and Inflammatory Disorders of the
Small Bowel, Gastrointestinal Polyposis Syndromes,
Epithelial Neoplasms of the Colorectum*

Dora M. Lam-Himlin, MD
Assistant Professor of Laboratory Medicine and
Anatomic Pathology
Mayo Medical School
Senior Associate Consultant in Gastrointestinal
Pathology
Mayo Clinic Arizona
Scottsdale, Arizona
*Non-Neoplastic and Neoplastic Disorders of the
Appendix*

Laura W. Lamps, MD
Associate Professor of Pathology
Director of Surgical Pathology
Department of Pathology
University of Arkansas for Medical Sciences
Little Rock, Arkansas
Infectious Diseases of the Colon

Marc R. Lewin, MD
Propath Dermatology
Dallas, Texas
*Epithelial Neoplasms of the Stomach,
Gastrointestinal Lymphoma*

Elizabeth Montgomery, MD
Professor of Pathology, Oncology, and Orthopedic
Surgery
Johns Hopkins Medical Institutions
Department of Pathology
Division of Gastrointestinal and Liver Pathology
Baltimore, Maryland
*Tumors of the Esophagus, Non-Neoplastic and
Inflammatory Disorders of the Small Bowel,
Gastrointestinal Mesenchymal Tumors,
Non-Neoplastic and Neoplastic Disorders of the
Appendix*

Roger Klein Moreira, MD
Assistant Professor
Department of Pathology and Cell Biology
Columbia University College of Physicians
and Surgeons
New York, New York
*Metabolic and Toxic Conditions of the Liver,
Inflammatory and Infectious Diseases of the Liver,
Liver Neoplasms*

Shiyama Mudali, MD
Department of Pathology
Johns Hopkins Medical Institutions
Baltimore, Maryland
Gastrointestinal Lymphoma

Thong Nguyen, DO
Associate Pathologist
Alegent Health System
Omaha, Nebraska
Gastrointestinal Mesenchymal Tumors

Jason Y. Park, MD, PhD, FCAP
Assistant Professor, Department of Pathology
University of Texas Southwestern Medical Center
Associate Director
Advanced Diagnostics Laboratory
Children's Medical Center
Dallas, Texas
Epithelial Neoplasms of the Stomach

M. Eugenia Rueda-Pedraza, MD, Col. USMC
Clinical Assistant Professor
Department of Pathology
Uniformed Services University of the Health Sciences
Bethesda, Maryland
Chief, Department of Pathology
Heidelberg Military Hospital
Heidelberg, Germany
Non-Neoplastic Disorders of the Esophagus

Chanjuan Shi, MD, PhD
Assistant Professor
Vanderbilt University
Department of Pathology
Nashville, Tennessee
Non-Neoplastic and Inflammatory Disorders of the Small Bowel

Leslie H. Sobin, MD
Department of Hepatic and Gastrointestinal Pathology
Armed Forces Institute of Pathology
Washington, DC
Idiopathic Inflammatory Bowel Disease

Michael Torbenson, MD
Associate Professor of Pathology
Department of Pathology
Johns Hopkins University School of Medicine
Baltimore, Maryland
Non-Neoplastic and Neoplastic Disorders of the Appendix

Athanasios C. Tsiatis, MD
Department of Pathology
Johns Hopkins Medical Institutions
Baltimore, Maryland
Molecular Diagnostics in Gastrointestinal Pathology

Kay Washington, MD, PhD
Professor, Department of Pathology
Vanderbilt University Medical Center
Nashville, Tennessee
Metabolic and Toxic Conditions of the Liver, Inflammatory and Infectious Diseases of the Liver, Liver Neoplasms

Foreword

The study and practice of anatomic pathology are both exciting and overwhelming. Surgical pathology, with all of the subspecialties it encompasses, and cytopathology have become increasingly complex and sophisticated, particularly with the incorporation of molecular pathology. It is simply not possible for any single individual to master all of the skills and knowledge required to perform these tasks at the highest level. Simply being able to make a correct diagnosis is challenging enough, but the standard of care has far surpassed merely providing a diagnosis. Pathologists are now asked to provide large amounts of ancillary information, both diagnostic and prognostic, often on small amounts of tissue, a task that can be daunting even to the most experienced surgical pathologist.

Although large general surgical pathology textbooks are useful resources, by necessity they could not possibly cover many of the aspects that pathologists need to know and include in their diagnostic reports. As such, the concept behind the *Foundations in Diagnostic Pathology* series was born. Given the success of the first series, we welcome the opportunity to update and improve all of the editions for the second series. *Foundations in Diagnostic Pathology* is designed to cover the major areas of surgical and cytopathology, and each edition is focused on one major topic. The goal of every book in this series is to provide the essential information that any pathologist, whether general or subspecialized, in training or in practice, would find useful in the evaluation of virtually any type of specimen encountered.

I am pleased that Drs. Christine Iacobuzio-Donahue and Elizabeth Montgomery agreed to edit this second edition of their book. Both of these individuals are superb gastrointestinal pathologists from Johns Hopkins Hospital, and they have edited an outstanding, state-of-the-art book on gastrointestinal pathology, which cuts to the essentials of what all pathologists want and need to know about diseases of the tubular gut, biliary tree, pancreas, and liver. The list of contributors is, as in the first edition, most impressive and includes nationally and internationally renowned pathologists who excel in their areas of expertise. The content in each chapter is practical, well organized, and well written, focusing on the thorough evaluation of biopsy and resection specimens and culminating in an accurate diagnosis using traditional morphology supported by immunohistochemical and molecular genetic techniques.

This edition of *Gastrointestinal and Liver Pathology* is organized in 21 chapters covering all of the major problems encountered in gastrointestinal pathology. There are separate chapters that describe the non-neoplastic and neoplastic conditions of the esophagus, stomach, small intestine, appendix, colon, and anus. Superb separate chapters on mesenchymal tumors of the gastrointestinal tract, infectious diseases of the colon, idiopathic inflammatory bowel disease, other inflammatory or iatrogenic colitides, and polyps and polyposis syndromes allow for the necessary depth to cover these broad topics. In addition, pathology of the gallbladder, extrahepatic bile ducts, and pancreas are covered in separate chapters, each of which provides the essential information and nuances of the organ that is covered. The last four chapters of the book cover metabolic and toxic conditions of the liver, inflammatory and infectious diseases of the liver, liver neoplasms, and gastrointestinal lymphomas. I know of no other book in the literature that covers all of these aspects of gastrointestinal pathology in such a concise manner. Moreover, many of the photomicrographs are new to this edition.

I wish to extend my sincere appreciation to Drs. Iacobuzio-Donahue and Montgomery, as well as all of the authors who contributed to this outstanding edition in the *Foundations in Diagnostic Pathology* series. As I was confident in the first edition series, I am completely confident that future editions in this series will be as thorough and as well done as their predecessors. I sincerely hope you enjoy this volume in the *Foundations in Diagnostic Pathology* series.

John R. Goldblum, MD

Preface

The practice of anatomic pathology, and of gastrointestinal pathology in particular, has undergone a dramatic transformation in the past decade. In addition to the multitude of diseases, syndromes, and clinical entities encountered in clinical practice every day, the increasing integration of molecular biology with gastrointestinal pathology is occurring at a fast pace, from large academic centers to community-based practices. Thus, the ability to feel current with the ever-expanding practice of pathology can be daunting. This challenge may be particularly overwhelming for residents just beginning their careers in the field of pathology, or any clinician attempting to remain informed about gastrointestinal pathology. For this reason, we are particularly pleased to have the opportunity to participate in the second edition of *Gastrointestinal and Liver Pathology* prepared for the *Foundations in Diagnostic Pathology* series. The information this book provides will be a valuable resource for all those interested in gastrointestinal pathology.

Although numerous excellent textbooks regarding the pathology and diseases of the gastrointestinal tract are available, we are especially proud of this edition for its novel format. First, the majority of images presented are new, and original material was prepared by the authors solely for this publication. Second, the format for each chapter follows a template to ensure ease of use, standardization of information presented, and completeness of each chapter. Finally, the many authors who contributed to this text were asked to participate based on their reputations as outstanding teachers and clinician educators. To all, we are deeply grateful.

ACKNOWLEDGMENTS

The editors acknowledge the tireless support and patience at Elsevier of Andy Hall, who has kept us on track, and Beth Hayes and Laura Slown, who went through each and every page of the text with great care.

Christine A. Iacobuzio-Donahue, MD, PhD
Elizabeth Montgomery, MD

Contents

Non-Neoplastic Disorders of the Esophagus

■ **Baojin Fu, MD** ■ **M. Eugenia Rueda-Pedraza, MD, Col. USMC**

Non-neoplastic disorders of the esophagus come in a great variety of forms, including structural abnormalities, inflammatory, infectious, traumatic, vascular, and those associated with systemic diseases. Some entities are mostly diagnosed by radiologic and endoscopic examination and, if examined via biopsy, they do not show specific histopathologic features; examples of these are esophageal rings and webs. Some others, however, require careful histopathologic examination, such as reflux, eosinophilic esophagitis, and infectious processes.

■ STRUCTURAL ABNORMALITIES

CONGENITAL

ESOPHAGEAL ATRESIA AND TRACHEOESOPHAGEAL FISTULA

CLINICAL FEATURES

These anomalies result from the failure of the foregut to completely divide into the esophagus and trachea. This separation occurs in the fourth week of gestation. This anomaly is slightly more common in males and occurs in 1 of every 4500 live births. The affected babies have food regurgitation, salivation, cyanosis, and aspiration. Sometimes they are associated with a trisomy (21, 18, and partial 13) or with the VACTERL (vertebral abnormalities, anal atresia, cardiac abnormalities, tracheoesophageal fistula and/or esophageal atresia, renal agenesis and dysplasia, and limb defects) association.

RADIOLOGIC FEATURES

Anteroposterior and lateral x-ray images of the chest and neck show a catheter inside the upper esophageal pouch while the distal esophagus and stomach contain air coming from the tracheoesophageal (TE) fistula.

ESOPHAGEAL ATRESIA AND TRACHEOESOPHAGEAL FISTULA—FACT SHEET

Definition
- Congenital anomalies resulting from failure of the foregut to divide into trachea and esophagus during the fourth week of embryonic development.

Incidence and Location
- Occurs in 1 of every 4500 live births.

Gender and Age Distribution
- Occurs in the newborn.
- Slight male predominance.

Clinical Features
- Food regurgitation, drooling, and aspiration.
- One form of tracheoesophageal (TE) fistula, the H shape, may be overlooked and diagnosed later in older children with repeated bouts of pneumonia.

Radiologic Features
- Anteroposterior and lateral x-ray films show the catheter in the upper esophageal blind pouch.
- When TE fistula exists, the distal esophagus and stomach are filled with air.

Prognosis and Therapy
- Excellent prognosis if diagnosis and surgical correction occur early.
- The presence of associated anomalies (trisomies) changes the outlook.

PATHOLOGIC FEATURES

GROSS FINDINGS

Esophageal atresias, with or without tracheoesophageal fistulas, are of five different types (Fig. 1-1). Type C is the most common, accounting for 85% of the cases

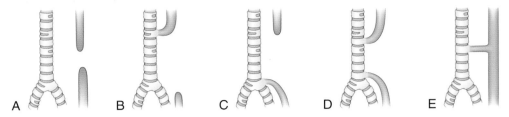

FIGURE 1-1
The five types of esophageal atresias.

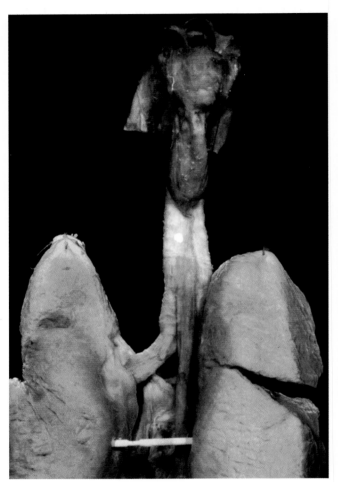

FIGURE 1-2
Esophageal atresia with tracheoesophageal (TE) fistula (posterior view). Blind pouch in the upper esophagus and distal TE fistula at the tracheal bifurcation. *(From Turk JL, ed. Royal College of Surgeons of England. Slide Atlas of Pathology. Alimentary Tract System. London, Gower Medical, 1986, with permission.)*

ESOPHAGEAL ATRESIA AND TRACHEOESOPHAGEAL FISTULA—PATHOLOGIC FEATURES

Gross Findings
- There are five types of atresia with or without tracheoesophageal fistula (see Fig. 1-1).
- The most common is type C, which occurs in 85% of the cases.

Differential Diagnosis
- Congenital esophageal stenosis may mimic atresia.
- Careful radiologic examination will differentiate them both.
- In congenital pyloric stenosis, the x-ray film will demonstrate esophageal integrity with air trapped in the stomach.

(Figs. 1-2 and 1-3). The E type (also known as H because of its shape) may be overlooked and diagnosed in older children with repeated bouts of pneumonia.

DIFFERENTIAL DIAGNOSIS

These entities should be differentiated from the less common congenital esophageal stenosis (Fig. 1-4). This anomaly demonstrates a significant narrowing of the midesophagus resulting from a web or muscular hypertrophy. Another entity, congenital pyloric stenosis, presents with projectile vomiting, and x-ray films show esophageal integrity and air trapped in the stomach.

PROGNOSIS AND THERAPY

Early diagnosis with prompt surgical repair confers an excellent prognosis. Associated anomalies such as trisomies change the outlook for these babies. Children born with the VACTERL association tend to fare better.

DUPLICATIONS AND CYSTS

These congenital anomalies are not always easy to differentiate from one another. Esophageal duplication accounts for 10% to 20% of all gastrointestinal duplications and is the result of a morphogenetic abnormality occurring around the fifth to eighth week of gestation.

Cysts can be classified as bronchogenic, enteric, or neuroenteric.

CLINICAL FEATURES

Patients experience feeding difficulties or respiratory distress during childhood. In some cases, the anomaly remains asymptomatic and is discovered during a routine chest x-ray examination.

ESOPHAGEAL DUPLICATIONS AND CYSTS—FACT SHEET

Definition

- Congenital anomalies caused by failure of normal development around the fifth to eighth week of gestation

Incidence and Location

- Duplications are seen in 1 in 8000 autopsies
- Accounts for 10% to 20% of all gastrointestinal duplications
- Located in lower third of esophagus, protruding into the posterior mediastinum
- Bronchogenic cysts protrude into the anterior mediastinum
- Enteric/neuroenteric cysts occupy the posterior mediastinum
- Neuroenteric cysts can have an hourglass configuration

Gender and Age Distribution

- No apparent gender preference
- Symptoms present in early childhood
- Some cases remain asymptomatic and are discovered on routine chest x-ray films

Clinical Features

- Feeding difficulties and respiratory distress

Radiologic Features

- Duplications are seen on x-ray films as intramural defects in the lower third of the esophagus
- Bronchogenic cysts show as a mass protruding into the anterior mediastinum.
- Neuroenteric cysts are associated with vertebral anomalies.

Prognosis and Therapy

- Good prognosis with adequate surgical resection

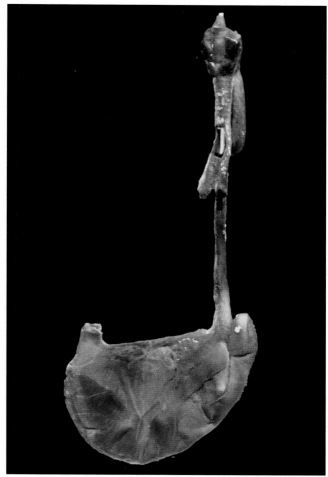

FIGURE 1-3

Esophageal atresia with tracheoesophageal fistula. Shows the stomach and distal esophagus connecting with the fistula at the tracheal bifurcation. *(From Turk JL, ed. Royal College of Surgeons of England. Slide Atlas of Pathology. Alimentary Tract System. London, Gower Medical, 1986, with permission.)*

RADIOLOGIC FEATURES

In duplication, the radiologic finding is that of an intramural defect, mostly in the lower third of the esophagus, protruding into the posterior mediastinum. Bronchogenic cysts occur anteriorly, while enteric or neuroenteric cysts appear in the posterior mediastinum, usually in association with hemivertebrae or spina bifida.

PATHOLOGIC FEATURES

GROSS FINDINGS

Duplications occur in the lower esophagus in 60% of cases; they are intramural and noncommunicating. Cysts measure on average 5 cm in diameter. Bronchogenic cysts present anteriorly and contain a rim of cartilage. Enteric/neuroenteric cysts sometimes have an hourglass shape, with one portion in the posterior mediastinum and the other inside the vertebral canal.

MICROSCOPIC FINDINGS

Duplications are located within the esophageal wall and have intact muscle layers (Fig. 1-5). The epithelial linings of either duplications or cysts may have squamous, cuboidal, or ciliated epithelium (Fig. 1-6). Most bronchogenic cysts contain cartilage in their walls.

DIFFERENTIAL DIAGNOSIS

Differential diagnosis includes acquired diverticula. These lesions occur in adults and always communicate with the esophageal lumen. The lining is squamous epithelial but may show erosions and ulcerations.

ESOPHAGEAL DUPLICATIONS AND CYSTS—PATHOLOGIC FEATURES

Gross Findings

- Duplication appears as an intramural mass in the lower esophagus.
- Cysts are on average 5 cm in diameter.
- Bronchogenic cysts may show a rim of cartilage on gross examination.
- Neuroenteric cysts may have an hourglass appearance with one component in the posterior mediastinum and the other inside the vertebral canal.

Microscopic Findings

- Duplications have a complete muscle layer.
- Bronchogenic cysts contain cartilage in their walls.
- Duplication cysts can be lined by squamous, cuboidal, or ciliated epithelium.
- Neuroenteric cysts are lined with intestinal epithelium or gastric mucosa.

Differential Diagnosis

- Diverticula are acquired conditions.
- Diverticula communicate with the esophageal lumen.
- Diverticula are lined by squamous epithelium.

PROGNOSIS AND THERAPY

Adequate surgical resection confers a good prognosis.

EPITHELIAL ECTOPIAS: GASTRIC HETEROTOPIA/ INLET PATCH AND HETEROTOPIC SEBACEOUS GLANDS

CLINICAL FEATURES

Gastric heterotopia is mostly asymptomatic and is found incidentally during endoscopy (4%). Sometimes it is associated with dyspepsia and a burning sensation. Less often, peptic ulceration and strictures develop. Rarely, malignant transformation occurs. Heterotopic sebaceous glands are asymptomatic.

GASTRIC HETEROTOPIA/INLET PATCH AND HETEROTOPIC SEBACEOUS GLANDS—FACT SHEET

Definition

- Heterotopic gastric mucosa in esophagus
- Heterotopic sebaceous glands in esophagus

Incidence and Location

- Meticulous autopsy studies have revealed a high incidence of heterotopic gastric mucosa (70%); at endoscopy they are present in 4% of individuals.
- Heterotopic gastric mucosa is mostly localized in the proximal esophagus.

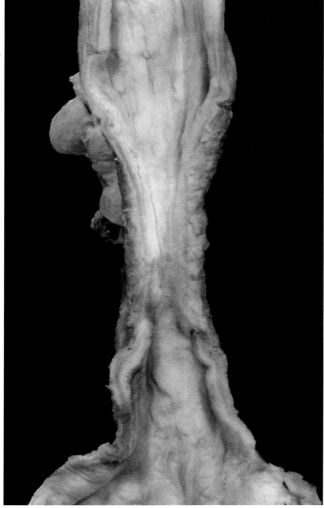

FIGURE 1-4
Esophagus with congenital esophageal stenosis. Note the narrowing of the middle segment. *(From Turk JL, ed. Royal College of Surgeons of England. Slide Atlas of Pathology. Alimentary Tract System. London, Gower Medical, 1986, with permission.)*

- Heterotopic sebaceous glands are present in 4% of individuals.
- Heterotopic sebaceous glands can be solitary or multiple.

Gender and Age Distribution

- No apparent gender preference
- Found in all age groups, but highest incidence in first year of life

Clinical Features

- Gastric heterotopia is mostly asymptomatic; occasionally it may cause dysphagia.
- Complications include ulcerations and strictures.
- Heterotopic sebaceous glands are asymptomatic.

Prognosis and Therapy

- Good prognosis. Treatment with antacids is indicated in symptomatic cases of gastric heterotopia.

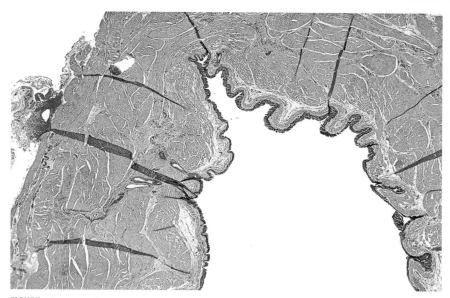

FIGURE 1-5

Esophageal duplication. Intact muscularis propria and cuboidal epithelium.

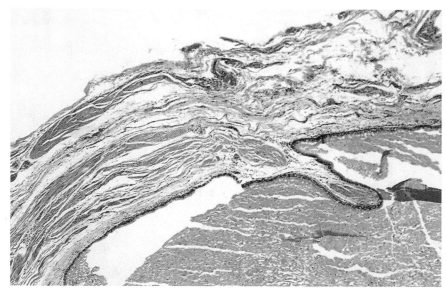

FIGURE 1-6

Esophageal cyst with columnar epithelium, luminal secretions, and attenuated muscle layer.

PATHOLOGIC FEATURES

GROSS FINDINGS

The gross endoscopic features reveal a well-demarcated round to oval patch of salmon-colored mucosa with sharp borders. This lesion is seen in the proximal portion of the esophagus. Meticulous autopsy studies have revealed a high incidence of heterotopic gastric mucosa (70%). Heterotopic sebaceous glands can be solitary or multiple, presenting as yellowish bumps.

MICROSCOPIC FINDINGS

Microscopic examination reveals gastric mucosa of the cardiac, fundic, or mixed type (Figs. 1-7 and 1-8). Acute inflammation and erosions can be seen. Heterotopic sebaceous glands look identical to their skin counterparts (Figs. 1-9 and 1-10).

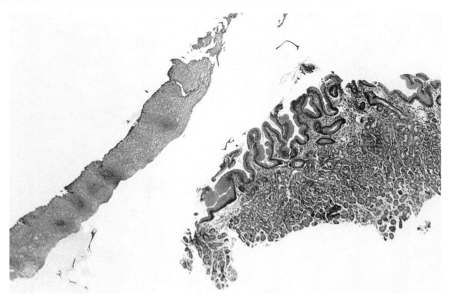

FIGURE 1-7

Gastric heterotopia inlet patch. Squamous epithelium and gastric-type mucosa.

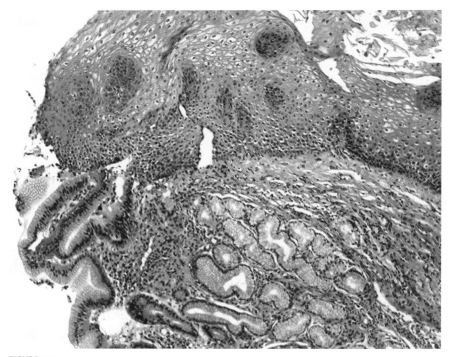

FIGURE 1-8

Gastric heterotopia inlet patch. Cardiac-type mucosa with inflammation.

DIFFERENTIAL DIAGNOSIS

Heterotopic gastric mucosa must be distinguished from Barrett's esophagus. The proximal location of the former distinguishes it from the latter. Heterotopic gastric mucosa rarely develops intestinal metaplasia. Multiple sebaceous heterotopias may look to the endoscopist similar to another asymptomatic entity called *glycogenic acanthosis*. The latter is characterized by white patches and histologically reveals excess glycogen in the mature squamous cells of the upper mucosal layers.

GASTRIC HETEROTOPIAS/INLET PATCH AND HETEROTOPIC SEBACEOUS GLANDS—PATHOLOGIC FEATURES

Gross Findings

- Gastric heterotopias are round to oval patches of salmon-colored mucosa in the proximal esophagus.
- Sebaceous heterotopias appear as single or multiple yellowish bumps.

Microscopic Findings

- Fundic, cardiac, or mixed mucosae are seen, sometimes inflamed or with erosions.
- Sebaceous glands are indistinguishable from their skin counterparts.

Differential Diagnosis

- The presence of gastric mucosa in the esophagus must be distinguished from Barrett's esophagus. Gastric heterotopia is mostly localized in the proximal esophagus and rarely shows intestinal metaplasia.
- Sebaceous heterotopia may be confused grossly with glycogenic acanthosis.

ACQUIRED

DIVERTICULA (ZENKER'S, MIDESOPHAGUS, AND EPIPHRENIC)

CLINICAL FEATURES

Clinical symptoms vary depending on the location of the lesion. Diverticulum, located in the uppermost portion of the esophagus (Zenker's), provokes dysphagia, regurgitation, halitosis, and aspiration. These symptoms usually present in middle-aged and older adults. A gurgling sound upon swallowing and a neck mass are sometimes present. No single etiologic mechanism has been found to explain its formation, but reduced upper esophageal sphincter compliance may be the cause. Midesophageal diverticulum may be asymptomatic and develops as a result of mediastinal inflammatory diseases such as tuberculosis. The epiphrenic diverticulum is located in the distal esophagus and is symptomatic due to its coexistence with hiatal hernia or diaphragmatic eventration. Disorders of the esophageal musculature appear to be the cause of middle and lower diverticula.

RADIOLOGIC FEATURES

These lesions are best demonstrated during barium esophagography. Zenker's diverticulum is best observed during the oropharyngeal phase of swallowing. Midesophageal diverticula are seen as outpouches during barium esophagography performed for other causes. The epiphrenic diverticulum is also easily diagnosed via barium esophagography.

DIVERTICULA—FACT SHEET

Definition

- Outpouchings of esophagus of acquired nature; localized in upper, middle, and lower esophagus

Incidence and Location

- Zenker's diverticulum is the most common (70%).
- Zenker's diverticulum is located at the junction between the pharynx and esophagus in an area called the *Killian triangle*.
- Midesophageal diverticulum is less common and occurs at the level of tracheal bifurcation.
- Epiphrenic diverticulum is located in the lower esophagus and accompanies hiatal hernia.

Gender and Age Distribution

- Mostly seen in middle-aged and older adults
- No gender preference

Clinical Features

- When the sac is small, it may be asymptomatic.
- In large Zenker's diverticulum, dysphagia, a gurgling sound, and a neck mass may develop.
- Regurgitation of food eaten several hours before is quite characteristic.
- Inflammatory diseases of the mediastinum sometimes accompany the midesophageal diverticulum; they are mostly asymptomatic.
- Hiatal hernia is seen in association with epiphrenic diverticulum.
- Motility abnormalities are the most acceptable causes of these lesions.

Radiologic Features

- Barium esophagography is the best technique to demonstrate the three types of diverticula.
- Esophagography during the oropharyngeal phase of swallowing is the best diagnostic procedure to demonstrate Zenker's diverticulum.

Prognosis and Therapy

- Prognosis depends on the size of the lesion and associated inflammatory conditions.
- Large diverticula are treated with surgical resection and myomectomy.
- Small asymptomatic ones are not treated surgically.

Differential Diagnosis

- Pseudodiverticula, either single or multiple (DEIP), are dilatations of submucosal glands and lack muscle wall of their own.

PATHOLOGIC FEATURES

GROSS FINDINGS

Zenker's diverticulum is a pouch located at the level of the pharyngoesophageal junction, a weak point in the wall between the inferior constrictor muscle of the pharynx and the fibers of the cricopharyngeal muscle. This

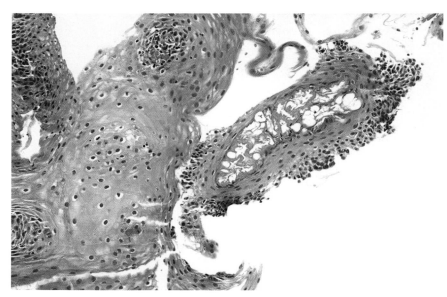

FIGURES 1-9
Heterotopic sebaceous glands, low-power view. Foamy sebaceous cells are present.

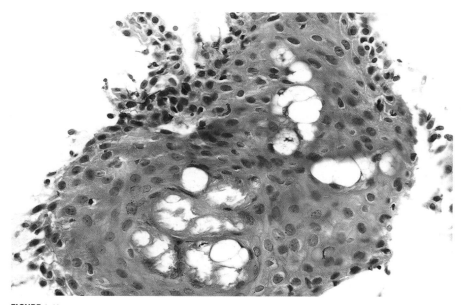

FIGURE 1-10
Heterotopic sebaceous glands, high-power view. Foamy sebaceous cells are present.

triangular area is known as the *triangle of Killian* (Fig. 1-11). The diverticula vary in size and may be filled with necrotic debris. The midesophageal diverticulum (also called *traction diverticulum*) is located at the level of the tracheal bifurcation, sometimes with adhesions to mediastinal lymph nodes involved with tuberculosis (Figs. 1-12 and 1-13). The epiphrenic diverticulum lies close to the diaphragm and is seen in association with a hiatal hernia.

MICROSCOPIC FEATURES

All three are true diverticula because they are lined with squamous epithelium and contain a muscle wall that is at times attenuated (Fig. 1-14). Inflammation with ulceration usually develops. Carcinoma has been seen in Zenker's diverticulum in 0.3% of the cases.

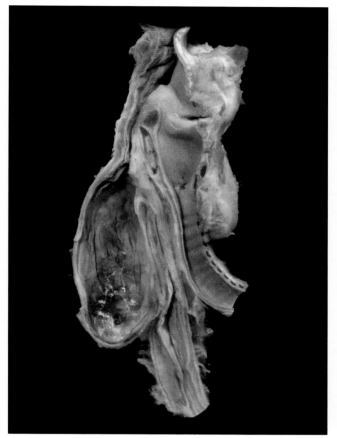

FIGURE 1-11

Zenker's diverticulum. Thin wall and luminal debris. *(From Turk JL, ed. Royal College of Surgeons of England. Slide Atlas of Pathology. Alimentary Tract System. London, Gower Medical, 1986, with permission.)*

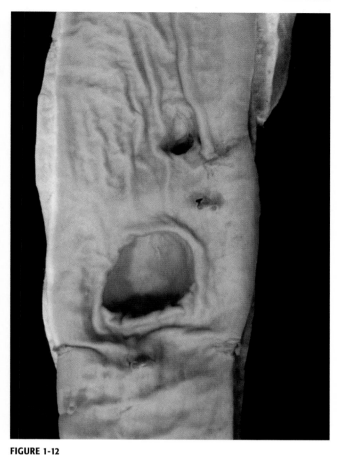

FIGURE 1-12

Midesophageal diverticulum (traction diverticulum; inside view). *(From Turk JL, ed. Royal College of Surgeons of England. Slide Atlas of Pathology. Alimentary Tract System. London, Gower Medical, 1986, with permission.)*

DIFFERENTIAL DIAGNOSIS

Diverticula should be differentiated from pseudodiverticula, which are cystic dilatations of submucosal glands, lacking a separate muscle coat. A peculiar entity called *diffuse esophageal intramural pseudodiverticulosis* (DEIP) is also in the differential diagnosis, presenting with dysphagia. The radiologic examination with contrast media shows multiple minute outpouchings in the esophageal wall. This entity is associated with diabetes, alcoholism, candidiasis, and chronic granulomatous disease.

PROGNOSIS AND THERAPY

Prognosis depends on the size of the diverticulum and on whether it is complicated by ulceration and hemorrhage. Large diverticula are treated with diverticulectomy and esophagomyotomy. Small ones do not require surgical intervention.

ESOPHAGEAL WEBS AND RINGS

These lesions are common and are mostly acquired, except for the rare congenital esophageal stenosis. They are concentric or eccentric narrowings of the esophageal lumen.

DIVERTICULA—PATHOLOGIC FEATURES

Gross Findings

- Zenker's diverticulum is a sac at the pharyngoesophageal junction.
- Mid-diverticulum occurs at the level of bifurcation of the trachea.
- Epiphrenic diverticulum occurs in the lower 10 cm of the esophagus.

Microscopic Findings

- Composed of all layers of the esophagus, but the muscle layer is attenuated.
- Lined by stratified squamous mucosa.
- Mucosa may become inflamed and ulcerated.
- In 0.3% of cases, carcinoma develops in Zenker's diverticulum.

CLINICAL FEATURES

Webs are found in 4% to 10% of autopsies. Clinically they are seen in 5% to 15% of patients presenting with dysphagia and choking sensation. Symptomatic webs occur in women older than 40 complaining of dysphagia and odynophagia. The now rare Plummer-Vinson syndrome consists of iron deficiency anemia, glossitis, cheilosis, and an upper esophageal web (Fig. 1-15).

Rings are found in 0.7% to 16% of autopsies, and their pathogenesis is debatable. Those found in the lower esophagus are called *Schatzki's ring.*

RADIOLOGIC FEATURES

These lesions are seen on a full-column barium examination. They form notches, curvilinear shadows, or thin membranous filling defects. Lower rings are seen in association with hiatal hernias.

PATHOLOGIC FEATURES

GROSS FINDINGS

Endoscopic examination reveals rings and webs as mucosal foldings or indentations of a pale, pink color. Ulceration is sometimes seen.

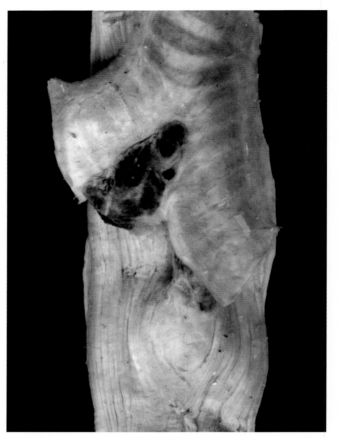

FIGURE 1-13
Midesophageal diverticulum (traction diverticulum; outside view). Adhesions between the lymph nodes and diverticulum. *(From Turk JL, ed. Royal College of Surgeons of England. Slide Atlas of Pathology. Alimentary Tract System. London, Gower Medical, 1986, with permission.)*

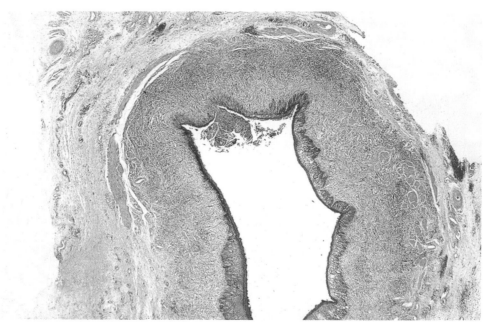

FIGURE 1-14
Zenker's diverticulum. Muscularis propria and squamous epithelial lining.

ESOPHAGEAL WEBS AND RINGS—FACT SHEET

Definition
- Acquired disorders provoking concentric or eccentric narrowing of the esophageal lumen

Incidence and Location
- Rings and webs are common abnormalities of the esophagus.
- Autopsy incidence of rings is 10%; that of webs is 16%.
- Webs are more common in the upper portion, rings in the lower.

Gender and Age Distribution
- More common in women older than age 40 years

Clinical Features
- Mostly asymptomatic
- Dysphagia and odynophagia are common symptoms.
- Upper esophageal webs are associated with the now rare Plummer-Vinson syndrome.

Radiologic Features
- Notches or curvilinear shadows seen in a full-column barium examination

Prognosis and Therapy
- Generally good prognosis
- Change of dietary habits in mild cases; dilation or surgery in more symptomatic cases

ESOPHAGEAL WEBS AND RINGS—PATHOLOGIC FEATURES

Gross Findings
- Mucosal foldings or indentations seen on endoscopic examination
- Lower rings show mucosal pallor and sometimes ulceration.

Microscopic Findings
- Webs are covered by squamous mucosa, sometimes inflamed.
- Lower rings have squamous mucosa on the proximal side and columnar epithelium on the distal side.
- Some lower rings show localized muscular thickening.

Differential Diagnosis
- Main differential diagnosis is postinflammatory stenosis resulting from reflux or lye strictures.
- Significant scarring fibrosis is found in these entities.

MICROSCOPIC FINDINGS

Webs are covered by squamous mucosa with edematous, inflamed submucosa. Lower rings and webs have squamous mucosa on their proximal side and columnar epithelium on the distal side. Still others are the result not of mucosal foldings but of localized annular muscular thickenings.

DIFFERENTIAL DIAGNOSIS

Postinflammatory stenosis, occurring after a long-standing reflux or a stenosis secondary to corrosive agents, is in the differential diagnosis. Lye strictures are mostly located at the level of the tracheal bifurcation, whereas reflux is mostly in the lower esophagus. Marked submucosal fibrosis in both entities is a characteristic finding.

PROGNOSIS AND THERAPY

Mild symptoms can be treated with dietary modifications. Dilation is the treatment of choice, and surgical therapy is left to those refractory to dilation.

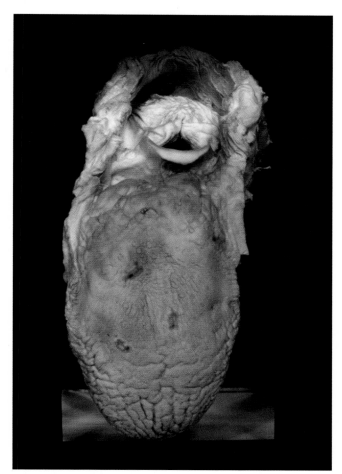

FIGURE 1-15
Upper esophageal web with glossitis. (From Turk JL, ed. Royal College of Surgeons of England. Slide Atlas of Pathology. Alimentary Tract System. London, Gower Medical, 1986, with permission.)

■ MOTILITY DISORDERS

Normal esophageal motility is a complex mechanism requiring intact, coordinated autonomic innervation. Inadequate function leads to dysmotility disorders, which can be divided into the spastic variety and achalasia. Spastic disorders are now commonly encountered with the increased use of endoscopy. Achalasia is relatively uncommon, with a prevalence of less than 10 cases per 10^5 population.

CLINICAL FEATURES

Clinical symptoms depend on the underlying peristaltic abnormality. Spastic disorders such as episodic dysphagia with an angina-like chest pain occur in two types of motility disorders. One, occurring primarily in men, consists of repetitive, high-amplitude, nonperistaltic contractions of the esophageal smooth muscle; the other is called *nutcracker esophagus* and consists of peristaltic, high-amplitude contractions. A third entity, characterized by diffuse esophageal spasms *(corkscrew esophagus)*, also causes severe dysphagia. In achalasia, the abnormality consists of aperistalsis, lack of lower esophageal sphincter (LES) relaxation and increased intraesophageal pressure. Patients are 20 to 40 years of age and complain of progressive dysphagia, regurgitation, and aspiration. Systemic disorders such as scleroderma, muscular dystrophies, amyloidosis, and Chagas disease also affect the normal peristaltic mechanism. The incidence of squamous cell carcinoma is increased in patients with achalasia.

RADIOLOGIC FEATURES

Barium swallow studies with videofluoroscopy and manometry demonstrate variable degrees of spasticity and dilatation of the esophageal lumen, depending on the underlying dysmotility disorder.

PATHOLOGIC FEATURES

GROSS FINDINGS

Endoscopic examination in cases of achalasia shows dilatation of the lumen, prominent vascularity, and pooled debris adherent to the wall (Figs. 1-16 and 1-17). In some cases, reflux changes and strictures are present. Spastic disorders reveal atypical contractions.

MOTILITY DISORDERS—FACT SHEET

Definition
- Disease entities affecting the normal coordination of swallowing and peristalsis

Incidence and Location
- Motility disorders affect the entire esophageal length.
- Spastic disorders are recognized with the increased use of manometric studies in patients complaining of noncardiac chest pain.
- Achalasia is an uncommon disorder with a prevalence of fewer than 10 cases per 10^5 population.

Gender and Age Distribution
- Achalasia patients are 20 to 40 years of age, and both sexes are affected equally.
- Spastic disorders occur mainly in men.

Clinical Features
- Severe episodic dysphagia and angina-type chest pain are typical of spastic disorders.
- Achalasia presents with progressive dysphagia, regurgitation, aspiration, and weight loss.

Radiologic Features
- In achalasia, contrast swallow discloses progressive dilatation of the esophagus with lack of relaxation at the LES and a characteristic beaklike deformity in the distal esophagus.
- The same method is used for spastic disorders to help differentiate them.

Prognosis and Therapy
- Prognosis depends on early diagnosis and treatment.
- Treatment modalities for achalasia include botulinum toxin injections and pneumatic dilation.
- Treatment for spastic disorders includes nitrates, sedatives, botulinum toxin, and pneumatic dilation.
- Careful follow-up is recommended for achalasia patients resulting from their increased risk for developing squamous cell carcinoma.

MICROSCOPIC CHANGES

Achalasia is characterized by a progressive loss of myenteric plexus caused by chronic inflammation of the ganglion cells (Fig. 1-18). The LES also shows a decrease in the number of these cells, but to a lesser degree. The occasional presence of wallerian degeneration and Lewy bodies indicates that this disease is the result of primary neuropathy. Hypertrophy of the muscle layer is also a feature.

Ganglion cell inflammation is sometimes seen in spastic disorders. In cases of diffuse esophageal spasm, one finds diffuse muscular hypertrophy.

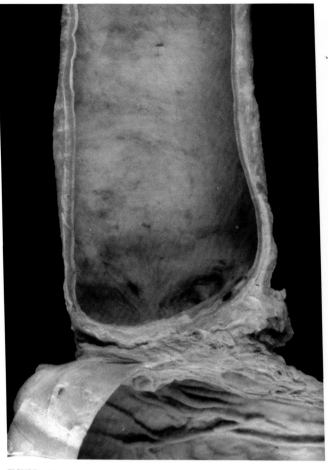

FIGURE 1-16

Achalasia. Marked lumen dilatation. *(From Turk JL, ed. Royal College of Surgeons of England. Slide Atlas of Pathology. Alimentary Tract System. London, Gower Medical, 1986, with permission.)*

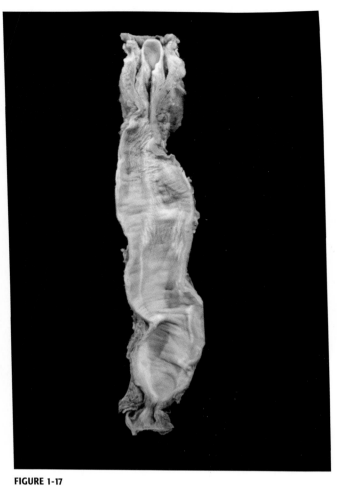

FIGURE 1-17

Achalasia. Tortuous esophagus and narrow distal segment. *(From Turk JL, ed. Royal College of Surgeons of England. Slide Atlas of Pathology. Alimentary Tract System. London, Gower Medical, 1986, with permission.)*

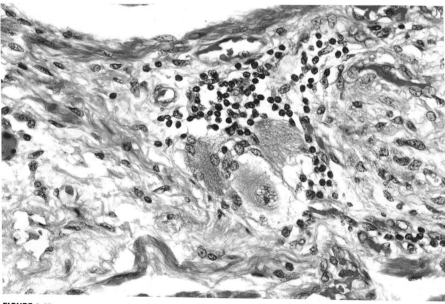

FIGURE 1-18

Achalasia. Myenteric plexus with chronic inflammation (ganglionitis).

MOTILITY DISORDERS—PATHOLOGIC FEATURES

Gross Findings

- In achalasia, endoscopic examination reveals a dilated lumen, pooled debris, prominent vascularity, and a lack of normal relaxation of the LES.
- Spastic disorders reveal abnormal motility on endoscopic examination.

Microscopic Findings

- Chronic ganglionitis with myenteric plexus destruction in the dilated portion of the esophagus is seen in achalasia.
- Wallerian degeneration and Lewy bodies are sometimes seen in ganglion cells.
- Spastic disorders can also have ganglionitis.
- Diffuse esophageal spasm shows marked and extensive hypertrophy of the inner muscle layer.

Differential Diagnosis

- Primary achalasia should be differentiated from secondary achalasia caused by scleroderma, Chagas disease, amyloidosis, and so on.
- Careful clinical/serologic correlation will clarify the different pathologic entities.

FERENTIAL DIAGNOSIS

disorders can mimic angina pectoris. Idiopathic should be differentiated from secondary acha- lting from scleroderma (Fig. 1-19), amyloidosis, dystrophy, and Chagas disease (Fig. 1-20). In a, there is marked intimal fibrosis of blood ciated with atrophy and fibrosis of the mus- ia. Amyloidosis reveals deposits of congo- d in arterioles of the lamina propria. In s disease, it has been demonstrated that isms produce a substance toxic to the he microorganisms, however, are seldom examination.

HERAPY

early diagnosis. In achalasia two : botulinum toxin injections and veral studies have demonstrated h pneumatic dilation (80%). r spastic disorders include cal- edatives, nitrates, and pneu-

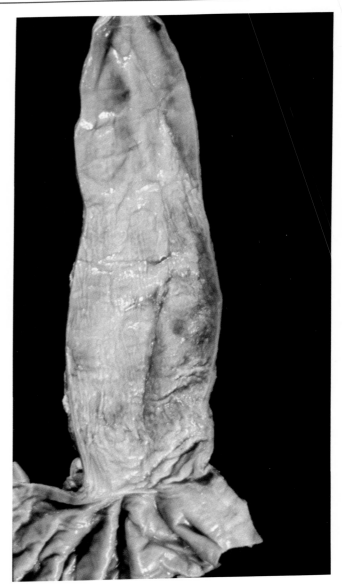

FIGURE 1-19

Scleroderma. Luminal dilatation and thinning of muscle wall. *(From Turk JL, ed. Royal College of Surgeons of England. Slide Atlas of Pathology. Alimentary Tract System. London, Gower Medical, 1986, with permission.)*

■ INFLAMMATORY AND INFECTIOUS DISORDERS

REFLUX ESOPHAGITIS

Reflux esophagitis, also known as *gastroesophageal reflux disease* (GERD), is one of the most common non-neoplastic disorders of the esophagus. Although the incidence of *Helicobacter pylori* infection, gastric carcinoma, and peptic ulcers has decreased in the Western hemisphere, gastroesophageal reflux disease has been on

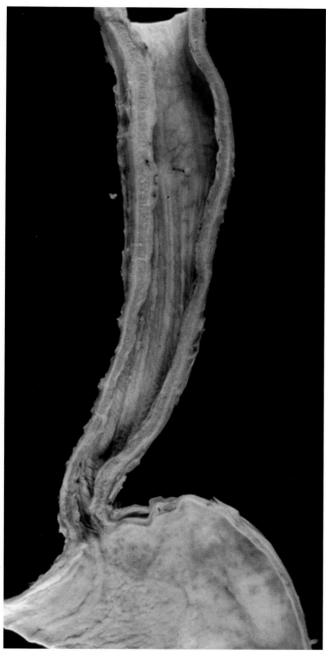

FIGURE 1-20

Chagas disease. Moderate luminal dilatation. *(From Turk JL, ed. Royal College of Surgeons of England. Slide Atlas of Pathology. Alimentary Tract System. London, Gower Medical, 1986, with permission.)*

REFLUX ESOPHAGITIS—FACT SHEET

Definition
- Inflammation of the lower esophagus, resulting from damage caused by acid reflux from the stomach

Incidence and Location
- The most common form of esophagitis, with an incidence of 10% in the population
- Localized in the lower portion of the esophagus

Gender and Age Distribution
- Affects both sexes and all age-groups

Clinical Features
- Heartburn and regurgitation are the typical symptoms.
- Atypical presentation includes angina-like pain, hoarseness, asthma, and hiccups.
- Some individuals are asymptomatic.

Prognosis and Therapy
- Prognosis depends on the degree of LES pressure.
- Early detection prevents complications.
- If left untreated, severe ulcerations, strictures, Barrett's esophagus, and adenocarcinoma may develop.
- Treatment includes lifestyle modifications, proton pump inhibitors, and surgical procedures (Nissen fundoplication) in severe cases.

CLINICAL FEATURES

Reflux occurs at all ages and in both sexes. Typical symptoms include heartburn and regurgitation, occurring more frequently after consumption of fat-rich foods and aggravated while in the recumbent position. Atypical symptoms include angina-like chest pain, chronic hoarseness, asthmatic episodes, and protracted hiccups. If left untreated, it may lead to complications such as erosive esophagitis, strictures, Barrett's esophagus, and malignancy.

It is important to emphasize that a number of individuals with reflux do not manifest symptoms, yet later present with adenocarcinoma arising from Barrett's esophagus.

The most important diagnostic procedures to detect reflux include ambulatory prolonged pH monitoring, endoscopy, and biopsy.

PATHOLOGIC FEATURES

GROSS FINDINGS

Endoscopic examination in cases of reflux is variable, depending on the severity and the chronicity of the symptoms. In mild cases, results of endoscopy may be negative;

---

the rise. There is circumstantial evidence that *H. pylori* infection protects against gastroesophageal reflux disease. The prevalence of GERD is approximately 11% in the U.S. population, with a higher proportion among pregnant women. The pathophysiologic hallmark of reflux is the presence of LES dysfunction.

REFLUX ESOPHAGITIS—PATHOLOGIC FEATURES

Gross Findings

- Reddish, hyperhemic areas at the squamocolumnar junction
- Erosions, either focal or circumferential
- Deep ulcers followed by strictures
- Barrett's esophagus (salmon-colored mucosal tongues) may be present in long-standing cases.

Microscopic Findings

- Intraepithelial edema, necrosis, and leukocyte infiltrate are seen in acute cases.
- Chronic cases have basal cell hyperplasia (> 15% of epithelial thickness), elongation of papillae (> 60% of epithelial thickness), and intraepithelial eosinophils.
- Number of intraepithelial T-lymphocytes is increased.
- More severe cases show ulceration, granulation tissue, and submucosal fibrosis.

Differential Diagnosis

- Reflux must be distinguished from eosinophilic esophagitis because the treatments are completely different.
- Infectious esophagitis includes *Candida,* herpes, and CMV esophagitis.
- Special stains for fungi (GMS and PAS) are recommended.
- For viral esophagitis, hematoxylin and eosin stain findings are sufficient most of the time for diagnosis.
- Immunostains for herpes virus and CMV may be indicated in doubtful cases.

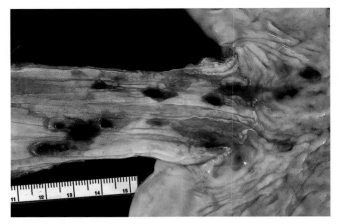

FIGURE 1-21
Esophagitis. Severe, with hemorrhagic erosions. *(Courtesy of Dr. P. Vasallo.)*

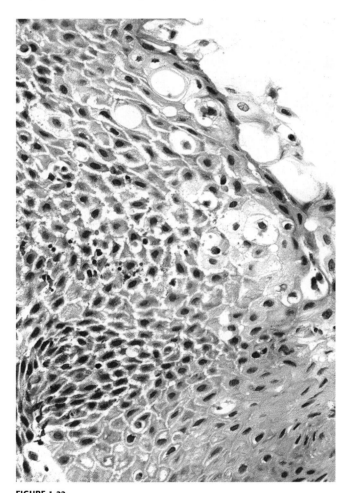

FIGURE 1-22
Reflux esophagitis. Intercellular edema and balloon cells.

in more severe cases, the sharp squamocolumnar junction is interrupted by reddish, congested mucosa. The presence of erosions, either focal or circumferential, indicates a more severe form. Deep ulcerations, bleeding, and strictures are seen in extreme cases (Fig. 1-21).

MICROSCOPIC FINDINGS

Microscopic findings depend on the severity of the lesion and can be divided into acute and chronic. In the acute form, the mucosa shows intraepithelial edema with areas of necrosis and balloon cells and increased intramucosal lymphocytes (Figs. 1-22 and 1-23). As the reflux becomes chronic, other changes occur to include basal cell hyperplasia (> 15 % of epithelial thickness), elongation of the papillae (> 60 % of epithelial thickness), and intraepithelial eosinophils (Figs. 1-24 and 1-25). A large number of intraepithelial T-lymphocytes percolate between squamous cells and adopt elongated shapes (squiggle cells). All these findings are seen in the lower esophagus and tend to disappear in more proximal biopsy samples.

DIFFERENTIAL DIAGNOSIS

Eosinophilic esophagitis, infectious esophagitis, and pill esophagitis are in the differential diagnosis. In eosinophilic esophagitis, the eosinophilic infiltrate is more severe, with clumps of eosinophils dispersed along the entire thickness of the mucosa, frequently congregating in the uppermost portion of the mucosa. Although reflux changes tend to disappear in proximal areas of the esophagus, findings in eosinophilic esophagitis remain the same at different levels of the mucosa.

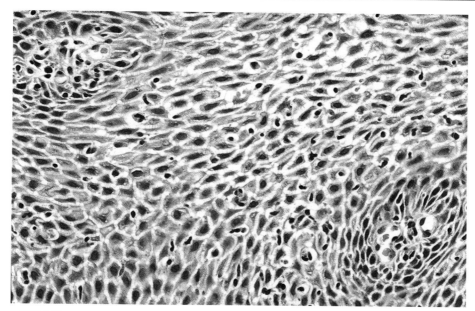

FIGURE 1-23
Reflux esophagitis. Increased number of intraepithelial lymphocytes.

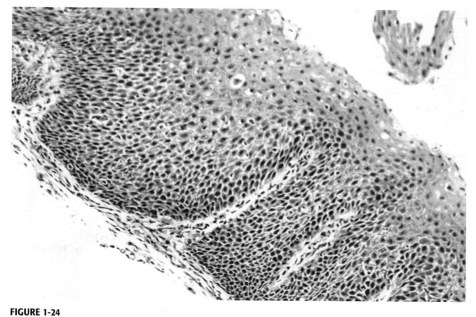

FIGURE 1-24
Reflux esophagitis. Basal cell hyperplasia, elongation of papillae, and focal cell necrosis.

Infectious esophagitis such as that caused by *Candida,* herpes virus, and cytomegalovirus (CMV) infections shows specific features. *Candida* esophagitis reveals yeast and pseudohyphal forms that invade the mucosa and are accompanied by severe acute inflammation. Herpes infection shows multinucleated giant cells with molding of nuclei and margination of chromatin. CMV changes are best appreciated in submucosal capillaries where large, infected cells show intranuclear and intracytoplasmic viral inclusions. Pill esophagitis reveals ulcerations and florid

granulation tissue. These changes are nonspecific, so they need to be analyzed in light of the clinical presentation.

PROGNOSIS AND THERAPY

Prognosis depends on the degree of LES pressures. Extremely low pressures (6 mm Hg) predict a more severe degree of reflux and worse prognosis. Early diagnosis before complications is essential for the best outcome of

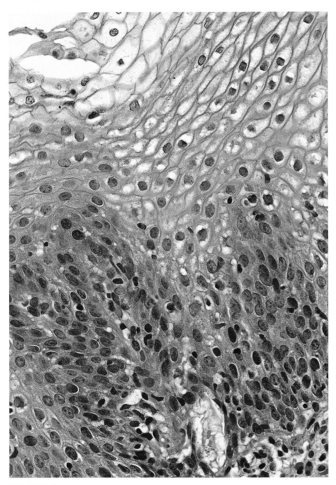

FIGURE 1-25
Reflux esophagitis. Intraepithelial eosinophils.

the patient. Conservative therapy is indicated with significant lifestyle modifications to include diet, elevation of the head of the bed, avoiding recumbence after meals, and avoidance of tobacco and alcohol consumption. Medications include proton pump inhibitors. If these methods fail, endoscopic therapies are indicated to include endoscopic luminal gastroplasty, biopolymer augmentation, or oral Nissen fundoplication.

EOSINOPHILIC ESOPHAGITIS

CLINICAL FEATURES

Eosinophilic esophagitis is a primary clinicopathologic disorder of the esophagus with a significant increase in recognition over the past decades. It occurs in all ages, but is seen more frequently in young children with atopic symptoms such as eczema, asthma, and food allergies. Symptoms manifest differently in different age groups: infants and young children often present with feeding difficulties, whereas older children and adults usually complain of dysphagia and food impaction. Eosinophilic esophagitis can progress to odynophagia and stenosis if not recognized early.

PATHOLOGIC FEATURES

GROSS FINDINGS

Endoscopic examination shows classic mucosal rings, furrows, granularity, exudates, and mucosal fragility (Figs. 1-26 and 1-27). However, in some patients the endoscopic findings can be normal. In long-standing cases, stricture formation may be seen.

MICROSCOPIC FINDINGS

Biopsies show a marked eosinophilic infiltrate with a heterogeneous mucosal distribution. Eosinophils tend to concentrate in the luminal aspect of the epithelium and may be associated with eosinophilic microabscesses (Fig. 1-28). Because the eosinophilic infiltrates are not distributed uniformly at different locations and/or levels, it is generally recommended that 20 or more eosinophils per high-power field in the most densely populated areas be a diagnostic cut-point for eosinophilic esophagitis (Fig. 1-29). Eosinophilic infiltrates involve both the distal and proximal segments of the esophagus with some indications of a more proximal involvement. Other findings include basal zone hyperplasia, elongation of

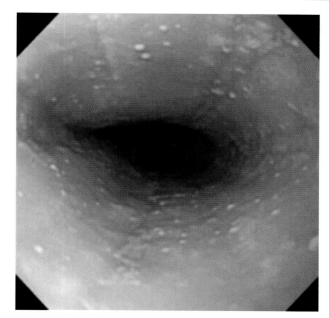

FIGURE 1-26
Eosinophilic esophagitis—endoscopy. Mucosal granularity. *(Courtesy of Dr. J. Gramling.)*

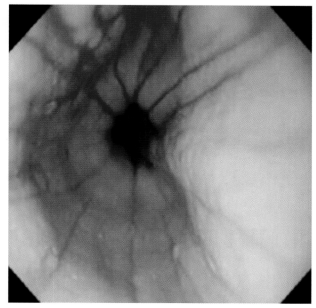

FIGURE 1-27
Eosinophilic esophagitis—endoscopy. Typical furrows and rings. *(Courtesy of Dr. J. Gramling.)*

EOSINOPHILIC ESOPHAGITIS—PATHOLOGIC FEATURES

Gross Findings
- Endoscopic examination reveals mucosal erythema, granularity, and furrows.
- In long-standing cases, strictures are seen.

Microscopic Findings
- Mucosa is heavily infiltrated with eosinophils (more than 20 per high-power field)
- Eosinophils tend to concentrate in surface layer of the epithelium and involve both the distal and proximal segments of esophagus. The infiltrates may be more prominent in the proximal as compared with the distal esophagus.
- Additional findings including basal zone hyperplasia, elongation of the vascular papillae, intercellular edema, congestion, and hemorrhage.

Differential Diagnosis
- Reflux esophagitis and viral and fungal infections are in the differential diagnosis.
- Reflux changes are mostly seen in biopsy samples from the distal esophagus or gastroesophageal junction.
- In eosinophilic gastroenteritis, eosinophils are also present in other segments of the GI tract.
- Special stains (GMS and PAS) help disclose hyphal and yeast forms of *Candida* infection.
- CMV and herpes have characteristic viral cytopathic changes.

DIFFERENTIAL DIAGNOSIS

Eosinophilic esophagitis must be distinguished mainly from reflux and infectious esophagitis because the treatment is entirely different. In reflux esophagitis, the changes are prominent in the lower esophagus and tend to disappear in more proximal biopsy samples. In infectious cases, the changes involve more of a polymorphonuclear infiltrate with necrotic debris. Viral cytopathic effects characterize herpes and CMV infections. In *Candida* esophagitis one sees yeast and pseudohyphae forms permeating the esophageal mucosa, accompanied by necrotic debris. Special stains (Gomori methenamine silver [GMS], periodic acid–Schiff [PAS]) are sometimes necessary to show them better.

PROGNOSIS AND THERAPY

The prognosis is excellent when treatment is given promptly. Progression of the disease is seen when an incorrect diagnosis of reflux is rendered. Therapy includes dietary elimination of offending foods and swallowing of topical steroids. Improvements are sometimes dramatic.

the vascular papillae to greater than 50% the thickness of the squamous epithelium, intercellular edema, congestion, and hemorrhage. In adults, T-lymphocytes and mast cells are increased along with an elevation of interleukin-5, tumor necrosis factor-α, and immunoglobulin E–mediated inflammation.

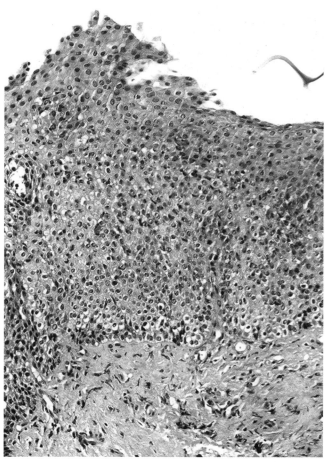

FIGURE 1-28
Eosinophilic esophagitis. Intense eosinophilic infiltrate.

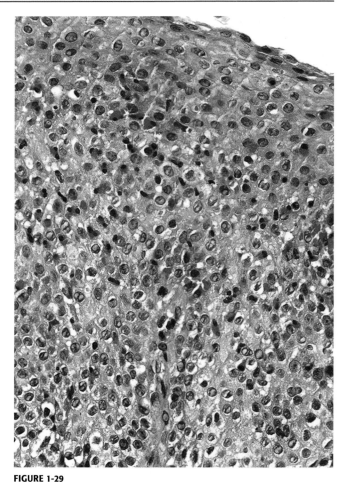

FIGURE 1-29
Eosinophilic esophagitis. Intraepithelial eosinophils (more than 20 per high-power field).

■ PILL ESOPHAGITIS

Esophageal ulcerations occur when medications taken with little or no water attach to and damage the mucosa. Drugs provoking this condition range from antibiotics to nonsteroidal anti-inflammatory agents.

CLINICAL FEATURES

This clinical presentation can occur at any age but seems to be more frequent in older adults, especially in women. The main symptoms are sudden retrosternal pain and painful swallowing.

In rare cases hematemesis occurs. Symptoms subside in a few days. Some patients present with atypical symptoms, suggesting a myocardial infarct or regular reflux disease. Some medications such as sodium valproate, ferrous sulfate, and aspirin-caffeine compounds have been associated with esophageal perforation and mediastinitis.

PILL ESOPHAGITIS—FACT SHEET

Definition
- Damage of the esophagus when pills adhere to the mucosal wall and release their content
- Occurs when pills are taken with little or no water

Incidence and Location
- Four cases per 100,000 population per year
- The lesions are mostly localized at the level of the aortic arch

Gender and Age Distribution
- Occurs mostly in older adults
- Females are more affected than males at a ratio of 2.2:1

Clinical Features
- Sudden onset of retrosternal pain and odynophagia
- Hematemesis and perforations are rare complications.

Prognosis and Therapy
- Patients recuperate within a few weeks after discontinuation of the drug.
- Antireflux therapy and swallowing of topical anesthetics are recommended.

PATHOLOGIC FEATURES

GROSS FINDINGS

Endoscopic examination reveals the presence of one or more discrete ulcers. Residual pill fragments sometimes can be seen. The lesions are more commonly seen at the level of the aortic arch but can present in any area of the esophagus. Other findings have been reported in cases associated with the ingestion of slow-release drugs. In such cases a more dramatic endoscopic finding is observed, with nodularity and abundant exudates, suggesting a neoplastic process.

MICROSCOPIC FINDINGS

Histologic findings are nonspecific and include superficial erosions or ulcerations with marked acute inflammation and florid granulation tissue (Figs. 1-30 and 1-31). Foreign material is sometimes present in the ulcer.

DIFFERENTIAL DIAGNOSIS

Ulcerations caused by herpes or *Candida* infection show characteristic findings that include pseudohyphal forms (in *Candida*) or the typical intranuclear inclusions and multinucleated giant cells (in herpes simplex virus [HSV]).

Ulceration caused by neoplastic processes is in the differential diagnosis, but careful histologic examination will disclose the real nature of the process.

PILL ESOPHAGITIS—PATHOLOGIC FEATURES

Gross Findings
- Discrete ulcerations occur mostly at the level of the aortic arch.
- Sometimes granularity and excessive exudates mimic a neoplastic condition.

Microscopic Findings
- Nonspecific erosions and ulcerations are seen with florid granulation tissue
- Sometimes foreign material is found.

Differential Diagnosis
- Infectious processes include as *Candida,* herpes, and CMV infections.
- Neoplastic lesions need to be excluded.

PROGNOSIS AND THERAPY

In most cases, patients recuperate ad integrum a few weeks after cessation of the drug. Antireflux therapy and swallowing of topical anesthetics is recommended. Cases of repeated injury may lead to strictures requiring dilation.

■ INFECTIOUS ESOPHAGITIS

Bacteria, fungi, viruses, and parasites can cause infections in the esophagus. The most common ones are *Candida*, HSV, and CMV. In South America, infection

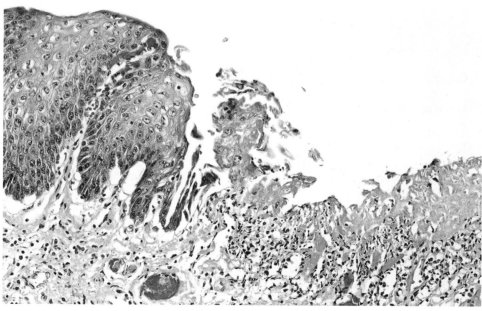

FIGURE 1-30

Pill esophagitis. Esophageal mucosa with ulceration.

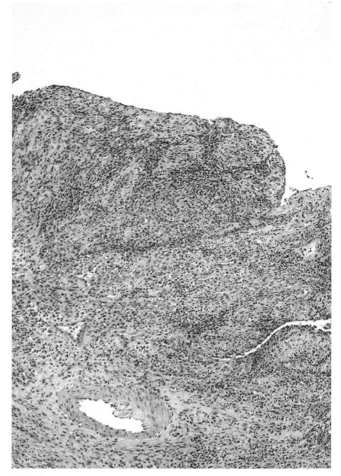

FIGURE 1-31

Pill esophagitis. Ulcer granulation tissue.

by *Trypanosoma cruzi* is the cause of esophageal disease leading to megaesophagus, megacolon, and dilated cardiomyopathy. This section addresses candidiasis, HSV, and CMV.

CLINICAL FEATURES

These three infectious processes affect mainly a patient who is immunocompromised due to either chemotherapy or human immunodeficiency virus disease. Patients undergoing bone marrow transplantation are also at risk. Herpes esophagitis can occur in healthy children or young adults presenting with fever and malaise. HSV type 1 is implicated in esophageal infection. *Candida* species are the most common fungal pathogens. *Candida albicans* is by far the most frequent, followed by *C. tropicalis, C. glabrata, C. dublenis,* and *C. parapsilosis.* CMV esophagitis is the third most common infection and is not seen in normal individuals. Dysphagia, chest pain, and odynophagia are the most common symptoms in all three infections. Some individuals with candidiasis may remain asymptomatic.

RADIOLOGIC FEATURES

Before the development of endoscopy, barium studies were used. They have been replaced by endoscopic examination. In barium studies, diffuse irregularities in the esophageal wall are observed in candidiasis, whereas discrete ulcerations are seen in both CMV and herpes infections.

PATHOLOGIC FEATURES

GROSS FINDINGS

In candidiasis, the endoscopic picture is that of numerous white plaques distributed along the esophageal length. Larger plaques sometimes obstruct the lumen, but ulcers are uncommon. Herpes infection reveals numerous ulcers of varying shape and size (Fig. 1-32), whereas CMV infection shows deep ulcers covered by yellow exudates mostly in the distal esophagus.

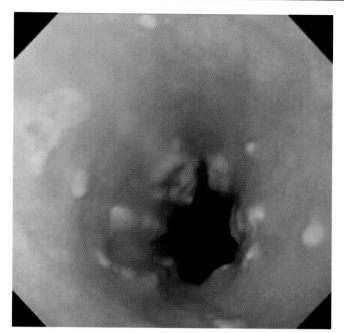

FIGURE 1-32

Herpes esophagitis—endoscopy. Ulcers and white exudates. *(Courtesy of Dr. J. Gramling.)*

MICROSCOPIC FINDINGS

Either esophageal brushings or biopsies have been used in the diagnosis of these infections. Brushings are more sensitive than biopsy specimens. Candidiasis affects the superficial mucosa and invades the deeper layers. An abundant infiltrate of neutrophils and debris are present. The organisms show typical yeast and pseudohyphal forms. Special stains (GMS and PAS) are sometimes necessary to reveal the microorganisms (Figs. 1-33 through 1-35).

In brushes stained with Papanicolaou, the hyphae and yeasts have an intense red color (Fig.1-36). The herpetic ulcers contain the characteristic multinucleated giant cells, with nuclear molding and margination of chromatin (Figs. 1-37 through 1-39). The classic Cowdry A inclusion bodies are also present. They are large, red intranuclear inclusions with a halo (Fig. 1-40); acute inflammation is commonly present. In CMV infection, the lesions appear as deep ulcers, and the infected cells are best seen in endothelial and mesenchymal cells. The characteristic finding is that of a large cell with intracytoplasmic basophilic inclusions and a large red intranuclear inclusion that gives the characteristic "owl's eye" (Figs. 1-41 through 1-43).

INFECTIOUS ESOPHAGITIS—PATHOLOGIC FEATURES

Gross Findings

- White plaques with exudates in candidiasis
- May involve the whole length of the esophagus
- Shallow ulcers of variable size, with widespread location in herpes cases
- CMV ulcers are located mostly in the distal esophagus.

Microscopic Findings

- The squamous epithelium is acutely inflamed and contains yeast and pseudohyphal forms characteristic of *Candida* infection.
- Multinucleated giant cells with nuclear molding and margination of chromatin are characteristic of herpes infection. The Cowdry A type of viral inclusion is also seen.
- Submucosal capillary endothelial and mesenchymal cells show large cells with both intracytoplasmic and intranuclear inclusions in cases of CMV infection.

Immunohistochemistry

- Specific stains are only used in difficult cases when the diagnosis is in doubt. The typical monoclonal antibody immunostain demonstrates positive intranuclear inclusions.

Differential Diagnosis

- In typical cases, the diagnosis is not difficult.
- Severe reflux and pill-induced esophageal injury are in the differential diagnosis.
- Viral cytopathic effects of varicella zoster are identical to those of HSV; immunostains and viral cultures are indicated to exclude this possibility.

ANCILLARY STUDIES

Most of the time there is no need for ancillary studies. Sometimes, however, when the diagnosis is not clear, the use of immunoperoxidase stain is necessary. Tissue culture for herpes and CMV is also recommended.

DIFFERENTIAL DIAGNOSIS

Severe reflux esophagitis and pill-induced esophageal injury are in the differential diagnosis. In reflux or pill injury, there is no evidence of either cellular cytopathic effect or fungal organisms. Varicella zoster infection shows an identical cytopathic effect, but these patients also present with skin vesicles. When in doubt, immunostains are required and viral cultures are recommended.

PROGNOSIS AND THERAPY

Prognosis depends on the underlying disease. *Candida* esophagitis is treated initially with oral azole medications (ketoconazole, fluconazole), reserving the intravenous treatment for refractory cases. Acyclovir is the therapy

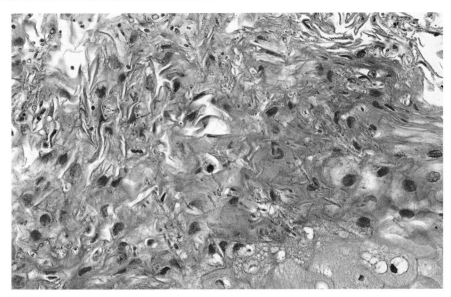

FIGURE 1-33

Candida esophagitis. Invasive pseudohyphae in squamous mucosa.

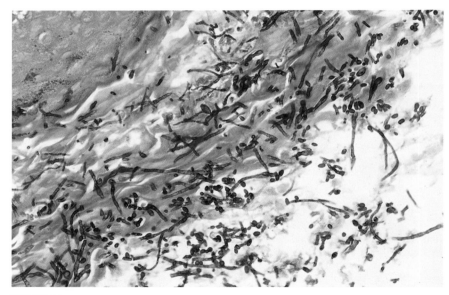

FIGURE 1-34

Candida esophagitis (periodic acid-Schiff).

of choice for herpetic infections. CMV infections require intravenous treatment with ganciclovir or cidofovir.

■ CAUSTIC ESOPHAGEAL INJURY

Caustic injuries in children are a public health problem, with over 5000 cases reported yearly in the United States. It is less common in adults, with an incidence of 1 in 100,000, of which 61% are the result of suicidal attempts. Children younger than 3 years

are the most frequent victims of accidents involving common household products such as bleaches, detergents, and alkalis.

CLINICAL FEATURES

The symptoms are quite variable, and there is little correlation between the severity of symptoms and the degree of esophageal damage. Dysphagia and odynophagia are the main symptoms, with chest and back pain presenting to a lesser extent. Patients complaining of oropharyngeal burns have no associated lesions in the

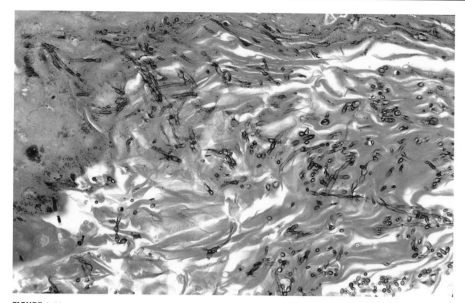

FIGURE 1-35

Candida esophagitis (Gomori methenamine silver).

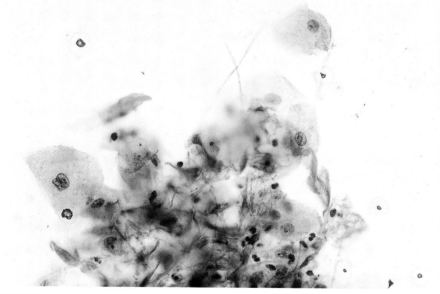

FIGURE 1-36

Candida esophagitis. Papanicolaou stain; esophageal brush showing hyphae and squamous cells. *(Courtesy of Dr. B. Crothers.)*

esophagus in 70% of the cases. When the corrosive agent reaches the stomach, abdominal pain and hematemesis are present. In severe cases, the entire esophageal mucosal cast is extruded (Fig. 1-44). In the most extreme cases, esophageal and gastric perforation with mediastinitis and peritonitis occur. Alkali ingestions are more severe than those caused by acids.

RADIOLOGIC FEATURES

A chest x-ray examination is essential to rule out pulmonary infiltrates, pneumothorax, pneumomediastinum, and subcutaneous emphysema. In follow-up cases, barium swallow will disclose the degree of stenosis.

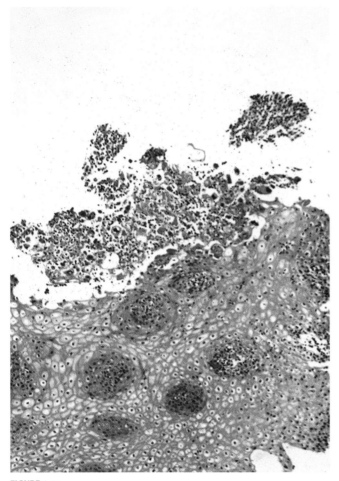

FIGURE 1-37
Herpes esophagitis. Infected cells and necroinflammatory debris.

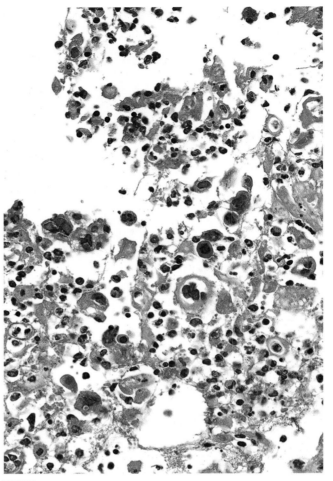

FIGURE 1-38
Herpes esophagitis. Multinucleated giant cells with molding and margination of the chromatin.

CAUSTIC ESOPHAGEAL INJURY—FACT SHEET

Definition
- Injury to the esophagus due to accidental or suicidal ingestion of acids or alkali

Incidence and Location
- More than 5000 cases of accidental caustic injuries to children occur annually in the United States
- Among the adult population the incidence is 1 in 100,000
- In adults, 61% of cases are the result of suicide attempts
- Lesions are located throughout, but mostly at the level of the aortic arch

Gender and Age Distribution
- Seen mostly in children younger than 3 years of age (accidents)
- Seen in adults as suicide attempts
- No gender preference

Clinical Features
- Clinical presentation can be deceiving
- Severe dysphagia and odynophagia with chest and back pain

- If the stomach is involved, perforation and peritonitis may develop
- Severe cases may present with perforation and mediastinitis

Radiologic Features
- Chest imaging is essential to rule out pulmonary infiltrates, pneumomediastinum, and subcutaneous emphysema
- In follow-up cases barium swallow will demonstrate degrees of stenosis

Prognosis and Therapy
- Prognosis will depend on the severity of the lesion
- Alkali lesions are more serious than acid lesions
- Treatment includes intravenous fluids, total parenteral nutrition, steroids, and antibiotics
- Dilation is required in cases of significant stenosis
- Surgery is required in cases of perforation

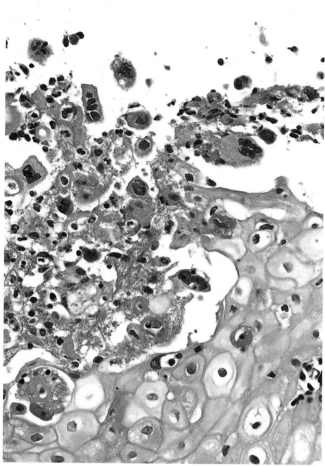

FIGURE 1-39

Herpes esophagitis. Multinucleated giant cells.

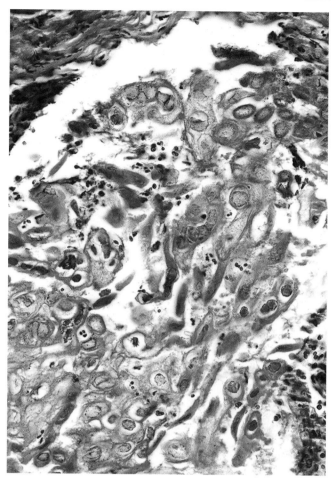

FIGURE 1-40

Herpes esophagitis. Cowdry B type cells.

PATHOLOGIC FEATURES

GROSS FINDINGS

Endoscopic findings vary depending on the severity of the case. A grading system exists similar to the one in skin burns. First-degree cases have superficial edema and erythema. Second-degree cases have muscular involvement with ulceration and necrosis. Third-degree cases have transmural lesions with possible extraesophageal extension (Fig. 1-45).

MICROSCOPIC FINDINGS

Variable degrees of injury occur depending on the offensive agent. Lesions caused by alkali are more severe than those by acids. Areas of coagulative necrosis, diffuse ulceration, and hemorrhage are characteristic.

CAUSTIC ESOPHAGEAL INJURY—PATHOLOGIC FEATURES

Gross Findings

- Findings include mucosal erythema, edema, and friability or ulceration.
- Caustic agents provoke severe necrosis.
- First-degree lesions affect the mucosa only.
- Second-degree lesions affect the muscularis.
- Third-degree lesions are transmural and have a possible extraesophageal extension.

Microscopic Findings

- First-degree lesions show edema and superficial erosion.
- Second-degree lesions show coagulative necrosis and ulceration with muscular extension.
- Third-degree lesions show transmural ulceration and necrotic tissue.
- Lesions can be seen with or without acute or chronic inflammation.

Differential Diagnosis

- When the clinical history is not available, reflux and infectious esophagitis must be ruled out.

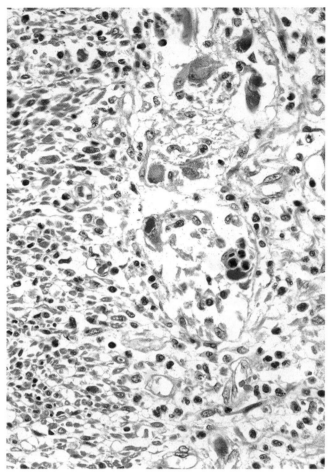

FIGURE 1-41

Cytomegalovirus esophagitis. Mesenchymal cells with cytopathic effect.

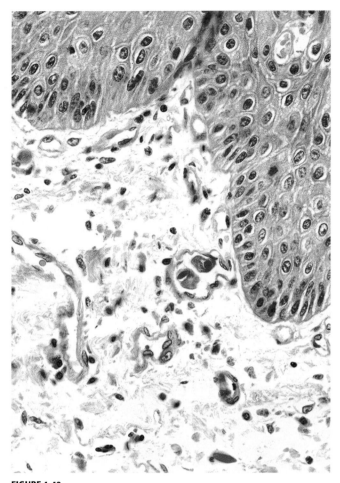

FIGURE 1-42

Cytomegalovirus esophagitis. Infected endothelial cells.

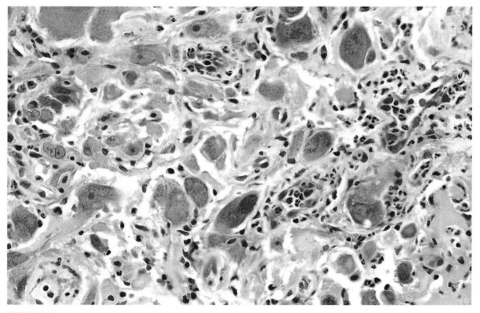

FIGURE 1-43

Cytomegalovirus esophagitis. Numerous bizarre cells with cytopathic effect, some with owl's eye nuclei.

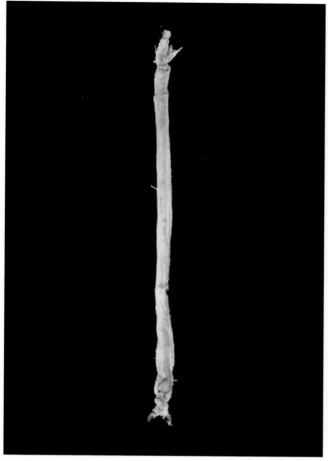

FIGURE 1-44

Esophageal mucosal cast. *(From Turk JL, ed. Royal College of Surgeons of England. Slide Atlas of Pathology. Alimentary Tract System. London, Gower Medical, 1986, with permission.)*

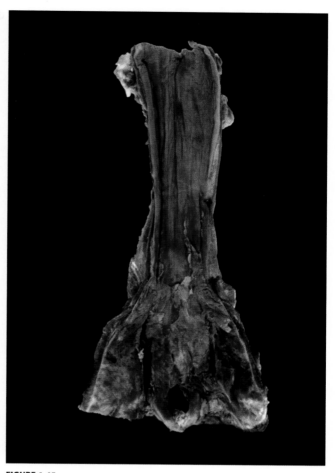

FIGURE 1-45

Caustic esophagitis. Necrosis and perforation. *(From Turk JL, ed. Royal College of Surgeons of England. Slide Atlas of Pathology. Alimentary Tract System. London, Gower Medical, 1986, with permission.)*

DIFFERENTIAL DIAGNOSIS

When the clinical history is not available, other entities enter into the differential diagnosis, including reflux and infectious esophagitis. In reflux, there is no evidence of coagulative necrosis. In infectious processes, either pseudohyphal forms or cytopathic viral effect is present.

PROGNOSIS AND THERAPY

Prognosis obviously depends on the severity of the lesion. Cases are always fatal when more than 6 mL of concentrated alkaline material is ingested. Intravenous fluids, total parenteral nutrition (if patients are unable to swallow), steroid therapy, and antibiotics are treatments of choice. Esophageal dilation is required if strictures develop. Follow-up is recommended resulting from an increased risk for squamous cell carcinoma 20 years after exposure.

■ RADIATION/CHEMOTHERAPY ESOPHAGITIS

These disorders are relatively common as a result of the increased use of radiation therapy to the chest and mediastinum. Some chemotherapeutic agents are capable of causing esophageal mucositis.

CLINICAL FEATURES

Esophageal symptoms in radiation injury depend on factors such as total dose, time period, and previous surgery. At doses of 60 Gy (6000 rads), the esophagus suffers irreversible damage. Acute radiation injury develops after 2 weeks of therapy and consists of dysphagia, odynophagia, and sometimes hematemesis and chest pain. These symptoms subside after radiation stops. Sequelae of radiation include strictures with dysmotility and dysphagia.

RADIATION/CHEMOTHERAPY ESOPHAGITIS—FACT SHEET

Definition
- Esophageal damage secondary to radiation or chemotherapy

Incidence and Location
- Not an infrequent clinical problem as a result of a high incidence of pulmonary and mediastinal neoplasms
- Lesion is seen in any part of the esophagus lying near a neoplastic process
- Sometimes the esophagus is the site of the neoplasm that undergoes radiation.

Gender and Age Distribution
- Affects both sexes
- Occurs mainly in adults and older adults

Clinical Features
- Dysphagia, odynophagia, and dysmotility
- Hematemesis and melena also can occur.

Prognosis and Therapy
- Irreversible damage occurs when the dose is 6000 rads or higher.
- Radiation and chemotherapy can potentiate each other.
- Dilation is used in cases of strictures.

RADIATION/CHEMOTHERAPY ESOPHAGITIS—PATHOLOGIC FEATURES

Gross Findings
- Findings include mucosal edema and acute confluent ulcers.
- Strictures are characteristic long-term complications.

Microscopic Findings
- Bizarre cytomegaly are seen in epithelial and stromal cells.
- Large pale nuclei and abundant vacuolated cytoplasm are seen in radiation esophagitis.
- Multinucleation is another feature.
- Parakeratosis, acanthosis, and blood vessel hyalinization are seen in more chronic cases.
- Chemotherapy can mimic neoplasia with large hyperchromatic nuclei.

Differential Diagnosis
- Neoplasia and viral infections are in the differential diagnosis.
- Neoplasia has a high N/C ratio, mitosis, and hyperchromatism.
- Sometimes neoplasia and radiation coexist in the same individual; immunostains are recommended.
- Multinucleation may be confused with HSV infection.
- Immunoperoxidase stains for HSV and CMV are recommended in difficult cases.

Symptoms are similar with different chemotherapeutic agents. When chemotherapy and radiation therapy are given, their synergistic effect provokes more severe damage with serious symptoms.

RADIOLOGIC FEATURES

In chronic cases, barium swallow reveals variable degrees of stenosis and dysmotility.

PATHOLOGIC FEATURES

GROSS FINDINGS

In acute cases, endoscopic examination reveals friable mucosa with edema and coalescent ulcers (mucositis). In chronic cases, strictures develop 13 to 21 months after therapy (Fig. 1-46).

MICROSCOPIC FINDINGS

Histologic examination in both cases shows significant atypia in epithelial and stromal cells. Enlarged, bizarre cells with pale nuclei and abundant vacuolated cytoplasm are commonly seen. Multinucleation is also a feature (Fig. 1-47). The diagnosis can be achieved with cytologic brush examination.

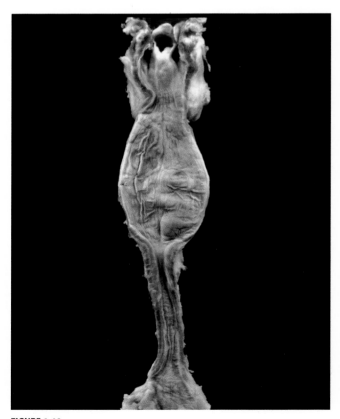

FIGURE 1-46

Esophageal stricture. *(From Turk JL, ed. Royal College of Surgeons of England. Slide Atlas of Pathology. Alimentary Tract System. London, Gower Medical, 1986, with permission.)*

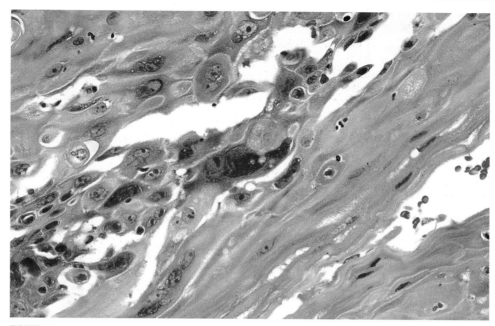

FIGURE 1-47

Radiation esophagitis. Cytomegaly with pale nuclei, abundant cytoplasm, and multinucleation.

DIFFERENTIAL DIAGNOSIS

The most important entities in the differential diagnosis are malignancy and viral esophagitis. Malignant epithelial cells and radiation/chemotherapy-induced damage can mimic each other and sometimes coexist in the same patient. Radiation-induced damage is characterized by uniform enlargement of the cell (cytomegaly), pale nuclei, and vacuolated cytoplasm. In more chronic cases, hyalinization of blood vessels, parakeratosis, and acanthosis are common. In malignancy, an increased nuclear/cytoplasmic (N/C) ratio is the norm, with hyperchromatic nuclei and condensed chromatin; mitotic activity is present. Changes caused by chemotherapy can closely resemble malignancy because mitosis and nuclear hyperchromatism can be present. When in doubt, immunostains for cytokeratin and proliferation markers should be performed.

Multinucleation can be confused with herpes infection, but there is no molding or margination of chromatin. Special immunostains for HSV are indicated to help in the differential diagnosis.

PROGNOSIS AND THERAPY

Prognosis depends on the radiation dose. Reversible damage occurs in doses lower than 6000 rads. A more serious prognosis is when the damage is the result of both radiation and chemotherapy. Esophageal dilation is indicated when stricture develops.

ESOPHAGEAL VARICES

Esophageal varices can be subdivided into uphill or downhill types. Uphill esophageal varices are a manifestation of portal hypertension. In the United States, portal hypertension is mostly due to alcoholic cirrhosis. Worldwide, other causes such as viral hepatitis with cirrhosis and schistosomiasis are more common. Other less common causes are secondary to portal vein thrombosis. When portal hypertension occurs, blood is diverted through the gastric coronary veins and esophageal submucosal plexus to the azygos vein, thus returning to the systemic circulation. Downhill esophageal varices are the result of superior vena cava obstruction due to bronchogenic carcinoma with mediastinal metastasis.

CLINICAL FEATURES

A patient with esophageal varices may not show any symptoms until they rupture, provoking massive hematemesis, melena, shock, and subsequent hepatic coma. In 60% of the cases the first episode is fatal.

RADIOLOGIC FEATURES

The radiologic technique called *mucosal relief* shows the varicose veins as polypoid or serpiginous shadows in the lower or upper esophagus.

ESOPHAGEAL VARICES—FACT SHEET

Definition

- Varicose veins in lower esophagus are the result of portal hypertension caused by cirrhosis (uphill varices).
- Varicose veins in upper esophagus are the result of superior vena cava obstruction (downhill varices).

Incidence and Location

- A frequent complication of alcoholic cirrhosis in the United States
- Worldwide, the result of schistosomiasis and viral hepatitis with cirrhosis
- Mainly localized in the lower esophagus

Gender and Age Distribution

- Occurs in both sexes with a slight male predominance
- Mostly a disease of adults

Clinical Features

- A patient with esophageal varices may be asymptomatic.
- When they rupture, massive hematemesis occurs.
- Most patients succumb after the first episode (60%).

Radiologic Features

- Varices appear as polypoid or serpiginous shadows.

Prognosis and Therapy

- Prognosis is poor if associated with cirrhosis.
- Prognosis is better if the cause is portal vein thrombosis.
- Sclerotherapy is the treatment of choice.

PATHOLOGIC FEATURES

GROSS FINDINGS

Endoscopic examination reveals tortuous bluish bumps protruding into the esophageal lumen. Red spots on the mucosa are associated with an increased risk for bleeding (Figs. 1-48 and 1-49).

ESOPHAGEAL VARICES—PATHOLOGIC FEATURES

Gross Findings

- Endoscopic examination reveals bluish veins protruding into the esophageal lumen.
- Red spots on the mucosal surface are associated with a high risk for rupture.

Microscopic Findings

- Postmortem histology shows markedly ectatic veins and venules in the submucosa. Sometimes the sclerosing agent appears as a brown substance in a vacuole.

Differential Diagnosis

- No other entity looks like esophageal varices, but radiologically they may be confused with submucosally infiltrating esophageal carcinomas.

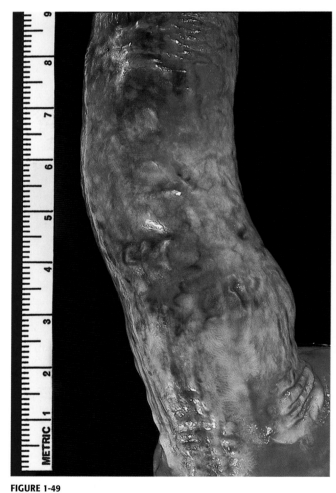

FIGURE 1-49

Esophageal varices. Prominent tortuous veins. *(Courtesy of Dr. P. Vasallo.)*

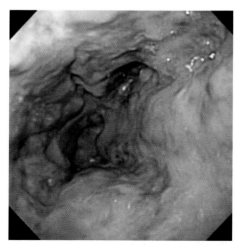

FIGURE 1-48

Esophageal varices—endoscopy. Varices with impending bleed. *(Courtesy of Dr. E. Frizzell.)*

Microscopic Findings

Specimens from postmortem examination show ectatic submucosal veins and venules (Fig. 1-50) with occasional thrombosis. Sometimes the sclerosing agent can be seen as a brown substance with a vacuole.

Differential Diagnosis

The endoscopic examination is so characteristic that no other disease comes to mind in the differential diagnosis.

Prognosis and Therapy

Prognosis is serious in cases of cirrhosis because 60% of patients die after the first episode of bleeding. The prognosis is better when caused by portal vein thrombosis. Sclerotherapy is the treatment of choice while the patient awaits a liver transplant.

ESOPHAGEAL PERFORATIONS AND TEARS

These rather dramatic lesions can be subdivided into spontaneous (Boerhaave's syndrome), iatrogenic, posttraumatic, and esophageal tears (Mallory-Weiss syndrome).

Clinical Features

A sudden increase in intraesophageal pressure can cause "spontaneous" perforation. The classic clinical presentation occurs in middle-aged men after alcohol and food overindulgence. This syndrome is also seen in hyperemesis gravidarum, heavy weight lifting, and so forth. Iatrogenic (instrumental) tearing is the most common cause, representing 48% of the cases. Endoscopy associated with dilatation increases the risk for perforation. Posttraumatic causes account for 8% to 15%. Blunt trauma (rare) is seen in motor vehicle accidents. Penetrating injuries are more common (11% to 17%), resulting from knife or gunshot wounds. Foreign bodies are the cause in 7% to 14% of posttraumatic cases. Symptoms and signs include severe chest and upper abdominal pain, nausea, subcutaneous emphysema, and shock. Esophageal tears (Mallory-Weiss) happen spontaneously or as a result of repeated episodes of vomiting in alcoholics; hematemesis and melena are the most common symptoms.

ESOPHAGEAL PERFORATIONS AND TEARS—FACT SHEET

Definition
- Spontaneous, iatrogenic, or traumatic lesions that result in perforation or tears in the esophagus

Incidence and Location
- Iatrogenic cases account for 48% of all perforations.
- Traumatic cases account for 33%.
- Spontaneous cases (Boerhaave's syndrome) are the least common (8%).
- Tears (Mallory-Weiss syndrome) probably have a higher incidence overall.
- Perforations occur most commonly in the lower esophagus.

Gender and Age Distribution
- Boerhaave's syndrome occurs in men abusing food and alcohol.
- Iatrogenic perforations occur at any age and in both sexes.
- Mallory-Weiss syndrome presents in adults with a history of alcoholism.

Clinical Features
- Symptoms and signs include severe chest pain, vomiting, and subcutaneous emphysema.
- In iatrogenic cases, pain appears right after an endoscopic procedure.
- Hematemesis and melena are characteristic of Mallory-Weiss syndrome.

Radiologic Features
- Posteroanterior and lateral chest x-ray films show pneumomediastinum, pleural effusion, and subcutaneous emphysema.
- Barium esophagography shows the site of perforation in 90% of the cases.
- Tears of Mallory-Weiss syndrome do not have radiologic findings.

Prognosis and Therapy
- High mortality rate in spontaneous or iatrogenic perforations if the diagnosis is delayed (15% to 29%).
- Prognosis is better for Mallory-Weiss syndrome.
- Treatment in most cases is surgical repair.
- Endoscopic hemostasis and thermal therapy are treatments of choice in Mallory-Weiss syndrome.

Radiologic Features

Posteroanterior, lateral chest, and upright abdominal radiographs show pneumomediastinum, pleural effusions, and subcutaneous emphysema. These changes usually appear 1 hour after the initial symptoms. Barium esophagography will detect 90% of surgically confirmed perforations. The tears of Mallory-Weiss syndrome do not have any radiologic findings.

Pathologic Features

Gross Findings

In cases of spontaneous rupture, the lesion is mostly in the distal esophagus. The average size of the lesion is 2 cm; hematomas are present around the tear. Endoscopic

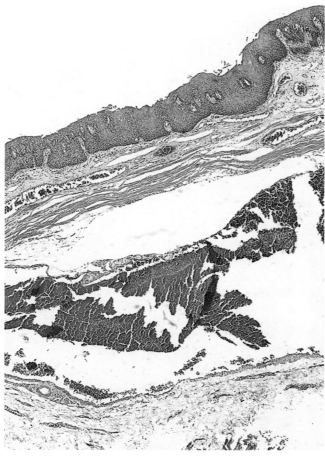

FIGURE 1-50
Esophageal varices. Dilated vessel beneath hyperplastic mucosa.

ESOPHAGEAL PERFORATIONS AND TEARS—PATHOLOGIC FEATURES

Gross Findings

- A full-thickness tear is most commonly seen in the distal esophagus.
- Average size is 2 cm.
- Hematoma surrounds the perforation.
- Abscess formation is seen in cases when the diagnosis is delayed.
- Endoscopic findings in Mallory-Weiss syndrome show longitudinal red tears extending across the Z line.

Microscopic Findings

- They confirm the gross appearance.
- Mallory-Weiss syndrome is never examined via biopsy. In fatal cases the tears demonstrate mucosal dehiscence, edema, and hemorrhage.

Differential Diagnosis

- Endoscopically, Mallory-Weiss may be confused with severe reflux or an ulcerated neoplasm. Reflux will show basal cell hyperplasia, elongation of papillae, and intramucosal eosinophils. An ulcerated neoplasm shows the malignant cells infiltrating and destroying the mucosa and other layers of the esophagus.

DIFFERENTIAL DIAGNOSIS

Clinically a large number of diseases can be confused with rupture, including perforated peptic ulcer, myocardial infarct, pancreatitis, and mesenteric thrombosis.

PROGNOSIS AND THERAPY

Spontaneous and iatrogenic perforations have a poor prognosis with a high mortality rate (15% to 24%) if diagnosis is delayed. Most cases are treated with surgery within 24 hours of diagnosis. Some, however, are treated conservatively with intravenous fluids and antibiotics if the perforation is contained. Mallory-Weiss tears are treated conservatively with thermal therapy and have a good prognosis.

findings in Mallory-Weiss syndrome reveal longitudinal red tears extending across the Z line.

MICROSCOPIC FINDINGS

In fatal cases there is extensive hemorrhage adjacent to the perforation, sometimes with abscess formation.

2

Tumors of the Esophagus

■ **Elizabeth Montgomery, MD**

■ FIBROVASCULAR POLYPS OF THE ESOPHAGUS

CLINICAL FEATURES

These lesions may not be truly neoplastic but are included here as tumefactions that are occasionally encountered in clinical practice. Fibrovascular polyps are extremely rare submucosal tumors of the esophagus that have been variably classified as "lipomas," "fibromas," and "fibrolipomatous" polyps. There is only one such case in the "in-house" surgical pathology files at The Johns Hopkins Hospital between the years 1984 and 2009. Indeed, although the dramatic presentation of these polyps has resulted in about 50 (including hypopharyngeal cases) individual patients reported in the English-language literature between 1969 and the present, only a single case-series of 16 fibrovascular polyps has been compiled: from cases seen at the Armed Forces Institute of Pathology (AFIP).

Most patients with esophageal fibrovascular polyps are middle-aged or older men, although children, infants, and women are rarely affected. In all age-groups, common presenting complaints include dysphagia, substernal discomfort, and sensation of a mass. In the series of Levine and colleagues, all 16 patients with giant fibrovascular polyps were symptomatic; dysphagia was the most common complaint (present in 87 %), followed by respiratory symptoms (25 %) and regurgitation of the polyp into the pharynx or mouth (12 %). Although that series did not show examples of asphyxiation, this is a feared complication that can result in sudden death from impingement of the mass on the larynx. The patient who was seen at our hospital had intermittent airway obstruction that occurred during episodes of vomiting and caused syncope.

The duration of symptoms from giant esophageal polyps has varied greatly among the reported cases. In the AFIP series of Levine and colleagues, the mean duration of symptoms was 17 months, and only 44 % of the patients reported symptoms for 6 months or less.

FIBROVASCULAR POLYPS OF THE ESOPHAGUS—FACT SHEET

Definition
■ Submucosal-based tumors of the esophagus composed of an admixture of adipose tissue, vessels, and fibrous connective tissue

Incidence and Location
■ Very rare; arise anywhere in the esophagus

Morbidity and Mortality
■ May cause morbidity and rare mortality based on obstruction of the esophagus or aspiration, but they are not malignant.

Gender, Race, and Age Distribution
■ Male predominance
■ No known racial predilection

Clinical Features
■ Present with dysphagia, mass sensation, and retrosternal discomfort

---

However, as noted, some patients present emergently and others have had symptoms for 2 months or less.

Most clinically recognized fibrovascular polyps of the esophagus merit the term "giant" when discussed in clinical reports. Lesions reaching 17 and 25 cm in length have been reported. They usually arise in the cervical esophagus, near the region of the cricopharyngeal muscle, which accounts for their tendency to prolapse into the mouth and their ability to impinge on the larynx. The characteristically elongated architecture of these polyps is believed to result from traction created during peristalsis and swallowing.

RADIOLOGIC FEATURES

Chest radiographs reveal a right-sided superior mediastinal mass and anterior tracheal bowing, or both. Barium studies show smooth but variably lobulated intraluminal masses that originate in the lower cervical esophagus, with variable sizes and distal extents, and an average length of about 15 cm. Depending on the amount of fat and fibrovascular tissue in the lesion, computed tomography reveals a heterogeneous appearance in most cases, with some lesions consisting of predominantly fat density and other of predominantly soft tissue density.

PATHOLOGIC FEATURES

GROSS FINDINGS

On gross examination, these are sausage-like pedunculated polyps arising from the wall of the esophagus. Their surface is covered by squamous mucosa, and their cores consist of an admixture of grossly identifiable adipose tissue and firm whitish connective tissue.

MICROSCOPIC FINDINGS

Fibrovascular polyps are histologically uniform lesions composed of variable admixtures of mature adipose tissue lobules, collagenous and sometimes myxoid tissue, and prominent vasculature, all surrounded by mature squamous epithelium (Figs. 2-1 and 2-2).

FIBROVASCULAR POLYPS OF THE ESOPHAGUS—PATHOLOGIC FEATURES

Gross Findings
- Sausage-shaped mucosa-covered mass arising from wall esophageal submucosa protruding into lumen

Microscopic Findings
- Mucosa-covered fibrovascular lesion with adipose tissue

Differential Diagnosis
- Occasionally confused with liposarcoma, which is even rarer in esophagus

DIFFERENTIAL DIAGNOSIS

The appearance of these lesions is relatively unique. Some examples display degenerative atypia in zones of adipose tissue, which may raise the possibility of a well-differentiated liposarcoma, but the latter tumor type is even more rare in the esophagus. However, there are occasional cases that can be diagnosed as such (Figs. 2-3 through 2-5).

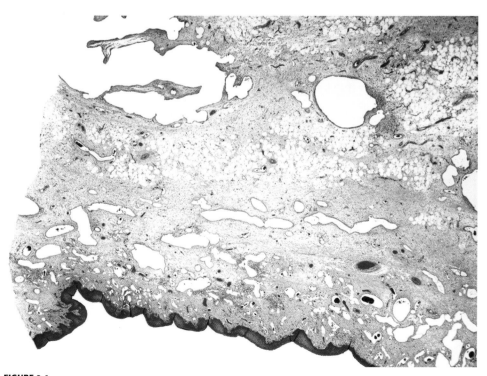

FIGURE 2-1
Fibrovascular polyp, low magnification. It consists of fat, fibrous tissue, and vessels.

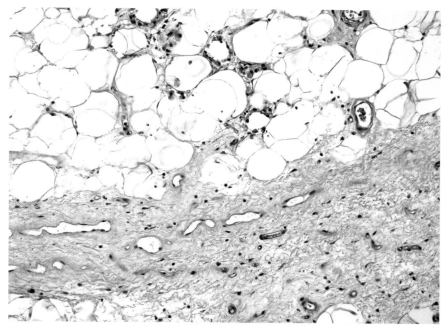

FIGURE 2-2

Fibrovascular polyp.

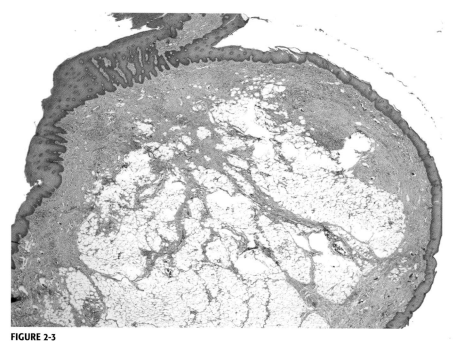

FIGURE 2-3

Well-differentiated liposarcoma of esophagus. Note the enlarged hyperchromatic nuclei. There is no need to see lipoblasts to diagnose well-differentiated liposarcoma.

PROGNOSIS AND THERAPY

Despite their often dramatic clinical presentation and their potential for morbidity and even sudden death, giant fibrovascular polyps of the esophagus should be recognized as uniformly benign lesions; local excision is curative. Depending on their size and the estimated risk of airway impingement, a variety of methods can be employed for resection. If the stalk can be visualized endoscopically, endoscopic ligation can be performed. Endoscopic polypectomy is the ideal management. However, in many other cases, surgical excision is required because of poor visualization, the site of attachment of the stalk, or impending respiratory compromise.

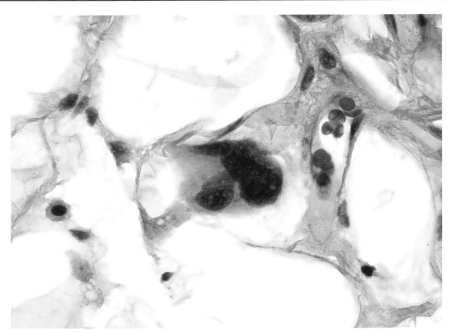

FIGURE 2-4
Well-differentiated liposarcoma of esophagus, high magnification. Note the opaque chromatin.

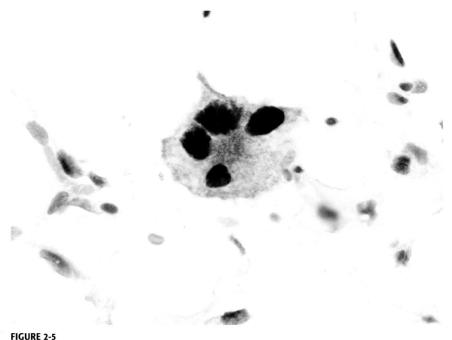

FIGURE 2-5
Well-differentiated liposarcoma of esophagus, MDM2 immunohistochemistry. Nuclear staining correlates with MDM2 amplification in well-differentiated liposarcomas.

Although there are rare instances of recurrence, metastasis has never been reported from these lesions. Secondary tumors such as squamous cell carcinoma arising within a fibrovascular polyp are exceptional.

■ SQUAMOUS PAPILLOMAS

CLINICAL FEATURES

These are uncommon lesions that are usually incidental findings at endoscopy. They usually occur in adults (rare examples are reported in children) and most

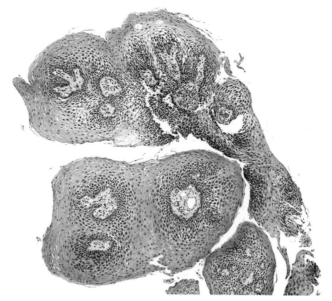

FIGURE 2-6
Squamous papilloma of esophagus. Most such tumors are incidental and unassociated with human papillomavirus.

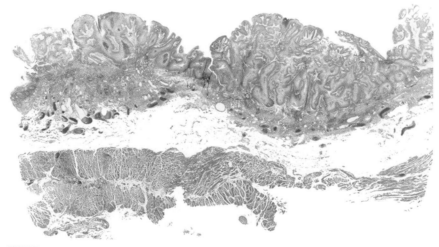

FIGURE 2-7
Esophageal papillomatosis in a young patient with tracheal papillomatosis associated with human papillomavirus.

(85%) are solitary, although some patients have multiple papillomas. They are usually found in the distal esophagus. In Western populations, their presence is associated with reflux disease but this may be coincidental. In the United States, most lesions arise in the distal esophagus, whereas in Japan, they are more likely to arise in the midesophagus.

PATHOLOGIC FEATURES

GROSS FINDINGS

Squamous papillomas are grossly seen as tiny polyps at endoscopy. Mucosal biopsy samples appear as small whitish nodules.

MICROSCOPIC FINDINGS

These lesions are simply composed of bland polypoid squamous mucosa with fibrovascular cores (Fig. 2-6). Exceptional cases display viral cytopathic effects (Figs. 2-7 and 2-8).

ANCILLARY STUDIES

IMMUNOHISTOCHEMISTRY

Because the appearance of these polyps has led to the concern that they are related to human papillomavirus (HPV), several studies have evaluated the presence of

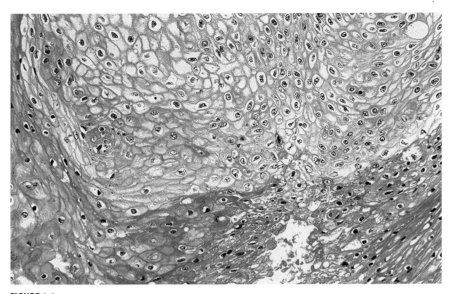

FIGURE 2-8
Human papillomavirus (HPV)-associated papilloma of esophagus showing koilocytotic atypia in keeping with an HPV-associated process.

SQUAMOUS PAPILLOMA OF ESOPHAGUS—FACT SHEET

Definition
- Small, usually incidental nodules of the esophagus composed of proliferated squamous epithelium

Incidence and Location
- Uncommon (estimated, 0.01% to 0.4%) and usually found in the distal esophagus

Morbidity and Mortality
- Essentially none except in rare examples that are associated with laryngeal papillomatosis, which may result in obstruction based on being numerous and uncontrollable

Gender, Race, and Age Distribution
- Sporadic small papillomas are more common in women, usually whites, with a wide age range, but most often in women in their early 40s

Clinical Features
- Incidental finding at endoscopy

SQUAMOUS PAPILLOMA OF ESOPHAGUS—PATHOLOGIC FEATURES

Gross Findings
- Small nodule seen at endoscopy

Microscopic Findings
- Small nodular squamous proliferation aligned in papillary configuration with fibrovascular cores and squamous coating

Immunohistochemistry
- Immunohistochemical, polymerase chain reaction, and in situ hybridization studies for HPV are negative in most series but occasional positive cases are reported

Differential Diagnosis
- Readily separated from squamous cell carcinoma in most cases on the basis of extremely bland cytology

---

DIFFERENTIAL DIAGNOSIS

The diagnosis is seldom a problem. Theoretically the differential diagnosis includes squamous epithelial dysplasia/intraepithelial neoplasia, but in practice the features of these lesions are so bland that there is no difficulty in distinguishing between diagnoses.

PROGNOSIS AND THERAPY

Squamous papillomas of the esophagus do not appear to "degenerate" into esophageal malignancies (or if they do it is a very rare event), and no dysplasia is seen histologically.

HPV in these lesions by both immunohistochemistry and in situ hybridization. The results have been negative in most cases, although a subset (<10%) appears to be associated with HPV. However, a subset of patients with HPV-associated laryngeal papillomatosis has HPV-related squamous papillomas of the esophagus, and occasional esophageal examples have been reported unassociated with laryngeal lesions.

Evidence of recurrence is unusual, but synchronous or metachronous carcinomas of the ororespiratory tract have been described. Many reports suggest a role for mucosal injury and regeneration in the pathogenesis of these lesions. The association with other malignancies may be significant.

■ BARRETT'S ESOPHAGUS, "GOBLET CELLS AT THE GASTROESOPHAGEAL JUNCTION," DYSPLASIA IN BARRETT'S ESOPHAGUS

CLINICAL FEATURES

The prototype patient with Barrett's esophagus is a 55-year-old white man who is overweight and has long-term symptomatic gastroesophageal (GE) reflux disease. He is less likely than controls to have *Helicobacter pylori* gastritis. Barrett's esophagus is distinctly uncommon in African Americans.

The presence of Barrett's mucosa in the esophagus does not in and of itself cause symptoms beyond the symptoms caused by the associated gastroesophageal reflux. The major importance of Barrett's esophagus lies in its status as a preneoplastic condition that predisposes to the development of esophageal adenocarcinoma. There is a well-defined metaplasia-dysplasia-adenocarcinoma sequence in Barrett's esophagus. From

---

BARRETT'S ESOPHAGUS—FACT SHEET

Definition
- A change of any length that is found in the esophagus and is shown to have intestinal metaplasia on biopsy (US definition). In Japan and the United Kingdom, intestinal metaplasia is not required.

Incidence and Location
- Common; found in 5% to 8% of individuals with gastroesophageal reflux disease.

Morbidity and Mortality
- Barrett's esophagus in and of itself does not result in mortality but is a strong risk factor for esophageal adenocarcinoma, with an estimated annual rate of transformation of approximately 0.5%.

Gender, Race, and Age Distribution
- Strong white male predominance with median age in the early 50s.

Clinical Features
- Symptomatic reflux usually leads to biopsy, but the Barrett's esophagus itself is asymptomatic; in fact, once metaplasia occurs, reflux symptoms are said to decrease.

---

a histologic standpoint, dysplasia is recognized when there is abnormal hyperchromatism, enlargement, crowding, and stratification of nuclei of the columnar-lining cells; dysplasia is categorized as low-grade and high-grade. Dysplastic Barrett's mucosa does not appear any different from nondysplastic Barrett mucosa on routine endoscopy, and the condition is defined histologically.

The pathogenesis of Barrett's esophagus is not clear. It is associated with chronic, severe reflux in most cases. It is unlikely that squamous epithelium directly undergoes metaplasia into columnar epithelium. Rather, it is considered more likely that destruction of the squamous epithelium first occurs from injury by acid or alkaline gastroesophageal reflux, followed by re-epithelialization by columnar epithelium, perhaps first with a hybrid-type epithelium that some have termed *multilayered epithelium* (Fig. 2-9). It is possible that the acid component sets up initial erosions and that the alkaline component may inform the reparative process (epidemiologically, bile is a carcinogen).

RADIOLOGIC FEATURES

There are no specific features of Barrett's esophagus, but the presence of a hiatal hernia on imaging studies is a clue, because this condition is a risk factor.

PATHOLOGIC FEATURES

GROSS FINDINGS

During the endoscopic procedure, Barrett's mucosa appears as tongues and patches of reddish salmon-colored mucosa (in contrast to the normal pearly gray-pink color of the squamous epithelium) that extend from the GE junction for varying distances up into the tubular esophagus. Short-segment Barrett's esophagus is defined as less than 3 cm of metaplastic columnar epithelium (Fig. 2-10), and long-segment Barrett's esophagus is defined as greater than 3 cm of metaplastic columnar epithelium (Fig. 2-11). This distinction is important because, although short-segment Barrett's esophagus is more common, it is less likely than long-segment Barrett's esophagus to give rise to esophageal adenocarcinoma.

MICROSCOPIC FINDINGS

Barrett's esophagus is defined as the replacement of the normal squamous epithelial lining of the tubular esophagus by columnar epithelium. In the past, this metaplastic columnar mucosa was classified as one of three types: (1) cardiac-type mucosa, (2) oxyntic-type mucosa, and (3) distinctive-type mucosa (also called

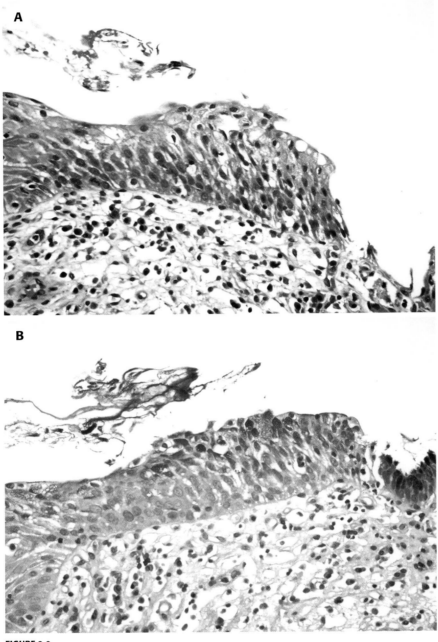

FIGURE 2-9

A, Multilayered epithelium (H&E), demonstrating features of both squamous and columnar mucosa. **B,** Multilayered epithelium (PAS/Alcian blue). There is alcianophilic mucin similar to that seen in goblet cells.

specialized Barrett's mucosa). Distinctive-type mucosa is columnar mucosa that contains goblet cells (normally present only in the small bowel and colon); typically these goblet cells are admixed with gastric-type lining cells, and this type of metaplasia is termed *incomplete* (Figs. 2-12 and 2-13). Distinctive-type Barrett mucosa is the most important of these three types; in fact, in current practice, Barrett's esophagus is equated with the

presence of distinctive-type mucosa in conjunction with endoscopic findings of Barrett's in the United States and Germany. However, in Japan and much of Europe and the United Kingdom, goblet cells are not required to diagnose Barrett's esophagus and it is thus an endoscopic rather than histologic diagnosis. The U.S. and German requirement for goblet cells is based on the assumption that patients with distinctive-type Barrett's esophagus

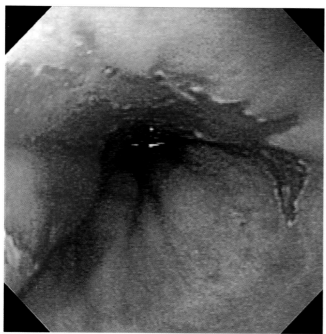

FIGURE 2-10

Barrett's esophagus, endoscopic appearance. Note the tongues of salmon-colored epithelium extending into the grayish squamous mucosa.

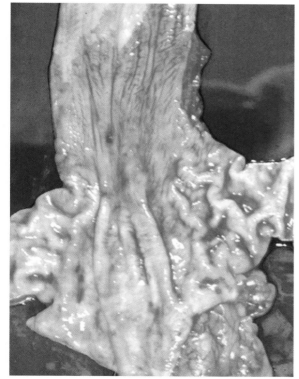

FIGURE 2-11

Long-segment Barrett's esophagus, resection specimen, showing velvet-like mucosa above the anatomic junction of the esophagus and stomach. This esophagus was excised in 1996 because there was extensive high-grade columnar epithelial dysplasia. Today many such lesions would be managed endoscopically.

BARRETT'S ESOPHAGUS—PATHOLOGIC FEATURES

Gross Findings

- Salmon-colored velvety mucosa in the esophagus
- Originates distally and progresses proximally

Microscopic Findings

- Usually incomplete intestinal metaplasia (goblet cells interspersed with cells resembling gastric foveolar cells)
- Examples: epithelial changes graded as indefinite for dysplasia, low-grade dysplasia, or high-grade dysplasia

Immunohistochemistry

- CK7+, Das1+, racemase+, CDX2+, MUC2+, variable MUC 5AC, and MUC6

Differential Diagnosis

- With intestinal metaplasia of the gastric cardia; requires clinico-pathologic correlation

---

are most susceptible to development of dysplasia and adenocarcinoma. However, there is evidence that any columnar mucosa can be associated with neoplasia and the criteria may change.

Alcian blue (pH 2.5) may be used to highlight goblet cells, but other cell types can display a blue staining that is not indicative of intestinal metaplasia. Esophageal submucosal glands are nearly always Alcian blue–positive, as are some gastric foveolar cells.

SUMMARY OF DEFINITION OF BARRETT'S ESOPHAGUS

According to the 2008 definition of the American College of Gastroenterology, Barrett's mucosa is a change in the esophageal epithelium of any length that (1) can be recognized at endoscopy and (2) is confirmed to have intestinal metaplasia by biopsy. As a result, pathologists cannot make the diagnosis of Barrett's mucosa in the absence of endoscopic findings, and regardless of the endoscopic findings, in the United States, Barrett's mucosa is diagnosed only when there are goblet cells—a definition that may be modified over time.

DYSPLASIA IN BARRETT'S ESOPHAGUS

GRADING DYSPLASIA IN BARRETT'S ESOPHAGUS—ALGORITHM

The algorithm outlined is based on four major mucosal features in Barrett's esophagus, but with additional histologic features aimed at helping observers better distinguish among indefinite for dysplasia (IND), low-grade dysplasia (LGD), and high-grade dysplasia (HGD). The algorithm presupposes that the biopsy in question is

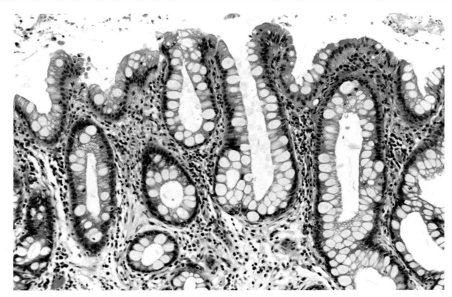

FIGURE 2-12

Barrett's esophagus. This biopsy specimen came from the tubular esophagus and shows intestinal metaplasia.

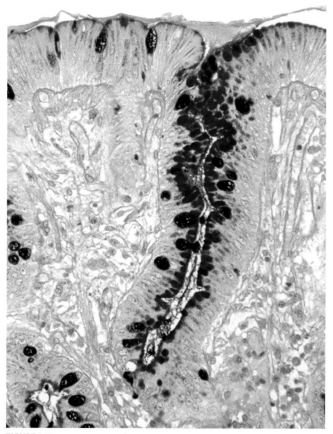

FIGURE 2-13

Barrett's esophagus (PAS/AB stain). Note the blue goblet cells with interposed cells displaying neutral mucin, imparting a magenta color on the PAS stain. This feature is more like the pattern of gastric foveolar cells rather than intestinal absorptive cells, and this combination of cell types is sometimes termed *incomplete intestinal metaplasia*.

taken from the esophagus containing compatible endoscopic features of Barrett's esophagus and that intestinal metaplasia is found. However, the same criteria can be used without intestinal metaplasia.

There are four features:

1. *Surface maturation* in comparison with the underlying glands
2. *Architecture* of the glands on the biopsy
3. *Cytologic features* of the proliferating cells
4. *Inflammation and erosions/ulcers*

Each feature may vary, and they are combined to arrive at a diagnosis.

SURFACE MATURATION

Surface maturation is assessed at low magnification and confirmed at high magnification. In nondysplastic Barrett's esophagus, the proliferating nuclei in the most basal layers of the glands are larger, more hyperchromatic, and more stratified than those at the surface, which are generally arranged in a monolayer with polarized basal nuclei. The glands in Barrett's esophagus are characteristically mildly atypical, especially when viewed in comparison with adjacent nonmetaplastic gastric fundic or cardiac-type glands. Thus, an eye-catching feature when scanning a biopsy at low magnification is the tinctorial comparison between the deep portions of the biopsy and the surface. This may be one of the following: the glands have proportionally larger nuclei, the glands and surface are similar as to nuclear size, or the surface has proportionally larger nuclei.

ARCHITECTURE

Architecture is also best assessed at low magnification. The glandular architecture of a biopsy is the relation between the glands and the lamina propria and also encompasses the outline of the glands. Architectural abnormalities encompass both increased numbers of glands and changes in their shape. In the nondysplastic setting, the glands tend to be round with little budding and are surrounded by abundant laminae propria. Crowding of normal-appearing glands is considered a mild architectural abnormality. Crowding of abnormal glands is a feature of dysplasia. Cribriform glands, cystic dilation, and necrotic luminal debris are considered severe architectural abnormalities.

CYTOLOGIC FEATURES

Cytologic features are mostly assessed at high magnification in zones selected as abnormal during the assessment of surface maturation and architecture. Some degree of nuclear enlargement and atypia are inherent in Barrett's metaplasia in the absence of dysplasia, especially in the basal zone. In summary, cytologic atypia in Barrett's esophagus can be caused by dysplasia, in which case it should be cytologically and architecturally unequivocal; reactive changes, particularly associated with inflammation; or inherent changes in the deeper glands of Barrett's esophagus, in which case the changes are mild and mature toward the surface. Dysplastic cells are generally hyperchromatic, and once the cells have been interpreted as dysplastic, assigning a low- and high-grade category reflects a matter of degree along a morphologic continuum, a point emphasized in the 2001 criteria. Also included in the assessment of cytologic features is the assessment of the relationship of nuclei, one to another, referred to as *nuclear polarity*. In "normal polarity," the long axis of the nucleus remains perpendicular to the basement membrane and the nuclei are aligned parallel one to another, whereas "loss of nuclear polarity" refers to loss of this perpendicular orientation and a random "jumbled" appearance of the nuclei in relation to the basement membrane and one another.

INFLAMMATION AND EROSIONS/ULCERS

Inflammation and erosions add difficulty and are assessed at both scanning and high magnification. They can obscure a truly malignant lesion or impart worrisome cytologic alterations that are attributable to a reparative process.

With application of the algorithm, the classification of dysplasia follows.

BARRETT'S ESOPHAGUS, NEGATIVE FOR DYSPLASIA

In Barrett's esophagus without dysplasia (Figs. 2-12 and 2-14), the surface appears more mature than the underlying glands in that the nuclear-to-cytoplasmic ratio of surface cells is lower than that of the deeper glands. The architecture is normal, with abundant laminae propria between glands. The cytologic features are normal; mitoses may be present in deeper glands, and there may be nuclear stratification. The individual nuclei should have smooth nuclear membranes, and nucleoli, if present, should be small with smooth outlines. Nuclear polarity should be maintained in deep and superficial aspects of the biopsy. If inflammation is a component, reparative features may be present. In this setting, nuclear membranes should remain smooth, although the cells may display nuclear-to-cytoplasmic enlargement

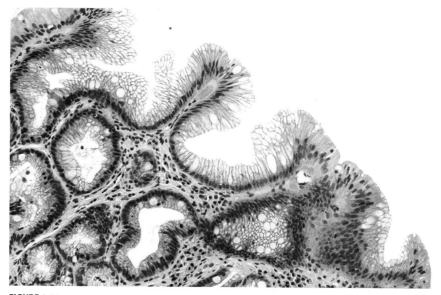

FIGURE 2-14
Barrett's esophagus, negative for dysplasia.

and nucleoli may become more prominent but retain smooth contours. The surface should show maturation compared with the deeper glands but there may be some loss of surface mucin.

Barrett's Esophagus, Indefinite for Dysplasia

By using the algorithm, we include cases that have deeper cytologic changes suggestive of dysplasia but that show surface maturation in IND category (Fig. 2-15). Cases in the IND category could have normal architecture or some degree of glandular crowding. On cytologic evaluation, lesions could have hyperchromasia, nuclear membrane irregularities, and increased mitoses in the deeper aspects and all of these matured to the surface. Loss of nuclear polarity is not a feature of IND. In the presence of inflammation, more striking architectural abnormalities can be included in the IND category. A helpful feature in separating IND from low-grade dysplasia is the presence of an abrupt "clonal" demarcation of the epithelial changes as seen in Figure 2-16. The presence of surface maturation is a helpful feature in separating potentially reactive lesions from truly neoplastic (dysplastic) ones, but some dysplastic lesions do display surface maturation, either as a result of tangential embedding or because they are early. The term *basal crypt dysplasia* has been applied to this appearance (Fig. 2-17).

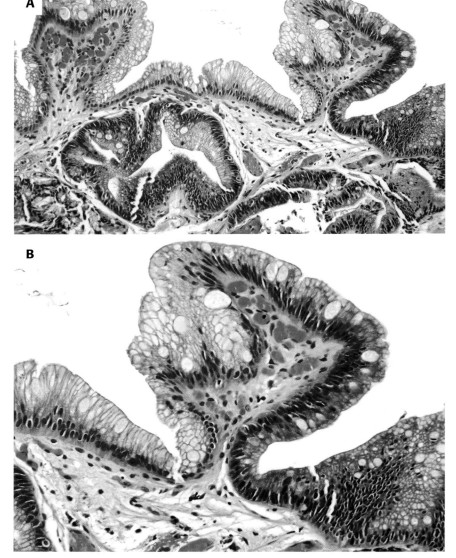

FIGURE 2-15

Columnar epithelial changes, indefinite for dysplasia. **A,** In this biopsy specimen, there are stratified epithelial cells in the deeper glands and on the surface at the right of the field. These areas gradually transition with the more clearly mature cells at the surface on the left, where the nuclei form a monolayer. **B,** Higher magnification.

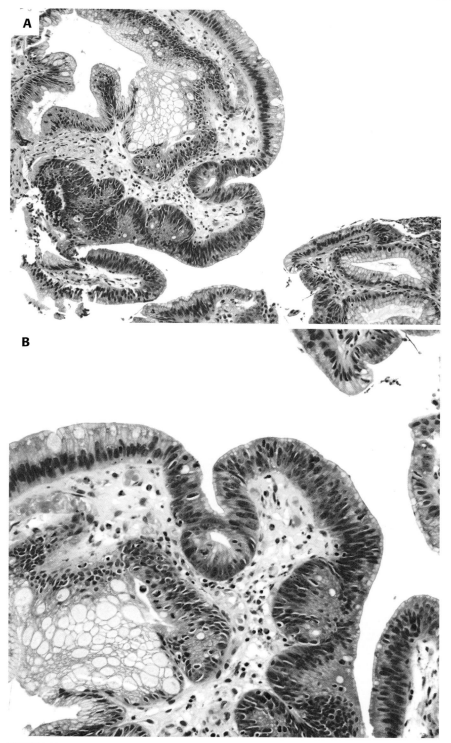

FIGURE 2-16

Low-grade dysplasia in Barrett's esophagus. **A,** The lower right contains an area of surface eptihelial changes that transition abruptly at the center of the field. **B,** Higher magnification of the transition point.

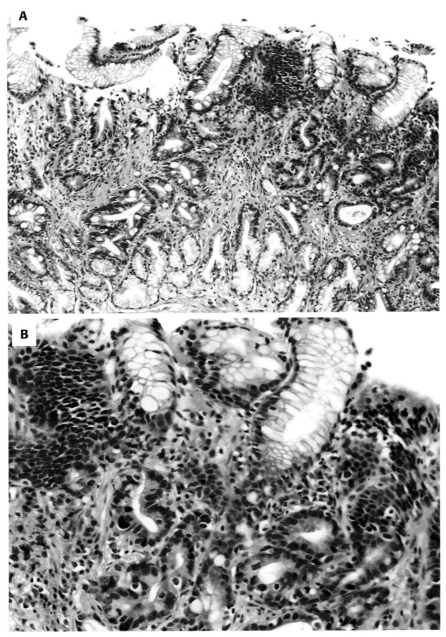

FIGURE 2-17

Dysplasia with surface maturation (basal crypt dysplasia). **A,** Usually surface maturation is a sign of reparative changes but occasional examples of dysplasia show the epithelial changes restricted to deeper glands, sometimes as a result of tangential embedding. **B,** Higher magnification.

BARRETT'S ESOPHAGUS, LOW-GRADE DYSPLASIA

In Barrett's esophagus with low-grade dysplasia, the surface appears similar to the underlying glands at low magnification or displays only slight maturation (see Fig. 2-16). The architecture may be mildly to markedly distorted with glandular crowding, although lamina propria should be identifiable between glands. The cytologic features are important and the changes should extend at least focally to the surface, although rare cases display a "basal crypt" pattern as noted earlier. There is nuclear hyperchromasia with some chromatin clumping. The nuclei show nuclear membrane irregularities but not pronounced nuclear enlargement. Nucleoli are not prominent in LGD, and loss of nuclear polarity is not a feature of LGD, although nuclear stratification similar to that seen in colonic adenomas may be present at the surface. Inflammation is typically minimal; cases with abundant inflammation and the other features of LGD are usually best classified in the IND category. If tangential embedding precludes evaluation of the surface, LGD can be diagnosed if there are dysplastic features in the deep aspects in the absence of inflammation (see Fig. 2-17), provided that the features of HGD are lacking.

BARRETT'S ESOPHAGUS, HIGH-GRADE DYSPLASIA

In HGD, surface maturation is lacking (Fig. 2-18). The architecture may show crowding of cytologically abnormal glands or be markedly distorted with prominent glandular crowding and little intervening lamina propria. If the cytologic features are sufficiently dysplastic, lesser architectural distortion is acceptable. Nuclei are hyperchromatic and nuclear membranes irregular. Cells may have either delicately clumped dark heterochromatin and inconspicuous nucleoli or prominent irregular nuclei with irregularly clumped chromatin and irregular nucleoli. Markedly enlarged hyperchromatic cells are a feature of HGD, and these may extend to the surface. Loss of nuclear polarity is seen in HGD. Mitoses are readily identifiable. Inflammation is typically minimal but some examples have dense inflammation. Some cases also show numerous small glands with a monolayer of hyperchromatic nuclei rather than stratified nuclei (Fig. 2-19). This pattern has been referred to as *nonadenomatous dysplasia*. There is evidence to suggest that the finding of HGD with an associated ulcer is highly suspicious for nearby invasive carcinoma.

INTRAMUCOSAL CARCINOMA

The distinction between HGD and the earliest intramucosal carcinoma (defined as invasion through the basement membrane into the lamina propria or muscularis mucosae but not beyond) remains difficult (Figs. 2-20 through 2-22). In general, these cases begin to demonstrate an effacement of lamina propria architecture and a syncytial growth pattern, extensive back-to-back microglands, and an intermingling of single cells and small clusters within the lamina propria. Typically, desmoplasia is absent to incompletely developed at this stage, hence its recognition is difficult and subjective. In carcinoma that has invaded more deeply (into the submucosa), desmoplasia and a clearly infiltrative growth pattern become readily apparent, although tangentially embedded and scarred tissue can pose diagnostic problems. In the upper gastrointestinal tract, invasion into the lamina propria is more significant than in the colon because the colon lamina propria lacks significant lymphatic access. In the colon, invasion into the lamina propria is biologically equivalent to HGD, whereas in the esophagus, invasion into the lamina propria can lead to metastatic disease.

ANCILLARY STUDIES

IMMUNOHISTOCHEMISTRY

Most examples of Barrett esophagus are CK7 reactive with surface CK20. Based on intestinal differentiation, CDX2 stains Barrett mucosa.

There is variable expression of MUC1, MUC6, MUC5AC, and MUC2. Das-1 Antibody (modestly named for Kiron M. Das) is also believed to stain Barrett's metaplasia strongly with less staining in gastric intestinal metaplasia. Markers for dysplasia that have been best explored include p53 and Ki-67, both of which demonstrate increased labeling in dysplasia. One laboratory has found α-methylacyl-coenzyme A racemase (AMACR) in labeling dysplasia but this has not been consistently useful in other laboratories. Promotor methylation of a host of genes has been noted and is believed to predict progression in nondysplastic Barrett mucosa.

DIFFERENTIAL DIAGNOSIS

The differential diagnosis of Barrett's esophagus includes gastric carditis with intestinal metaplasia, which requires clinicopathologic correlation with endoscopic findings. This distinction may be less critical than was believed in the past because gastric cardiac carcinomas seem to be associated with the same risk factors as esophageal adenocarcinomas.

The following scenarios cover most situations; the informal comments were developed by members of the Gastrointestinal Pathology Society:

1. **Any gastric-type mucosa with no goblet cells**: This is stomach. If it is cardia, it is highly likely that it has inflammation. **Most mild carditis has no known cause,** especially if the *H. pylori* status is unknown as it usually is. In such cases, the appropriate diagnosis is either **"Carditis of unknown etiology"** or **"No significant abnormality."** However, much evidence points to reflux as a cause of "carditis."
2. **Goblet cell–containing mucosa** from **endoscopic tongues** that the endoscopist thinks are Barrett's: Diagnose as **"Barrett's mucosa"** with the appropriate dysplasia designation (none, indefinite, low-grade, high-grade).
3. **Goblet cell–containing mucosa,** but there are **no endoscopic tongues,** although there may be a prominent endoscopic Z line (the squamocolumnar junction): Diagnose as **"Goblet cells at the cardia."**
4. **Goblet cell–containing mucosa,** but there is **endoscopic uncertainty;** that is, the endoscopist is not sure whether there are tongues or only a prominent Z line: Diagnose as **"Goblet cell–containing**

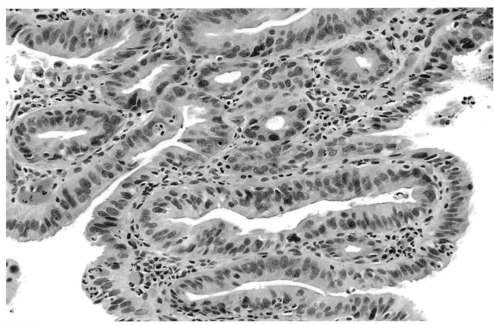

FIGURE 2-18

High-grade dysplasia in Barrett's esophagus.

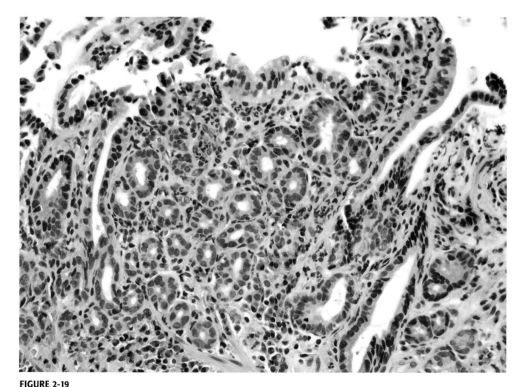

FIGURE 2-19

High-grade dysplasia in Barrett's esophagus. This example has numerous small glands with cells forming a monolayer (rather than stratified). These small tubules are composed of hyperchromatic nuclei.

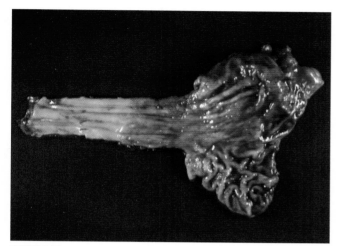

FIGURE 2-20

Esophagectomy from a patient with an early invasive adenocarcinoma.

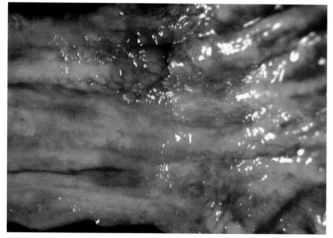

FIGURE 2-21

The subtle nodule in the distal esophagus corresponded to an early invasive adenocarcinoma.

mucosa, either Barrett's mucosa or goblet cells at the cardia," with the appropriate dysplasia designation. If the endoscopist is uncertain whether there is Barrett's mucosa, then pathologists cannot be certain.

PROGNOSIS AND THERAPY

Guidelines for surveillance intervals have been developed by the American College of Gastroenterologists as in Table 2-1. These do not specify segment length.

Because the purpose of surveillance is to detect the earliest lesions, it is important for pathologists handling these biopsy specimens to recognize them. Unfortunately, biopsy interpretation is plagued by problems with intraobserver and interobserver reproducibility, which probably accounts in part for the wide range of progression rates in various series, particularly at the lower ends of the spectrum. Among many surrogate markers explored to improve prognostication, flow cytometry and assessment of p53 may be useful adjuncts in identifying patients at highest risk or even in identifying endoscopic foci of interest for follow-up in patients who are undergoing endoscopic mapping. Sampling error can also be a serious problem in monitoring these patients, but the use of supravital dyes (inexpensive) or newer techniques such as confocal laser endoscopy (expensive) and other methods for "optical biopsy" to identify the best sites to biopsy can be useful.

However, despite substantial limitations inherent in interpretation of biopsies, grade of dysplasia correlates well with progression to invasive carcinoma, and it

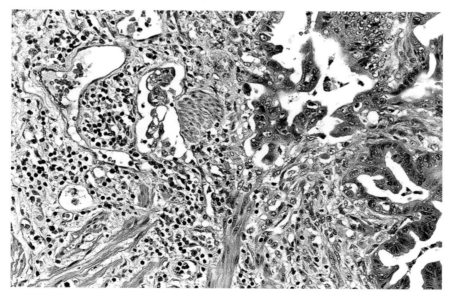

FIGURE 2-22

This adenocarcinoma invades only into the muscularis mucosae ("intramucosal adenocarcinoma," Stage T1a) but has already achieved vascular invasion.

TABLE 2-1

ACG Guidelines for Follow-up of Barrett's Esophagus

Dysplasia	Documentation	Follow-up
None	Two EGDs with biopsy within a year	Endoscopy every 3 years
Low-grade	Highest grade on repeat EGD with biopsies within 6 mos Expert review	1-year interval until two negative EGD with biopsy
High-grade	Repeat EGD with biopsies within 3 months to exclude carcinoma Expert review	Endoscopic mucosal resection Surveillance every 3 months or intervention based on individual patient

EGD = esophagogastroduodenoscopy

remains the foundation of clinical decision making. For example, in our series, grade on initial biopsy correlated significantly with progression to invasive carcinoma (log rank $P = .0001$). Rates of progression in a few series are tabulated (Table 2-2).

In the past, esophagectomy was recommended for HGD but this is no longer the case. There are now excellent data on endoscopic ablation using photodynamic therapy, radiofrequency ablation, and endoscopic mucosal resections. There had been a concern that these techniques would leave "buried Barrett" dysplasia (Fig. 2-23) that would progress to carcinoma, but this seems not to be an issue in practice.

■ ADENOCARCINOMA

CLINICAL FEATURES

Esophageal carcinoma currently has the most rapidly increasing tumor incidence in the United States. It is often diagnosed at a late stage despite an established association with a precursor lesion (Barrett's esophagus).

ESOPHAGEAL ADENOCARCINOMA—FACT SHEET

Definition
- A carcinoma displaying glandular differentiation arising in the esophagus, often in the setting of Barrett's esophagus.

Incidence and Location
- The overall incidence of esophageal cancer in the United States is 4.8 cases per 100,000 persons; it is not clear what percentage is adenocarcinoma, but probably more than half
- The rate of adenocarcinoma has increased by 450% among white males in the past 20 years; most examples are in the distal esophagus with overlapping features with so-called gastric cardiac carcinoma

Morbidity and Mortality
- Overall 5-year survival rate is poor (about 15%), but low-stage lesions have an excellent prognosis; however, most patients present at high stage

Gender, Race, and Age Distribution
- The mean age at diagnosis is in the mid-60s with a strong white male prevalence

Clinical Features
- In most cases, dysphagia and odynophagia at presentation
- Weight loss is common
- Some patients have symptomatic reflux

TABLE 2-2

Follow-up of Barrett's Esophagus According to Grade of Dysplasia

Series: Surveillance Protocol?	Fraction: Percent Progressing to Cancer—No Dysplasia	Indefinite	Low-Grade	High-Grade
Montgomery—No	0/44-0%	4/22-18%	4/26-15%	20/33-60%
Reid—Yes	5/129-3.8%	1/79-1.2%	3/43-6.9%	33/76-59%
Sampliner (summary data—No)	5/150-3%		8/45-18%	21/61-34%
Schnell—Yes*				12/75-16%
Weston—Yes			5/48-10.4%	

*Data from one Veterans Administration hospital (Hines, VA).

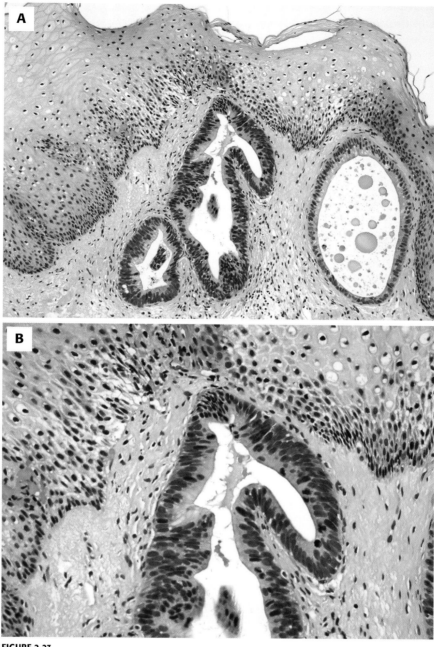

FIGURE 2-23

A, This focus of high-grade dysplasia is under the squamous mucosa ("buried Barrett," "pseudoregression pattern").
B, Higher magnification of the lesion.

Adenocarcinomas of the esophagus arise in the setting of Barrett's esophagus and often areas of dysplastic Barrett's mucosa are found near the carcinoma. According to some experts, approximately 10% of patients with Barrett's esophagus have or will develop adenocarcinoma. However, this percentage includes those patients who have their adenocarcinoma diagnosed at the time of their first endoscopy (prevalent carcinomas), as well as those patients who develop adenocarcinoma at some point subsequent to their diagnosis of Barrett's esophagus (incident carcinomas). The risk to patients who have only Barrett's esophagus is, therefore, much lower than 10%.

In addition to Barrett's esophagus, other predisposing factors for the development of esophageal adenocarcinoma include male gender, white race, and obesity. Approximately 90% of adenocarcinomas occurring in association with Barrett's esophagus occur in white

ESOPHAGEAL ADENOCARCINOMA—PATHOLOGIC FEATURES

Gross Findings

- Mass lesion typically involving the lower one third of the esophagus
- Often, associated Barrett's mucosa is seen in resected esophagus.

Microscopic Findings

- Malignant neoplasm with glandular differentiation
- May assume any of a variety of patterns, including signet cell pattern
- Associated Barrett's metaplasia should be sought

Immunohistochemistry

- Not specific; often CK7+, variable CDX2, MUC5AC, or MUC 6

Differential Diagnosis

- When poorly differentiated, lymphoma and melanoma can be differentiated by immunohistochemistry

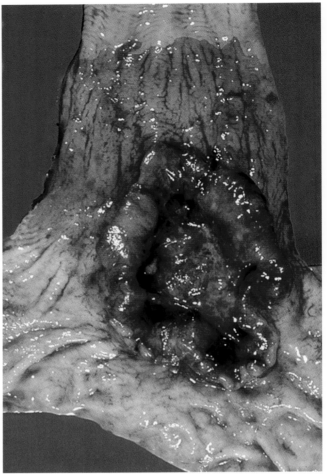

FIGURE 2-24

Esophageal adenocarcinoma, resection specimen. Note the background of Barrett's esophagus.

males, typically middle-aged white men with a median age in the late 50s. As with esophageal squamous cell carcinomas, smoking and alcohol consumption are predisposing factors for adenocarcinoma.

Because Barrett's mucosa begins at the gastroesophageal junction and extends superiorly for varying distances into the tubular esophagus, adenocarcinomas are also most common in the distal one third of the esophagus (in contrast to squamous cell carcinomas, which are most commonly found in the middle one third).

RADIOLOGIC FEATURES

Other than their presentation as a mass lesion in the distal one third of the esophagus, the imaging characteristics of esophageal adenocarcinomas are not specific.

PATHOLOGIC FEATURES

GROSS FINDINGS

Esophageal adenocarcinomas are seen at esophagectomy as firm whitish lesions, usually involving the distal one third. Often residual Barrett's mucosa can be recognized by its salmon color and "velvety appearance" (Fig. 2-24).

MICROSCOPIC FINDINGS

Recognizing esophageal adenocarcinomas is generally not a challenge because these lesions appear as other adenocarcinomas; that is, they are composed of malignant cells with glandular differentiation (Figs. 2-25 and 2-26), either in the form of ductal structures or mucin production. Overall, their patterns have been classified as papillary, tubular, and signet-ring cell types. Some display endocrine cells, Paneth cells, or a predominance of mucin production. Tumors displaying adenosquamous features (Fig. 2-27), and even adenoid cystic and mucoepidermoid lesions, are known. On small biopsies the presence of desmoplasia helps distinguish high-grade dysplasia from invasive carcinoma (see Fig. 2-26).

Although poorly differentiated adenocarcinomas behave more aggressively than well-differentiated ones, more important than histologic typing is proper staging. For this it should be noted that T1 includes tumors invading the lamina propria or the submucosa, whereas T2 encompasses those invading the muscularis propria. Because the muscularis mucosae of the esophagus tends to either thicken or duplicate (Figs. 2-28 and 2-29) as a reparative response, careful attention to correct identification of the layers of the esophageal wall is important.

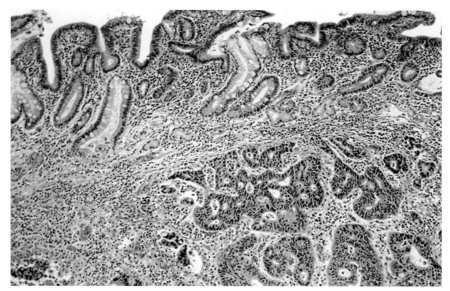

FIGURE 2-25

Esophageal adenocarcinoma. Note the overlying Barrett's esophagus in this field.

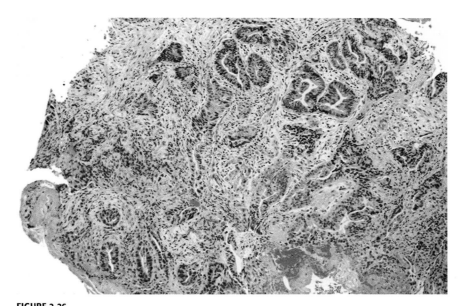

FIGURE 2-26

Esophageal adenocarcinoma. Note the prominent desmoplasia in clearly invasive carcinoma; its presence can be a helpful feature in biopsy diagnosis as in this case.

ANCILLARY STUDIES

Reported molecular genetic alterations include: p53 mutation and deletion; deletion of Rb, p16, and APC; overexpression of epidermal growth factor receptor (EGFR) and transforming growth factor-α; and clonal DNA aneuploidy. There is no important role for ras gene mutations. Promoter methylation for numerous genes has been reported.

DIFFERENTIAL DIAGNOSIS

The differential diagnosis is the same as with other adenocarcinomas (e.g., direct extension from pulmonary primaries). When carcinomas are poorly differentiated, they may assume spindle cell morphology and an immunohistochemical panel is advised to exclude spindle cell tumors (see subsequent section on Melanoma of the Esophagus). In the past, distinction from gastric cardiac carcinomas

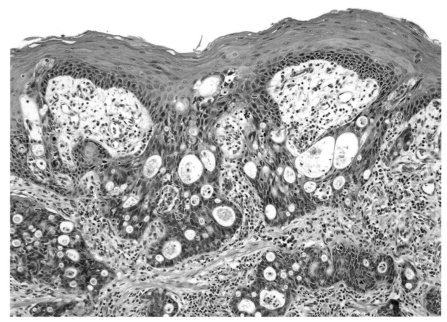

FIGURE 2-27
Adenosquamous carcinoma of the esophagus showing both squamous and columnar differentiation.

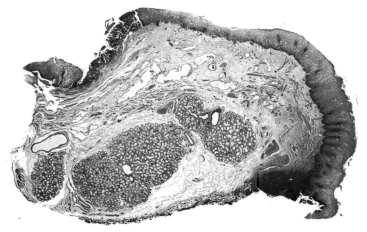

FIGURE 2-28
Endoscopic mucosal resection sample showing duplication of the muscularis mucosae. There are large submucosal glands at the bottom of the field, proving that the deepest portion of the sample is submucosal. Above the submucosal glands are strips of muscularis mucosae, and above those strips are dilated lamina propria vessels. However, note that there is a more slender collection of smooth muscle bundles still closer to the epithelium, the duplicated muscularis mucosae, situated just beneath the columnar epithelial lesion.

has been an issue, but this should be ameliorated by the AJCC 7th edition staging, which states: "The staging of carcinomas of the esophagogastric/gastroesophageal junction is based on the following TNM rule: a tumor the epicenter of which is within 5 cm of the GE junction and also extends into the esophagus is classified and staged using the esophageal carcinoma scheme. Tumors with an epicenter in the stomach greater than 5 cm from the GE junction or those within 5 cm of the esophagogastric junction without extension in the esophagus are classified and staged using the gastric carcinoma scheme."

PROGNOSIS AND THERAPY

Preoperative neoadjuvant chemotherapy and radiotherapy followed by esophagectomy is the preferred treatment; there is an especially poor prognosis when the patient presents with symptoms in the absence of surveillance for early detection. The overall 5-year survival is poor (about 15 %); the few patients with a good outcome tend to be those with early lesions detected in surveillance.

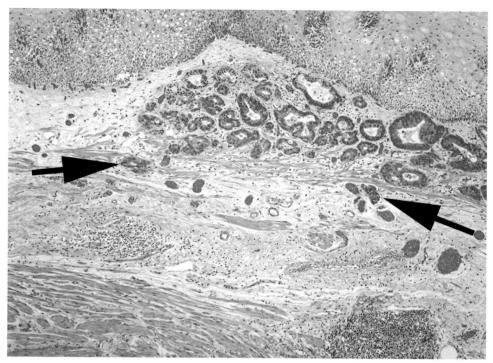

FIGURE 2-29
Intramucosal carcinoma showing invasion of the inner (duplicated) muscularis mucosae. The outer thicker original muscularis mucosae is at the bottom of the field. This is a T1a lesion.

■ SQUAMOUS CELL CARCINOMA

CLINICAL FEATURES

As with adenocarcinomas, most patients with squamous carcinomas are male and most are adults at least in their 50s. Unlike adenocarcinomas, which typically affect white males, there is a predominance of squamous carcinoma among African American males.

The incidence of squamous cell carcinoma is decreasing relative to that of esophageal adenocarcinomas in the United States. However, squamous carcinomas have a high incidence in "developing" countries, for example, in southern Africa and China.

There are many etiologic associations with squamous carcinoma, but any factor that causes chronic irritation and inflammation of the esophageal mucosa appears to predispose to squamous cell carcinoma of the esophagus. Substantial alcohol intake, especially in combination with smoking, greatly increases the risk of squamous cell carcinoma (but not adenocarcinoma), and may account for most cases of squamous cell carcinoma of the esophagus in the developed world (Fig. 2-30). The combination of smoking and alcohol abuse is associated with a similarly increased risk of head and neck cancer.

Clinically unsuspected squamous cell carcinoma of the esophagus is discovered incidentally in 1% to 2% of patients with head and neck cancers.

Other causes of chronic esophageal irritation include achalasia and esophageal diverticula, in which food is retained and decomposes, thereby releasing various chemical irritants. In several countries, frequent consumption of extremely hot beverages appears to increase the incidence of squamous cell carcinoma. Persons who have ingested lye or other caustic fluids should be monitored carefully for the development of this cancer.

Nonepidermolytic palmoplantar keratoderma (tylosis), a rare autosomal dominant disorder defined by a genetic abnormality at chromosome 17q25, is the only recognized familial syndrome that predisposes patients to squamous cell carcinoma of the esophagus. It is characterized by hyperkeratosis of the palms and soles and thickening of the oral mucosa. It confers up to a 95% risk for squamous cell carcinoma of the esophagus by the age of 70 years.

In a subset of patients who flush after drinking alcohol (typically Asian individuals), this phenomenon is triggered mainly by severe acetaldehydemia in individuals possessing inactive aldehyde dehydrogenase (ALDH). These persons have a polymorphism that enhances the risk for esophageal squamous cancer in light to heavy drinkers.

ESOPHAGEAL CANCER, BRITTANY, FRANCE (CORREA, 1984)

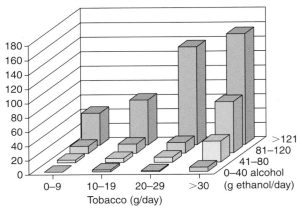

FIGURE 2-30

Squamous cell carcinoma of the esophagus. Additive influence of tobacco and alcohol consumption.

Squamous cell carcinoma (but not adenocarcinoma) is also linked to low socioeconomic status. Deficiency syndromes associated with this cancer, such as the Plummer-Vinson syndrome (dysphagia, iron-deficiency anemia, and esophageal webs), are becoming increasingly rare in the developed world as overall nutrition improves. Squamous carcinomas are most common in the middle one third of the esophagus.

ESOPHAGEAL SQUAMOUS CARCINOMA—FACT SHEET

Definition
- Malignant neoplasm of the esophagus showing squamous differentiation, usually with keratinization

Incidence and Location
- The overall incidence of esophageal cancer in the United States is 4.8 cases per 100,000 persons; it is not clear what percentage is squamous, but probably less than one half
- In contrast to the rate of adenocarcinoma, the rate of squamous cell carcinoma is decreasing in the United States; most examples are in the midesophagus

Morbidity and Mortality
- The overall prognosis for these tumors is poor, similar to that for adenocarcinoma.

Gender, Race, and Age Distribution
- These tumors predominate in African American men in their 60s
- Tobacco and alcohol are strong risk factors

Clinical Features
- Similar to adenocarcinoma—dysphagia, odynophagia, weight loss

RADIOLOGIC FEATURES

The presence of an esophageal mass in the middle one third of the esophagus is in keeping with squamous cell carcinoma, but there are no specific radiologic features of this type of tumor.

PATHOLOGIC FEATURES

GROSS FINDINGS

At esophagectomy, these tumors are firm white mucosal-based masses usually involving the middle one third of the esophagus, although the proximal esophagus may be affected (Fig. 2-31).

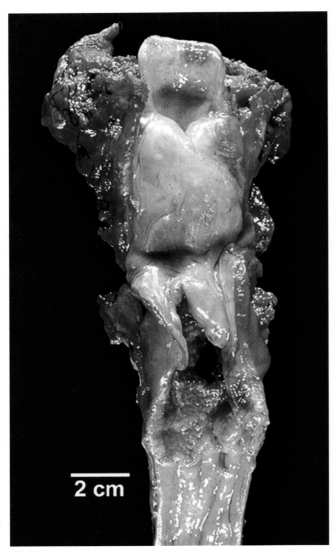

FIGURE 2-31

Squamous carcinoma of the esophagus. This lesion is proximal (most involve the midesophagus).

ESOPHAGEAL SQUAMOUS CARCINOMA—PATHOLOGIC FEATURES

Gross Findings

- Mass lesion most often in the middle one third of the esophagus

Microscopic Findings

- Carcinoma with squamous differentiation (keratinization is common)
- Associated in situ squamous carcinoma often seen
- Example: Spindle cell morphology, which tends to be exophytic

Immunohistochemistry

- May display CK5/6, P63 (as well as other keratins)

Differential Diagnosis

- Most are not a diagnostic problem; spindled examples can usually be resolved with immunohistochemistry or additional sampling to detect an in situ component

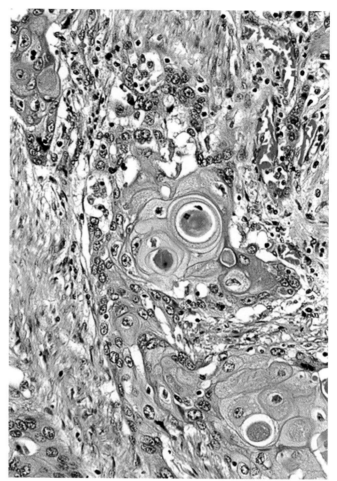

FIGURE 2-32

Typical keratinizing squamous cell carcinoma of the esophagus.

MICROSCOPIC FINDINGS

Squamous carcinoma of the esophagus appears similar to squamous carcinomas elsewhere (Fig. 2-32). It is usually well-differentiated squamous carcinoma with prominent keratinization. Background squamous epithelial dysplasia (intraepithelial neoplasia) including "carcinoma in situ" (high-grade dysplasia/intraepithelial neoplasia) is frequent at the periphery of invasive tumors (Fig. 2-33). Dysplasia alone without invasion is uncommon. Some squamous carcinomas assume a prominent spindle cell appearance. This latter subtype tends to present as a polypoid mass. Short-term survival of such tumors is better than that for flat typical carcinomas, owing to their exophytic growth, but long-term follow-up erases an apparent survival advantage.

ANCILLARY STUDIES

IMMUNOHISTOCHEMISTRY

Squamous cell carcinomas of the esophagus, like squamous carcinomas elsewhere, express CK5/6 and p63 and the host of epithelial markers.

FINE-NEEDLE ASPIRATION BIOPSY

Cytologic preparations of squamous carcinoma of the esophagus mirror those of squamous cell carcinoma of other sites.

OTHER STUDIES

Reported molecular genetic abnormalities include p53 mutations and deletion; deletion of Rb and p16; amplification of EGFR; c-*myc*, int-2/hst-1, and cyclin D1; overexpression of EGFR and insulin-like growth factor receptor-1.

DIFFERENTIAL DIAGNOSIS

Most examples are not a diagnostic problem. When spindled, melanomas and sarcomas must be excluded. The best way to do this is by sampling as much of the overlying squamous mucosa as possible in order to detect an in situ component. Otherwise, S-100 protein and various keratins are most useful. Primary sarcomas of the esophagus are extremely rare.

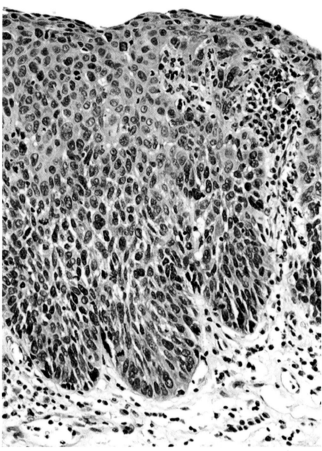

FIGURE 2-33
Esophageal squamous carcinoma in situ.

GRANULAR CELL TUMOR OF THE ESOPHAGUS

CLINICAL FEATURES

Granular cell tumors in general are rare and overall most common in the tongue and the skin. A subset is multicentric and rare examples are malignant. Granular cell tumors of the esophagus form about 1% to 2% of granular cell tumors. There are fewer than 100 reports of esophageal granular cell tumors in the literature and most are reported as isolated cases. The AFIP amassed only 24 cases for their series. In our own material from a high-volume hospital, we have encountered only 25 "in-house" esophageal granular cell tumors in the past 20 years. Most are found in the distal esophagus and about 10% are multicentric. There is a female predominance, and these tumors are over-represented in African Americans compared with whites. Rare malignant examples have been reported in the esophagus.

RADIOLOGIC FEATURES

Radiologic features vary with the size of the lesion, but the tumors may be found in any portion of the esophagus (most are distal) and are submucosal based. They are most likely to be assessed by endoscopic ultrasonography and, on this modality, appear as well-marginated masses. Associated concentric narrowing can also be found.

PATHOLOGIC FEATURES

GROSS FINDINGS

Cut surfaces of these tumors show whitish, firm, well-marginated submucosal-based lesions.

MICROSCOPIC FINDINGS

The microscopic features of granular cell tumor in the esophagus are identical to those in other sites. Tumors are well marginated but not encapsulated, and they are composed of plump neoplastic cells with abundant lightly amphophilic granular cytoplasm, which displays retention of periodic acid–Schiff (PAS) staining on diastase digestion. The cells are typically closely packed and clustered in the submucosa, with minor extensions into mucosa and muscularis propria. Nuclei are small to pyknotic with occasional nucleoli. Some lesions display squamous ("pseudoepitheliomatous") hyperplasia in the overlying mucosa, which can raise the possibility of squamous cell carcinoma on superficial biopsy specimens (Fig. 2-34).

PROGNOSIS AND THERAPY

Unfortunately, squamous carcinomas usually present late clinically, after extension into periesophageal soft tissue is already present. Esophageal obstruction; extension of carcinoma into mediastinal and intrathoracic structures (tracheobronchial tree, aorta, and lung); and mediastinal lymph node metastases are more frequent clinical problems than distant metastases.

Radiotherapy or chemotherapy is the usual treatment, sometimes with esophagectomy; this is usually palliative rather than curative. Esophageal squamous carcinoma has a dismal prognosis—the 5-year survival rate is 5% to 10%.

MESENCHYMAL TUMORS

Neural tumors, leiomyoma, and gastrointestinal stromal tumors are discussed in Chapter 7.

GRANULAR CELL TUMOR OF ESOPHAGUS—FACT SHEET

Definition

- Tumor displaying nerve sheath differentiation and peculiar granular cytoplasm on hematoxylin and eosin staining

Incidence and Location

- Rare tumor that typically affects the tongue but that may be found in the esophagus approximately 1% of the time
- In the gastrointestinal tract, the esophagus is the most common site
- Most tumors affect the distal esophagus, and approximately 5% to 10% of reported lesions are multicentric (this is probably a high estimate)
- Rare examples are malignant

Morbidity and Mortality

- Most lesions are incidental and treated by endoscopic excision

Gender, Race, and Age Distribution

- There is a female predominance and African Americans are disproportionally affected
- These lesions are most common in young adults

Clinical Features

- Usually found incidentally

GRANULAR CELL TUMOR OF ESOPHAGUS—PATHOLOGIC FEATURES

Gross Findings

- Nodule seen endoscopically

Microscopic Findings

- Well-marginated tumors composed of plump neoplastic cells with abundant lightly amphophilic granular cytoplasm
- Typically, closely packed cells centered in the submucosa with minor extensions into mucosa and muscularis propria
- Small to pyknotic nuclei with occasional nucleoli
- Squamous ("pseudoepitheliomatous") hyperplasia in the overlying mucosa, which can raise the possibility of squamous cell carcinoma on superficial biopsy samples

Immunohistochemistry

- Granular cell tumors are reactive with S-100 protein, calretinin, inhibin α, myelin basic protein, nestin, and CD68/Kp1 but lack muscle markers and melanoma markers

Differential Diagnosis

- Rhabdomyoma, melanoma, alveolar soft part sarcoma (ASPS)
- Immunohistochemistry generally resolves questions about melanomas and rhabdomyomas, but with ASPS, both granular cell tumor and ASPS may display nuclear expression of TFE3, initially believed specific for ASPS

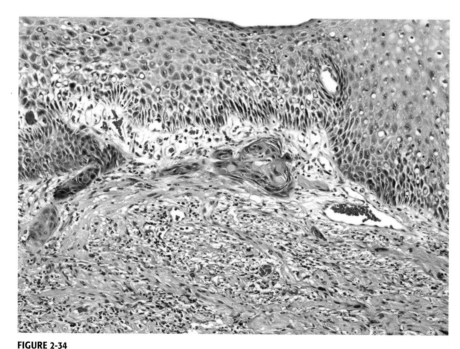

FIGURE 2-34
Granular cell tumor of the esophagus with overlying "pseudoepitheliomatous" hyperplasia.

ANCILLARY STUDIES

ULTRASTRUCTURAL FINDINGS

On ultrastructural examination, cells are arranged in small clusters delimited by basement membrane material. Most mature cells are distended with granules that obliterate the usual cellular organelles such as Golgi complex, rough endoplasmic reticulum, and mitochondria. Granules are membrane limited with electron-dense contents or larger vesicles. Unmyelinated axons course between cells.

IMMUNOHISTOCHEMISTRY

Granular cell tumors are reactive with S-100 protein (Fig. 2-35), calretinin, inhibin α, myelin basic protein, nestin, and CD68/Kp1 but lack muscle markers and melanoma markers. Unfortunately, like alveolar soft part sarcoma (ASPS), they can also react with TFE3 antibodies.

FINE-NEEDLE ASPIRATION BIOPSY

These tumors are seldom diagnosed by fine-needle aspiration (FNA), but FNA shows granular cells with a low nucleus-to-cytoplasm ratio and cases are reported in the literature with prospective cytologic diagnosis.

DIFFERENTIAL DIAGNOSIS

The differential diagnosis is the same as with rhabdomyoma and ASPS. Both diseases are rare at this anatomic site. Rhabdomyoma differs by expression of skeletal muscle and pan-muscle markers. ASPS differs by having an alveolar pattern, rich vascularity, PAS-reactive crystals that may assume a rhomboid shape, and the presence of a nucleolus in almost every cell. Unfortunately, both ASPS and granular cell tumors may have reactivity with antibodies to TFE3, initially believed to be specific for ASPS.

PROGNOSIS AND THERAPY

Most granular cell tumors behave in a benign fashion. Those rare examples that have metastasized typically displayed prominent cytologic alterations or mitotic activity.

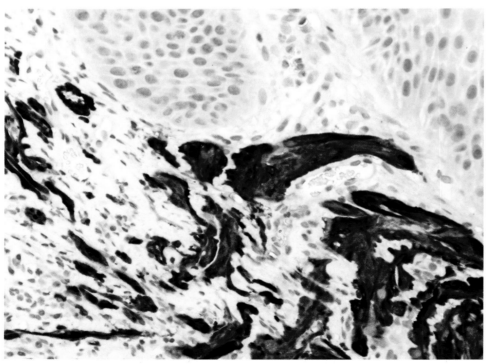

FIGURE 2-35
Granular cell tumor (S-100 stain).

■ MELANOMA OF THE ESOPHAGUS

CLINICAL FEATURES

It is difficult to accept melanomas as primary lesions in the gastrointestinal tract with the exception of the anus and esophagus where melanocytes are normally present. Primary melanoma of the esophagus is quite rare, with fewer than 300 cases reported. The affected patients are adults, with a mean age of approximately 60 years. Men are more commonly affected than women, but there is no racial predominance. Lesions are more common in the distal than in the proximal esophagus. At endoscopy, lesions are polypoid and pigment is seen in about 85% of cases.

RADIOLOGIC FEATURES

Imaging studies show bulky polypoid masses that bulge intraluminally without resultant obstruction.

PATHOLOGIC FEATURES

GROSS FINDINGS

Lesions have their epicenter near the surface and bulge intraluminally. Many lesions are pigmented, an obvious diagnostic clue. Otherwise, the lesions are whitish and poorly marginated.

MELANOMA OF THE ESOPHAGUS—FACT SHEET

Definition
- Lesion with features identical to cutaneous melanoma but affecting the esophagus

Incidence and Location
- Esophageal melanomas are rare lesions and usually affect the distal esophagus

Morbidity and Mortality
- Highly lethal neoplasm

Gender, Race, and Age Distribution
- No racial predilection (in contrast to cutaneous melanoma) is apparent
- Patients are generally in their 60s and there is a male predominance

Clinical Features
- Mass lesion of esophagus that may be pigmented and typically bulges intraluminally

MICROSCOPIC FINDINGS

The findings in esophageal melanomas are similar to those discussed elsewhere (Figs. 2-36 and 2-37). Examples regarded as primary may display an in situ component. Obviously, finding this is extremely useful in establishing the esophagus as the primary site. Otherwise, cells are spindled to epithelioid with variable pigment, prominent nucleoli, and prominent intranuclear pseudoinclusions.

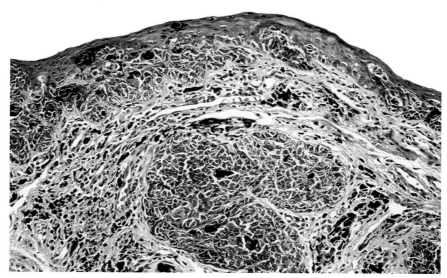

FIGURE 2-36
Esophageal melanoma. This lesion displays a junctional component, so it can be confidently diagnosed as a primary lesion.

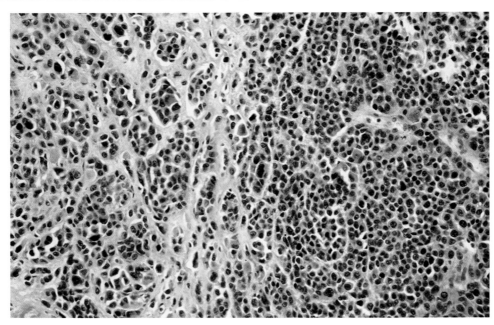

FIGURE 2-37
Esophageal melanoma displaying features akin to those of primary skin lesions.

MELANOMA OF THE ESOPHAGUS—PATHOLOGIC FEATURES

Gross Findings
- Polypoid mass, which is often pigmented

Microscopic Findings
- Similar to cutaneous melanomas with a possible junctional component

Immunohistochemistry
- Like its cutaneous counterpart, expresses S-100 protein and stains with melanoma-specific preparations (HMB45, MART, MITF, and Melan A).

Differential Diagnosis
- Other poorly differentiated neoplasms (poorly differentiated carcinomas and lymphomas)

ANCILLARY STUDIES

IMMUNOHISTOCHEMISTRY

Immunohistochemistry can be extremely helpful in establishing the diagnosis, in that melanomas of the esophagus label in the same manner as melanomas at other anatomic sites; that is, with S-100 protein, melanoma antigen recognized by T cells (MART), HMB45, MITF, and Melan A (related to MART.)

DIFFERENTIAL DIAGNOSIS

The differential diagnosis is with poorly differentiated carcinoma, which is more likely, and with high-grade lymphomas. These congeners are usually excluded with a panel including lymphoid markers (including CD30 for anaplastic lymphoma) and pankeratins. Sarcomas are rarely a component of the differential diagnosis, but a spindled melanoma may lack melanoma markers other than S-100 protein. In the case of a spindle cell tumor that is strongly S-100 protein reactive, cellular (benign) schwannoma is also a part of the differential diagnosis; the distinction is on cytologic grounds with attention to nuclear pleomorphism and large nucleoli, features of melanoma but not of cellular schwannoma.

PROGNOSIS AND THERAPY

Primary melanomas of the esophagus have a dismal prognosis. Only rare patients whose tumors present early can be cured.

3

Non-Neoplastic Disorders of the Stomach

■ **Baishali Bhattacharya, MD, MPH**

■ ACUTE EROSIVE/HEMORRHAGIC GASTRITIS (STRESS GASTRITIS)

Acute erosive/hemorrhagic gastritis is characterized by an acute gastric injury with an abrupt onset of abdominal pain and bleeding, usually associated with intake of alcohol, nonsteroidal anti-inflammatory drugs (NSAIDs), or low hemodynamic state following major trauma, presenting with multiple superficial erosions in the gastric mucosa and histologically characterized by hemorrhage, mucosal defect, and superficial necrosis (Fig. 3-1).

CLINICAL FEATURES

Patients present with abrupt onset of abdominal pain (burning epigastric pain), nausea, vomiting, and gastrointestinal (GI) bleeding with melena, hematemesis, or occult bleeding. Bleeding can be minimal and self-resolving or life threatening. Box 3-1 lists various etiologic agents (Figs. 3-2 through 3-6). Patients with aspirin- or alcohol-induced injury usually make a quick recovery, whereas hypoperfusion-related gastritis (stress ulcers) is associated with greater morbidity and mortality. Studies have found acute erosive gastropathy as the cause of upper GI bleeding

---

ACUTE EROSIVE/HEMORRHAGIC GASTRITIS (STRESS GASTRITIS)—FACT SHEET

Definition
- Abrupt onset of abdominal pain and bleeding associated with intake of alcohol, NSAIDs, or low hemodynamic state following major trauma, and presenting with multiple erosions in the gastric mucosa

Morbidity and Mortality
- Bleeding can be minimal and self-resolving or life-threatening.
- Patients with comorbid condition such as liver disease have higher morbidity and mortality rates.

Gender, Race, and Age
- Patients are mostly older: age range, 29 to 87 years.

Clinical Features
- Abrupt onset of abdominal pain, vomiting, and GI bleeding

Prognosis and Therapy
- Most cases have an uneventful course with full recovery within a short period
- Intravenous fluids and blood transfusion
- Stop the offending agent
- H_2 blockers, proton pump inhibitors, prostaglandin analogues
- Fatal bleeding may require surgical intervention

ACUTE EROSIVE/HEMORRHAGIC GASTRITIS (STRESS GASTRITIS)—PATHOLOGIC FEATURES

Gross Findings
- Stress-related ulcers are present in the fundus and body
- NSAID-related erosions are present in the antrum
- Multiple superficial, round, dark erosions, few millimeters in diameter
- The intervening gastric mucosa is edematous and hyperemic

Microscopic Findings
- Histologic findings depend on the biopsy interval
- Superficial lamina propria hemorrhage, mucosal sloughing, neutrophil infiltration, and mucosal necrosis.
- Changes limited to the mucosa
- The healing phase is associated with regenerative epithelium with dark enlarged nuclei with prominent nucleoli, and syncytial glandular architecture
- These changes should not be mistaken for malignancy

Differential Diagnosis
- Mallory-Weiss tear, peptic ulcers, esophageal variceal bleeding
- Nasogastric tube trauma
- Chronic active *Helicobacter pylori* gastritis
- Dysplasia, intramucosal carcinoma
- Chemical gastropathy
- Biopsy forceps trauma (artifact)

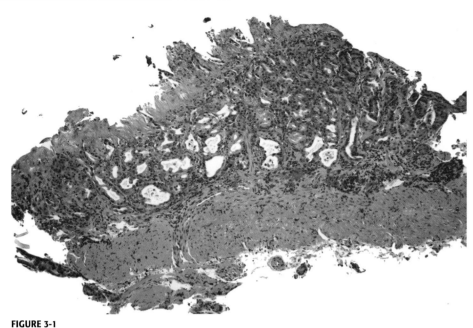

FIGURE 3-1
Acute erosive gastritis with mucosal necrosis and hemorrhage.

BOX 3-1
Associations with Erosive Gastritis

- Aspirin, nonsteroidal anti-inflammatory drugs
- Steroids
- Alcohol (see Fig. 3-2)
- Potassium chloride
- Phenylbutazone
- Iron pills (Fig. 3-3)
- Colchicine
- Sodium polystyrene sulfonate (Kayexalate) in sorbitol (see Figs. 3-4 and 3-5)
- Cocaine, "crack"
- Corrosives, acid and alkali ingestion
- Radiation (see Fig. 3-6)
- Chemotherapy
- Hypoperfusion type injury
- Major trauma, stress ulcers
- Head injury, Cushing ulcer
- Severe burn, Curling ulcer
- Sepsis, postoperative stage

in 6% to 34% of cases; the other important causes of bleeding are peptic ulcer disease, esophageal varices, and Mallory-Weiss tear. Although more often affecting older patients, the reported age range is 29 to 87 years.

The pathogenesis of acute hemorrhagic gastritis reflects an imbalance between mucosal irritants such as acid, pepsin, bile salts, NSAIDs, and other chemicals versus mucoprotective factors such as mucin, bicarbonates, prostaglandins, epidermal growth factors, mucosal blood flow, and the remarkable ability of gastric mucosa to re-epithelialize.

1. Direct irritant action of chemical agents such as NSAIDs and alcohol resulting in mucosal erosion, necrosis, and hemorrhage.

2. Additional injury by acid, pepsin, and bile salts that gain entry resulting from the disrupted mucosal barrier.

3. NSAIDs with their cyclo-oxygenase–inhibiting action inhibit prostaglandins, which in turn reduces bicarbonate and mucin secretions that have protective roles on the mucosal surface.

4. In cases of hypoperfusion-related stress ulcers, the pathogenesis is related to reduced gastric mucosal blood flow, vasoconstriction, and reperfusion injury with release of free oxygen radicals.

PATHOLOGIC FEATURES

GROSS AND ENDOSCOPIC FINDINGS

Endoscopic examination has superseded radiologic tests in diagnosis and management. Stress-related ulcers are mostly distributed in the fundus and body, whereas NSAID-related erosive gastropathy is present in the antrum. The gastric erosions are multiple, 2 to 5 mm in diameter, superficial, round, and dark. The intervening mucosa is edematous and hyperemic with petechial hemorrhage.

MICROSCOPIC FINDINGS

Histologic findings may or may not be impressive owing mostly to the remarkable capacity of stomach mucosa to re-epithelialize. Hence, depending on the interval of the gastritis with the endoscopic biopsy, histologic changes range from subepithelial hemorrhage/superficial lamina propria hemorrhage, mucosal sloughing and necrosis, to neutrophil infiltration.

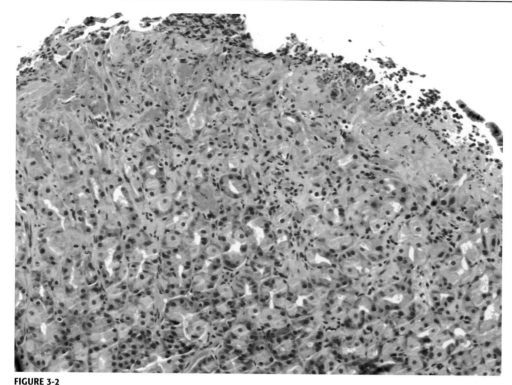

FIGURE 3-2
Hemorrhagic gastritis caused by an alcoholic binge characterized by superficial necrosis with congestion and fibrinopurulent exudate.

Gastric erosions are limited to the mucosa and do not extend beyond the muscularis mucosae. Gastric ulcers, on the other hand, are deep, with extension beyond the submucosa. The healing phase is associated with regenerative epithelium with increased mitotic activity, dark enlarged nuclei with prominent nucleoli, amphophilic cytoplasm (a feature of active RNA synthesis), and syncytial glandular architecture (Fig. 3-7). These changes can be alarming and should not be mistaken for malignancy. The presence of superimposed ulcer or erosion with active neutrophilic exudates is a feature that should caution against making a diagnosis of malignancy.

DIFFERENTIAL DIAGNOSIS

- Mallory-Weiss tear, peptic ulcers, esophageal variceal bleeding: clinical differentials of upper GI bleeding.
- Trauma related to nasogastric tube.
- Chronic active *Helicobacter pylori* gastritis: Onset is not acute as the name suggests. Associated with superficial diffuse lymphoplasmacytic inflammation with neutrophilic cryptitis. Modified Giemsa stain highlights the organisms.
- Dysplasia, intramucosal carcinoma: True dysplastic change is present on the surface with nuclear stratifi-

cation, hyperchromasia, and increased mitoses. There may be intestinal metaplasia in the surrounding mucosa. Regenerative epithelial change is present in a setting of erosion/ulcers, and the features are limited to deeper areas with presence of surface maturation. The regenerative epithelial cells have abundant amphophilic cytoplasm, prominent nucleoli, and smooth nuclear membrane.
- Chemical gastropathy: chronic change associated with bile reflux, NSAIDs with mucosal elongation, smooth muscle hyperplasia in the lamina propria, and regenerative change.
- Biopsy forceps trauma: commonly seen in mucosal biopsies and should not be mistaken for acute hemorrhagic gastropathy. Histologically characterized by superficial lamina propria congestion without signs of injury or significant inflammation.

PROGNOSIS AND THERAPY

Most patients make an uneventful recovery within a short time period. Depending on the hemodynamic state, management consists of supportive measures such as intravenous fluids and blood transfusion; stopping the offending agent, H_2 blockers, proton pump inhibitors (PPIs), prostaglandin analogues, and so forth. In cases of life-threatening bleeding, surgical intervention may be necessary.

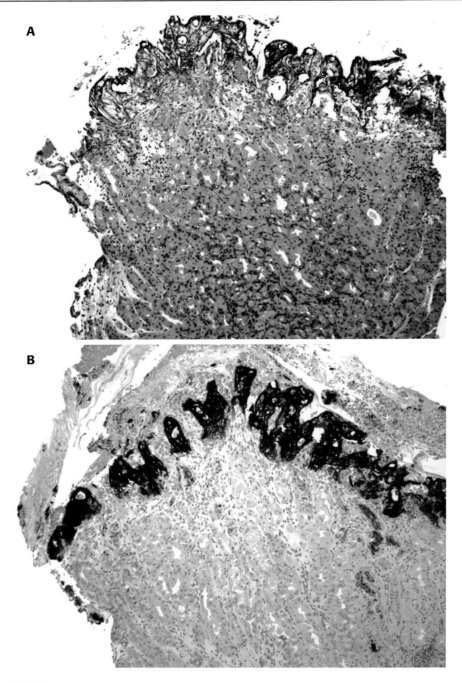

FIGURE 3-3

Brownish-yellow crystalline deposits **(A)** in the erosion are seen in iron pill gastritis and special staining for iron (Prussian blue) is positive **(B).**

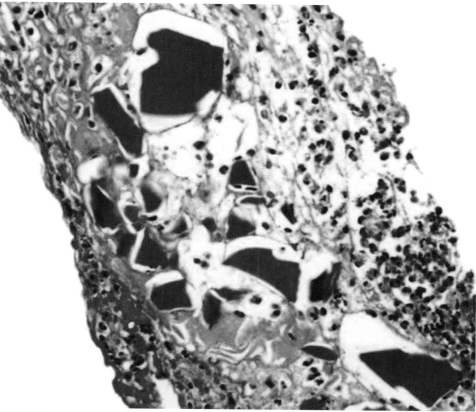

FIGURE 3-4

Kayexalate crystals (sodium polystyrene sulfonate) admixed in exudates on H&E stain appear as basophilic/magenta crystals with a fish-scale (mosaic) pattern. Kayexalate in sorbitol is used to treat hyperkalemia and known to cause colonic necrosis, as well as mucosal damage in the upper gastrointestinal tract including the stomach mucosa. Interestingly, the kayexalate crystals are "innocent bystanders" and the damage is due to the hyperosmotic action of sorbitol.

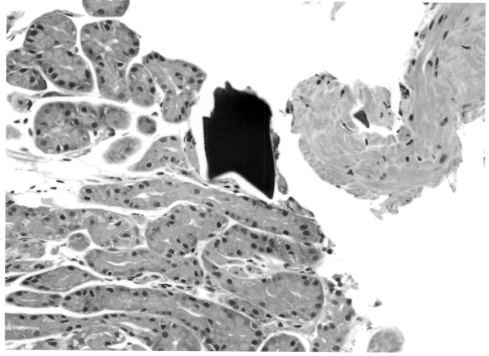

FIGURE 3-5

Cholestyramine crystals, which can mimic Kayexalate, are rhomboid and opaque but do not have the mosaic appearance.

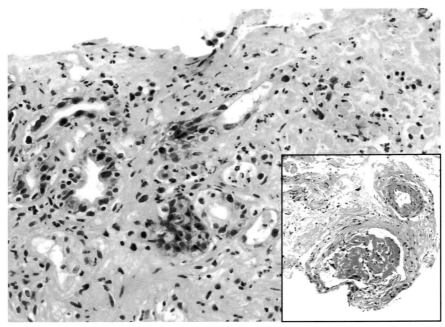

FIGURE 3-6
Radiation gastritis with superficial necrosis and lamina propria hyalinization with reactive glandular changes mimicking ischemic gastritis. Notice the vascular thrombi *(inset)*.

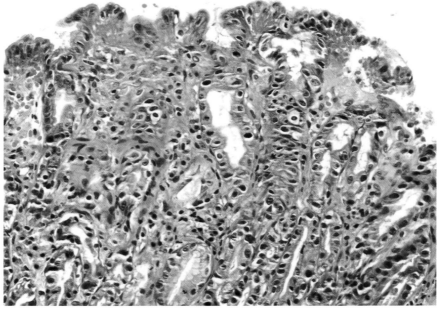

FIGURE 3-7
Healing erosive gastritis with marked regenerative epithelial changes with amphophilic cytoplasm and enlarged nuclei. There appears to be surface maturation.

■ CHEMICAL (REACTIVE) GASTROPATHY

Chemical gastropathy is a chemical-induced damage characterized by foveolar hyperplasia, regenerative epithelial changes, smooth muscle proliferation in the lamina propria, and vascular congestion of the gastric antral mucosa. Chemical gastropathy is synonymous with type C gastritis, reactive gastritis, reactive gastropathy, and alkaline or bile reflux gastritis.

CLINICAL FEATURES

Chemical gastropathy is a fairly common diagnostic entity in gastric biopsies. Symptoms range from vague upper abdominal pain to nausea, vomiting, gastroduodenal

CHEMICAL (REACTIVE) GASTROPATHY—FACT SHEET

Definition
- Chemical-induced damage of the gastric antral mucosa characterized by foveolar hyperplasia, regenerative epithelial changes, smooth muscle proliferation in the lamina propria, and vascular congestion

Morbidity and Mortality
- May cause GI bleeding and ulcers

Gender, Race, and Age
- Mean age group is 66 years (range, 22 to 88 years)

Clinical Features
- Vague upper abdominal pain, nausea, vomiting, gastroduodenal ulcers, and GI bleeding
- Etiologies include long-term aspirin use, NSAID use, and bile reflux following gastroenterostomies

Prognosis and Therapy
- Treatment involves PPIs and discontinuing offending agents such as NSAIDs

CHEMICAL (REACTIVE) GASTROPATHY—PATHOLOGIC FEATURES

Endoscopic Findings
- Erythema and erosions in the gastric antrum
- Visible bile reflux on endoscopic examination

Microscopic Findings
- Changes are limited to the antrum and prepyloric area
- Marked foveolar hyperplasia characterized by villiform change of the surface foveola, and elongation and tortuosity of the gastric pits resembling a corkscrew
- Reactive surface foveolar epithelium with depleted mucin
- Smooth muscle proliferation and vascular congestion in the lamina propria
- Paucity of inflammatory cells; focal erosions may be associated with small pockets of neutrophils and eosinophils

Immunohistochemistry
- Giemsa stain for *Helicobacter pylori* is negative

Differential Diagnosis
- Hyperplastic polyp
- Gastric antral vascular ectasia
- Mucosa adjacent to ulcers

erosions or ulcers, and GI bleeding. Mean age is 66 years (range, 22 to 88 years), and both sexes show equal predilection. Etiologies include chronic aspirin or other NSAID use, bile reflux following gastroenterostomies, vagotomy, and pyloroplasty. In nonsurgical patients, bile reflux may be due to an incompetent pyloric sphincter or gastric dysmotility. Other putative causes include alcohol intake and smoking. The pattern of injury in chemical gastropathy reflects chronic repetitive bouts of injury followed by attempts at regeneration and repair.

PATHOLOGIC FEATURES

GROSS AND ENDOSCOPIC FINDINGS

The endoscopic findings are usually nonspecific, consisting of erythema and erosions in the gastric antrum. Visible gastric bile staining on endoscopic examination can be helpful in diagnosis.

MICROSCOPIC FINDINGS

The antral mucosa shows foveolar hyperplasia characterized by villiform change of the surface epithelium and elongation and tortuosity of gastric pits with a corkscrew appearance (Fig. 3-8). The surface epithelial cells are immature with cuboidal shape, depleted mucin, and enlarged nuclei, which, when marked, can be mistaken for dysplasia. The lamina propria shows smooth muscle proliferation and vascular congestion. There is usually a paucity of inflammatory cells. Focal erosions may be associated with small pockets of neutrophils and eosinophils. The changes are limited to the antrum. Chronic chemical gastropathy may also be associated with intestinal metaplasia in the gastric antrum, which is thought to be the result of ulcer repair. Oxyntic mucosa occasionally may show reactive changes of the surface, but the findings are usually subtle. Bile reflux gastropathy following Billroth I-II surgery with antrectomy is present in the body or fundus.

ANCILLARY STUDIES

HISTOCHEMISTRY

- Giemsa (or immunohistochemical) stain for *H. pylori* is negative
- Periodic acid-Schiff (PAS)/alcian blue at pH 2.5 is helpful (but not necessary for diagnosis) in demonstrating depleted foveolar surface mucin

DIFFERENTIAL DIAGNOSIS

- Hyperplastic polyp: The marked foveolar hyperplasia in chemical gastropathy may resemble hyperplastic polyps. On the other hand, small/early hyperplastic polyps with focal foveolar hyperplasia may resemble chemical gastropathy. The endoscopic appearance of a polyp/nodule is important in making the distinction.
- Gastric antral vascular ectasia (GAVE): The typical endoscopic appearance of watermelon stomach and vascular thrombi in the lamina propria differentiate this entity.

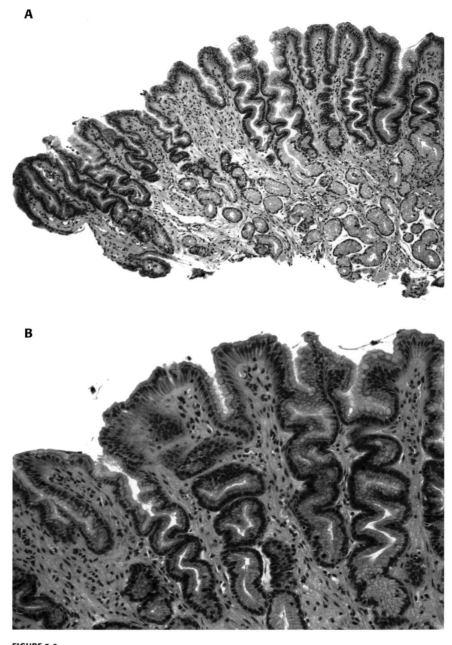

FIGURE 3-8

Chemical gastropathy. Biopsy of antral mucosa showing foveolar hyperplasia and corkscrew appearance of gastric pits. Note the depleted surface mucin and lamina propria with smooth muscle proliferation and paucity of inflammatory cells.

- Mucosa adjacent to an ulcer with foveolar hyperplasia and edema (Fig. 3-9) can histologically resemble chemical gastropathy. The clinical context of an ulcer is important in distinguishing between these entities.
- Mixed chemical/reactive gastropathy and chronic gastritis: This pattern can coexist in biopsy samples and consists of a mild inflammation in the lamina propria and a disproportionate degree of foveolar hyperplasia and edema. This mixed pattern may suggest an overlap of chemical gastropathy in a background of mild chronic gastritis. Foveolar hyperplasia, by itself, is not specific to chemical gastropathy and can also be seen with chronic *H. pylori* gastritis. However, the moderate to severe inflammation in *H. pylori*–associated gastritis is absent in chemical gastropathy.

PROGNOSIS AND THERAPY

This is a benign entity and management involves discontinuing the offending agents such as NSAIDs and medical management with antisecretory drugs such as PPIs.

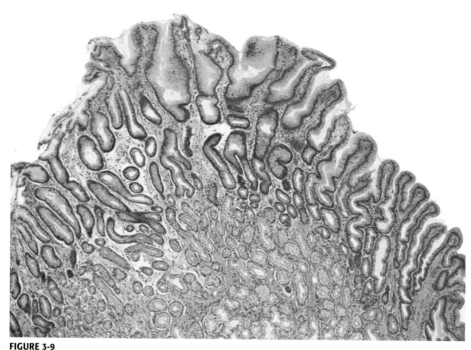

FIGURE 3-9
Foveolar hyperplasia and edema near an ulcer resembling chemical gastropathy.

■ *HELICOBACTER PYLORI* GASTRITIS

First described by Australian scientists J. Robin Warren and pathologist Barry J Marshall in 1982, *H. pylori* gastritis is a chronic infectious form of gastritis caused by spiral, flagellated gram-negative rods and characterized by superficial chronic active gastritis. *H. pylori* gastritis is synonymous with *Campylobacter pylori* gastritis, diffuse antral gastritis, chronic superficial gastritis, and type B gastritis.

CLINICAL FEATURES

Signs and symptoms include abdominal pain, nausea, vomiting, dyspepsia, weight loss, iron deficiency anemia, and ulcer-related bleeding. *H. pylori* gastritis is a universal infection prevalent in 50% of the world's population. It is more prevalent in developing countries, where up to 75% of population older than 25 years of age is infected, the prevalence reaching 80% to 90%. Most people acquire infection during childhood. Transmission of infection is human to human, with poor sanitary conditions and overcrowding being risk factors. In developed countries, the overall prevalence is 25% to 30%, and the seroprevalence ranges from 5% to 27% in early childhood and exceeding 50% to 60% in adults older than 60 years of age. In the United States, African Americans, Asian Americans, and Hispanics have a higher prevalence than whites (70% versus 35%).

HELICOBACTER PYLORI GASTRITIS—FACT SHEET

Definition
- Chronic infectious form of gastritis caused by curved, flagellated gram-negative rods—*Helicobacter pylori*—and characterized by superficial chronic active gastritis

Incidence and Location
- Universal infection
- In developing countries, up to 75% of the population older than 25 years are infected, with the prevalence reaching 80% to 90%
- In developed countries, the overall prevalence is 25% to 30%; the seroprevalence ranges from 5% to 27% in early childhood and exceeds 50% to 60% in adults older than 60 years of age
- In the United States, African Americans and Hispanics have a higher prevalence than whites (70% vs. 35%)

Morbidity and Mortality
- Ulcer-related bleeding
- Association with peptic ulcer disease, gastric lymphoma, and carcinoma
- Definite or group I human carcinogen (World Health Organization)

Clinical Features
- Abdominal pain, nausea, vomiting, dyspepsia, weight loss, iron deficiency anemia, and ulcer-related bleeding

Prognosis and Therapy
- Triple therapy for 14 days consisting of either bismuth or PPIs combined with two antibiotics such as metronidazole, clarithromycin, tetracycline, or amoxicillin
- Cure rate of greater than 95% is achieved
- Short treatment courses of 1 to 5 days may be effective with an eradication rate of 89% to 95%

HELICOBACTER PYLORI GASTRITIS—PATHOLOGIC FEATURES

Gross (Endoscopic) Findings

- Gastric mucosal erythema, erosions, granularity, and nodularity
- For optimal evaluation at least two mucosal biopsies, each from the antrum and body are recommended

Microscopic Findings

- Chronic active gastritis with marked lymphoplasmacytic inflammation and neutrophils
- The inflammation is predominantly in the superficial aspect (luminal) of mucosal biopsy
- Active or neutrophilic inflammation is prominent in the gastric pits, causing pititis
- Foveolar hyperplasia, features of degeneration, and, in severe cases, erosion, hemorrhage, and mucosal necrosis
- Prominent lymphoid aggregates
- The organisms appear as slightly curved seagull wing–shaped rods, most prominent in the gastric mucin and the lining surface foveolar epithelium and gastric pits
- The organisms can be visible on H&E examination, especially when numerous, but adjunct, stains are used to confirm their presence
- Active inflammation is usually a marker for the presence of *Helicobacter* organisms; organisms are often absent in cases of atrophy or intestinal metaplasia

Immunohistochemical Findings

- Special stains utilized:
  - Modified Giemsa stain and Diff-Quik are popular, quick, cheap, and easy to perform
  - Silver stains: Warthin-Starry, Genta stain
  - Immunohistochemistry for *Helicobacter*

Differential Diagnosis

- *H. heilmannii* gastritis
- Gastric marginal zone B-cell lymphoma
- Focal active gastritis: gastric Crohn's disease
- Autoimmune gastritis
- Non–*H. pylori* bacteria

H. pylori is a curved, gram-negative rod with S-shaped or seagull wing appearance. It is motile, using single polar flagellum. It is a microaerophilic bacillus 0.5 µm in width and 2.5 µm in length. This organism has a tropism for gastric mucosa or metaplastic gastric mucosa in organs such as the duodenum. The pathogenesis depends on its ability to colonize gastric epithelium via adhesins such as BabA, SabA, urease; virulence factors such as Cag A, Vac A, and urease, which in turn generates cytokines such as interleukin-8 to attract neutrophils.

The discovery of the *Helicobacter* organism and its association with peptic ulcer disease, gastric mucosa–associated lymphoid tissue (MALT) lymphoma, and carcinoma has revolutionized modern understanding of disease processes and influenced patient management. Warren and Marshall became the recipients of the Nobel Prize in Physiology or Medicine in 2005 for this significant discovery. The World Health Organization has classified *H. pylori* as a group I human carcinogen of gastric cancer. Infected persons have a three- to six-fold greater risk of developing gastric cancer over that of uninfected persons.

PATHOLOGIC FEATURES

ENDOSCOPIC FINDINGS

Endoscopic findings are variable and include gastric mucosal erythema, erosions, granularity, and nodularity. The endoscopic appearance may even be normal, placing emphasis on the value of histologic examination. There may be associated gastric and duodenal ulcers. Mucosal nodularity simulating gastric lymphoma or carcinoma can be present. The nodularity is usually caused by florid lymphoid hyperplasia (Fig. 3-10). For optimal evaluation, at least two mucosal biopsy specimens, one each from the antrum and body, are recommended. Sampling of a single site may reduce the test sensitivity.

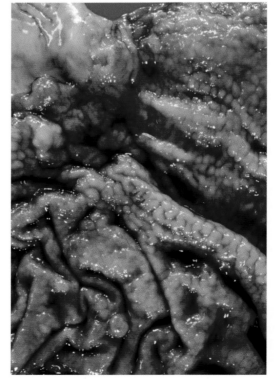

FIGURE 3-10

Gastric mucosal nodularity simulating lymphoma or carcinoma. Such a nodularity as this is often present in *Helicobacter* gastritis, caused by the florid lymphoid hyperplasia. *(Courtesy of Shriram Jakate, MD, Rush Medical College, Chicago.)*

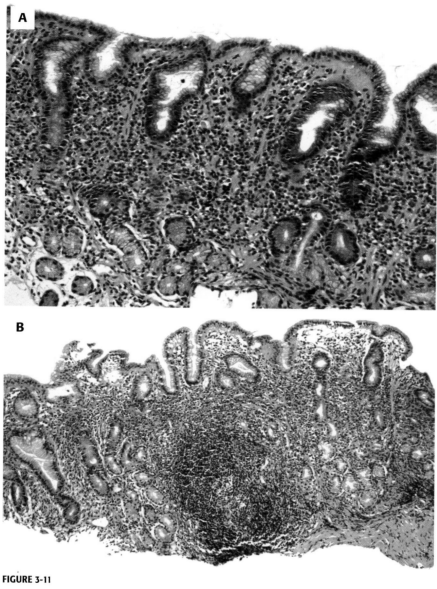

FIGURE 3-11

Helicobacter gastritis, antral biopsy. **A,** A diffuse band of superficial lymphoplasmacytic inflammation. **B,** Prominent lymphoid follicles.

MICROSCOPIC FINDINGS

H. pylori commonly colonizes both antrum and body mucosa. In severe infection, the organisms can be present in biopsy samples of the cardia. The inflammation is prominent in the superficial gastric mucosa and characterized by intense lymphoplasmacytic inflammation admixed with neutrophils (Fig. 3-11). Active or neutrophilic inflammation is prominent in the surface epithelium and gastric pits, with pititis and crypt abscesses (Fig. 3-12). Additional histologic features include foveolar hyperplasia (not just limited to reactive gastropathy), degenerative changes, erosion, hemorrhage, and lymphoid follicles (see Fig. 3-11B).

The organisms appear as slightly curved seagull wing–shaped rods, most prominent in the gastric mucus, overlying surface epithelium, and gastric pits. The organisms may be visible on hematoxylin and eosin (H&E) examination (Fig. 3-13A), but adjunct stains are used and

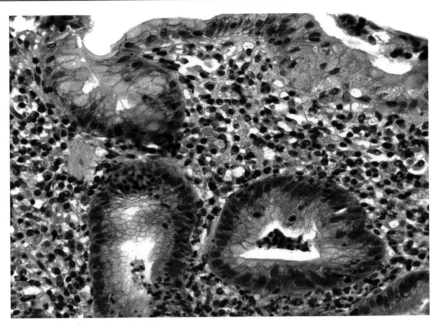

FIGURE 3-12

Helicobacter gastritis. High-power view showing active neutrophilic inflammation and a crypt abscess.

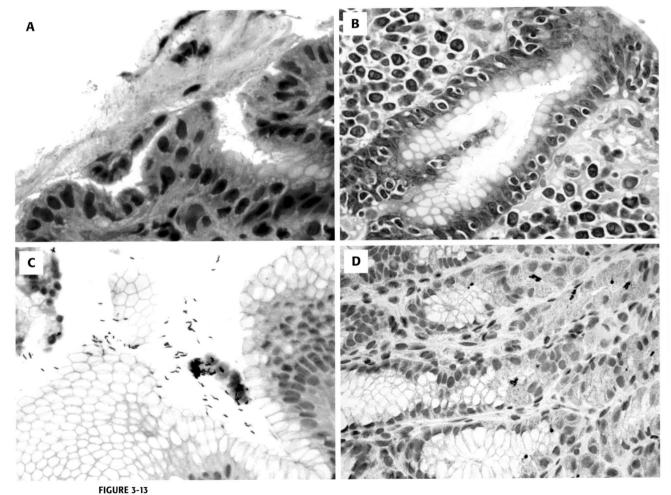

FIGURE 3-13

A, *Helicobacter pylori* organisms seen on H&E stain, admixed in surface mucin. Notice the curved shapes. **B,** *Helicobacter* gastritis. Diff-Quik stain highlights the slightly curved seagull wing–shaped *H. pylori* organisms in the gastric pits lining the foveolar epithelium. **C,** Immunostain for *H. pylori* shows the organisms lining the gastric foveolae. **D,** Coccoid, deep, intracellular location of *H. pylori* is visible as highlighted by this immunostain.

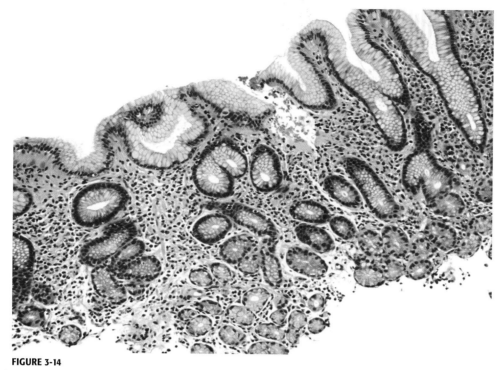

FIGURE 3-14

Chronic inactive gastritis in a patient recently treated for *Helicobacter pylori* infection. Note the lamina propria with plasma cells but without active inflammation.

recommended to confirm their presence (see Fig. 3-13B through D). Active neutrophilic inflammation is usually a marker for the presence of *Helicobacter* organisms. Table 3-1 highlights other manifestations that may be attributed to *H. pylori* infection (Fig. 3-14).

Because of the widespread use of PPIs, it is not uncommon to find the *Helicobacter* organisms in the body/ fundus, but not in the antral mucosa: The changing microenviroment and gastric pH may have a role to play. Often, the organisms are impossible to locate by histochemical staining because of the coccoid shape and deep or even intracellular location within glands, making it necessary to perform immunohistochemistry (see Fig. 3-13D). This phenomenon also emphasizes the need

TABLE 3-1

Histologic Manifestations Indicative of Present or Past *Helicobacter pylori* Infection

Acute *Helicobacter* gastritis	This is the acute manifestation when the infection is initially acquired and almost never comes to medical attention and therefore is not biopsied. In fact, the best evidence came from Dr. Marshall himself, who drank from a Petri dish containing the organisms from the culture of a patient with *H. pylori* infection and suffered from acute gastritis with nausea, vomiting, and halitosis.
Chronic inactive gastritis	Characterized by clusters of plasma cells in the lamina propria (see Fig 3-14). Lacks active inflammation and may reflect past *Helicobacter* infection.
Lymphocytic gastritis and follicular gastritis	Lymphocytic gastritis contains prominent intraepithelial lymphocytosis and follicular gastritis contains florid lymphoid follicles; both entities are seen with *H. pylori* infection.
Granulomatous gastritis	*Helicobacter* infection may have a more important role to play in gastric granulomas than it is credited for.
Hyperplastic polyp	May be a marker of *H. pylori* infection in the nonpolypoid gastric mucosa.
Environmental atrophic metaplastic gastritis (EMAG), multifocal atrophic gastritis, or type B gastritis	*H. pylori* is an important cause of EMAG, a precursor to gastric dysplasia and carcinoma. Characterized by gradual loss of normal glands and multifocal intestinal metaplasia, predominantly in the gastric antrum but also present in the body and cardia. Unlike in autoimmune gastritis, the gastrin level in EMAG is either low or normal. The antrum is normal in autoimmune gastritis, which is not the case in EMAG.

to educate GI specialists to obtain biopsy samples of the antrum and body, and to discontinue PPIs 2 weeks before the endoscopy, or else the infection may be missed.

ANCILLARY STUDIES

See Table 3-2.

DIFFERENTIAL DIAGNOSIS

- *Helicobacter heilmannii* gastritis (*Gastrospirillum hominis*): Rare cause of *Helicobacter* gastritis responsible for approximately 0.3% cases. Caused by a tight spiral bacterium that is 5 to 6 μm in length, which is longer than *H. pylori* (Fig. 3-15A and B). It is also seen in cats and

TABLE 3-2
Helicobacter pylori Tests

	INVASIVE TESTS	
Biopsy, special stains	Modified Giemsa, Diff-Quik, silver stains—Warthin-Starry, Genta stain	Diff-Quik and modified Giemsa are preferred over silver stains (cost). Sensitivity 84% to 99% and specificity 90% to 99%.
Immunostain for *H. pylori*	Especially useful in demonstrating variant forms of *H. pylori,* such as the coccoid forms (see Fig. 3-13D) that can occur in partially treated cases, patients on antibiotics or proton-pump inhibitors (PPIs), and resistant forms. PPI therapy can drive the organisms into the parietal cells when they become visible by immunostains.	Costly compared with special stains such as Diff-Quik; performed when the findings of special stains are questionable. Immunostain is also positive in *H. heilmannii* gastritis.
Biopsy-based rapid urease tests	Biopsy tissue is placed on urea medium and positive test is indicated by color change caused by an increase in pH as a result of urea breakdown into ammonia catalyzed by urease produced by all strains of *Helicobacter* organisms.	CLOtest, hpfast, PyloriTek. Sensitivity 89% to 98% and specificity up to 93% to 98%. Sensitivity depends on organism load in the biopsy tissue and number of biopsy samples used. Less sensitive in pediatric population.
Culture	Incubation in nonselective mediums such as chocolate or blood agar for 5-7 days.	Sensitivity is 77% to 92%, and specificity is 100%. Not used routinely but may gain importance in the future owing to the emergence of resistant strains.
Molecular tests	Polymerase chain reaction (PCR)-based detection of *H. pylori* using various genetic targets such as 23S ribosome, vac A, ureA, and cag A gene.	
	NONINVASIVE TESTS	
Serology	Detect IgG antibodies in serum or even whole blood to *H. pylori* antigens using enzyme-linked immunosorbent assay (ELISA)	Screening test used to detect current or past infection. Performance varies with the different commercial kits with an overall sensitivity and specificity of 88% to 92% and 86% to 95%, respectively. Reduced sensitivity in HIV-infected individuals. Patients with *H. heilmannii* may have a negative test to anti–*H. pylori* IgG assays. Serologic results can stay positive for a very long time, making them less useful for follow-up. Follow-up serology to test for eradication should be done only after 6 months.
Urea breath test (UBT)	Patient is given radioactively labeled urea to drink. The urease produced by *Helicobacter* organisms will break down urea and the labeled CO_2 is detected in the exhaled breath.	Sensitivity is 90% to 100% and specificity is 98% to 100%. UBT is used as a follow-up for patients who continue to be symptomatic.
Stool antigen test	*H. pylori* antigens is detected from fecal sample by enzyme immunoassay.	Sensitivity is 89% and specificity 94%. Like UBT, this test can also be used to confirm eradication.

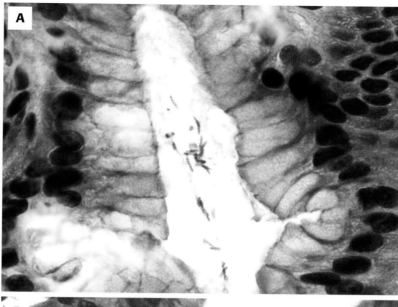

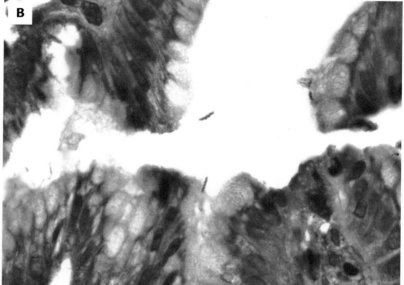

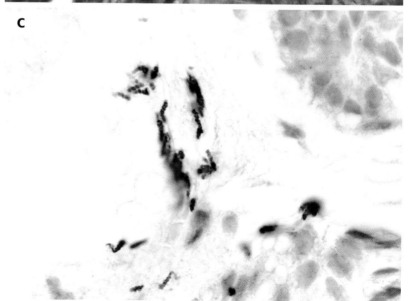

FIGURE 3-15

A, Unlike *Helicobacter pylori, Helicobacter heilmannii* organisms are longer, tightly spiraled, present in the lumen, and less tightly adherent to surface foveolar cells (H&E). **B,** *H. heilmannii* in (MGS). **C,** The antibody for *H. pylori* also stains *H. heilmannii.*

dogs, raising the possibility of an animal source of infection. Because of their larger size, they can be seen on H&E examination and are present in the gastric mucus and lumen of gastric pits without coming in close contact with the epithelium. They are seen intracellularly as well. Immunostain for *H. pylori* also stains *H. Heilmannii* (see Fig. 3-15C), and treatment is also the same.

- Gastric marginal zone B-cell lymphoma or low-grade MALT lymphoma: The florid lymphoid hyperplasia in *Helicobacter* gastritis can be mistaken for low-grade MALT lymphoma. However, immunostains for CD20 and CD3 demonstrate a reactive pattern consisting of mixed T and B lymphocytes (CD20-positive in the germinal center B-cells and mantle cuff, CD3-positive in peripheral T-lymphocytes). Unlike MALT lymphoma, which is characterized by monomorphic B-cells extending below the muscularis mucosae, *Helicobacter* gastritis causes superficial inflammation and lacks destructive lymphoepithelial lesions. The neoplastic lymphoid cells in MALT lymphoma coexpress CD20 and CD43 and may show light chain restriction. The intraepithelial lymphocytes in *Helicobacter* gastritis are mostly CD3-positive T-lymphocytes, unlike the CD20-positive neoplastic B-cells in gastric MALT lymphomas. A word of caution: Features such as lymphoepithelial lesion and dense B-cell aggregates can also be seen in gastritis. Studies have shown a clonal population of lymphoid cells in reactive germinal centers associated with *Helicobacter*, so one needs to be cautious about interpreting molecular studies.
- Conditions that can be associated with focal active gastritis: Crohn's disease, erosions in chemical gastropathy.
- Autoimmune gastritis: The antrum is normal or may show mild chemical gastropathy. The body shows atrophy with reduced to absent oxyntic glands, intestinal metaplasia, and enterochromaffin-like (ECL) cell hyperplasia. Patients have antibodies to intrinsic factor and parietal cells leading to hypochlorhydria, vitamin B_{12} deficiency, and hypergastrinemia. Hypergastrinemia also occurs in *Helicobacter* gastritis, although not to the extent seen in autoimmune gastritis.
- Non–*H. pylori* bacteria: Occasionally, gastric biopsy samples may contain colonies of bacteria that are not *H. pylori* but that are likely oral contaminants; these are often seen in ulcer beds or atrophic gastritis. These are recognized as follows: (1) coccoid or rod shape and *not* spirals or curved; (2) size smaller than *H. pylori*; (3) bunching together; (4) no close association with foveolar epithelium; (5) negative immunolabeling for *H. pylori*.

PROGNOSIS AND THERAPY

Triple therapy for 14 days consisting of either bismuth or a PPI combined with two antibiotics has been the most popular regimen, achieving up to a 95% cure rate. The recommended antibiotics are metronidazole, clarithromycin, and tetracycline or amoxicillin.

However, recent studies have shown that short treatment courses of 1 to 5 days may be equally effective with an eradication rate of 89% to 95% with better compliance, reduced cost, and fewer adverse effects.

◼ GASTRIC PEPTIC ULCER DISEASE

1. Benign gastric ulceration caused by acid-pepsin damage.
2. In the United States, peptic ulcer disease develops in 500,000 people each year; 70% of patients are between 25 and 64 years old.
3. Common locations of peptic ulcer disease are stomach and proximal duodenum; duodenum is a more common site.
4. Less common sites of ulceration are lower esophagus, distal duodenum/jejunum, and ectopic gastric mucosa of Meckel's diverticulum.
5. Causes
   a. *H. pylori* infection and NSAIDs are the leading cause of peptic ulcers in 60% to 70% and 24% of cases, respectively, in the United States.
   b. *H. pylori* infection: Increased gastrin production, virulence factors such as CagA and mucosal damage by inflammation are all attributed to ulcer development.
      (1) *H. pylori* treatment reduces ulcer recurrence in both gastric and duodenal ulcer.
   c. NSAIDs: In patients without *H. pylori* infection, NSAIDs are the most common cause of peptic ulcer. NSAID ulcers are on the rise as the prevalence of *H. pylori* infection is declining in the United States.
   d. Medications, such as steroids.
   e. Rare causes: Zollinger-Ellison syndrome.
6. Clinical feature
   a. Severe epigastric pain exacerbated by food intake.
   b. Duodenal ulcer pain is relieved by food intake.
   c. Vomiting, weight loss, hematemesis, melena, and gastric outlet obstruction caused by scarring and pyloric stenosis; peritonitis caused by perforation.
7. Gross findings
   a. Gastric ulcers are usually present in the lesser curvature, 2 to 4 cm, and round to oval ulcers with a smooth base and regular, perpendicular edges (Fig. 3-16), unlike the irregular heaped-up borders of malignant ulcers.
8. Histology
   a. Mucosal defect extending below the muscularis mucosae with extension into the submucosa and muscularis propria.
   b. Early ulcers are associated with fibrinoid necrosis, inflammation, and granulation tissue reaction.
   c. Chronic ulcers are associated with fibrosis and scarring (Fig. 3-17).

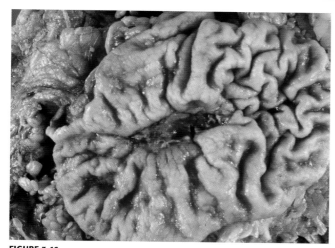

FIGURE 3-16

Benign gastric ulcer with a smooth base and regular borders.

9. Management
   a. Eradication of *H. pylori* infection is key to successful ulcer healing and will reduce the risk of recurrence or rebleeding.
   b. Acid suppressors, especially PPIs.
   c. Endoscopic treatment modalities such as epinephrine injection, coagulation, or clipping of bleeding sites.
   d. Stopping intake of NSAIDs and prostaglandin analogues such as misoprostol.
   e. Surgical management in cases of perforation.
   f. Discontinuing smoking, alcohol, and illicit drug use.

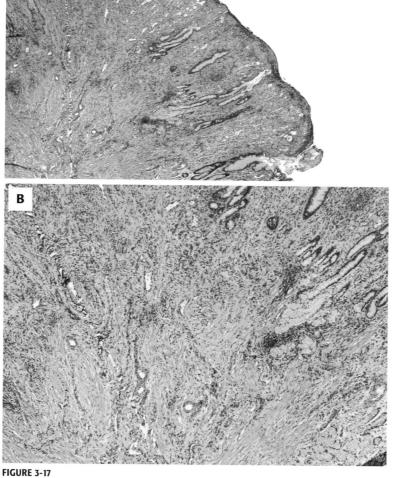

FIGURE 3-17

Unlike erosions, gastric ulcers are deep with extension below the muscularis mucosae **(A).** Chronic ulcers are characterized by fibrosis and stricture **(B).**

■ AUTOIMMUNE GASTRITIS (AUTOIMMUNE METAPLASTIC ATROPHIC GASTRITIS)

Autoimmune gastritis is an immune-mediated chronic gastritis in which the antibodies are directed against gastric parietal cells and intrinsic factor, resulting in loss of oxyntic cells, hypochlorhydria, achlorhydria, and vitamin B_{12} deficiency. Autoimmune gastritis is synonymous with type A gastritis, diffuse corporal atrophic gastritis, atrophic gastritis, autoimmune chronic gastritis, and autoimmune-associated gastritis.

CLINICAL FEATURES

First described by Thomas Addison in 1849, autoimmune gastritis affects nearly 2% of the population older than 60 years old and is responsible for less than 5% of chronic gastritis. It was classically described in individuals of northern European or Scandinavian descent but is now known to be equally represented in African Americans and Latin Americans. White females in their 50s and 60s are affected more (male-to-female ratio, 1:3). Autoimmune gastritis is an immune-mediated injury to the gastric oxyntic mucosa, and serum analysis frequently demonstrates antiparietal cell antibodies targeted against H^+/K^+-ATPase in 60% to 85% and intrinsic factor antibodies in 30% to 50% (Table 3-3). Patients present with abdominal pain, weight loss, diarrhea, malabsorption, and neurologic complications, such as peripheral neuropathy and subacute combined degeneration of spinal cord related to severe vitamin B_{12} deficiency. Iron deficiency anemia can be seen in 20% to 40% of patients, whereas pernicious anemia is seen in 15% to 25% of patients. Reduced gastric acid plays a role in iron deficiency because gastric acid is necessary to release iron from bound protein, as well as reduce ferric iron to ferrous state necessary for absorption. Pernicious anemia is characterized by macrocytosis, megaloblasts, pancytopenia, atrophic glossitis, low serum B_{12} concentration, and normal folate level. Pernicious anemia is a late manifestation of autoimmune gastritis, taking 20 to 30 years to develop, and is caused by progressive loss of parietal cells, which are necessary for intrinsic factor production, as well as autoantibody targeted at intrinsic factor preventing the formation of B_{12}-intrinsic factor complex. Patients may have other autoimmune disorders such as insulin-dependent diabetes mellitus, Hashimoto's thyroiditis, adrenal insufficiency, Graves' disease, vitiligo, or myasthenia gravis.

TABLE 3-3
Pertinent Laboratory Findings in Autoimmune Gastritis

Antiparietal cell antibodies	Positive (target H^+/K^+ATPase): 60% to 85%
Intrinsic factor antibodies	Positive: 30% to 50%
Serum gastrin	Elevated
Gastric pH	Alkaline or neutral
Vitamin B_{12} level	Reduced
Serum pepsinogen I	Reduced (loss of chief cells)
Schilling test	Positive and corrected by vitamin B_{12} injection
Helicobacter pylori serology	Usually negative
HLA haplotypes	HLA −B8, DR-3

Helicobacter infection can also be associated with autoantibody formation, with studies implicating antibodies against *H. pylori* directed at H^+/K^+-ATPase of the parietal cells, as are the antiparietal cell antibodies in autoimmune gastritis.

PATHOLOGIC FEATURES

GROSS AND ENDOSCOPIC FINDINGS

Autoimmune gastritis affects the gastric body and fundus and spares the antrum. On endoscopic examination, the body mucosa appears shiny and red, resulting from effacement of rugal folds, with a prominent submucosal vascular pattern, which becomes visible as a result of mucosal atrophy. Patients may present with multiple pseudopolyps that represent preserved islands of oxyntic mucosa surrounded by flattened body mucosa. Other associations include hyperplastic polyps (most common polyps), multiple carcinoids, and even adenocarcinoma.

MICROSCOPIC FINDINGS

The histologic findings are limited to the body/fundic mucosa with normal antral findings and consist of (1) chronic gastritis with prominent lymphocytic and plasma cell infiltration of the lamina propria directed at oxyntic glands (the chronic inflammation often being more prominent in the deeper mucosa), (2) loss of oxyntic glands (i.e., chief and parietal cells), (3) pseudopyloric metaplasia (glands that resemble mucous glands in the antrum but lack gastrin cells), and (4) intestinal metaplasia with goblet and Paneth cells (Fig. 3-18AB).

AUTOIMMUNE GASTRITIS (AUTOIMMUNE METAPLASTIC ATROPHIC GASTRITIS)—FACT SHEET

Definition

- Immune-mediated form of chronic gastritis resulting in loss of oxyntic cells, hypochlorhydria, achlorhydria, and vitamin B_{12} deficiency

Incidence and Location

- Affects nearly 2% of people older than 60 years
- No racial predilection (in the past, there was a belief that Northern Europeans were preferentially affected)

Gender, Race, and Age

- Patients are usually older white women in their 50s and 60s
- Male-to-female ratio of 1:3

Clinical Features

- Abdominal pain and discomfort, weight loss, pernicious anemia, and rarely subacute combined degeneration of spinal cord
- Patients may have other immune-related disorders such as insulin-mediated diabetes mellitus, Hashimoto's thyroiditis, or adrenal insufficiency
- Serum analysis frequently positive for antiparietal cell antibodies and intrinsic factor antibodies
- Elevated serum gastrin
- Reduced B_{12}; positive Schilling test corrected by administering intrinsic factor
- *Helicobacter* serology is usually negative

Prognosis and Therapy

- 2% to 9% prevalence of gastric carcinoids and a twofold to threefold increase in gastric carcinomas
- Medical management includes vitamin B_{12} injections
- Surgical management for multiple carcinoids includes endoscopic polypectomies, total gastrectomy, or antrectomy
- Screening is not advocated at present given the high cost-benefit ratio

AUTOIMMUNE GASTRITIS (AUTOIMMUNE METAPLASTIC ATROPHIC GASTRITIS)—PATHOLOGIC FEATURES

Gross Findings

- Affects gastric body and fundus and spares the antrum
- Endoscopic and gross features consist of thinning of body mucosa with effacement of rugal folds and prominent submucosal vascular pattern, which become visible as a result of mucosal atrophy
- Associated findings include hyperplastic polyps (most common polyps), multiple carcinoids, and even adenocarcinoma

Microscopic Findings

- Histologic findings are limited to the body and fundic mucosa with normal antral findings
- Chronic gastritis with prominent lamina propria lymphocytic and plasma cell infiltration directed at oxyntic glands
- Loss of oxyntic glands (i.e., chief and parietal cells)
- Pseudopyloric metaplasia, intestinal metaplasia, and pancreatic metaplasia
- Findings may be variable depending on the stage of the disease
- Linear and nodular ECL hyperplasia in the body mucosa

Immunohistochemical Features

- Gastrin and chromogranin A

Differential Diagnosis

- Environmental atrophic metaplastic gastritis (diffuse antral or multifocal atrophic gastritis caused by *Helicobacter pylori* infection)
- Pernicious anemia related to autoimmune polyglandular syndrome type I

Pancreatic acinar metaplasia and mild active inflammation may be present. Findings may vary depending on the stage of the disease. Biopsy specimens taken during early stages show chronic gastritis and some loss of oxyntic glands, but intestinal metaplasia may be lacking. It is not unusual to see parietal cell pseudohypertrophy in this early active stage. In late stages, the oxyntic mucosa can resemble small intestine complete with villi lined by absorptive, goblet, and Paneth cells (so-called complete intestinal metaplasia). The low serum B_{12} in pernicious anemia can cause megaloblastoid change of the foveolar epithelium.

The antral mucosa is not atrophic and usually has chemical gastropathy or a mild chronic gastritis (Fig. 3-19A). The low acid state created by the loss of parietal cells stimulates gastrin cell hyperplasia in the antrum (see Fig. 3-19B), which in turn causes nodular and linear hyperplasia of the enterochromaffin-like (ECL) cells in the body responsible for histamine secretion. These appear as linear hyperplasias (linear arrangement of five or more neuroendocrine cells) or small neuroendocrine nodules at mucosal base (see Fig. 3-18C). Patients may also have multiple carcinoid tumors, mostly in the body. However, hyperplastic polyps are the most common polyps seen.

ANCILLARY STUDIES

IMMUNOHISTOCHEMISTRY

Gastrin immunostain is useful in distinguishing body mucosa (lacks G cells; see Fig. 3-18D) from the antral mucosa, which contains G cells. In autoimmune gastritis, when the body mucosa becomes "antralized" resulting from destruction of oxyntic glands and pseudopyloric metaplasia, gastrin immunostain can be useful to check the biopsy location, especially when unspecified in the requisition form. Gastrin highlights the G-cell hyperplasia in the antrum (see Fig. 3-19B). Rare gastrin-positive cells may be seen in foci with intestinal metaplasia.

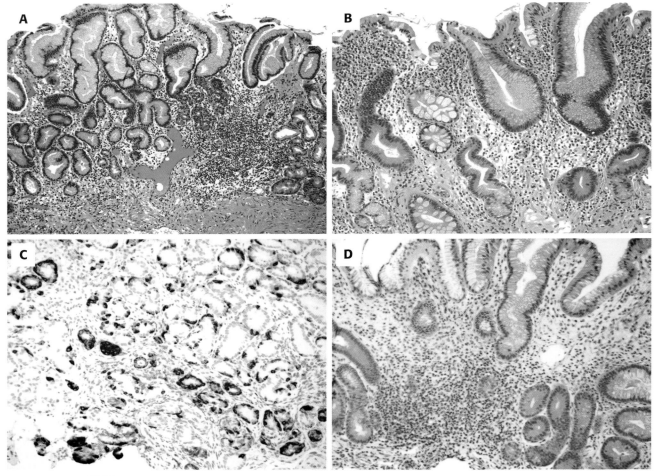

FIGURE 3-18

A, Autoimmune gastritis. Gastric body biopsy sample showing loss of oxyntic glands, chronic lymphoplasmacytic infiltrate more in the deeper aspect, and pyloric metaplasia. **B,** Body biopsy with loss of oxyntic glands and intestinal metaplasia. **C,** Autoimmune gastritis. Chromogranin immunostain highlighting linear and nodular enterochromaffin-like (ECL) cell hyperplasia in the body mucosa. **D,** Gastrin immunostain in the body is negative. Based on this, some observers refer to the presence of metaplastic antral type glands as *pseudopyloric metaplasia* because the glands do not produce gastrin (see Fig. 3-19B).

Chromogranin A highlights the linear and nodular ECL cell hyperplasia (see Fig. 3-18C), as well as gastric carcinoids.

H. pylori stains are negative.

DIFFERENTIAL DIAGNOSIS

- Environmental metaplastic atrophic gastritis (Table 3-4).
- Pernicious anemia related to autoimmune polyglandular syndrome type I: Rare disorder presenting in childhood and characterized by a generalized loss of GI endocrine cells including gastrin cells, caused by antibodies directed against endocrine cells. Patients have a low serum gastrin and do not have antiparietal cell antibody. The gastric body can resemble autoimmune gastritis, and the loss of parietal cells is

a result of the low serum gastrin (a trophic factor for parietal cells).

PROGNOSIS AND THERAPY

Autoimmune gastritis carries a 2% to 9% prevalence of gastric carcinoids and a twofold to threefold increase in the prevalence of gastric adenocarcinomas. Gastric carcinoid tumors associated with autoimmune gastritis are usually indolent.

Medical therapies include administering vitamin B_{12} injections. In patients with multiple carcinoids, management includes endoscopic polypectomies with close surveillance or antrectomy. Antrectomy has been shown to cause resolution of the hypergastrinemic state, leading to reduction in the size of carcinoids. Screening is not advocated at present given the high cost-benefit ratio.

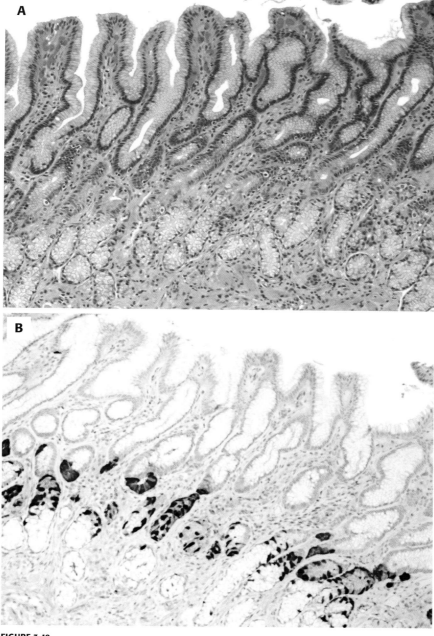

FIGURE 3-19

A, Antral biopsy specimen from an autoimmune gastritis case showing mild reactive gastropathy and lack of metaplasia.
B, Gastrin immunostain of the antrum highlights prominent G-cells.

■ GRANULOMATOUS GASTRITIS

Granulomatous gastritis is an uncommon form of gastritis, comprising 0.27% to 0.35% of all gastritis and characterized by granulomatous infiltrate in the stomach. It encompasses a wide spectrum of diseases that have mucosal or submucosal granulomas in the stomach as the defining histologic feature. Granulomas consist of a nodular, circumscribed collection of epithelioid histiocytes admixed with lymphocytes, eosinophils, giant cells, and even neutrophils, with or without central necrosis and a lymphoid cuff.

TABLE 3-4

Features of Autoimmune versus Environmental Atrophic Gastritis

	Autoimmune Metaplastic Atrophic Gastritis (AMAG)	Environmental Metaplastic Atrophic Gastritis (EMAG)
Synonyms	Type A gastritis Diffuse corporal gastritis	Type B gastritis Diffuse antral gastritis Multifocal atrophic gastritis
Population affected	Northern European and Scandinavian descent	Worldwide
Sex	Female predominance	No sex predilection
Etiology	Immune mediated	*H. pylori* infection
H. pylori colonization	<20%	90% to 100%
Location	Body and fundus	Antrum predominantly with extension to body, multifocal
Antiparietal cell antibody	Positive	Negative
Anti-intrinsic factor antibody	Positive	Negative
Vitamin B_{12} level	Low	Normal
Serum gastrin	Very high	Normal or low

TABLE 3-5

Differential Diagnoses of Granulomatous Gastritis

Gastric Crohn's disease—52%

Sarcoidosis-1—21%

Foreign body granuloma-food, suture material, barium, mucin—10%

Isolated granulomatous gastritis—25%

Tumor-associated granulomas—7%

Infections (tuberculosis, histoplasmosis, schistosomiasis Whipple's disease, leprosy, syphilis)

Vasculitis associated granulomas (Churg Strauss disease)

Helicobacter pylori gastritis

Data from Ectors NL, Dixon MF, Geboes KJ, et al: Granulomatous gastritis: a morphological and diagnostic approach. Histopathology 1993; 23:55-61; and Shapiro JL, Goldblum JR, Petras RE: A clinicopathologic study of 42 patients with granulomatous gastritis: is there really an "idiopathic" granulomatous gastritis? Am J Surg Pathol 1996; 20:462-470.

The final diagnosis depends on the clinical, radiologic, endoscopic, microbiological, and histologic findings and treatment response (Table 3-5). When a granuloma is seen on H&E examination, additional studies such as the use of polarized light to rule out foreign body, special stains such as AFB, GMS, and PAS become a vital part of the assessment.

GASTRIC CROHN'S DISEASE

In the Western world gastric Crohn's disease accounts for 17% to 55% of cases of granulomatous gastritis. Approximately 30% of patients with Crohn's disease have upper GI findings; patients with both small and large bowel involvement are at increased risk. Patients are younger, often in the pediatric age group. Symptoms consist of abdominal pain, nausea, and vomiting. Patients may present with coexisting lower GI symptoms such as chronic diarrhea and weight loss.

RADIOLOGIC FINDINGS

Radiologic findings include ulcers, strictures, and gastric outlet obstruction.

PATHOLOGIC FEATURES

GROSS AND ENDOSCOPIC FINDINGS

Findings range from normal mucosa to erythema, aphthoid-type erosions, superficial or deep ulcers, nodules, thickened folds, and stenosis. Findings are usually predominant in the antrum.

MICROSCOPIC FINDINGS

Gastric biopsies in patients with Crohn's can range from normal to *H. pylori*–negative mild chronic gastritis, or patchy chronic active gastritis (Fig. 3-20). The finding of granulomas is very helpful in establishing the diagnosis of Crohn's disease, although granulomas are present in only 7% to 34% cases. Foveolar isthmi are common sites for Crohn's granulomas, and they consist of small loose clusters of epithelioid histiocytes. Granulomas are usually seen in younger patients and often correspond to the nodules or aphthoid erosions seen on endoscopy. Granulomas

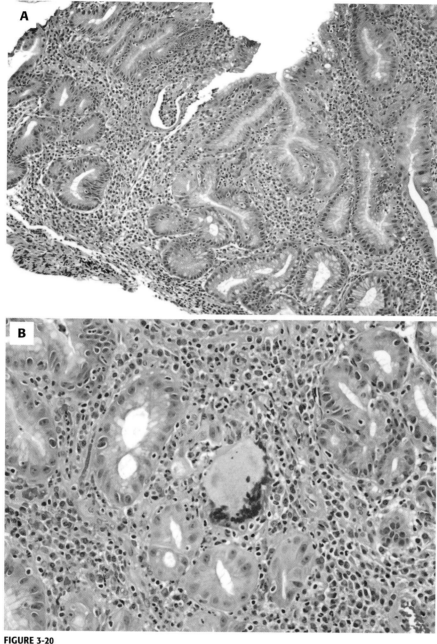

FIGURE 3-20

Gastric Crohn's showing lymphoplasmacytic infiltrate and crypt abscess **(A)** and giant cell **(B).** Immunostain for *Helicobacter pylori* was negative.

can also be present in normal gastric mucosa, thus emphasizing the importance of sampling normal mucosa for biopsy. Other histologic findings include pit abscesses and focal active gastritis or focally enhanced gastritis, which is composed of a focal lymphohistiocytic cluster with admixed acute inflammation. Focally enhanced gastritis is not limited to Crohn's, however, and can be seen in ulcerative colitis and graft versus host disease.

On gastric resections, the diagnosis of Crohn's disease is easier, and histologic features such as linear fissures, undermining ulcers, transmural inflammation with lymphoid follicles, granulomas, and neural hyperplasia are all helpful.

Taking multiple biopsy samples, using jumbo forceps, and examining multiple serial sections increase the chances of finding granulomas in Crohn's disease.

Ruling out *H. pylori* infection by special stains is important. Ten percent to 15% of Crohn's patients may have *H. pylori* gastritis.

GASTRIC SARCOIDOSIS

- Sarcoidosis is a multisystemic granulomatous disease, characterized by hypercalcemia and commonly affecting lungs and hilar lymph nodes.
- Affects young adults.
- Common in African Americans.
- Gastric antrum can be involved in 10% of patients with systemic disease.
- Grossly the gastric mucosa may be nodular (Fig. 3-21) with ulcers, thickening, and a segmental linitis plastica–like appearance.

- Patients may present with gastric outlet obstruction or bleeding.
- Sarcoid granulomas are compact noncaseating granulomas with a surrounding lymphocytic cuff (Figs. 3-22 and 3-23).
- It is a diagnosis of exclusion, and diagnosis is usually reached on clinical correlation and chest computed tomography findings.
- Patients respond to steroids.

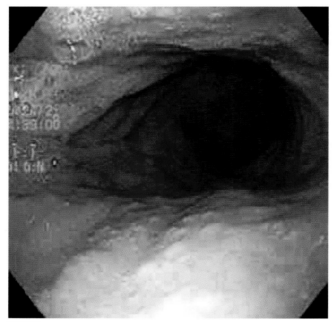

FIGURE 3-21

Gastric sarcoidosis with a nodular mucosal appearance on endoscopy.

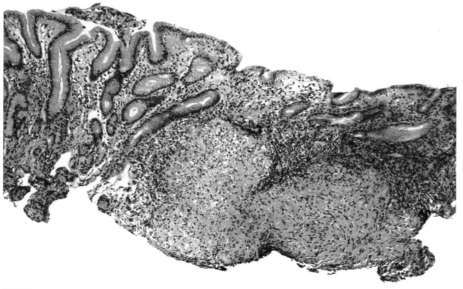

FIGURE 3-22

Antral mucosa showing noncaseating granulomas in the lamina propria in a patient with sarcoidosis.

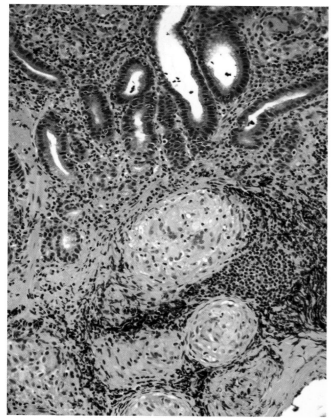

FIGURE 3-23

Compact noncaseating with lymphoid cuff granulomas in a patient with gastric sarcoidosis.

ISOLATED GRANULOMATOUS GASTRITIS

Idiopathic granulomatous gastritis was a term coined by Fahimi in 1963, after excluding known entities such as Crohn's disease and sarcoidosis. The granulomas are large and compact and are limited to the stomach. There have been a number of papers challenging this concept, and many authors link the granulomas to an inflammatory response to *H. pylori* infection. Miyamoto and colleagues reported disappearance of the granulomas following successful eradication of two such cases after treatment of *Helicobacter* infection. Another paper found an association with vasculitis. The conclusion seems to be that, in most cases, if we seek an etiology, we may be successful.

LYMPHOCYTIC GASTRITIS

Lymphocytic gastritis is an uncommon form of chronic gastritis, which was described by Haot and colleagues in 1988. It is characterized by marked intraepithelial lymphocytosis in the gastric surface and pit epithelium. Lymphocytic gastritis is synonymous with varioliform gastritis (refers to the endoscopic appearance) and chronic erosive verrucous gastritis.

CLINICAL FEATURES

Lymphocytic gastritis has a prevalence of 1% to 4% in upper GI endoscopies. Symptoms include dyspepsia, iron deficiency anemia, and diarrhea. It is seen in adults and children (age range, 1 to 89 years). A slight female predominance is present. According to Wu and colleagues, approximately 38% of lymphocytic gastritis patients have celiac disease and 29% have *H. pylori* gastritis. Other less common associations consist of varioliform gastritis, Crohn's disease, human immunodeficiency virus (HIV) infection, lymphocytic gastroenterocolitis, esophageal carcinoma, and gastric lymphoma. Lymphocytic gastritis is found in 33% of celiac patients who undergo gastric biopsies, and 4% of patients with *H. pylori* gastritis have lymphocytic gastritis. Celiac patients with lymphocytic gastritis may also have lymphocytic colitis (38%). Lymphocytic gastritis has also been described in patients with lymphocytic enterocolitis. This reiterates the importance of taking gastric, duodenal, and colonic biopsy samples for a complete evaluation of the histologic findings. Lymphocytic gastritis can present with Ménétrier's-like protein-losing gastropathy. Lymphocytic gastritis resolves with treatment for *H. pylori*.

RADIOLOGIC FEATURES

Nodules with central erosion give rise to classic volcano-like lesions on radiography. A double-contrast upper GI series shows discrete radiolucent halos with central barium flecks.

PATHOLOGIC FEATURES

GROSS AND ENDOSCOPIC FINDINGS

Endoscopic appearance may be normal or consist of mucosal nodules, erosions, and enlarged gastric folds. These latter gross appearances may mimic carcinoma or lymphoma. The nodules may contain central depression or erosion and are described as varioliform or aphthoid erosions.

MICROSCOPIC FINDINGS

Histologic findings include marked intraepithelial lymphocytosis of gastric surface and pit epithelium comprising more than 25 lymphocytes per 100 epithelial cells. Normal gastric controls have 3.5 lymphocytes per 100 cells, and diseased controls such as patients with *Helicobacter* gastritis have 5 lymphocytes per 100 cells. The deeper glandular epithelium is spared. The lamina propria is also expanded by lymphocytes and plasma cells (Fig. 3-24). The intraepithelial lymphocytes are

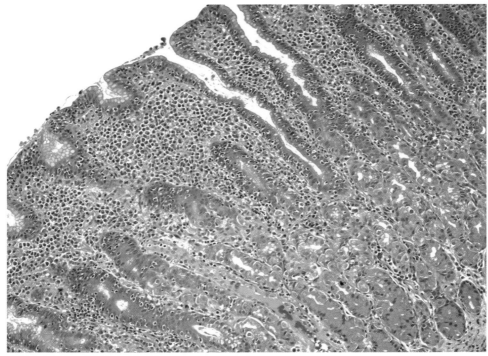

FIGURE 3-24

Lymphocytic gastritis. Oxyntic mucosa with marked increase in intraepithelial lymphocytes in the surface epithelium and gastric pits. The lamina propria is expanded by plasma cells and lymphocytes.

recognized by their condensed, dark nuclei surrounded by a clear halo (Fig. 3-25). The foveolar pits are slightly tortuous and elongated. Areas with erosions may contain active inflammation with neutrophils.

Lymphocytic gastritis can involve the gastric antrum, as well as the body. It is antrum predominant in celiac patients, whereas in *H. pylori* and varioliform gastritis, the body is commonly involved.

ANCILLARY STUDIES

IMMUNOHISTOCHEMISTRY

- The intraepithelial lymphocytes are CD3- and CD8-positive cytotoxic/suppressor T-lymphocytes.
- In gastric maltomas the neoplastic lymphocytes in lymphoepithelial lesions are CD20-positive B-cells.
- Stains for *Helicobacter* organisms.

DIFFERENTIAL DIAGNOSIS

GASTRIC MALT LYMPHOMA

This is a low-grade monoclonal B-cell lymphoma with CD20- and CD43-positive malignant B-lymphocytes infiltrating epithelial cells. There is significant epithelial and lamina propria destruction by the neoplastic

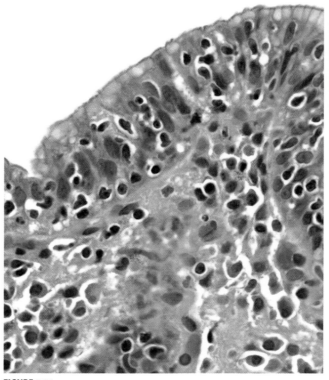

FIGURE 3-25

Lymphocytic gastritis. High-power view showing the condensed dark nuclei of intraepithelial lymphocytes surrounded by a clear halo.

lymphoid infiltrate with formation of characteristic lymphoepithelial lesions. The intraepithelial lymphocytes in lymphocytic gastritis are CD3-positive mature T-lymphocytes.

Chronic Active H. Pylori Gastritis

The histologic appearance is that of a superficial chronic active gastritis with neutrophils and plasma cells. The surface epithelium lacks the characteristic lymphocytosis that is seen in lymphocytic gastritis. Intraepithelial lymphocytes usually number 4 to 5 lymphocytes per 100 epithelial cells.

Gastric Endocrine Cell Hyperplasia

These can sometimes mimic lymphocytes. Stains for gastrin or chromogranin help differentiate the diagnoses.

PROGNOSIS AND THERAPY

Lymphocytic gastritis is an inflammatory condition. Treatment is directed at associated conditions such as celiac disease (gluten-free diet) or eradication of *Helicobacter* gastritis (antibiotics). Patients with lymphocytic gastroenterocolitis may be refractory to a gluten-free diet and need steroids. Patients with ulcers/erosions are also treated with PPIs.

■ INFECTIOUS GASTRITIS

The most common and important cause of infectious gastritis is *H. pylori* infection. The following sections discuss various other etiologies of gastric infections. As is true with most infections, these infections are more common in immunocompromised patients.

VIRUSES

- Cytomegalovirus (CMV): The inclusions in CMV gastritis are often present in gastric glandular epithelium along with the mesenchymal cells such as endothelial cells and fibroblasts. There are cytoplasmic and nuclear inclusions characterized by enlarged cells with eosinophilic nuclear inclusions, perinuclear halo, and cytoplasmic reddish granules (Figs. 3-26 and 3-27). Infection of vascular endothelial cells causes a picture similar to ischemic gastritis can be present on biopsies (Fig. 3-28). Immunostains (Fig. 3-29), molecular studies such as polymerase chain reaction, and viral cultures are helpful adjunctive studies. CMV infection can present in children with protein-losing enteropathy with enlarged gastric folds simulating Ménétrier's disease (MD). Endoscopic appearance consists of gastric ulcers, polypoid lesions

and may mimic an infiltrative process. Diagnostic yield is increased by taking multiple biopsies from the base as well as edge of an ulcer.
- Herpes: Can rarely cause erosions and gastritis in immunosuppressed patients. Nuclear inclusions with ground-glass appearance and the three Ms: multinucleation, margination, and moulding. Often associated with necrosis.

BACTERIA

- Mycobacteria tuberculosis: Still an important cause of infection in developing countries, the granulomas show central caseation with Langerhans giant cells and lymphocytes. Stains for acid-fast bacilli (often the organisms are very scarce, thus the need to use oil immersion) and tuberculosis cultures are important. Patients can present with weight loss, anorexia, night sweats, and indolent fever with symptoms of gastric outlet obstruction or bleeding from an ulcer.
- *Mycobacterium avium intracellulare* (MAI): Common opportunistic infection in patients with acquired immunodeficiency syndrome (AIDS); the stomach is only rarely involved. The gastric mucosa is expanded by foamy histiocytes stuffed with acid-fast bacilli (Fig. 3-30). Unlike tuberculosis, granulomas are not a feature of MAI infection.
- Syphilis: Presents with ulcers, thickened folds, and strictures (hourglass stomach). Intense plasma cell infiltration, mononuclear vasculitis, presence of spirochetes, *Treponema pallidum*. Silver stains such as Warthin-Starry are helpful.
- Whipple's disease

FUNGAL

- Histoplasma
- *Aspergillus, Mucor*: Immunocompromised state; invasive forms are almost always fatal.
- Candida: Fungal colonization can be seen in approximately 20 % of benign gastric ulcers. The fungal yeasts and pseudohyphae are usually admixed in the ulcer exudate and do not affect ulcer healing. Most ulcers heal with acid-suppressive medications and do not require antimycotics. Nonhealing ulcers may benefit from fluconazole.

PARASITES

- Anisakiasis: Caused by ingesting raw fish and seen in countries such as Japan and the Netherlands.
- *Strongyloides stercoralis* (Fig. 3-31): Nematode infection; biopsy often shows all stages of the worm

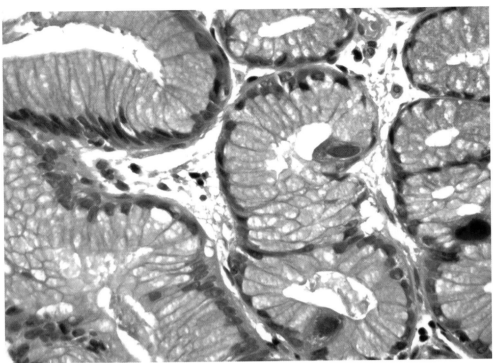

FIGURE 3-26
Cytomegalovirus gastritis. Gastric foveolar epithelial cells with cytomegalovirus inclusions. Note both nuclear and cytoplasmic inclusions.

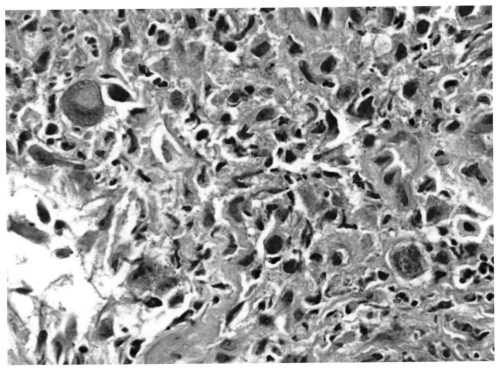

FIGURE 3-27
Endothelial cells and stromal cells. Cytomegalovirus cytopathic effect is shown (nuclear and reddish granular cytoplasmic staining).

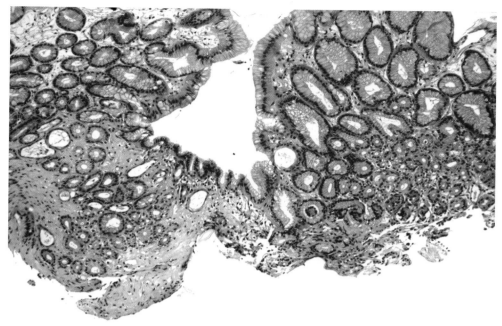

FIGURE 3-28
Gastric mucosal biopsy. Lamina propria condensation and glandular dropout consistent with ischemic change in a case of CMV gastritis.

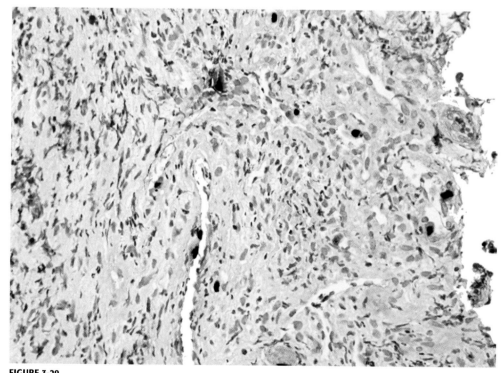

FIGURE 3-29
Positive immunohistochemistry for CMV. Demonstrated by dark brown nuclear staining. (Also note staining in endothelial cells.)

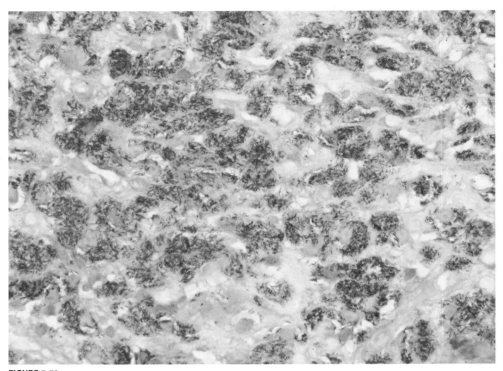

FIGURE 3-30
Mycobacterium avium intracellulare infection, showing macrophages stuffed with acid-fast bacilli (Fite stain).

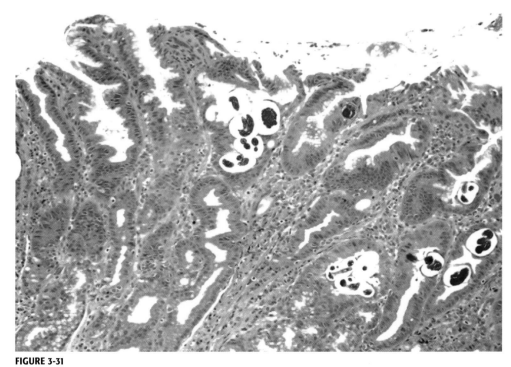

FIGURE 3-31
Strongyloides gastritis. Gastric antral mucosa. Note cross sections of *Strongyloides stercoralis* larvae in gastric pits.

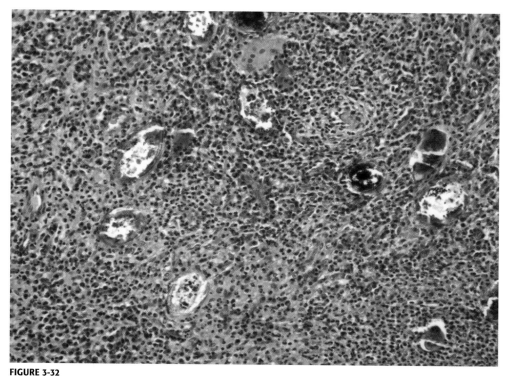

FIGURE 3-32
Numerous schistosome eggs. Some are calcified and associated with intense eosinophilic infiltration.

(adults, larva, eggs) embedded in crypts. Disseminated strongyloidiasis can be fatal.

- *Schistosoma mansoni* (Fig. 3-32).
- Cryptosporidiosis: Seen in patients with AIDS, although their prevalence is decreasing owing to better and more widespread use of antiretrovirals.
- Giardiasis: May rarely present in gastric mucosa with chronic atrophic gastritis and reduced gastric acidity. Invariably associated with intestinal giardiasis.

PHLEGMONOUS (SUPPURATIVE) GASTRITIS

This is an almost invariably fatal condition detected in emergency laparotomy resection of stomach or autopsy studies. Patients are usually older, alcoholic, and debilitated, with vague abdominal pain and fever. The causative organisms are bacteria such as streptococci, staphylococci, *Escherichia coli,* and *Proteus.* The histologic section of stomach shows predominantly submucosal and mural intense acute neutrophilic inflammation with necrosis and mucosal sloughing. Gram stain demonstrates numerous gram-positive and gram-negative bacteria. Acute emphysematous gastritis is a complication of phlegmonous gastritis, caused by gas-producing bacteria such as *Clostridium welchii.* Grossly the gastric wall is crepitant.

EOSINOPHILIC GASTRITIS

Eosinophilic gastritis is a manifestation of eosinophilic gastroenteritis (EG), a rare inflammatory condition characterized by intense eosinophilic infiltration of the GI tract. Synonyms include eosinophilic gastroenteritis and allergic gastroenteropathy.

CLINICAL FEATURES

The diagnostic criteria for eosinophilic gastroenteritis include (1) GI symptoms, (2) histologic evidence of eosinophilic infiltration of the GI tract, (3) absence of eosinophilic infiltration in extraintestinal organs, and (4) exclusion of known causes of eosinophilia, such as parasitic infestation or drug reaction. Patients also present with history of allergy (50%), asthma, food intolerance (52%), eczema, drug sensitivities, peripheral blood eosinophilia (80%), and elevated serum immunoglobulin E levels. Although food intolerance has been postulated as an etiologic factor, most cases lack a specific allergen and multiple allergens are cited as the cause. Cytokines such as IL-5, IL-3, and eotaxins play an important role in the proliferation and recruitment of eosinophils. EG may affect all races and any age group, although usually affecting adults between 20 and 50 years of age. There is no sex predominance. Pediatric involvement is common: 15% to 20% of cases are in children. Any part of the GI tract from the esophagus to the rectum can be involved, and stomach antrum is the most common site of involvement. Esophagus and small bowel are also commonly involved. Eosinophilic proctocolitis is seen most often in infants (an important cause of bloody stool) and is usually attributed to cow's milk allergy.

Eosinophilic gastritis can show preferential involvement of the mucosa, muscle layer, or serosa (Klein classification). Symptoms depend on the site and extent of eosinophilic infiltration. Mucosal disease can present as abdominal pain, nausea, vomiting, diarrhea, weight loss, malabsorption, protein-losing enteropathy, and anemia caused by GI bleeding. Patients with involvement of submucosa and muscularis propria present with obstructive symptoms and symptoms mimicking pyloric stenosis. Serosal involvement is characterized by eosinophilic ascites, peripheral eosinophilia, and dramatic response to steroids. Rarely patients may present with an acute abdominal emergency and perforation necessitating emergency laparotomy.

RADIOLOGIC FEATURES

Radiographic studies may demonstrate marked edema and thickening of gastric mucosal folds, obstructive features (mural disease), or wall thickening.

PATHOLOGIC FEATURES

GROSS AND ENDOSCOPIC FINDINGS

Gastric mucosa may be normal on endoscopic examination or reveal erosions, ulcerations erythema, and nodularity.

MICROSCOPIC FINDINGS

Histologic examination is critical for diagnosis. Eosinophils are a normal cellular component of the GI mucosa. Eosinophilic gastritis is characterized by intense eosinophilic infiltration (>20 per high-power field) with prominent lamina propria eosinophils, intraepithelial eosinophils, and eosinophilic crypt abscesses (Fig. 3-33). The eosinophilic infiltration is accompanied by epithelial damage, regenerative change, and marked edema. Eosinophils are the dominant cell type and other inflammatory cells are not prominent. The presence of even small clusters of eosinophils in the submucosa, muscularis, or serosa is abnormal. The eosinophilic infiltrate can be patchy or diffuse, and mucosal biopsies can be nondiagnostic in up to 10% of cases. Multiple full-thickness and even open biopsies may be necessary to establish the diagnosis in cases with only muscle or serosal involvement.

EOSINOPHILIC GASTRITIS—FACT SHEET

Definition
- Eosinophilic gastritis is a rare inflammatory condition characterized by gastrointestinal symptoms and eosinophilic infiltration of the gastrointestinal tract

Morbidity and Mortality
- Rarely patients may present with acute abdominal emergency and perforation
- Gastrointestinal bleeding

Gender, Race, and Age
- Patients are usually 20 to 50 years old
- Pediatric involvement in 15% to 20% of cases
- Male-to-female ratio 1:1

Clinical Features
- History of allergy, asthma, food intolerance, eczema, drug sensitivities, peripheral blood eosinophilia, and increased immunoglobulin E levels
- Symptoms depend on the site and extent of eosinophilic infiltration
- Mucosal disease can present as abdominal pain, nausea, vomiting, diarrhea, weight loss, malabsorption, protein-losing enteropathy, and gastrointestinal bleeding
- Patients with submucosal and muscularis propria involvement present with obstructive symptoms
- Eosinophilic ascites with serosal involvement
- Other causes of tissue eosinophilia such as parasitic infestation, drug reaction, and hypereosinophilic syndrome should be excluded.

Radiologic Features
- Marked edema and thickening of the gastric wall

Prognosis and Therapy
- Dramatic improvement with steroids
- Surgery in obstructive or refractory cases

DIFFERENTIAL DIAGNOSIS

- Parasitic infestation: Parasitic infestation is associated often with intense eosinophilic infiltration surrounding parasitic ova, larvae, or nematode such as anisakiasis, *Strongyloides*, and *Ascaris*. Careful histologic examination for ova and parasites and stool examination is important.
- Drugs such as gold, azathioprine, carbamazepine, enalapril, and co-trimoxazole can also cause eosinophilia in the GI tract.
- Hypereosinophilic syndrome: Fatal disease characterized by peripheral eosinophilia (>1500/mm^3) and diffuse infiltration of eosinophils in various organs such as myocardium, lungs, and GI tract.
- Eosinophils can be focally prominent in gastric Crohn's disease, gastric carcinomas, lymphomas,

EOSINOPHILIC GASTRITIS—PATHOLOGIC FEATURES

Gross Findings

- Gastric mucosa may be normal or contain erosions, ulcerations, erythema, and nodules

Microscopic Findings

- Histologic examination is critical for diagnosis
- Gastric antral mucosa commonly involved
- Intense eosinophilic infiltration with prominent lamina propria eosinophils, eosinophilic crypt abscesses, and epithelial damage
- Eosinophils are the dominant cell type
- Eosinophilic infiltrate can be patchy or diffuse, and mucosal biopsies can be nondiagnostic in up to 10%
- Multiple, full-thickness, and even open biopsies may be necessary to establish the diagnosis in cases with only muscle or serosal involvement

Differential Diagnosis

- Parasitic infestation
- Hypereosinophilic syndrome
- Eosinophils can be focally prominent in gastric Crohn's disease, gastric carcinomas, lymphomas, connective tissue disorder, and peptic ulcer disease
- Langerhans cell histiocytosis
- Eosinophilic granuloma
- Mast cell disease
- Churg-Strauss vasculitis
- Drugs such as gold, azathioprine, carbamazepine, enalapril, co-trimoxazole
- Inflammatory fibroid polyp

connective tissue disorder, vasculitis such as Churg-Strauss disease, and peptic ulcer disease.

- Langerhans cell histiocytosis: Seen mostly in children; eosinophils are intermixed with Langerhans histiocytes with elongated bean-shaped nuclei. These are positive for CD1a and S-100 and show intracytoplasmic Birbeck granules on electron microscopy.
- Mast cell disease: Eosinophils can mask mast cells, which are positive for mast cell tryptase, CD117, and CD25. Special stains such as toludine blue and Giemsa also highlight the cytoplasmic granules. History of skin urticaria may be helpful.
- Inflammatory bowel disease (IBD): Eosinophils can be a prominent component of IBD; more prominent in colonic biopsies.
- Inflammatory fibroid polyp: This is characterized by a prominent eosinophilic infiltration but presents as a mass lesion.

PROGNOSIS AND THERAPY

Patients with eosinophilic gastroenteritis show an excellent response to steroids. Discontinuation may be followed by relapse. Patients have also shown good response to oral sodium chromoglycate. Surgical resection may be necessary in patients with obstruction or in refractory cases.

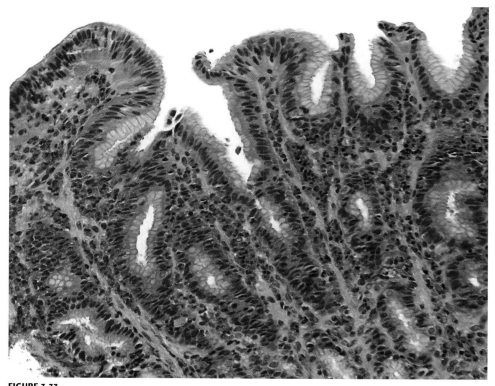

FIGURE 3-33

Intense eosinophilic infiltration in a case of eosinophilic gastritis. Notice surface regenerative changes and glandular infiltration by eosinophils.

■ COLLAGENOUS GASTRITIS

First described by Colletti and Trainer in 1989, collagenous gastritis is a rare entity consisting of subepithelial collagen deposition in superficial gastric mucosa exceeding 10 μm, surface epithelial damage, and lymphoplasmacytic inflammation of the lamina propria.

CLINICAL FEATURES

Since its first description in 1989, around 36 cases of collagenous gastritis have been described in the literature. A slight female predominance is seen. Both children and adults are affected; the age range is 8 to 80 years. Clinical manifestations include chronic diarrhea, anorexia, nausea, vomiting, abdominal pain, weight loss, anemia, and bleeding. Other associations with collagenous gastritis may include collagenous colitis, lymphocytic colitis, celiac sprue, collagenous sprue, lymphocytic gastritis, and inflammatory bowel disease. According to Lagorce-Pages and colleagues, patients with collagenous gastritis fall into two sub-

sets: (1) children and young adults presenting with anemia, nodular gastric mucosal pattern in endoscopy, and disease limited to the gastric mucosa without colonic involvement, and (2) adults presenting with chronic watery diarrhea, often associated with collagenous colitis. In one study, the adult patients with collagenous gastritis often had associated autoimmune disorders, celiac sprue, collagenous colitis, collagenous sprue, or lymphocytic gastritis.

Little is known about the pathophysiology of this disease. Explanations provided include (1) excessive collagen deposition caused by reparative process following chronic inflammation and injury to the mucosa, as a result of autoimmune, toxic, or infectious agents; (2) collagen deposition by abnormal pericryptal fibroblasts; and (3) leakage of plasma proteins and fibrinogen with subsequent replacement by collagen.

PATHOLOGIC FEATURES

GROSS AND ENDOSCOPIC FINDINGS

Both the gastric antrum and body are affected. Endoscopic appearance consists of diffuse nodularity, erythema, and erosions.

COLLAGENOUS GASTRITIS—FACT SHEET

Definition
- A rare entity consisting of subepithelial collagen deposition of more than 10 μm, surface epithelial damage, and lymphoplasmacytic inflammation of the lamina propria

Incidence
- Rare entity described as case reports and short series

Morbidity and Mortality
- Benign inflammatory disorder
- Can cause chronic morbidity including anemia, chronic diarrhea, and significant weight loss

Gender, Race, and Age
- Slight female predominance
- Seen in adults and children: age range, 8 to 80 years

Clinical Features
- Clinical manifestations include chronic watery diarrhea, weight loss, anorexia, nausea, vomiting, abdominal pain, anemia, and bleeding
- Often associated with collagenous colitis, lymphocytic colitis, celiac sprue, collagenous sprue, lymphocytic gastritis, and inflammatory bowel disease

Prognosis and Therapy
- No definite treatment
- Prednisone, budesonide, azathioprine, and a gluten-free diet have been shown to improve symptoms and cause weight gain
- Important to biopsy the duodenum and colon to exclude celiac and collagenous sprue, as well as collagenous and lymphocytic colitis

---

COLLAGENOUS GASTRITIS—PATHOLOGIC FEATURES

Gross Findings
- Both the gastric antrum and body affected
- Endoscopic appearance consists of diffuse nodularity (common), diffuse or patchy erythema, and erosions

Microscopic Findings
- Superficial gastric mucosa shows a strikingly increased subepithelial collagen band, which is diffuse or patchy, averaging 30 to 40 μm in thickness
- The subepithelial collagen band also shows irregularity of the lower edge with trapping of capillaries and inflammatory cells
- The surface foveolar epithelium shows degenerative changes such as flattening or cuboidal changes, as well as epithelial stripping
- The lamina propria contains increased inflammation comprising mostly lymphocytes and plasma cells
- Features of lymphocytic gastritis may be present

Immunohistochemical Features
- Masson's trichrome stain highlights the subepithelial collagen band
- Amyloid stains such as Congo red or thioflavin T are negative
- The subepithelial collagen band is negative for collagen IV and laminin and positive for type I and III collagen

Differential Diagnosis
- Gastric amyloidosis
- Radiation gastritis
- Ischemic gastritis
- Scleroderma

MICROSCOPIC FINDINGS

Histologic findings in collagenous gastritis are similar to those of collagenous colitis. Superficial gastric antral and body mucosa show a diffuse or patchy distribution of strikingly increased subepithelial collagen band that is usually discontinuous in nature (Fig. 3-34). The collagen thickness is greater than 10 μm, ranging from 20 to 120 μm and averaging 30 to 40 μm. Normal thickness is less than 2 to 3 μm. Apart from quantitative increase, the subepithelial collagen also shows qualitative abnormality, including trapping of capillaries and inflammatory cells, and a ragged lower border similar to that seen in collagenous colitis. Surface foveolar epithelium shows degenerative changes such as flattening or cuboidal changes, mucin depletion, and epithelial stripping. The lamina propria contains increased inflammation comprising mostly lymphocytes and plasma cells but may also contain active inflammation. Other features may include lymphocytic gastritis with increased intraepithelial lymphocytosis, more than 20 lymphocytes per 100 epithelial cells. Unlike lymphocytic gastritis, which is often associated with *H. pylori* infection, most patients with collagenous gastritis test negative for *Helicobacter*.

ANCILLARY STUDIES

HISTOCHEMISTRY AND IMMUNOHISTOCHEMISTRY

- Masson's trichrome: Highlights the subepithelial collagen band (Fig. 3-35).
- Amyloid stains, such as Congo red or thioflavin T, are negative.
- CD3, CD20, κ and λ show a polyclonal population of lymphocytes and a predominance of T lymphocytes.
- The subepithelial collagen band is negative for collagen IV and laminin (composition of normal basement membrane), proving that the collagen is abnormal and consists of mainly types I and III collagen.

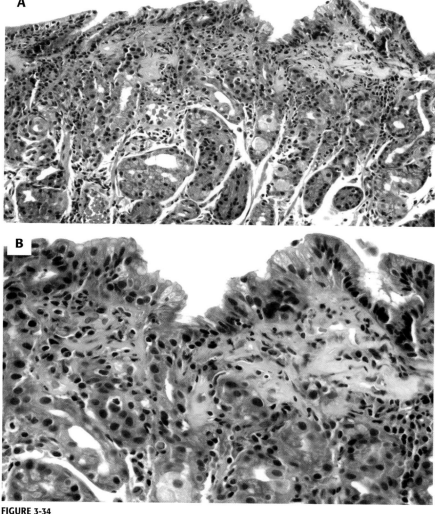

FIGURE 3-34

Collagenous gastritis. **A** and **B**, Note the increased subepithelial deposition of collagen in this body biopsy. *(Courtesy of Carlos Torres, MD, Pathology Partners, Irving, Texas.)*

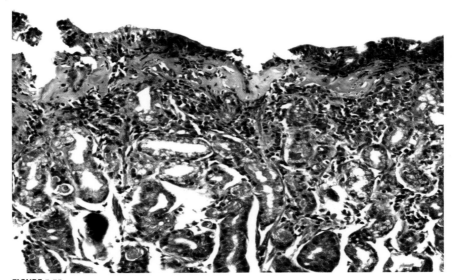

FIGURE 3-35
Trichrome stain. The subepithelial collagen is highlighted and stains blue.

DIFFERENTIAL DIAGNOSIS

- Gastric amyloidosis: Amyloid deposition can be superficial and may resemble a collagen band. However, the deposit is not just limited to the superficial mucosa as in collagenous gastritis but involves the submucosa. It is also seen in the walls of blood vessels. Congo red stain will show apple-green birefringence and trichrome is negative.
- Lamina propria fibrosis as in scleroderma, radiation gastritis, and ischemic gastritis: All of these conditions are characterized by increased fibrosis that is not limited to the subepithelial zone and is usually diffuse in nature. Scleroderma can involve the submucosa, muscularis propria, and even serosa. Radiation gastritis will also show fragile and hyalinized blood vessels apart from fibrosis (see Fig. 3-6).

PROGNOSIS AND THERAPY

Treatment is still empirical and includes budesonide (also used to treat collagenous colitis), prednisone, azathioprine, 5-aminosalicylates, nutritional supplements, and a gluten-free diet. Some studies have suggested improvement in patients' symptoms with steroids and a gluten-free diet. In most instances, despite symptomatic improvement, follow-up biopsies show a persistence of collagen. Considering the frequent association with other collagenous enterocolitides, it is important to biopsy the duodenum and colon in all cases of collagenous gastritis.

■ GASTRIC MUCOSAL CALCINOSIS (ALUMINOCALCINOSIS)

Gastric mucosal calcinosis (GMC) is infrequently encountered in biopsies and is associated with calcium deposition in the superficial gastric mucosa.

CLINICAL FEATURES

GMC can be classified as metastatic, dystrophic, and idiopathic. Dystrophic calcification is encountered in inflamed or damaged gastric mucosa. Metastatic calcification, the most frequent type of GMC, occurs in almost normal gastric mucosa in patients with abnormal biochemical milieu such as hypercalcemia and hyperphosphatemia. GMC is mostly seen in chronic renal failure, organ transplant patients, and patients taking aluminum-containing antacids or sucralfate. Other associations include hyperparathyroidism, sarcoidosis, multiple myeloma, tumor lysis syndrome, hypervitaminosis D, hypervitaminosis A, milk-alkali syndrome, and isotretinoin use. The overall incidence of GMC is less than 0.1% of all gastric biopsies. Studies have shown GMC to be present in 14% to 60% of gastric biopsies in selected patients with transplants and chronic renal disease. The incidence is 5% in nontransplant patients with gastric ulcers. The patients in one study were all women. Associated findings include chemical gastropathy, CMV infection, gastric ulcers, and cancers. Sometimes, however, an underlying etiology is not known. The deposits can occur in the fundus, body, or antrum. Patients may present with nausea, vomiting, dyspepsia, abdominal pain, anemia, or GI bleeding.

GASTRIC MUCOSAL CALCINOSIS (ALUMINOCALCINOSIS)—FACT SHEET

Definition
- Rare condition characterized by gastric mucosal deposits of calcium beneath the foveolar tips

Incidence and Location
- 14% to 60% of gastric biopsies from transplant patients
- 5% of gastric biopsies from nontransplant patients with gastric ulcers
- Fundus, antrum, or body

Morbidity and Mortality
- Usually seen in end-stage renal failure patients, organ transplant recipients, patients on dialysis, and patients on aluminum-containing antacids and sucralfate

Gender, Race, and Age
- Female predominance
- Adults

Clinical Features
- Nausea, vomiting, dyspepsia, abdominal pain, anemia, or GI bleeding.

Prognosis and Treatment
- Benign, of unknown clinical significance

GASTRIC MUCOSAL CALCINOSIS (ALUMINOCALCINOSIS)—PATHOLOGIC FEATURES

Endoscopic Findings
- Appear as whitish plaques

Microscopic Findings:
- Basophilic, extracellular deposits located beneath the foveolar tips or deep in lamina propria
- May be rimmed by macrophages
- Slightly refractile
- Do not polarize

Immunohistochemical Findings
- Negative CMV immunostain
- Positive Von Kossa and Alizarin red stain (calcium stains)

Differential Diagnosis
- CMV gastritis

PATHOLOGIC FEATURES

ENDOSCOPIC FINDINGS

GMC appears as whitish plaques or nodules smaller than 5 mm.

MICROSCOPIC FINDINGS

The gastric biopsies show basophilic extracellular deposits in the superficial gastric aspect, usually beneath the foveolar tips, but the deposits can also appear in the deeper aspect of the mucosa (Fig. 3-36). These calcium deposits are 50 to 500 μm in size, slightly refractile, and do not polarize. Occasionally the deposits may be rimmed by histiocytes and giant cells (Fig. 3-37). Background stomach may show foveolar hyperplasia with mucin depletion and reactive epithelial changes.

ANCILLARY STUDIES

ULTRASTRUCTURAL FEATURES

X-ray microanalysis has shown the deposits to contain calcium, aluminum, phosphorus, and chlorine.

HISTOCHEMISTRY

Specimens are positive on Von Kossa and Alizarin red staining.

DIFFERENTIAL DIAGNOSIS

The basophilic deposits are tinctorially similar to CMV inclusions and can be mistaken for such. CMV inclusions are seen in epithelial or endothelial cells and contain characteristic nuclear and cytoplasmic inclusions (see Figs. 3-26 and 3-27). Mucosal calcinosis consists of large, extracellular, basophilic deposits. The characteristic location underneath the foveolar tips is also diagnostically useful. This distinction is important because pathologists are frequently asked to rule out CMV gastritis in transplant settings.

PROGNOSIS AND THERAPY

The significance of GMC in mucosal biopsies is not clear. However, it is important to report the findings, given their frequent association to underlying medical conditions, such as chronic renal failure, and with history of transplantation. Metastatic calcium deposits in the stomach may also be an indicator of generalized deposits in other organs such as the heart.

■ MÉNÉTRIER'S DISEASE

Described first by Ménétrier in 1888, Ménétrier's Disease (MD) is a rare acquired disorder involving the gastric body and is associated with gastric rugal hypertrophy,

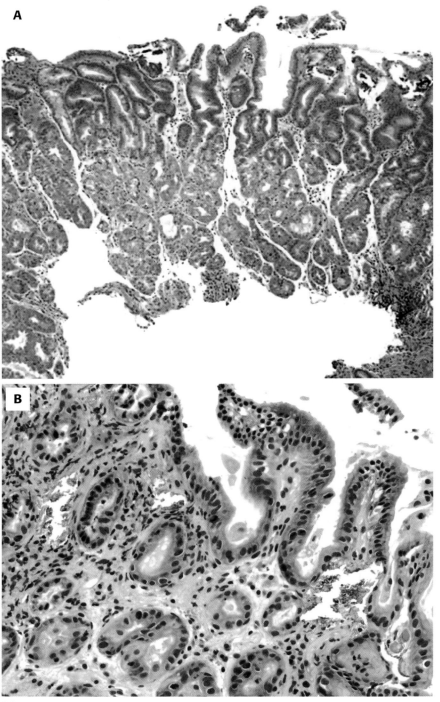

FIGURE 3-36

A, Gastric mucosal calcium deposits beneath the foveolar tips, appearing basophilic and refractile. **B,** Basophilic calcium deposits slightly deeper in the lamina propria.

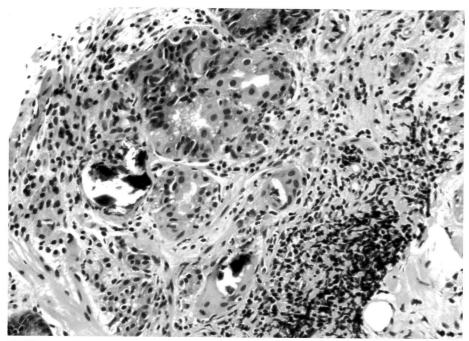

FIGURE 3-37
Mucosal calcium deposits associated with giant cell reaction and chronic gastritis.

protein-losing gastropathy, and hypochlorhydria. Synonymous are giant hypertrophic gastritis, hypoproteinemic hypertrophic gastropathy, and giant mucosal rugae.

CLINICAL FEATURES

MD is a rare disorder that has been described in adults and children (average age, fourth to sixth decades of life). It is more common in men than in women (ratio 3:1). The disease course is usually chronic, with an unfavorable prognosis. Patients present with hypoproteinemia resulting from nonselective protein loss across the gastric mucosal barrier and peripheral edema. Studies have shown loss of immunoglobulins, albumin, and transferrin. Other causes of protein loss caused by renal and liver disorders need to be ruled out. Patients may present with low or normal acid output. Symptoms appear insidiously and become progressive, consisting of epigastric pain, dyspepsia, anorexia, peripheral edema, hematemesis, and vomiting. The risk for developing carcinoma with MD is subject to debate. Approximately 15% of MD cases in the literature have been associated with carcinoma. In contrast to adults, children have a self-limited course and CMV infection has been frequently implicated. Overexpression of transforming growth factor-α (TGF-α) has a possible role in the pathogenesis of MD. Transgenic mice that overproduce TGF-α in the stomach have many features of MD, such as foveolar hyperplasia, increased mucin content, decreased parietal cell mass, and reduced acid production.

RADIOLOGIC FEATURES

A thickened gastric wall with marked enlargement of gastric mucosal folds is seen, along with a fine reticulated barium pattern resulting from mucus hypersecretion.

PATHOLOGIC FEATURES

GROSS AND ENDOSCOPIC FINDINGS

Gross findings consist of giant polypoid mucosal folds (1 to 3 cm in thickness) giving rise to an almost cerebriform, spongy appearance (Fig. 3-38). This mucosal hypertrophy is limited to the body, with relative sparing of the antrum. In children, the antrum is often involved.

This gross appearance is not limited to MD and can be seen in a number of other entities such as Zollinger-Ellison syndrome (ZES), gastric lymphoma, diffusely infiltrative signet ring carcinoma, *H. pylori* lymphocytic gastritis, CMV gastritis, granulomatous gastritis, eosinophilic gastritis, and gastric polyposis such as Cronkhite-Canada syndrome.

MICROSCOPIC FINDINGS

Microscopic features of MD consist of marked tortuosity and elongation of gastric foveolar epithelium lined by mucous cells and cystic dilatation of the deeper

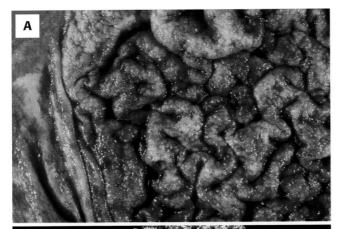

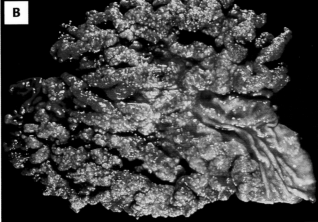

FIGURE 3-38

Ménétrier's disease. **A** and **B,** The giant mucosal hypertrophy of gastric body in Ménétrier's disease, with a cerebriform appearance in *A*. The antrum is spared. (**A,** *Courtesy of Shriram Jakate, MD, Rush Medical College, Chicago.*)

mucous glands (Fig. 3-39). Dilated mucous glands in the superficial submucosa may resemble gastritis cystica polyposa. The oxyntic glands are usually reduced and replaced by mucous glands. Inflammation can be variable and even absent. In a subset of cases, lymphocytic gastritis showing marked intraepithelial lymphocytosis may be seen. Intestinal metaplasia, ulcerations, and regenerative atypia are not features of MD.

Marked foveolar hyperplasia can be seen in chemical gastropathy, hyperplastic polyps, gastric ulcers, and at the postgastroenterostomy stomal site. Hence, the diagnosis of MD requires typical histologic findings in a full-thickness mucosal biopsy specimen in conjunction with the clinical presentation.

ANCILLARY STUDIES

IMMUNOHISTOCHEMISTRY

- Overexpression of TGF-α
- Immunostains for CMV and *H. pylori*

DIFFERENTIAL DIAGNOSIS

- ZES: Hyperplasia of parietal and chief cells with increased acid production as a result of increased gastrin secretion caused by gastrinomas. Associated with multiple gastric and duodenal ulcers. Not associated with protein loss or foveolar hyperplasia.
- Hyperplastic hypersecretory gastropathy: Hyperplasia of parietal and chief cells with normal or increased acid production, and without protein loss. Unlike ZES, gastrin level is normal.
- Hyperplastic polyps: Localized small (<2 cm) polyps. Unlike MD, inflammatory infiltrate and regenerative change is often prominent in hyperplastic polyps. More common in antrum. Uninvolved gastric mucosa usually shows chronic atrophy with intestinal metaplasia.
- Chronic *Helicobacter* or CMV gastritis may resemble MD. It is important to rule out these conditions because the management and outcomes are very different.
- Cronkhite-Canada syndrome: Diffuse GI polyposis with abnormal skin pigmentation and nail dystrophy.

PROGNOSIS AND THERAPY

In adults, the disease course is chronic with an unfavorable prognosis. Symptoms may improve with antibiotics, histamine H_2 blockers, anticholinergic agents that reduce gastric protein loss, corticosteroids, and octreotide (somatostatin analogue). One study reported marked improvement in symptoms such as vomiting and increased serum albumin following an experimental treatment with monoclonal antibody against epidermal growth factor receptor (EGFR). TGF-α is one of the ligands that binds to EGFR. Partial or total gastrectomy is reserved for refractory cases.

■ ZOLLINGER-ELLISON SYNDROME

First described in 1955, ZES is a triad consisting of hypergastrinemia caused by gastrin-secreting tumors (gastrinomas), increased acid production, and severe peptic ulcer disease.

CLINICAL FEATURES

ZES has an incidence of 0.1 to 3 per million population in the United States and comprises 0.1% of all duodenal ulcer patients. It affects adults and children (age

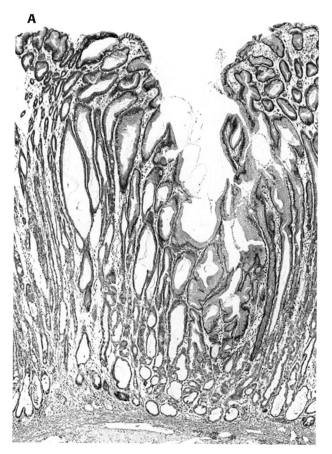

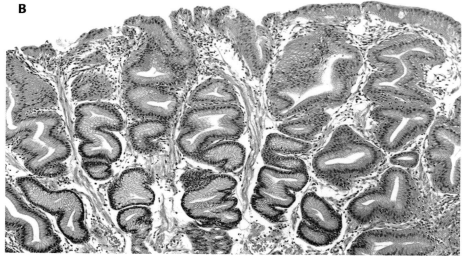

FIGURE 3-39

Low- and medium-power view of Ménétrier's disease. **A,** Shows marked tortuosity and elongation of gastric foveolar epithelium and cystic dilatation of the deeper mucous glands. **B,** The oxyntic glands are replaced by mucous glands.

range, 7 to 90 years; average age, 50 years). Males and females show an equal frequency. ZES is characterized by gastrinomas located usually in the duodenum, pancreas, or area adjacent to the common bile duct (gastrinoma triangle). Hypergastrinemia leads to persistent and massive secretion of acid and pepsin, giving rise to multiple and recurrent peptic ulcers, severe esophagitis, duodenojejunitis, epigastric pain, diarrhea, malabsorption, and weight loss. The massive acid output causes inactivation of pancreatic enzymes and bile salts, leading to symptoms including malabsorption and diarrhea. An elevated fasting serum gastrin level of greater than 1000 pg/mL is virtually diagnostic of ZES. Other clinical features include a positive secretin test result (secretin injection followed by elevation of gastrin greater than 200 pg/mL above basal level) and basal acid output greater than 10 mEq/hr. Gastrinomas are usually multifocal and are malignant in 50% to 60% of cases with lymph node and liver metastases.

Eighty percent of ZES patients have sporadic gastrinomas. In the remaining 20% of ZES patients, the gastrinomas are part of multiple endocrine neoplasia type I (MEN-I) syndrome. MEN-I is an autosomal dominant disorder resulting from mutations in the MEN-I gene on chromosome 11q13, which encodes for a 610–amino acid protein, menin. MEN-I is characterized by parathyroid hyperplasia, pancreatic endocrine tumors, pituitary adenomas, and adrenal adenomas.

RADIOLOGIC FEATURES

Imaging studies such as computed tomography (CT) and magnetic resonance imaging (MRI) demonstrate markedly thickened gastric folds. Imaging studies such as somatostatin receptor scintigraphy (gastrinomas have somatostatin type 2 receptors) and endoscopic ultrasonography have greater sensitivity in localizing gastrinomas. These along with abdominal CT and MRI are also used for staging.

PATHOLOGIC FEATURES

GROSS AND ENDOSCOPIC FINDINGS

ZES causes massive hypertrophy of gastric rugae in the body and fundus that can range from 0.6 to 4.5 cm in thickness (Fig. 3-40). The antral mucosa is often reduced in size.

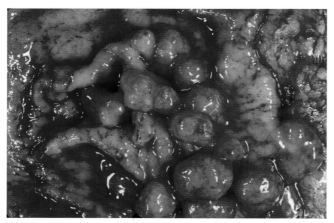

FIGURE 3-40

Zollinger-Ellison syndrome. Note the massive hypertrophy of gastric rugal folds with polypoid appearance. *(Courtesy of Shriram Jakate, MD, Rush Medical College, Chicago.)*

MICROSCOPIC FINDINGS

The trophic effect of gastrin causes increased thickness of oxyntic mucosa in ZES (Fig. 3-41). Parietal cells show hypertrophy and hyperplasia and extend up to the foveolar neck region (Fig. 3-42). Parietal cells often extend to the gastric antrum.

Gastrin also causes hyperplasia of ECL cells in the gastric fundus and body, leading to linear and nodular ECL hyperplasia. Carcinoid tumors of the oxyntic mucosa are present in 37% patients with MEN-I–associated ZES and none in patients with sporadic ZES.

ANCILLARY STUDIES

IMMUNOHISTOCHEMISTRY

- Gastrinomas stain for gastrin, chromogranin, and synaptophysin.
- ECL hyperplasia and gastric carcinoids stain for chromogranin and vesicular monoamine transporter, isoform 2 (VMAT-2), which regulates the intravesicular accumulation of histamine. The ECL cells are negative for gastrin, somatostatin, and serotonin.

DIFFERENTIAL DIAGNOSIS

- MD is associated with gastric rugal hypertrophy, protein-losing gastropathy, and hypochlorhydria. Acid secretion is reduced, and oxyntic cells are replaced by mucous cells in MD. MD is associated with giant foveolar hyperplasia and mucous glands in the gastric body, whereas ZES is associated with hypergastrinemia leading to hyperplasia of oxyntic mucosa and ECL cells in the gastric body.
- Chronic active *H. pylori* gastritis often results in antral G-cell hyperplasia, acid hypersecretion, and peptic ulcer disease. However, the presence of curved bacilli and superficial chronic active gastritis help distinguish it from ZES.
- Autoimmune metaplastic atrophic gastritis: This is an important cause of hypergastrinemia. However, unlike ZES, the gastric body shows atrophy rather than hypertrophy and hypochlorhydria or achlorhydria. Patients have antibodies to intrinsic factor and megaloblastic anemia caused by reduced vitamin B_{12}.

PROGNOSIS AND THERAPY

Patients with ZES require long-term medical therapy for adequate control of gastric hypersecretion with PPIs such as omeprazole or lansoprazole. Partial or total gastrectomy may be required for intractable cases. Patients with sporadic gastrinomas that are localized

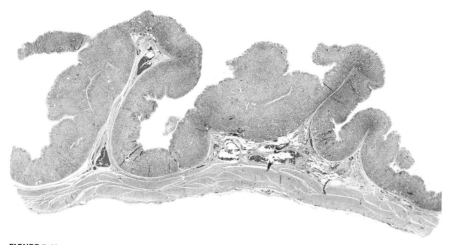

FIGURE 3-41

Low-power view shows the diffuse hyperplasia of gastric oxyntic mucosa in Zollinger-Ellison syndrome.

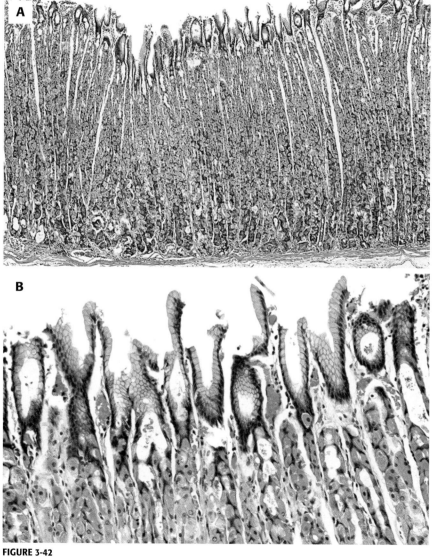

FIGURE 3-42

Zollinger-Ellison syndrome, medium-power view. **A** and **B,** Note the parietal cell hyperplasia and hypertrophy with parietal cells extending up to foveolar neck.

and without metastases are ideal candidates for surgical removal. Patients with hepatic or distant metastases are managed with chemotherapy, hormonal therapy, or surgical debulking. Achieving surgical cure in ZES patients with MEN-I is more difficult, and patients need to be on life-long acid suppressors. The need for family screening and screening for endocrine tumor elsewhere also is important.

ZES patients who have had successful tumor resection show a 60% to 100% survival rate at 10 years. Patients with unresectable tumors have a 40% survival rate at 5 years. MEN-I patients have better 5- and 10-year survival rates than do those with sporadic ZES (62% to 85% versus 40% to 70%).

■ GASTRIC HYPERPLASTIC POLYPS

Hyperplastic polyps of the stomach are common epithelial polyps of the stomach composed of dilated, elongated, and tortuous gastric foveolar epithelium and edematous lamina propria containing inflammatory cells. Gastric hyperplastic polyps are synonymous with inflammatory polyp, regenerative polyp, hyperplasiogenous polyp, and focal/polypoid foveolar hyperplasia.

CLINICAL FEATURES

In adults, gastric polyps have a prevalence rate of 3% to 6% at endoscopic examination. Hyperplastic polyps are common epithelial polyps making up 25% to 75% of stomach polyps. In one study in the United States, 77% of all gastric polyps were fundic gland polyps and 17% were hyperplastic polyps. The decreasing prevalence of hyperplastic polyps may be related to the increasing use of PPIs and declining rate of H. pylori infection. However, in studies from Brazil and Greece, hyperplastic polyps are still the most common gastric polyps. Hyperplastic polyps are antral predominant (60%), with the remaining involving the gastric body or fundus (30%) and the cardia. They are usually single but can be multiple in 20% of cases. A slight female predominance may be seen (male-to-female ratio 1:2.4), and adults in the sixth and seventh decades of life are commonly affected. Hyperplastic polyps were also the most common polyps in pediatric patients, accounting for 42% of gastric polyps in children. Hyperplastic polyposis is used to denote greater than 50 hyperplastic polyps in the stomach.

Clinical symptoms include bleeding, abdominal pain, anemia, nausea, vomiting, and weight loss. Large pedunculated polyps may produce gastric outlet obstruction. Smaller polyps are often incidental findings during surveillance.

Hyperplastic polyps may harbor foci of intestinal metaplasia (16%), dysplasia (4%), and rarely carcinoma (0.6%) within the polyp. According to Abraham and associates, gastric hyperplastic polyps are associated with abnormalities in the surrounding nonpolypoid mucosa in up to 85% of cases. These include intestinal metaplasia (37%), dysplasia (2%), synchronous or metachronous carcinoma (6%), H. pylori gastritis (25%), chemical gastropathy (21%), and autoimmune gastritis (12%). Other common associations include partial gastrectomies for ulcers, post-laser therapy for watermelon stomach (gastric antral vascular ectasia, or GAVE), and CMV gastritis. Gastric hyperplastic polyps have also been shown to be increased in transplant settings.

Given the frequent presence of background mucosal pathologies, hyperplastic polyps are most likely an exuberant regenerative response to mucosal injuries. Supporting this hypothesis are studies that have shown regression of hyperplastic polyps following H. pylori eradication. However, Carneiro and coworkers presented a family pedigree with hyperplastic polyposis and increased incidence of gastric carcinoma. Also, the presence of a point mutation in codon 12 of K-ras oncogene in all three concurrent hyperplastic polyps in a study conducted by Dijkhuizen and colleagues raises the possibility of clonal origin of these polyps.

PATHOLOGIC FEATURES

GROSS AND ENDOSCOPIC FINDINGS

Polyps can range in size from less than 1 cm to up to 12 cm, but most are less than 1 cm. They are mostly broad-based or sessile but can also be pedunculated. Very large polyps may be mistaken for a carcinoma. The polyps have a smooth, lobulated, and glistening surface, often containing areas of erosion, and they are soft (Fig. 3-43).

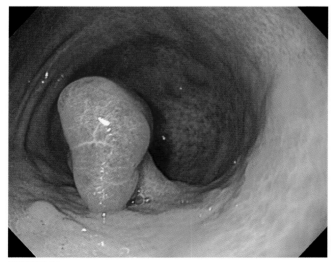

FIGURE 3-43

A single smooth and hyperemic gastric hyperplastic polyp with a stalk. *(Courtesy of Shriram Jakate, MD, Rush Medical College, Illinois.)*

GASTRIC HYPERPLASTIC POLYPS—FACT SHEET

Definition

- Common gastric epithelial polyps composed of dilated, elongated, branched, and tortuous foveolar epithelium and edematous stroma containing inflammatory cells

Incidence and Location

- Common gastric epithelial polyps make up 25% to 75% of stomach polyps
- Most are located in the antrum (60%), with the remaining found in the body or fundus (30%) and less often in the cardia

Morbidity and Mortality

- Majority are entirely benign
- Polyps harboring invasive carcinoma usually contain intramucosal carcinoma and have a good prognosis
- Large polyps may cause bleeding and gastric outlet obstruction

Gender, Race, and Age

- Slight female predominance (male-to-female ratio 1:2.4)
- Adults in their sixth to seventh decades of life are commonly affected

Clinical Features

- Patients can present with bleeding, iron deficiency anemia, abdominal pain, and dyspepsia
- Larger polyps can be mistaken for carcinoma and can present with gastric outlet obstruction
- Smaller polyps are often incidental findings during surveillance

Prognosis and Therapy

- Benign in most instances
- Small risk of harboring dysplasia or invasive carcinoma either within the polyp itself or in the nonpolypoid mucosa remains; thus all polyps should be completely submitted for histologic examination
- Treatment includes snare polypectomy, endoscopic mucosal resection, and treating associated conditions such as *Helicobacter* gastritis

GASTRIC HYPERPLASTIC POLYPS—PATHOLOGIC FEATURES

Gross Findings

- Polyps can range in size from a few millimeters up to 12 cm (average 1 cm)
- Polyps have a smooth, lobulated and glistening surface, often with areas of erosion
- Soft
- Usually sessile; can be pedunculated
- Multiple in 20% of cases

Microscopic Findings

- Dilated, elongated, branched, and tortuous foveolar epithelium, often with prominent globoid features
- Edematous and inflamed stroma
- Regenerative foci can look alarming with depleted mucin, hyperchromatic nuclei, and prominent nucleoli
- May contain foci of intestinal metaplasia, dysplasia, or invasive carcinoma. Larger polyps are more at risk of harboring such areas
- Often associated with mucosal pathologies in the nonpolypoid mucosa
- Biopsying the nonpolypoid mucosa is important so that treatment may be directed toward the underlying disease giving rise to these polyps

Differential Diagnosis

- Fundic gland polyps
- Peutz-Jehgers polyps
- Juvenile polyps
- MD
- Cronkhite-Canada syndrome
- Focal foveolar hyperplasia, polypoid foveolar hyperplasia
- Gastritis cystica glandularis

MICROSCOPIC FINDINGS

Histologically, the polyps are composed of hyperplastic, elongated, and tortuous gastric foveolae (Fig. 3-44). These glands frequently contain outpouchings and papillary infoldings. The foveolar cells often contain globoid features that can be mistaken for goblet cells or even signet cells (Fig. 3-45). Deeper mucous glands resemble pyloric type glands and contain gastric-type neutral mucin. The stroma is edematous, causing separation of glands and contains variable number of inflammatory cells such as lymphocytes, plasma cells, eosinophils, and even lymphoid aggregates. Larger polyps often contain wisps of smooth muscle bundles extending from muscularis mucosae into the lamina propria of the polyp. Areas with erosion may contain marked epithelial changes with depleted mucin, hyperchromatic nuclei, and prominent nucleoli. These regenerative areas should not be mistaken for dysplasia (Fig. 3-46). Unlike true dysplasia, surface maturation is present and the cells are reactive, appearing with prominent nucleoli, amphophilic cytoplasm (an indicator of active RNA synthesis), and usually associated with active inflammation containing neutrophils.

Hyperplastic polyps may contain foci of intestinal metaplasia (Fig. 3-47A), dysplasia (see Fig. 3-47B), or invasive carcinoma. Rarely the polyps may contain sneaky signet ring carcinoma. Dysplastic foci are characterized by lack of surface maturation, pseudostratified epithelium with enlarged hyperchromatic nuclei, and increased mitotic rate. High-grade dysplasia is characterized by loss of polarity, marked cytologic atypia, and architectural abnormalities such as cribriform glands (Fig. 3-47B).

ANCILLARY STUDIES

HISTOCHEMISTRY AND IMMUNOHISTOCHEMISTRY

- PAS/alcian blue or mucicarmine stains highlight acidic mucin in goblet cells and signet ring cell cancers. Also useful to demonstrate the neutral mucin in foveolar epithelium (which should stain pink as opposed to the blue of acidic mucin).

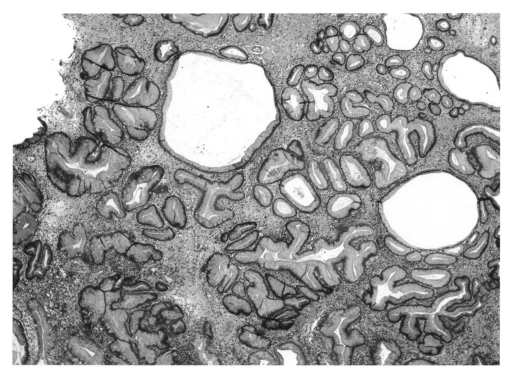

FIGURE 3-44

Dilated, tortuous gastric foveolar epithelium with frequent outpouchings and edematous stroma.

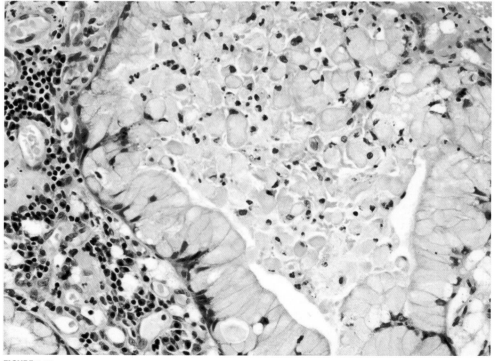

FIGURE 3-45

Globoid cells mimicking signet ring cells in a hyperplastic polyp.

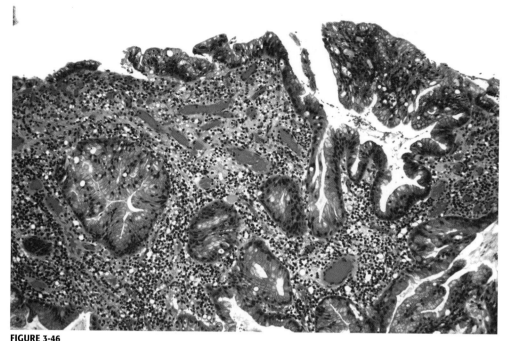

FIGURE 3-46
Regenerative focus. This is often present in gastric hyperplastic polyps and should not be mistaken for dysplasia.

- Stains for highlighting *H. pylori*.
- Immunostains for p53 and Ki-67: Increased and surface Ki-67 staining and overexpression of p53 staining may aid in confirming an H&E-based impression of dysplasia in difficult cases.

DIFFERENTIAL DIAGNOSIS

- Fundic gland polyps: These have a different histology, consisting of dilated cysts lined by chief and parietal cells, and lack significant inflammation. Unlike hyperplastic polyps, fundic gland polyps are associated with a normal mucosal background.
- Peutz-Jeghers polyps: More common in the small intestine, these polyps have a characteristic morphology with arborizing bundles of smooth muscle that cause mucosal splitting, along with clinical stigmata such as pigmentation around lips. However, gastric Peutz-Jeghers polyps may resemble hyperplastic polyps and frequently lack the arborizing muscle.
- Juvenile polyps: Common in children, juvenile polyps contain a smooth rounded surface that is frequently eroded with granulation tissue reaction. The stroma contains cystically dilated glands, often filled with neutrophils.
- Ménétrier's disease: Diffusely involves the gastric body and fundic mucosa with oxyntic glandular atrophy. Ménétrier's disease lacks significant inflammation, edema, and dramatic foveolar hyperplasia associated with protein-losing gastropathy.

- Cronkhite-Canada syndrome: Diffuse GI polyposis containing marked lamina propria edema. Clinical associations such as abnormal skin pigmentation and nail dystrophy are helpful in diagnosis. Gastric polyps in Cowden's disease may also resemble hyperplastic polyps. Correct diagnosis requires clinical and endoscopic correlation, and biopsy is often misleading.
- Focal foveolar hyperplasia, polypoid foveolar hyperplasia: Often seen adjacent to ulcers. As part of chemical gastropathy, these present as tiny sessile excrescences and consist of elongated superficial gastric foveolae.
- Gastritis cystica glandularis: Associated with post-Billroth gastrectomies and present near stomal sites with marked foveolar hyperplasia. Unlike hyperplastic polyps, these lesions contain prominent features of mucosal prolapse with cystically dilated glands often located in the submucosa and muscularis propria.

PROGNOSIS AND THERAPY

In most cases, hyperplastic polyps are benign lesions. A small risk of harboring dysplasia or invasive carcinoma either within the polyp itself or in the nonpolypoid mucosa remains. Polyps larger than 2 cm are at increased risk of harboring dysplasia or malignancy. Carcinoma arising in the polyp is mostly intramucosal and carries good prognosis. Thus complete removal by endoscopic snare polypectomy is recommended. In a series of 93 hyperplastic polyps in 56 patients

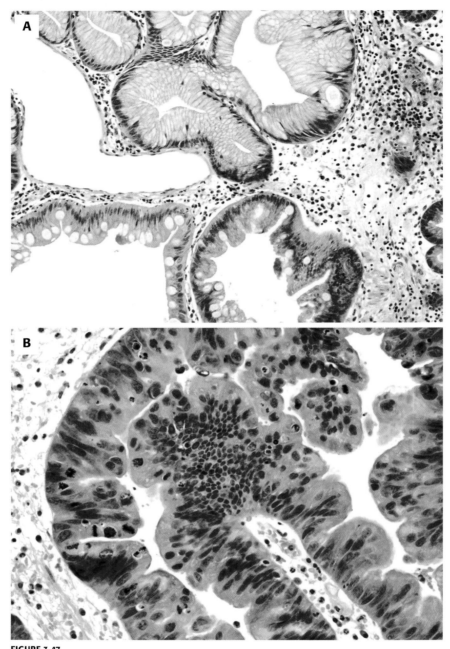

FIGURE 3-47

A, Intestinal metaplasia with goblet cells in a gastric hyperplastic polyp. **B,** High-grade dysplasia in a gastric hyperplastic polyp.

followed up by Kamiya and associates, two polyps became malignant 5 and 7 years after the first biopsy; 68% of polyps remained unchanged and 30% polyps were found to increase or decrease in size, or even completely disappear. Smaller polyps (a few millimeters in size) have been shown to regress or completely disappear following eradication of *H. pylori* infection. It is important to emphasize sampling the nonpolypoid mucosa for biopsy.

■ FUNDIC GLAND POLYPS

Fundic gland polyps (FGPs) are benign gastric epithelial polyps found in the gastric body and fundus, composed of oxyntic glandular hyperplasia and hypertrophy and dilated fundic cysts. FGPs are synonymous with fundic gland hyperplasia, cystic hamartomatous gastric polyp, cysts of glandular body, and Elster's glandular cysts.

CLINICAL FEATURES

FGPs are common gastric epithelial polyps making up 13% to 47% of gastric polyps. In the United States, these polyps have become the most common gastric polyps, comprising 77% of gastric polyps, the increased prevalence attributed to the decreasing *H. pylori* infection and widespread use of PPIs. FGPs occur in two different settings: sporadic and syndromic (familial adenomatous polyposis, or FAP). FGPs are present in 0.8% to 1.9% of non-FAP patients and are seen in 26% to 84% of FAP patients. FGPs are the most common cause of gastric polyposis, accounting for 70% of such cases, seen in not only syndromic FAP-related cases but also sporadic cases. Until 1977, patients with sporadic FGP polyposis underwent gastrectomy because the polyps were believed to be precancerous, until Elster and colleagues established their harmless nature. Most patients are 40 to 69 years of age, average 57 years. A female predominance is present, with a male-to-female ratio of 1:2 to 1:3. FGPs in syndromic settings occur in younger individuals in their 20s and 30s. They can be seen even in children and show an equal sex distribution. Patients are mostly asymptomatic or may present with mild abdominal pain, dyspepsia, or reflux. Unlike hyperplastic polyps, which almost never occur in normal stomachs, FGPs arise in normal gastric mucosa and are not associated with *H. pylori* infection or atrophy. There are conflicting reports about the association of long-term PPI therapy and FGPs, with some studies supporting and others refuting an association. Long-term PPI use has been associated with a fourfold risk of developing FGPs. Moreover, studies have shown complete regression of the FGPs upon cessation of the PPI therapy.

PATHOLOGIC FEATURES

GROSS AND ENDOSCOPIC FINDINGS

FGPs are present almost exclusively in the body or fundus and often are multiple occurring in clusters. In the syndromic setting, these polyps often carpet the gastric mucosa appearing in hundreds. They are soft, sessile, and hemispherical, with a smooth and translucent appearance (Fig. 3-48). FGPs are small ranging from 1 to 7 mm in size, with the smaller polyps appearing as mucosal "mammilations." Because of their small size, these polyps are often hidden by rugal folds and become visible when the stomach is fully distended. They are usually identical in color to the surrounding gastric mucosa. Unlike hyperplastic polyps, the surrounding gastric mucosa in FGPs is normal. During biopsy these polyps usually detach in toto.

FUNDIC GLAND POLYPS—FACT SHEET

Definition

- Fundic gland polyps are benign gastric epithelial polyps in the gastric body and fundus consisting of disordered proliferation of oxyntic mucosa and dilated fundic glands, often with glandular budding

Incidence and Location

- Prevalence ranges from 0.8% to 1.9% in non-FAP patients and 26% to 84% in FAP patients
- These polyps have become the commonest gastric polyps, comprising 77% of gastric polyps in the United States

Morbidity and Mortality

- Benign with no malignant potential

Gender, Race, and Age

- Patients are 40 to 69 years of age, average 57 years
- Female predominance with a male-to-female ratio of 1:2 to 1:3.
- FGPs in syndromic settings occur in younger individuals in their 20s and 30s and show an equal sex distribution
- FGPs in children are extremely rare and warrant a search for FAP

Clinical Features

- Most are asymptomatic

Prognosis and Therapy

- FGPs are entirely benign with no malignant potential
- The presence of multiple FGPs in a young patient may warrant additional studies to rule out FAP

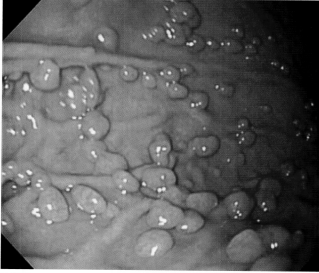

FIGURE 3-48

Fundic gland polyposis. Note the endoscopic appearance of multiple sessile fundic gland polyps in the body mucosa with a smooth and translucent appearance with identical color to the surrounding gastric mucosa. (*Courtesy of Shriram Jakate, MD, Rush Medical College, Chicago.*)

FUNDIC GLAND POLYPS—PATHOLOGIC FEATURES

Gross Findings

- Present exclusively in the body or fundus
- Often multiple occurring in clusters
- Soft, sessile, hemispherical, with a smooth and translucent appearance; small, ranging from 1 to 7 mm in size; usually identical in color to the surrounding gastric mucosa
- Normal surrounding nonpolypoid gastric mucosa

Microscopic Findings

- Disarrayed proliferation of oxyntic mucosa with cystically dilated fundic glands or microcysts lined by flattened oxyntic epithelium, mostly parietal cells and less often by chief cells and mucus neck cells
- Minimal or absent inflammation
- In syndromic (around 25%) and rarely even in sporadic settings, FGPs may contain low-grade dysplasia characterized by hyperchromasia, nuclear enlargement, pseudostratification, and loss of mucin of the surface epithelium

Molecular Features

- Sporadic FGPs: β-catenin mutations, 90%
- Syndromic FGPs: Somatic APC gene mutation, 50%

Differential Diagnosis

- Hyperplastic polyps
- Peutz-Jehgers polyps
- Juvenile polyps
- Gastritis cystica glandularis
- PPI effect
- Gastric adenomas

MICROSCOPIC FINDINGS

Histologically FGPs consist of proliferation of oxyntic mucosa with cystically dilated fundic glands or microcysts lined by attenuated parietal cells, chief cells, and mucus neck cells (Fig. 3-49). Glandular budding is commonly seen. The lamina propria lacks much inflammation and may contain mild edema. There may be slight hyperplasia of the surface foveolar epithelium with shallow to absent pits.

In syndromic (around 25%) and rarely even in sporadic settings (less than 1%), FGPs may contain low-grade surface epithelial dysplasia characterized by hyperchromasia, nuclear enlargement, pseudostratification, and loss of mucin (Fig. 3-50).

ANCILLARY STUDIES

MOLECULAR STUDIES

Studies have revealed molecular abnormalities in FGPs suggesting they are neoplastic rather than hamartomatous lesions, as was previously thought. FGPs associated with FAP and even sporadic FGPs with dysplasia

harbor somatic *APC* gene alterations in 50% of cases. Sporadic FGPs on the other hand show activating β-*catenin* mutations (up to 90%). *K-ras* gene mutations and microsatellite instability do not have much of a role in FGPs.

DIFFERENTIAL DIAGNOSIS

PPI THERAPY

Often biopsies of oxyntic mucosa from patients on PPI therapy show hypertrophic parietal cells with apical cytoplasmic protrusions and dilated glands (Fig. 3-51). The low-acid environment created by the H^+/K^+-ATPase inhibiting action of the PPIs causes gastrin stimulation, which in turn has a trophic effect on parietal cells, resulting in dilated intracytoplasmic canaliculi caused by the inspissated hydrogen ion. FGPs, on the other hand, show fundic cysts with flattened oxyntic lining.

HYPERPLASTIC POLYPS

Common epithelial polyps of the stomach are composed of dilated, elongated, and tortuous gastric foveolar epithelium, and edematous lamina propria containing inflammatory cells. These polyps are usually markers of associated mucosal pathology in the surrounding stomach.

PEUTZ-JEGHERS POLYPS

More common in the small intestine, these polyps have a characteristic morphology with arborizing bundles of smooth muscle that cause mucosal splitting, along with clinical stigmata such as pigmentation around lips.

JUVENILE POLYPS

Common in children, juvenile polyps contain a smooth rounded surface, which is frequently eroded with granulation tissue reaction. The stroma contains cystically dilated glands often filled with neutrophils.

GASTRITIS CYSTICA POLYPOSA/PROFUNDA

Occurs in gastroenterostomy stomal sites and consists of erosions, marked inflammation and marked foveolar hyperplasia. These lesions contain prominent features of mucosal prolapse with cystically dilated mucus glands located in the submucosa and muscularis propria.

CARCINOIDS

Carcinoid tumors are more of a gross differential diagnostic consideration than a microscopic one because they are small, often multiple and occur in the body/fundus region and also show a female predominance,

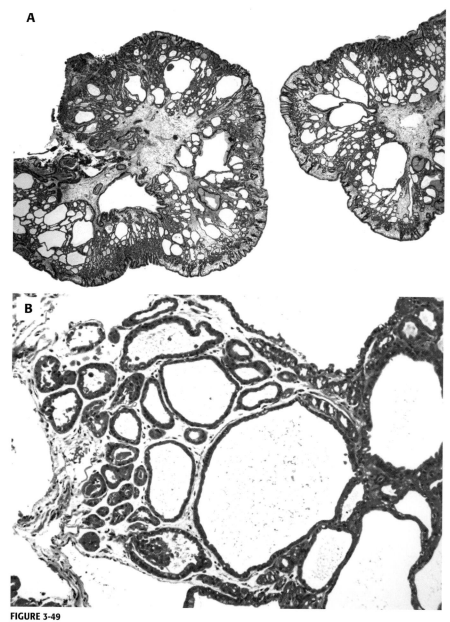

FIGURE 3-49

A and **B,** Fundic gland polyps with cystically dilated fundic glands lined by flattened parietal and chief cells.

similar to FGPs. However, grossly carcinoids are firm and yellowish and histologically show characteristic cords and nests of neuroendocrine cells. The surrounding gastric mucosa in FGPs is normal, whereas carcinoids occur in a background of autoimmune gastritis.

GASTRIC ADENOMAS

FGPs with low-grade dysplasia can be mistaken for an adenoma. The presence of microcysts lined by parietal and chief cells in FGPs will be useful in making the correct distinction. Gastric adenomas are more common in

the antrum, whereas FGPs are seen in the body and fundus. This distinction is important because FGPs with low-grade dysplasia carry virtually no risk of developing carcinoma, whereas adenomas carry a significant risk for malignancy.

PROGNOSIS AND THERAPY

FGPs are entirely benign with no malignant potential. Spontaneous regressions are known to occur. Finding multiple FGPs in a young patient may warrant additional

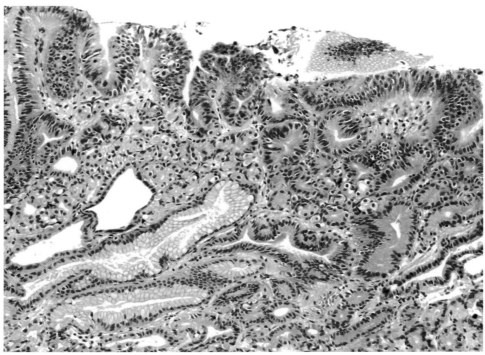

FIGURE 3-50
Low-grade surface epithelial dysplasia with hyperchromatic and pseudostratified nuclei in a sporadic fundic gland polyp.

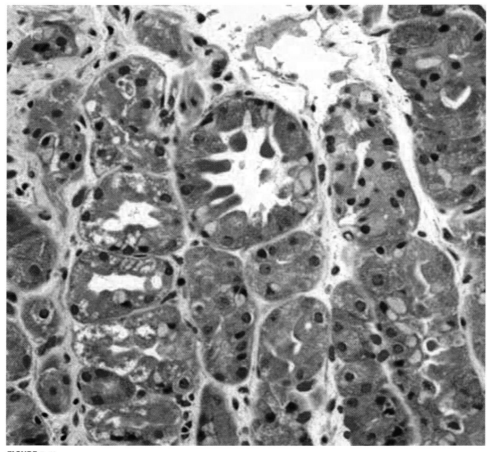

FIGURE 3-51
Biopsy of oxyntic mucosa from patient on PPI therapy. Such biopsies often show enlarged and hyperplastic parietal cells with snouts.

studies to rule out familial polyposis. Physicians may consider discontinuing PPI therapy in patients with large FGPs. Polyposis associated with sporadic FGPs has not been shown to cause adenocarcinoma. Even FGPs associated with surface epithelial dysplasia appear to behave in an indolent fashion with the need for surveillance very doubtful.

GASTRITIS CYSTICA POLYPOSA

Gastritis cystica polyposa is described as polypoid gastric lesions occurring near a gastroenterostomy stoma, characterized by dilated cystic glands in the mucosa and submucosa. Gastritis cystica polyposa is synonymous with gastritis cystica profunda, gastritis cystica superficialis, gastric cystic polyposis, stromal polypoid hypertrophic gastritis, and polypoid cystic gastritis.

CLINICAL FEATURES

Gastritis cystica polyposa is a rare lesion presenting near gastroenterostomy stomal sites several years after gastroenterostomies (Billroth I and II surgeries) for peptic ulcer disease. Gastritis cystica polyposa can develop 3 to 40 years following gastric operations. Patients are usually men in their 70s. Clinically patients are suspected of having stump carcinoma or an adenoma. Gastritis cystica polyposa shows histologic similarity to mucosal prolapse lesions elsewhere in the GI tract, such as solitary rectal ulcer, colitis cystica profunda, and colostomy and ileostomy sites. Anastomotic site changes including mechanical/ischemic injuries, mucosal prolapse, and bile reflux are thought to play a role in the pathogenesis. Unlike mucosal prolapse lesions in the colon, which are usually benign, gastritis cystica polyposa can be associated with dysplasia and gastric stump carcinoma.

RADIOLOGIC FEATURES

Multiple exophytic masses are seen around stomal sites in barium studies and CT scans, which can simulate malignancy.

PATHOLOGIC FEATURES

GROSS AND ENDOSCOPIC FINDINGS

Gastritis cystica polyposa presents as single or multiple, soft, sessile 1- to 3-cm polyps around gastric stomal sites. These polyps can present as confluent, circumferential masses around the stoma. The mucosa overlying the

---

GASTRITIS CYSTICA POLYPOSA—FACT SHEET

Definition
- Polypoid gastric lesions occurring near gastroenterostomy stomas, characterized by dilated cystic glands in the mucosa and submucosa

Gender, Race, and Age
- Men in their 70s

Radiologic Features
- Multiple exophytic masses around stomal sites in barium studies and CT scan

Prognosis and Treatment
- Benign condition
- Follow-up for cancer surveillance

GASTRITIS CYSTICA POLYPOSA—PATHOLOGIC FEATURES

Gross Findings
- Single or multiple, soft, sessile 1- to 3-cm polyps around gastric stomal sites
- Cut section shows thickened gastric wall containing numerous cystic glands

Microscopic Findings
- Foveolar hyperplasia, regenerative surface epithelial changes, cystically dilated pyloric-type glands in the mucosa, submucosa and even muscularis propria
- Lamina propria and submucosa displays scarring, fibrosis, and thickened and splayed muscle bundles
- Gastric remnant shows reduced oxyntic glands, edema, and chronic inflammation

Differential Diagnosis
- Invasive adenocarcinoma

---

polyp is usually smooth and resembles the surrounding gastric mucosa or may be red. Cut section shows thickened gastric wall containing numerous cystic glands.

MICROSCOPIC FINDINGS

Histologic features include foveolar hyperplasia, regenerative surface epithelial changes, and cystically dilated pyloric-type glands in the mucosa, submucosa, and even in the muscularis propria (Fig. 3-52). Depending on the location of the cystic glands, these lesions have been termed *gastritis cystica superficialis* or *gastritis cystica profunda*. Lamina propria and submucosa contain increased chronic inflammation, fibrosis, and scarring and often display thickened and splayed muscle bundles. The cystic glands are often in close

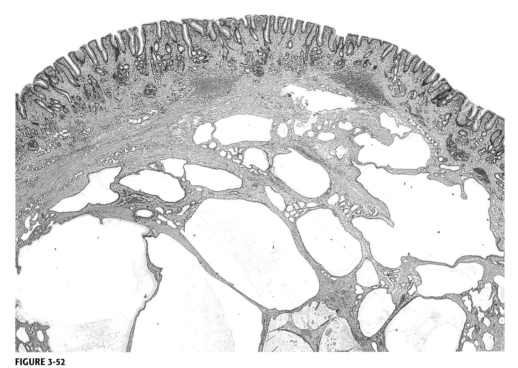

FIGURE 3-52

Gastritis cystica profunda showing cystically dilated glands extending into the submucosa. The overlying mucosa shows atrophic changes. *(Courtesy of Richard Lash, MD, Caris Diagnostics, Irving, Texas.)*

approximation with the smooth muscle bundles, a feature that can be mistaken for invasive adenocarcinoma. However, the glands lack atypia and desmoplastic reaction. Biopsy of the gastric remnant shows reduced oxyntic glands owing to the lack of gastrin caused by antrectomy, lamina propria edema, and chronic inflammation. There may be intestinal metaplasia and even dysplasia.

ANCILLARY STUDIES

IMMUNOHISTOCHEMISTRY

Stains for *H. pylori.*

DIFFERENTIAL DIAGNOSIS

Invasive adenocarcinoma: The presence of cystically dilated glands deep in the submucosa or even muscularis propria in gastritis cystica profunda can be mistaken for invasive adenocarcinoma. Unlike the malignant glands of adenocarcinoma, the cystic glands in gastritis cystica profunda lack pleomorphism and desmoplastic stroma and are often surrounded by lamina propria or smooth muscle bundles. This differentiation is especially important because patients with gastric stumps are at increased risk for developing gastric carcinomas.

PROGNOSIS AND THERAPY

Although benign, gastritis cystica polyposa can be associated with dysplasia and stump carcinoma. Thus regular follow-up is important.

■ PANCREATIC HETEROTOPIA

Pancreatic heterotopia is pancreatic tissue outside the normal pancreas with no vascular or anatomic continuity with the pancreas. It is synonymous with pancreatic rest and ectopic pancreas.

CLINICAL FEATURES

Pancreatic heterotopia is an uncommon lesion, the majority of which is seen in the stomach, duodenum, jejunum, and Meckel's diverticulum. Less common sites include lungs, gallbladder, mediastinum, mesentery, esophagus, bile ducts, and umbilical cord. Approximately 30% of pancreatic heterotopias occur in the stomach. In autopsy series, the incidence ranges from 0.5% to 13%. Stolte and coworkers diagnosed pancreatic heterotopia in 0.8% of more than 5000 gastric polyps. It can affect adult and pediatric patients, average age is 45 years, and a slight male predominance is seen (male-to-female ratio 1:0.7). Most

PANCREATIC HETEROTOPIA—FACT SHEET

Definition

- Heterotopic pancreas is pancreatic tissue outside the normal pancreas lacking any vascular or anatomic continuity with pancreas

Incidence and Location

- Gastric pancreatic heterotopias make up around 30% of all pancreatic heterotopias
- In autopsy series, the incidence ranges from 0.5% to 13%
- Stolte and colleagues diagnosed pancreatic heterotopia in 0.8% of more than 5000 gastric polyps

Morbidity and Mortality

- Benign non-neoplastic
- Large polyps in prepyloric region may cause gastric outlet obstruction
- Rare instances of developing pancreatitis, pancreatic cysts, islet cell tumor, or even ductal adenocarcinoma

Gender, Race, and Age

- Can affect adult and pediatric patients; average age is 45 years
- Slight male predominance (male-to-female ratio 1:0.7)

Clinical Features

- Most patients are asymptomatic
- Symptoms include abdominal pain, epigastric discomfort, nausea, vomiting, and bleeding
- Larger lesions may present with gastric outlet obstruction

Prognosis and Therapy

- Benign non-neoplastic lesions
- Superficial lesions are effectively treated with endoscopic resection
- Deeper lesions may require wedge resection using laporotomy or laparoscopy
- As pancreatic heterotopia often presents as a mass lesion, it is important for surgical pathologists to be aware of this entity during frozen sections.

PANCREATIC HETEROTOPIA—PATHOLOGIC FEATURES

Gross Findings

- 0.2 to 4 cm, usually solitary, hemispherical, well-demarcated intramural nodules mostly in the gastric antrum or prepyloric area
- Dome-shaped, smooth surfaced, intramural nodules with a central umbilication or erosion that represents the draining pancreatic duct
- Cut section shows well-circumscribed nodule based in the submucosa or muscularis propria with normal or ulcerated overlying mucosa
- Cut surface is tan-yellow and often lobulated, resembling normal pancreas

Microscopic Findings

- The heterotopic tissue contains admixture of pancreatic acinar tissue, ducts, and islet cells in varying proportion
- Because the lesion is often submucosal, superficial biopsies containing only the overlying mucosa may be nondiagnostic, thus necessitating deeper biopsies

Immunohistochemical Features

- Most cases are diagnosed based on the H&E stain
- Endocrine/islet cells—chromogranin A, somatostatin, insulin, glucagon
- Pancreas exocrine markers—trypsin, chymotrypsin, lipase, α-amylase, among others

Differential Diagnosis

- Invasive well-differentiated adenocarcinoma
- Gastritis cystica profunda
- Adenomyoma
- Pancreatic acinar metaplasia
- Paneth cell metaplasia
- Neuroendocrine tumor

---

patients are not symptomatic. When present, symptoms include abdominal pain, epigastric discomfort, nausea, vomiting, and bleeding. Large prepyloric lesions may present with gastric outlet obstruction. Rarely the heterotopic tissue may develop pancreatitis, pancreatic cysts, islet cell tumor, or even ductal adenocarcinoma. The heterotopic tissue is thought to originate during embryologic development from duodenal evaginations that persist in the intestinal wall.

PATHOLOGIC FEATURES

GROSS AND ENDOSCOPIC FINDINGS

Pancreatic heterotopias present as solitary (the large majority), 0.2- to 4-cm nodules in the gastric antrum or prepyloric area. Endoscopic appearance is characteristic consisting of a smooth surfaced, hemispherical, intramural nodule with a central dimple or erosion that represents the draining pancreatic duct (Fig. 3-53). On cut section, the lesion is well demarcated, located in the submucosa or muscularis propria with normal or ulcerated overlying mucosa. The cut surface is yellowish and lobulated, resembling normal pancreas.

MICROSCOPIC FINDINGS

The heterotopic tissue may contain an admixture of pancreatic acinar tissue (Fig. 3-54), ducts (Fig. 3-55), and islet cells in varying proportion and are divided into four Heinrich types: type I, total heterotopia (all cell types, most common variant); type II, canalicular heterotopia (ducts only); type III, exocrine heterotopia (acinar cells only), and type IV, endocrine heterotopia (islets only, rare).

Because the lesion is often submucosal, superficial biopsies containing only the overlying mucosa may be nondiagnostic. Thus deeper biopsies or endoscopic removal are important for a precise diagnosis.

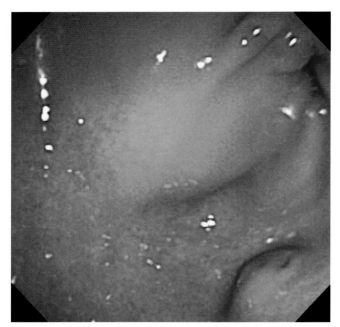

FIGURE 3-53

Pancreatic heterotopia, endoscopic view: Smooth surfaced submucosal nodule with a central dimple. *(Courtesy of Shriram Jakate, MD, Rush Medical College, Chicago.)*

ANCILLARY STUDIES

IMMUNOHISTOCHEMISTRY

Although not necessary for diagnosis, immunostains are useful to delineate the endocrine/islet cells—chromogranin A, somatostatin, insulin, glucagon; and pancreas exocrine markers—trypsin, chymotrypsin, lipase, and α-amylase.

DIFFERENTIAL DIAGNOSIS

The submucosal location of the lesion brings about a macroscopic differential of GI stromal tumors, lipomas, and leiomyomas, which is resolved on histologic examination.

INVASIVE WELL-DIFFERENTIATED ADENOCARCINOMA

This is an important differential considering that most pancreatic heterotopias arise in deep submucosa or muscularis and can be mistaken for adenocarcinoma, especially during frozen sections. The key to correctly recognizing pancreatic heterotopia is the lobulated arrangement of acinar and duct structure (like in normal pancreas), lack of malignant cytoarchitectural features, and lack of desmoplastic stromal response. In pancreatic heterotopia, the various elements are admixed with smooth muscle bundles.

ADENOMYOMA

Type III pancreatic heterotopia with only ductal elements can be difficult to distinguish from adenomyomas.

GASTRITIS CYSTICA PROFUNDA

Occurs in gastroenterostomy stomal sites and consists of erosions, marked inflammation, and marked foveolar hyperplasia. These lesions contain prominent features of mucosal prolapse with cystically dilated mucus glands located in the submucosa and muscularis propria. The finding in pancreatic heterotopias of acinar and islet tissue can be especially helpful.

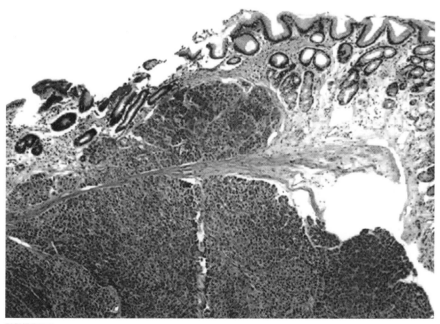

FIGURE 3-54

Medium-power view of pancreatic heterotopia. This well-circumscribed submucosal nodule consists of pancreatic acinar tissue.

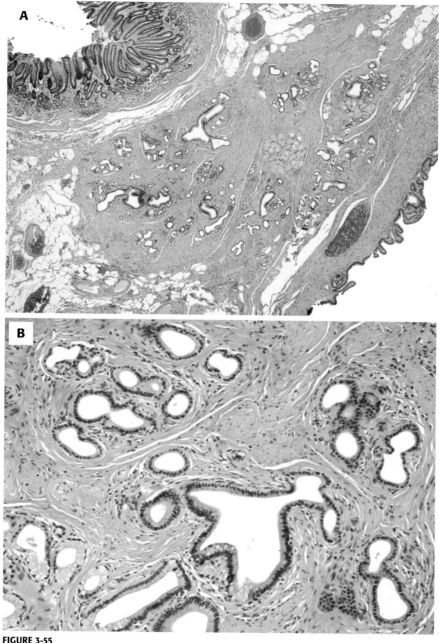

FIGURE 3-55

Heterotopic pancreatic tissue is composed of pancreatic ducts and rare acini interspersed among smooth muscle bundles.

PANCREATIC ACINAR METAPLASIA

This is a relatively common incidental finding in gastric biopsies, especially the cardia (Fig. 3-56). Unlike pancreatic heterotopia, which presents as a mass, pancreatic metaplasia consists of microscopic foci of pancreatic acini and is usually seen in association with inflammatory processes such as reflux esophagitis. Pancreatic metaplasia lacks ducts and islets, although some observers believe that the pancreatic foci found in the esophagus are also heterotopic.

PANETH CELL METAPLASIA

This is usually accompanied with intestinal metaplasia seen in chronic atrophic gastritis and autoimmune gastritis. Paneth cells have larger refractile red granules, whereas pancreatic acinar cells have finer basophilic granules at the base and reddish granules at the apex.

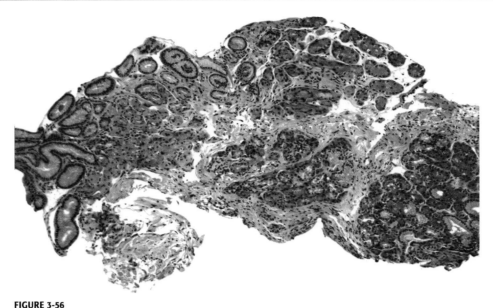

FIGURE 3-56
Biopsy samples of gastric cardia. Such samples often contain pancreatic acinar metaplasia/heterotopia.

NEUROENDOCRINE TUMOR

Pure endocrine heterotopia (the rarest among the pancreatic heterotopias) may present a diagnostic challenge with neuroendocrine tumors. Endocrine heterotopias present as small microscopic nests scattered in the submucosa and muscularis and are not associated with any stromal response. Neurondocrine tumors present as mass lesions with the tumor cells arranged as trabeculae, tubules, and rosettes.

PROGNOSIS AND THERAPY

Pancreatic heterotopias are benign non-neoplastic lesions. There have been reports of islet cell tumors or even ductal adenocarcinomas developing in the heterotopic tissue, but this is extremely rare. Symptomatic lesions are effectively treated by endoscopic resections if the lesion is superficial. Deeper lesions may require wedge resection using laporotomy or laparoscopy. Because pancreatic heterotopia often presents as a mass lesion, it is important for surgical pathologists to be aware of this entity during frozen sections.

■ GASTRIC XANTHOMAS (XANTHELASMAS)

Described first by Lubarsch and Borchardt in 1929, who called these lesions *lipid islands in gastric mucosa*, gastric xanthomas consist of loose collections of lipid-laden macrophages in the lamina propria. Synonyms include stomach lipidosis, xanthelasma, and gastric xanthomas.

CLINICAL FEATURES

The stomach is a common site of xanthomas. These lesions rarely occur in the esophagus, small intestine, and colon. Gastric xanthomas present as sessile, single, or multiple, 1- to 5-mm, yellowish white mucosal nodules or plaques. Although found anywhere in the stomach, it is more common in the antrum, especially the prepyloric area, lesser curvature, and adjacent to gastric stoma. Males are affected more than females, with a 3:1 male predominance. Adults in their 60s are commonly affected. Gastric xanthomas usually do not show any relation to skin xanthelasmas or hyperlipidemia but have been associated with cholestasis, and some studies have implied an underlying dyslipidemia. Endoscopic studies have shown an incidence ranging from 0.3% to 3.9%. Japanese series have found a higher frequency with one autopsy series reporting 58% incidence in 193 consecutive autopsies. Gastric xanthomas are seen in association with gastric ulcers, carcinomas, chemical gastropathy, postgastroenterostomies, chronic atrophic gastritis with intestinal metaplasia, and *H. pylori* gastritis (48% in one study). The frequent association with gastric pathologies point to a reparative response to various injuries. The increased frequency after Billroth gastrectomies and bile-reflux gastropathy supports the hypothesis of impaired mucosal transport of lipids following bile reflux.

PATHOLOGIC FEATURES

GROSS AND ENDOSCOPIC FINDINGS

Small, sessile, yellowish white nodules or plaques, usually multiple, and 1 to 5 mm in size (Figs. 3-57 and 3-58).

GASTRIC XANTHOMAS (XANTHELASMAS)—FACT SHEET

Definition

- Loose non-neoplastic collection of lipid-laden macrophages in gastric lamina propria

Incidence and Location

- Gastric antrum, prepyloric area, lesser curvature, and stoma
- Autopsy series show an incidence ranging from 1.9% to 58%
- Endoscopic series show 0.3% to 3.9% frequency

Morbidity and Mortality

- Benign and non-neoplastic lesions
- Associated with gastric ulcers, bile-reflux gastropathy, post-Billroth gastrectomies, and chronic gastritis, among others
- Although of little significance by itself, gastric xanthomas are a reflection of past or concurrent gastric pathology.

Gender, Age, and Race Distribution

- Male predominance, 3:1.
- Adults, average age sixth decade of life

Clinical Features

- Associated with symptoms of bile reflux such as dyspepsia, abdominal pain, nausea, vomiting
- Most cases are not associated with skin xanthomas or hyperlipidemia

Prognosis and Treatment

- Of no clinical significance by itself
- May regress without treatment
- Treat associated conditions such as bile reflux gastropathy or *Helicobacter* infection

GASTRIC XANTHOMAS (XANTHELASMAS)—PATHOLOGIC FEATURES

Gross Findings

- Small, sessile, single or multiple yellowish white nodules
- 1 to 5 mm in size

Microscopic Findings

- Lipid-laden macrophages in gastric lamina propria
- Macrophages contain foamy cytoplasm with centrally placed bland nuclei
- No increase in mitoses

Immunohistochemistry

- Positive for Sudan black, Oil Red O, CD68
- Negative for mucicarmine, PAS, cytokeratins, S-100

Differential Diagnosis

- Signet ring cell carcinoma
- Granular cell tumor
- Clear cell carcinoid
- MAI infection
- Whipple's disease
- Malacoplakia
- Lepromatous leprosy

MICROSCOPIC FINDINGS

Histologically gastric xanthomas consist of a loose cluster of lipid-laden macrophages in the lamina propria. The macrophages show abundant foamy cytoplasm containing cholesterol and neutral fats with central bland nondescript nuclei (Fig. 3-59). The surrounding gastric mucosa may show chemical/bile reflux gastropathy,

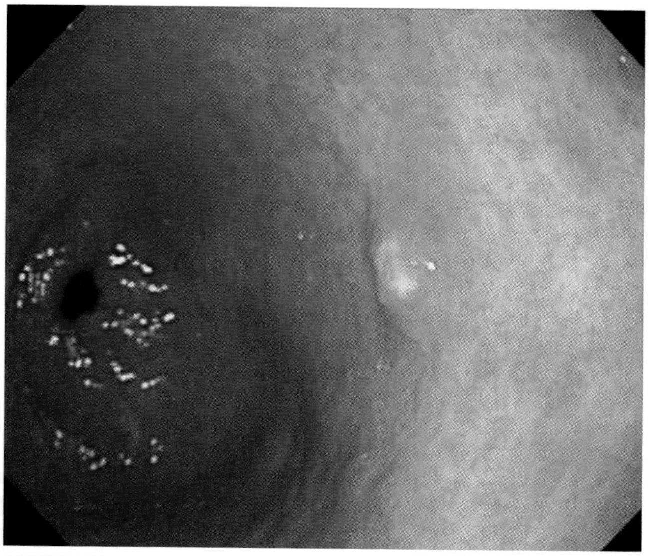

FIGURE 3-57

The typical endoscopic appearance of a gastric xanthoma. It usually consists of a small, sessile yellowish nodule or plaque. *(Courtesy of Shriram Jakate, MD, Rush Medical College, Chicago.)*

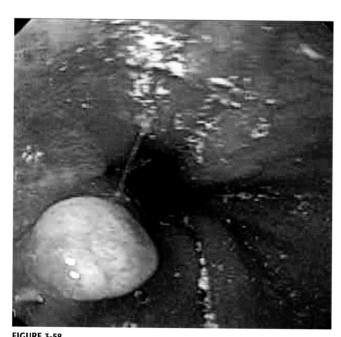

FIGURE 3-58

A case of gastric xanthoma presenting as a yellowish nodule.

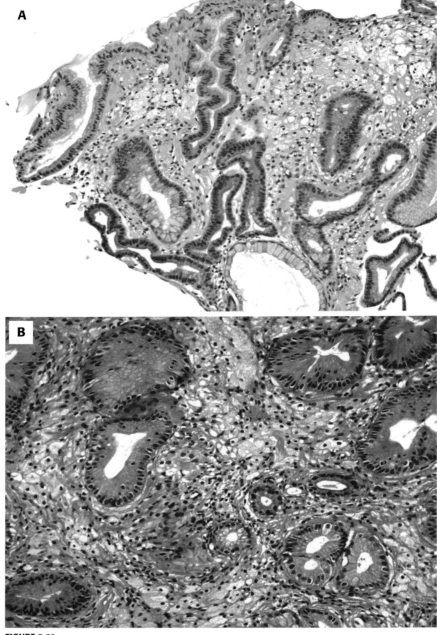

FIGURE 3-59

A, Gastric xanthoma in a patient who had undergone Billroth surgery and presented with bile reflux gastropathy.
B, High-power view. Note the foamy lipid-laden macrophages in the lamina propria with a central bland nuclei.

chronic gastritis with intestinal metaplasia, or *Helicobacter* gastritis.

ANCILLARY STUDIES

HISTOCHEMISTRY AND IMMUNOHISTOCHEMISTRY

POSITIVE STAINS

Sudan Black, Oil red O, CD68 (Fig. 3-60A).

NEGATIVE STAINS

PAS (see Fig. 3-60B), mucicarmine, cytokeratins, S-100.

DIFFERENTIAL DIAGNOSIS

- Signet ring cell carcinoma: This is an important differential diagnosis. Signet ring cells contain cytoplasmic mucin vacuoles, hyperchromatic eccentrically placed malignant nuclei, frequent mitoses, and

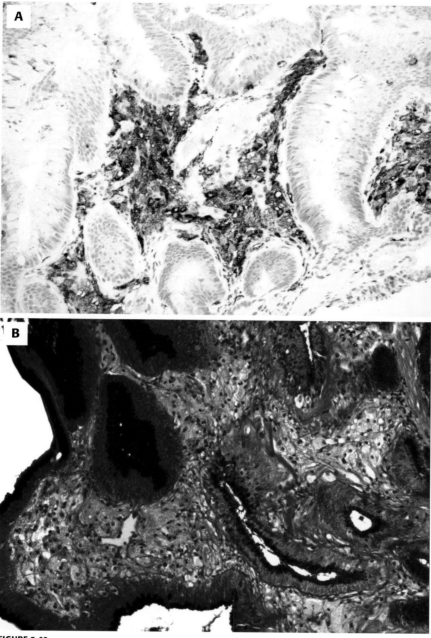

FIGURE 3-60
A, CD68 is strongly positive in the gastric xanthoma cells. **B,** PAS stain is negative in xanthoma cells owing to their lipid content.

positive staining with cytokeratins (CAM 5.2), mucin stains, and PAS.
- Granular cell tumor: Clusters of cells in the lamina propria and submucosa with abundant polygonal, eosinophilic granular cytoplasm, centrally placed nuclei, and positive staining with S-100 and CD68.

- Clear cell carcinoid tumor: Apart from being histologic mimics, these can grossly resemble xanthomas, appearing as yellow nodules. Immunonohistochemistry for chromogranin and synaptophysin are positive in carcinoids.
- MAI infection: Patients with AIDS. Positive for acid-fast bacilli stain.

- Malacoplakia: Xanthogranulomatous reaction to gram-negative bacterial infections such as *Escherichia coli.*
- Characteristic Michaelis-Guttman bodies that stain with calcium stains such as Von Kossa.
- Whipple's disease: Pertinent clinical history of multisystemic involvement. Microscopically the foamy macrophages are stuffed with bacillary forms of *Trophyrema whipplei* and show positive staining with PAS (intensely positive) and Whipple immunostain.
- Lepromatous leprosy: Acid-fast positive bacilli in foamy macrophages.

PROGNOSIS AND THERAPY

Benign non-neoplastic lesions that may regress with time. Treatment is directed at associated gastric pathologies.

■ GASTRIC AMYLOID

GI amyloidosis is an almost universal finding in systemic amyloidosis and consists of extracellular deposition of insoluble, fibrillary β-pleated protein sheets in the mucosa, submucosa, muscularis propria, or serosa.

CLINICAL FEATURES

The older classification of amyloidosis consisted of localized and generalized, or primary (AL) and secondary (AA). Localized amyloidosis generally does not involve the GI tract. However, systemic amyloidosis almost universally involves the gut. Other common sites of amyloid deposition include heart, kidney, liver, and spleen, with patients presenting with restrictive cardiomyopathy, nephrotic syndrome, hepatosplenomegaly, neuropathy depending upon the site and extent of amyloid deposition. The old classification has been replaced by the new classification, which is based on the precursor protein responsible for amyloid production (Table 3-6).

Except for the familial forms, amyloidosis is seen in older adults with an average age of 60s. GI manifestations consist of hemorrhage, prolonged nausea and vomiting, weight loss, malabsorption, gastric outlet obstruction, gastroparesis, and stasis-related change such as bacterial overgrowth and diarrhea. Amyloid deposits in the blood vessels make the vessels fragile and leaky, leading to hemorrhage. Muscle and nerve deposits cause motility problems. Mucosal deposits lead to malabsorption and diarrhea. Rarely gastric amyloidosis may present as a tumoral mass and can be mistaken for a carcinoma. Diagnosis is achieved through tissue biopsy of the GI tract. The rectum and stomach are preferred biopsy sites with a high yield.

TABLE 3-6
Classification of Gastric Amyloids

Classification	Precursor Protein, Disease Associations, and Clinical Feature
AA amyloidosis	Serum amyloid-A protein (SAA) and secondary amyloidosis Chronic illnesses (e.g., rheumatoid arthritis, tuberculosis, bronchiectasis, Crohn's disease, familial Mediterranean fever/ nephrotic syndrome, cardiomyopathy)
AL amyloid	Immunoglobulin light chains-κ or λ, primary amyloidosis Plasma cell neoplasm, lymphomas and cardiomyopathy, hepatosplenomegaly, macroglossia
ATTR amyloid	Transthyretin: Autosomal-dominant, cardiomyopathy, neuropathy Wild-type TTR causes senile amyloidosis with cardiomyopathy
β_2 Microglobulin amyloid	β_2 microglobulin, renal failure, and long-term hemodialysis and musculoskeletal issues
$\alpha\beta$ Amyloid	β-Precursor protein, Alzheimer's disease
AIAPP	Islet amyloid polypeptide, type 2 diabetes mellitus

Biopsy samples must be adequate and contain submucosal vessels in order to increase the diagnostic yield because superficial mucosal biopsies may completely and easily miss the deposits.

RADIOLOGIC FEATURES

Bowel walls are thickened and less pliable. Rarely amyloidosis can present as a mass lesion leading to gastric outlet obstruction. Scintigraphy with serum amyloid P component can demonstrate systemic amyloid deposits especially in solid organs such as the liver, kidney, and spleen.

PATHOLOGIC FEATURES

GROSS AND ENDOSCOPIC FINDINGS

Endoscopic appearance consists of mucosal erosions, ulcers, thickened folds, and tumoral mass (Fig. 3-61). Resection specimens with massive amyloid deposition have thick and rigid walls with waxy appearance.

MICROSCOPIC FINDINGS

The distribution of amyloid in the gut can be patchy or diffuse. Amyloid presents as a dense, homogenous, acellular, eosinophilic extracellular deposits in the

GASTRIC AMYLOID—FACT SHEET

Definition

- GI amyloidosis is an almost universal finding in systemic amyloidosis, consisting of extracellular deposition of insoluble, fibrillary β-pleated protein sheets

Morbidity and Mortality

- GI amyloidosis can cause fatal bleeding

Gender, Race, and Age

- Patients are usually older except in hereditary cases
- AL amyloidosis may affect young adults

Clinical Features

- GI hemorrhage, prolonged nausea and vomiting, weight loss, malabsorption
- Gastric outlet obstruction, gastroparesis, stasis-related change, diarrhea

Prognosis and Therapy

- Depends on the type and extent of deposits and on the vital organs involved
- AL amyloidosis has the worst prognosis with less than a year survival without treatment
- Microscopic deposits in older adults may be of little clinical significance
- Therapy is directed at reducing the supply of precursor proteins

GASTRIC AMYLOID—PATHOLOGIC FEATURES

Gross Findings

- Mucosal erosions, ulcers, thickened folds, tumoral mass
- Thick and rigid walls with waxy appearance

Microscopic Findings

- Dense, homogenous, acellular, eosinophilic extracellular deposits in the lamina propria, submucosa, muscularis propria, nerve trunks, and vascular wall
- Amyloid in the lamina propria can appear as globular deposits
- Tumoral deposits replace the normal gastric mucosa and submucosa

Ultrastructural Features

- Nonbranching fibrils 7.5 to 10 nm in diameter

Immunohistochemical Findings

- Congo red—characteristic apple-green birefringence on polarized light
- Thioflavin T—fluorescent dye
- Immunostains—CD138, κ, λ, antibodies directed against the different precursor proteins

Differential Diagnosis

- Vascular arteriosclerosis
- Systemic sclerosis
- Ischemic gastritis and other causes of lamina propria fibrosis

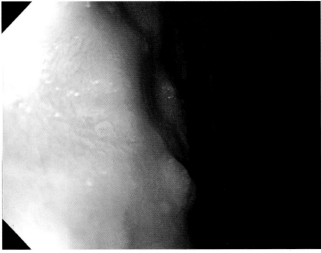

FIGURE 3-61
Endoscopic appearance of gastric amyloidosis appearing as thickened, vaguely nodular mucosa. *(Courtesy of Shriram Jakate, MD, Rush Medical College, Chicago.)*

lamina propria, submucosa, muscularis propria, nerve trunks, and vascular wall (Fig. 3-62). Amyloid deposits often show cracking with slitlike spaces as a result of tissue processing artifact. Amyloid in the lamina propria can appear as globular deposits (see Fig. 3-62B). AA amyloid deposits are usually present in

the lamina propria. Massive amyloid accumulation in the muscularis propria and submucosa is usually associated with AL amyloidosis.

ANCILLARY STUDIES

ULTRASTRUCTURAL FEATURES

Electron microscopy reveals non-branching fibrils 7.5 to 10 nm in diameters. The fibrils are composed of β-pleated sheets of amyloid proteins.

HISTOCHEMISTRY AND IMMUNOHISTOCHEMISTRY

- Congo red stain: This cotton dye remains the stain of choice for diagnosing amyloid. On normal light the amyloid is stained brick red (Fig. 3-63A) and with polarized light, amyloid shows the characteristic apple-green birefringence (see Fig. 3-63B).
- AL amyloid is resistant to potassium permanganate pretreatment, and AA amyloid is sensitive to potassium permanganate treatment before Congo red staining.
- Sirius red and Sirius supra scarlet: Also cotton dyes that stain amyloid red.
- Thioflavin T: Fluorescent dye.

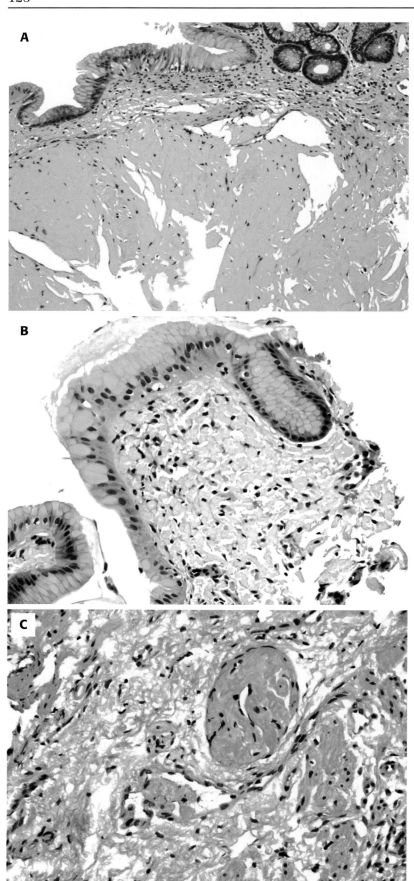

FIGURE 3-62

A, Gastric amyloid, consisting of eosinophilic, acellular deposits with cracking artifact appearing as a tumoral mass. **B,** Notice the globular amyloid deposits beneath the foveolar epithelium. **C,** Vascular amyloid deposits.

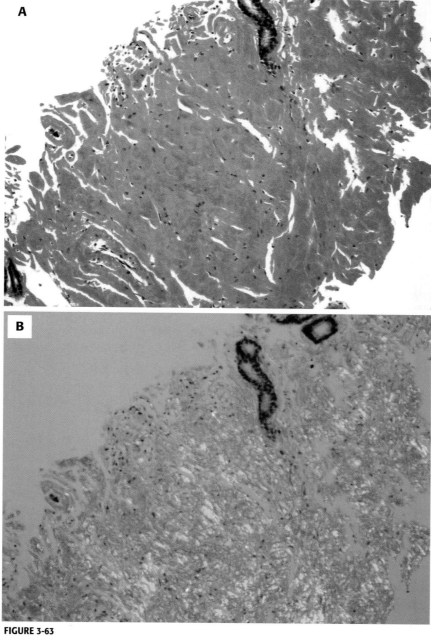

FIGURE 3-63

Same area as in Figure 3-62A stained with Congo red. The amyloid appears brick red using standard illumination light **(A)** and, with polarization **(B),** showing bright-green birefringence.

- Immunostains: κ, λ, plasma cell marker such as CD138, antibodies directed against the various precursor proteins such as AA, transthyretin, and β_2 microglobulin.

DIFFERENTIAL DIAGNOSIS

- Arteriosclerosis of vessels with hyalinization may be mistaken for amyloid deposits. Masson's trichrome will stain the sclerosis blue and Congo red stain will be negative.

- Systemic sclerosis: Connective tissue disorder such as scleroderma resulting in fibrosis of muscularis and submucosa, which may be mistaken for amyloid. Masson's trichrome will stain the collagen blue and Congo red will be negative.

- Ischemic gastritis and other causes of lamina propria fibrosis: Amyloid deposits in the lamina propria appear as eosinophilic, dense globular extracellular deposits. Vascular amyloid deposits are nearly always present. Ischemic injury will be associated with mucosal erosions, exudate, and micocrypts.

PROGNOSIS AND THERAPY

Prognosis depends upon the type, extent, and severity of amyloid deposit, organs involved, presence of cardiomyopathy, and severity of the underlying disease. Microscopic focal deposits in older adults may be of no clinical significance, but widespread deposition can be a progressive and even fatal disease. AL amyloidosis with cardiac involvement has the worst prognosis with untreated patients surviving less than a year. AA amyloid patients survive 2 to 4 years, and ATTR amyloid patients may survive 15 years. Therapy is mostly directed at reducing the supply of precursor proteins, correcting bleeding problems, and enhancing motility. Liver transplantation is curative in hereditary ATTR amyloidosis because the mutated TTR is produced by the liver.

■ INFLAMMATORY FIBROID POLYP

First described by Vaněk in 1949, inflammatory fibroid polyps (IFPs), named by Helwig and Ranier in 1952, are benign submucosal polyps composed of bland spindle cells admixed with blood vessels and inflammatory cells rich in eosinophils. Synonyms include Vaněk polyp, gastric submucosal granuloma with eosinophilic infiltration, eosinophilic granuloma, fibroma, and eosinophilic pseudotumor.

CLINICAL FEATURES

IFPs can arise anywhere in the GI tract, although the stomach is the most frequent site (70%). Other sites in decreasing order of frequency are the ileum, colon, jejunum, duodenum, and esophagus. In the stomach, IFPs make up approximately 3% to 4% of all gastric polyps. It is mostly seen in adults, the mean age being 64 years (range, 7 to 92 years). Females show a slight predominance (male-to-female ratio 1:1.2). Most are located in the antrum (67.3%), followed by the body (8.2%), pylorus (2.4%), incisura (1.7%), and cardia and fundus (1%). Clinical presentation depends on the size and can vary from incidental findings at endoscopy, to obstructive symptoms, bleeding, abdominal pain, nausea, vomiting, and weight loss. Multiple and recurrent IFPs have been described in three generations of a family in Devon, England (Devon polyposis syndrome). Earlier studies suggested a reparative response to an injurious agent such as microbial agent or a physical or chemical irritant. However, IFPs have been shown to harbor activating *PDGFRA* (platelet-derived growth receptor alpha) mutations in exons 12 and 18, thus raising the possibility of IFPs being neoplastic rather than reactive as was previously thought.

INFLAMMATORY FIBROID POLYP—FACT SHEET

Definition
- Benign submucosal based polypoid lesion comprising proliferating spindle cells with edematous stroma containing blood vessels and inflammatory cells

Incidence and Location
- 3% to 4% of stomach polyps
- Mostly in the antrum

Morbidity and Mortality
- Benign non-neoplastic lesion
- Large polyps may cause gastric outlet obstruction and bleeding resulting from surface ulceration

Gender, Race, and Age
- Slight female predominance
- Affects adults
- Average age, 60s

Clinical Features
- Most cases are incidentally found on upper endoscopy
- Larger lesions may cause obstructive symptoms such as abdominal pain, nausea, and vomiting

Prognosis and Therapy
- Benign, cured by local excision

PATHOLOGIC FEATURES

GROSS AND ENDOSCOPIC FINDINGS

Sessile or polypoid, mostly submucosal-based masses, IFPs range in size from less than 1 cm to 12 cm; average size is 1.5 cm. Most lesions are single and rarely multiple. They are well demarcated but unencapsulated with a gray-tan firm surface. The overlying gastric mucosa is smooth or ulcerated (Fig. 3-64).

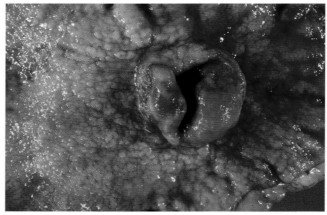

FIGURE 3-64

Inflammatory fibroid polyp. Gastric resection specimen showing a broad-based submucosal polypoid mass with central ulceration. *(Courtesy of Shriram Jakate, MD, Rush Medical College, Chicago.)*

INFLAMMATORY FIBROID POLYP—PATHOLOGIC FEATURES

Gross Findings

- Sessile or polypoid submucosal mass
- Tan gray, firm, with smooth or ulcerated mucosal surface

Microscopic Findings

- Submucosally based lesion consisting of a myxoid stroma with bland spindle stromal cells concentrically arranged around blood vessels, prominent small and large blood vessels and inflammatory cells, especially eosinophils
- Atypical mitoses and necrosis are absent
- Frequently extends to the overlying mucosa causing reactive change in the glandular epithelium
- Rarely, may contain adenoma or carcinoma of the overlying gastric epithelium

Ultrastructural Features

- Myofibroblastic

Immunohistochemical Features

- CD34 and Vimentin positive
- May also show positive staining for α-smooth muscle actin, muscle-specific actin, and CD68
- Negative for cytokeratins, EMA, CD117, and S-100

Differential Diagnosis

- GI stromal tumors
- Schwannoma, leiomyoma, solitary fibrous tumor, perineurioma
- Eosinophilic disorders: parasitic infestation, EG

MICROSCOPIC FINDINGS

IFPs are usually submucosal based, often splaying the muscularis mucosae, and expanding the base of the mucosa. Muscularis propria and subserosa are not involved, unlike for GI stromal tumors (GISTs). IFPs consist of a proliferation of spindle or stellate stromal cells in an edematous or myxoid stroma containing prominent vasculature and inflammatory cells consisting of eosinophils, lymphocytes, plasma cells, and mast cells (Fig. 3-65). Eosinophils are usually striking. Slightly older lesions may be less myxoid with a more collagenous appearance. Nodular lymphoid aggregates are often present. The stromal cells have oval or spindle nuclei with finely granular chromatin, small nucleoli, and eosinophilic cytoplasm. The stromal cells are arranged in a perivascular or periglandular pattern with a whorl-like "onion skin" appearance (Fig. 3-66A). Multinucleated giant cells, with floret-like arrangement can be frequently encountered (Fig. 3-66B). Mitotic figures are scarce with no atypical mitotic figures. The vascular network consists of prominent capillaries, and medium to large vessels with hyalinized walls. Rarely, polyps may be accompanied by adenoma or carcinoma of the overlying mucosa.

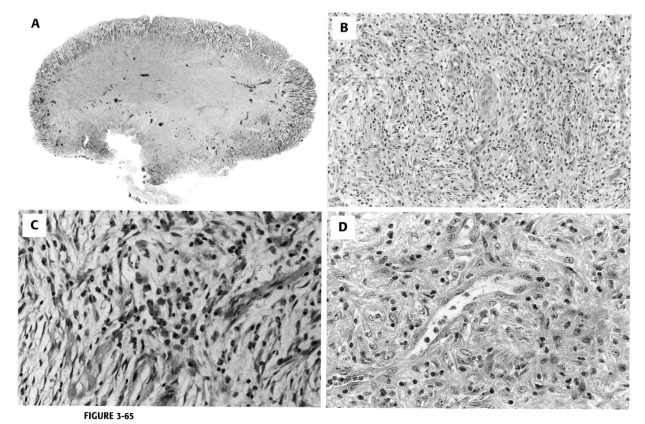

FIGURE 3-65

A, Low-power view showing the typical submucosal location of an inflammatory fibroid polyp. **B,** The lesion consists of spindle cells in a myxoid stroma containing prominent vasculature and inflammatory cells, especially eosinophils. Note the onion skin–like arrangement of stromal cells around vasculature. **C** and **D,** High-power view showing eosinophils in a myxoid stroma.

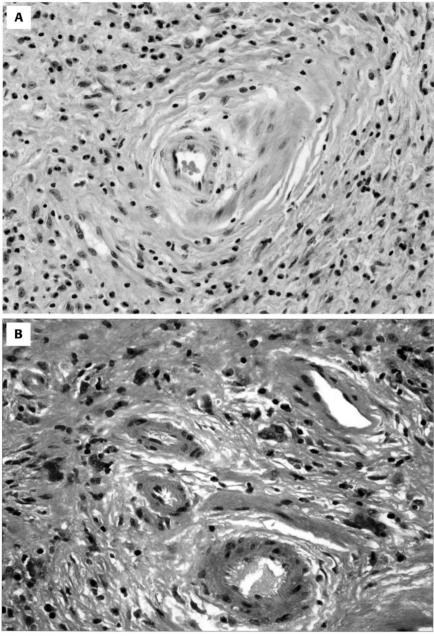

FIGURE 3-66

A, Stromal edema, eosinophils, and characteristic perivascular "onion skin" arrangement of the spindle cells in an inflammatory fibroid polyp (IFP). **B,** Note the giant cells scattered in the stroma of an IFP.

ANCILLARY STUDIES

ULTRASTRUCTURAL FEATURES

Myofibroblastic differentiation with abundant rough endoplasmic reticulum, bundles of cytoplasmic filaments focally associated with dense bodies.

IMMUNOHISTOCHEMISTRY

See Table 3-7.

DIFFERENTIAL DIAGNOSIS

Benign mesenchymal tumors such as schwannoma, leiomyoma, solitary fibrous tumor, and perineurioma can be distinguished by lack of eosinophils, typical

TABLE 3-7
Pattern of Immunostaining in IFPs

Positive Stains	Negative Stains
Vimentin	CD117 or CKIT
CD34	S-100
α-Smooth muscle actin (26%)	Cytokeratins
Muscle-specific actin or HHF-35 (20%)	Desmin
Calponin	Factor VIII
CD68 (KP-1—37%)	EMA
Cyclin D1	Type IV collagen
Fascin	Bcl-2
	Anaplastic lymphoma kinase
	HMB-45
	EBER, HHV-8
	DOG1
	Ki-67

morphology, and positive immunostains for S-100 (schwannoma), desmin (leiomyoma), Bcl-2 (solitary fibrous tumor), and EMA, Glut-1, and claudin-1 (perineurioma), respectively.

GASTROINTESTINAL STROMAL TUMORS

The discovery that IFPs commonly harbor *PDGFRA* mutations may suggest that GISTs and IFPs may be more closely linked then was previously thought. *PDGFRA* mutations have been found in GISTs lacking *KIT* mutations. IFPs are also strongly positive for CD34, which is also the case in most GISTs. However distinguishing IFPs from GISTs is important because unlike GISTs, IFPs behave in a benign fashion and do not recur or metastasize. The loose edematous stroma rich in inflammatory cells (especially eosinophils), concentrically arranged stromal cells around blood vessels, and negative CD117 immunostain are all helpful in differentiating IFPs from GISTs. IFPs can contain occasional mitoses but no atypical mitoses.

EOSINOPHILIC GASTROENTERITIS

Eosinophilic gastroenteritis does not present as a single mass. Histologic findings include patchy eosinophilic infiltrate of mucosa, submucosa, muscularis propria, or serosa. History of peripheral eosinophila, asthma, and younger age at presentation are also distinguishing clinical features.

PARASITIC INFECTION

Schistosomiasis, anisakiasis, or strongyloides can cause intense granulomatous reaction with eosinophils and may be mistaken for an IFP. Findings such as schistosome egg or strongyloides larvae will rule out an IFP.

PROGNOSIS AND THERAPY

IFPs are benign lesions cured by local excision.

■ GASTRIC ANTRAL VASCULAR ECTASIA (WATERMELON STOMACH)

Gastric antral vascular ectasia (GAVE) is an uncommon but important cause of acute and chronic, occult GI bleeding, typically in older females, and is characterized endoscopically by linear vascular stripes in the gastric antrum.

CLINICAL FEATURES

GAVE is an uncommon condition that is increasingly recognized as an important cause of acute or chronic unexplained GI blood loss giving rise to iron deficiency anemia. The anemia can be severe and refractory to iron replacement therapy, often requiring blood transfusion. GAVE primarily affects women (76%), with a mean age of 69 years (range, 42 to 89 years). Clinical presentations include iron deficiency anemia (88%), heme-positive stool (42%), melena (15%), and rarely hematemesis (3%) and hematochezia (1%). GAVE is commonly associated with autoimmune and connective tissue disorders such as Raynaud's phenomenon, sclerodactyly, autoimmune gastritis, hypothyroidism, primary biliary cirrhosis, autoimmune liver disease, and diabetes mellitus. Other associations include cirrhosis (important to differentiate from portal hypertensive gastropathy [PHG]), chronic renal failure, and cardiovascular disease. The pathogenesis of GAVE is unknown. It has been proposed that traumatic gastric peristalsis and subsequent prolapse of antral mucosa through the pylorus may cause vascular elongation and ectasia. Humoral factors such as hypergastrinemia, proliferation of neuroendocrine cells secreting vasoactive intestinal polypeptide (VIP), and 5-hydroxy tryptamine (serotonin) have also been implicated.

PATHOLOGIC FEATURES

GROSS AND ENDOSCOPIC FINDINGS

In 1984, Jabbari and colleagues coined the phrase "watermelon stomach" to describe the characteristic endoscopic appearance of GAVE consisting of parallel, intensely red vascular stripes situated at the crests of mucosal folds traversing the gastric antrum and converging on the pylorus (Fig. 3-67). A surgical resection specimen shows a thickened antral wall with prominent submucosal vessels running in a longitudinal direction toward the pylorus.

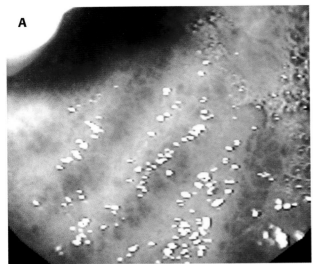

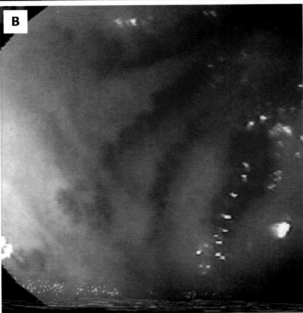

FIGURE 3-67

Characteristic endoscopic appearance of gastric antral vascular ectasia. Note the parallel, intensely red vascular stripes resembling watermelon, in two separate patients (**A** and **B**). (A, *Courtesy of Shriram Jakate, MD, Rush Medical College, Chicago, Illinois.*)

MICROSCOPIC FINDINGS

The characteristic histologic appearance consists of foveolar hyperplasia, dilated mucosal capillaries with fibrin thrombi, and fibromuscular hyperplasia of lamina propria with minimal or absent inflammation. The presence of fibrin thrombi is important for diagnosis (Fig. 3-68). The submucosal vessels are also dilated and tortuous. The gastric body may show atrophic gastritis with intestinal metaplasia.

DIFFERENTIAL DIAGNOSIS

See Table 3-8.

GASTRIC ANTRAL VASCULAR ECTASIA (WATERMELON STOMACH)—FACT SHEET

Definition

- GAVE is an uncommon but important cause of acute or chronic unexplained bleeding, characterized endoscopically by linear vascular stripes in the gastric antrum

Morbidity and Mortality

- Related mainly to GI blood loss
- May give rise to severe anemia refractory to iron replacement therapy, requiring blood transfusions

Gender, Race, and Age

- Female predominance (76% are women)
- Mean age 69 years (range, 42 to 89 years)

Clinical Features

- Iron deficiency anemia (88%), heme-positive stool (42%), melena (15%), and rarely hematemesis (3%) and hematochezia (1%)
- Commonly associated with autoimmune and connective tissue disorders such as Raynaud's phenomenon, sclerodactyly, autoimmune gastritis, hypothyroidism, primary biliary cirrhosis, autoimmune liver disease, and diabetes mellitus
- Other associations include cirrhosis, chronic renal failure, post bone marrow transplantation, and cardiovascular disease

Prognosis and Therapy

- Treatment is dictated by the rate of blood loss
- Conservative management includes iron supplement or blood transfusion, which may be insufficient
- Various endoscopic treatment modalities include laser, heater probe therapy, bipolar electrocautery, and injection sclerotherapy
- Surgical antrectomy offers definitive therapy but carries a mortality rate of 7.4%

GASTRIC ANTRAL VASCULAR ECTASIA (WATERMELON STOMACH)—PATHOLOGIC FEATURES

Gross Findings

- Located in the antrum
- Characteristic endoscopic appearance consisting of intensely red, linear, vascular stripes situated at the crests of mucosal folds traversing the gastric antrum and converging on the pylorus
- Appearance resembles the stripes of watermelon
- Resection specimen shows thickened antral wall with dilated and tortuous submucosal vessels

Microscopic Findings

- Dilated mucosal capillaries with fibrin thrombi, fibromuscular hyperplasia of lamina propria with minimal or absent inflammation
- Fibrin thrombi are a characteristic feature
- The submucosal vessels are also dilated and tortuous
- Stomach body may show atrophic gastritis with intestinal metaplasia

Differential Diagnosis

- Portal hypertensive gastropathy

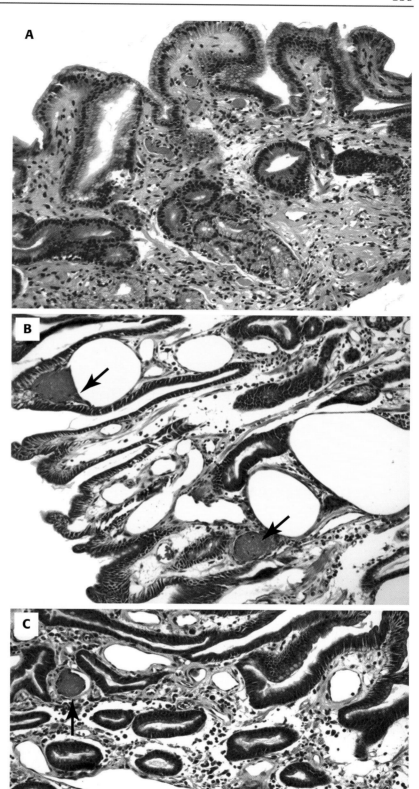

FIGURE 3-68

Gastric antral vascular ectasia. Antral biopsy samples showing foveolar hyperplasia, dilated mucosal capillaries with fibrin thrombi, and fibromuscular hyperplasia of lamina propria. Note the fibrin thrombi *(arrows)* that are important for diagnosis.

TABLE 3-8

Comparison of Distinction between Gastric Antral Vascular Ectasia and Portal Hypertensive Gastropathy

	GAVE	Portal Hypertensive Gastropathy
Location	Predominantly antrum	Predominantly body
Endoscopic appearance	Linear red stripes resembling watermelon	Diffuse mosaic vascular pattern, cherry red spots, scarlatina rash
Endoscopic ultrasound	Thin atrophic gastric wall with thickening limited to antral region	Diffusely thickened gastric wall with dilated veins
Characteristic histology	Dilated mucosal capillaries with thrombi	Vascular ectasia, perivascular stromal thickening
Associated conditions	Autoimmune and connective tissue diseases, also cirrhosis	Cirrhosis with portal hypertension
Management	Endoscopic laser therapy, antrectomy	Portal decompression, shunting

PROGNOSIS AND THERAPY

Treatment is based mainly on the rate of blood loss. Conservative management with iron supplement or blood transfusion may be insufficient. Various endoscopic modalities are available and include laser, heater probe therapy, bipolar electrocautery, and injection sclerotherapy. Excellent results have been shown with laser therapy. Surgical antrectomy offers definitive therapy but carries a mortality rate of 7.4%.

■ PORTAL HYPERTENSIVE GASTROPATHY

The term *portal hypertensive gastropathy* (PHG) is used to describe the vascular manifestations of portal hypertension in the stomach consisting of a mosaic-like pattern with or without red spots on endoscopy. Synonyms include congestive gastropathy and congestive gastroenteropathy.

CLINICAL FEATURES

PHG is seen in patients with cirrhotic or noncirrhotic portal hypertension. Patients usually present with mild bleeding, and unlike GAVE, anemia or transfusion requirement is less common. The stomach is most often involved, but the small intestine and colon can also show manifestations of portal hypertension (portal hypertensive intestinal vasculopathy, portal colopathy). PHG can affect adults and children, and a male predominance is present.

The pathogenesis of PHG is thought to be hemodynamic alterations and increased splenic circulation resulting in increased gastric mucosal blood flow caused by portal hypertension. Patients who have undergone sclerotherapy or banding for their esophageal varices are at higher risk of developing PHG.

PATHOLOGIC FEATURES

GROSS AND ENDOSCOPIC FINDINGS

PHG involves the proximal stomach (an important distinction from GAVE). The endoscopic appearance of PHG ranges from diffuse fine pink speckling or "scarlatina" rash with a mosaic pattern resembling snake skin (Fig. 3-69) to severe gastropathy with cherry-red spots and diffuse hemorrhagic gastropathy.

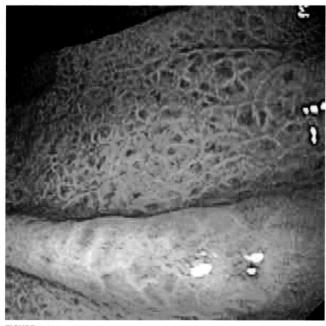

FIGURE 3-69

"Mosaic" or snake skin appearance of the gastric body mucosa in a patient with portal hypertensive gastropathy.

PORTAL HYPERTENSIVE GASTROPATHY—FACT SHEET

Definition
- PHG is used to describe the vascular manifestations of portal hypertension in the stomach consisting of a mosaic-like pattern with or without red spots on endoscopy

Morbidity and Mortality
- Morbidity is related to the low-volume blood loss
- Not a significant cause of mortality

Gender, Race, and Age
- Affects adults and children
- Male predominance

Clinical Features
- Seen in patients with cirrhotic or noncirrhotic portal hypertension
- Mild bleeding
- Patients who have undergone sclerotherapy or banding for their esophageal varices are at higher risk of developing PHG

Prognosis and Therapy
- Transjugular intrahepatic portosystemic shunt and shunt surgery
- Nonselective β-blockers such as propranolol

PORTAL HYPERTENSIVE GASTROPATHY—PATHOLOGIC FEATURES

Gross Findings
- PHG involves the fundus and body
- Endoscopic appearance ranges from diffuse fine pink speckling or "scarlatina" rash with a mosaic pattern resembling snake skin, to severe gastropathy with cherry-red spots and diffuse hemorrhagic gastropathy

Microscopic Findings
- Marked congestive vasculopathy with dilated mucosal capillaries and venules
- Changes are more prominent in submucosal veins, which show marked congestion, intimal thickening, and tortuosity
- Fibrin thrombi are not seen
- Mucosal biopsies often have low yield

Differential Diagnosis
- Gastric antral vascular ectasia

MICROSCOPIC FINDINGS

The histologic findings consist of marked congestive vasculopathy with dilated mucosal capillaries and venules (Figs. 3-70 and 3-71). Changes are more promi-nent in submucosal veins, which show marked conges-tion, intimal thickening, and tortuosity. The ectatic vessels are accompanied by perivascular stromal fibro-sis, lamina propria edema, and scant or absent inflam-mation. Fibrin thrombi are not seen.

Mucosal biopsies often have low yield given the predominantly submucosal vascular abnormalities, and endoscopists are reluctant to get deeper biopsies given the coagulation abnormalities in these cirrhotic patients.

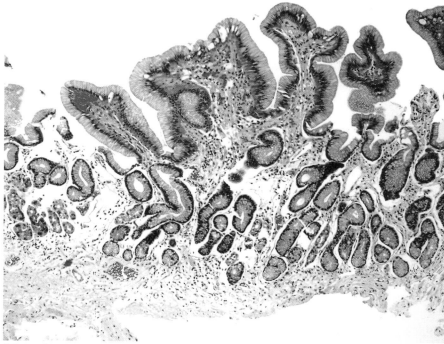

FIGURE 3-70
Gastric mucosal biopsy in a portal hypertensive gastropathy with dilated mucosal capillaries and congestion. Note the absence of fibrin thrombi.

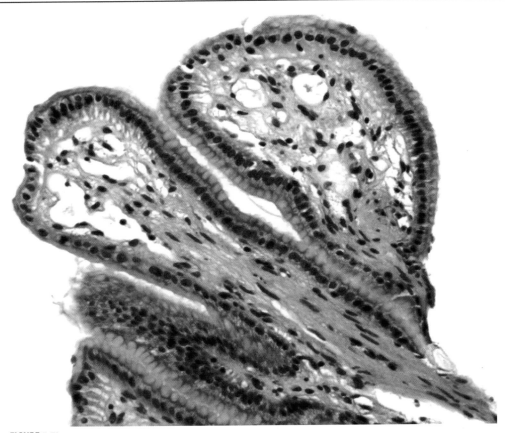

FIGURE 3-71
High-power view showing prominent and dilated mucosal capillaries in PHG.

DIFFERENTIAL DIAGNOSIS

- GAVE (see Table 3-8): Unlike PHG, GAVE is infrequently associated with portal hypertension. GAVE involves the gastric antrum, has a characteristic endoscopic appearance (watermelon stomach), and has biopsy findings of dilated mucosal capillaries with fibrin thrombi. Unlike GAVE, the endoscopic and biopsy findings of PHG are not highly specific.
- Mucosal congestion caused by biopsy artifact should not be mistaken for PHG.

PROGNOSIS AND THERAPY

Portal decompression procedures such as transjugular intrahepatic portosystemic shunt (TIPS) and shunt surgery are effective in resolving the gastropathy and bleeding. Nonselective β-blockers such as propranolol have shown promise in preventing bleeding.

■ DIEULAFOY'S LESION (CALIBER PERSISTENT ARTERY)

Named for Paul Georges Dieulafoy, a French surgeon, who described three cases in 1898, Dieulafoy's lesion is an uncommon cause of recurrent and often massive upper GI bleeding. It consists of a small mucosal defect overlying an artery of persistent large caliber in the mucosa. Synonymous with exulceratio simplex, cirsoid aneurysm, gastric arteriosclerosis, and submucosal arterial malformation.

CLINICAL FEATURES

Dieulafoy's lesion or caliber persistent artery typically presents as recurrent, often massive upper GI bleeding without preceding symptoms. Patients present with hematemesis, melena, and anemia frequently needing red cell transfusions. Symptoms such as abdominal pain, anorexia, and dyspepsia are not common. History of NSAID use, peptic ulcer, or alcohol abuse is notably absent.

DIEULAFOY'S LESION (CALIBER PERSISTENT ARTERY)—FACT SHEET

Definition

- Dieulafoy's lesion is an uncommon cause of upper GI bleeding consisting of a small mucosal defect overlying an artery of persistent large caliber in the mucosa

Incidence and Location

- Incidence as a cause of GI bleeding varies from 0.3% to 6.7%
- The lesion is typically present in the proximal fundus within 6 cm of the gastroesophageal junction, along the lesser curvature
- Apart from stomach, other sites such as duodenum, jejunum, large intestine, and rectum can also be involved

Morbidity and Mortality

- Current endoscopic therapeutic modalities have considerably reduced morbidity and mortality
- In the pre-endoscopic era the mortality rate was as high as 80% owing to massive bleeding from undiagnosed lesions

Gender, Race, and Age

- It is slightly more common in males, male-to-female ratio of 2:1
- Median age 54 years: range, 16 to 91 years

Clinical Features

- Typically presents as recurrent, often massive upper GI bleeding without preceding symptoms
- Symptoms include hematemesis, melena, and anemia frequently needing red cell transfusions
- Symptoms such as abdominal pain, anorexia, or dyspepsia are not common
- History of NSAID use, peptic ulcer, or alcohol abuse is notably absent

Radiologic Features

- Almost 80% of the lesions are identified by endoscopy, sometimes requiring multiple endoscopies
- Angiography and endoscopic ultrasonography are useful to identify lesions not detected by endoscopy
- Barium studies are not very helpful

Prognosis and Therapy

- Endoscopic therapeutic modalities are the first line of treatment
- Therapeutic interventions consist of electrocoagulation, hemoclipping, banding, epinephrine injection, and injection sclerotherapy
- Recurrent bleeding may warrant surgical therapy, which includes gastrotomy with ligation of the responsible vessel and proximal gastric resection

DIEULAFOY'S LESION (CALIBER PERSISTENT ARTERY)—PATHOLOGIC FEATURES

Gross Findings

- The typical gross or endoscopic appearance consists of a 2- to 5-mm mucosal defect with a protruding vessel

Microscopic Findings

- Histology consists of a large-caliber muscular artery with a tortuous course through the submucosa focally extending to the mucosa and into the gastric lumen
- The large-caliber vessel may show partial disruption with the overlying mucosa showing erosion, hemorrhage, and blood clots; however, the vessel lacks arteriosclerosis, calcification, aneurysmal dilatation, or vasculitis
- The surrounding gastric mucosa is essentially normal

Differential Diagnosis

- Other causes of bleeding, such as Mallory Weiss tear, peptic ulcer disease, angiodysplasia, chemical gastropathy, and gastric antral vascular ectasia, need to be ruled out
- The characteristic location of this lesion in the proximal fundus with a large-caliber, otherwise histologically unremarkable vessel protruding through a mucosal defect, essentially normal adjacent mucosa, and absence of NSAID intake or alcohol abuse are all helpful distinguishing features

RADIOLOGIC FEATURES

The majority (80%) of the lesions are identified by endoscopy, sometimes requiring multiple endoscopies. Angiography and endoscopic ultrasonography are useful to identify lesions not detected by endoscopy. Barium studies are not helpful. Lesions in the colon are not as amenable to endoscopic diagnosis.

PATHOLOGIC FEATURES

GROSS AND ENDOSCOPIC FINDINGS

The endoscopic appearance consists of a 2- to 5-mm mucosal defect with a protruding vessel. The mucosa may look normal between bleeding episodes. Dieulafoy's lesion should be seriously considered in the differential diagnosis when a patient presents with massive GI bleeding without an endoscopically identifiable source of bleeding because this lesion may be difficult to visualize resulting from its proximal fundic location.

MICROSCOPIC FINDINGS

The characteristic histology on resection or autopsy specimens consists of a large-caliber muscular artery with a tortuous course through the submucosa, focally

The lesion is usually found in the proximal fundus within 6 cm of the gastroesophageal junction, along the lesser curvature. Apart from stomach, other sites such as the duodenum, jejunum, large intestine, and rectum can be involved. It is slightly more common in males, (male-to-female ratio 2:1), with a median age of 54 years (range, 16 to 91 years).

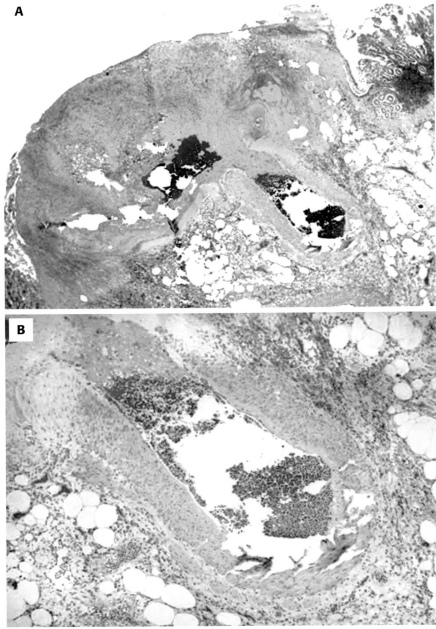

FIGURE 3-72
Notice a large caliber artery in the submucosa extending to the mucosa with overlying thrombi and ulceration seen at low
(A) and high **(B)** magnification.

extending to the mucosa and communicating with the gastric lumen. The vessel may show partial disruption, with the overlying mucosa showing erosion, hemorrhage, and blood clots (Fig. 3-72). The vessel lacks arteriosclerosis, calcification, aneurysmal dilatation, or vasculitis. The surrounding gastric mucosa is essentially normal. There is no evidence of deep ulceration or disruption of the muscularis propria.

ANCILLARY STUDIES

Elastic stain of the vessel is helpful but not essential for diagnosis.

DIFFERENTIAL DIAGNOSIS

Other causes of bleeding such as Mallory-Weiss tear, peptic ulcer disease, angiodysplasia, chemical gastropathy, and gastric antral vascular ectasia need to be ruled out. The characteristic location of this lesion in the proximal fundus with a large-caliber, otherwise histologically unremarkable vessel protruding through a mucosal defect; essentially normal adjacent mucosa; and absence of NSAID intake or alcohol abuse are all helpful distinguishing features.

PROGNOSIS AND THERAPY

Endoscopic therapeutic modalities are the first line of treatment and have reduced mortality considerably provided that the lesion is identified and treated early. In the pre-endoscopic era, the mortality reached up to 80% resulting from massive bleeding from undiagnosed lesions. Therapeutic interventions consist of electrocoagulation, hemoclipping, banding, epinephrine injection, and injection sclerotherapy. Recurrent bleeding may warrant surgical therapy, which includes gastrotomy with ligation of the responsible vessel or proximal gastric resection.

4

Epithelial Neoplasms of the Stomach

■ **Jason Y. Park, MD, PhD, FCAP** ■ **Hubert H. Fenton, MD**
■ **Marc R. Lewin, MD** ■ **H. Parry Dilworth, MD**

Gastric carcinomas have a variety of precursors that can be identified histologically. Precursor lesions can be broadly classified into categories of either gastric epithelial dysplasia (GED) for *flat* (grossly normal) lesions or gastric adenoma for lesions that are raised or polypoid. Microscopic examination alone cannot always distinguish between a flat or polypoid process, and therefore correlation with endoscopic or gross appearance is helpful in the evaluation of gastric dysplasia.

Adenocarcinomas are the most common type of carcinomas of the stomach, and these may be broadly divided into intestinal and diffuse subtypes. Overall, the prognosis of gastric carcinomas is poor. The role of the pathologist is to identify precursor lesions before they have progressed to invasive carcinoma. The early identification of precursor lesions can lead to complete resection and prevent the development of invasive carcinoma.

Neuroendocrine tumors are epithelial neoplasms that are rarely encountered in the stomach and have prognoses that span from indolent to aggressive. Microscopic examination of neuroendocrine tumors with consideration for the clinical history and appearance of the background gastric mucosa can be helpful for determining the expected prognosis.

■ GASTRIC EPITHELIAL DYSPLASIA

CLINICAL FEATURES

It is widely recognized that gastric epithelial dysplasia (GED) is a precancerous lesion with the ability to progress to gastric carcinoma. GED is associated with 40% to 100% of early gastric cancers and 5% to 80% of advanced carcinomas. In addition, approximately 60% of gastric cancers are discovered following a diagnosis of dysplasia.

Most cases of GED occur in males in the fifth to seventh decade of life. It is primarily observed in the gastric antrum. Western populations demonstrate a prevalence of GED up to 3.75% with peaks of 20% in high-risk areas such as Japan and Eastern Europe. Other risk factors for the development of GED include pernicious anemia or familial adenomatous polyposis.

GASTRIC EPITHELIAL DYSPLASIA—FACT SHEET

Definition

- Dysplasia of flat gastric epithelium that has the potential for transformation to invasive carcinoma

Incidence

- More common in Westernized countries
- Prevalence ranges between 0.5% and 3.75%, up to 20% in high-risk areas
- Higher incidences reported for patients with familial adenomatous polyposis

Morbidity and Mortality

- Related to risk of neoplastic progression
- Associated with 40% to 100% of early gastric cancers and 5% to 80% of advanced carcinomas
- More than half of gastric cancers are discovered after rendering a diagnosis of dysplasia

Gender, Age, and Race Distribution

- Male predominance
- Fifth to seventh decade of life
- No known racial predominance

Clinical Features

- No associated clinical symptoms
- May arise in a background of intestinal metaplasia

Prognosis

- Approximately 50% of low-grade dysplasias will undergo regression
- Twenty percent to 30% of monitored low-grade dysplasias show persistence of the lesion without progression
- Fifteen percent of cases of low-grade dysplasia show progression to carcinoma
- Progression of high-grade dysplasia to carcinoma is seen in 80% to 85% of cases

---

GASTRIC DYSPLASIA—PATHOLOGIC FEATURES

Gross Findings

- Normal appearance endoscopically

Microscopic Findings

- Glandular crowding, branching, and budding
- Crowded, enlarged nuclei with prominent nucleoli
- Decreased apical mucin
- Frequent mitoses
- High-grade dysplasia associated with crowding of glands, cribriform glands, loss of intervening stroma, and complete loss of nuclear polarity

Differential Diagnosis

- Reactive epithelial changes

In half of all cases of low-grade GED diagnosed by either biopsy or resection specimens, regression of the low-grade dysplasia may be encountered. This observation raises the possibility that low-grade dysplasia may be a reactive lesion. However, approximately 15% of patients with low-grade GED progress to either high-grade dysplasia or carcinoma.

PATHOLOGIC FEATURES

GROSS FINDINGS

These lesions are grossly unremarkable and are often not recognized by standard endoscopy. They are often referred to as flat dysplasias.

MICROSCOPIC FINDINGS

The diagnosis and grading of dysplasia in the stomach has historically differed between Japanese and Western pathologists. A consensus approach led to the Vienna classification of gastrointestinal epithelial neoplasia. The categories of dysplasia in the Vienna classification include: negative for dysplasia, indefinite for dysplasia, non-invasive low-grade dysplasia, non-invasive high-grade dysplasia (including carcinoma in situ), and invasive carcinoma (including both intramucosal carcinoma and submucosal carcinoma).

Architectural changes of low-grade dysplasia include mild to moderate crowding, branching, and budding of the gastric glands (Fig. 4-1A). Cytologically, the dysplastic cells exhibit nuclear crowding and hyperchromatism but otherwise retain their nuclear basal orientation and polarity. In high-grade dysplasia, the architectural changes become pronounced, seen as a loss of intervening stroma and back to back orientation of the dysplastic glands (see Fig. 4-1B). In addition, the marked glandular dilatation, branching, and intraluminal folding develops into complex forms such as cribriforming.

Cytologic elements associated with higher-grade lesions include loss of nuclear polarity with marked stratification of the nuclei extending to the luminal aspect of glands. There is a marked increase in the nuclear to cytoplasmic ratio, with the cells developing a more rounded nuclear form. Mitoses are prominent, and intraluminal necrotic material may be seen. When an early infiltrating carcinoma confined to the lamina propria is identified within gastric epithelial dysplasia, it is termed intramucosal carcinoma (see Fig. 4-1C and D).

DIFFERENTIAL DIAGNOSIS

The main differential diagnosis of GED is reactive or regenerative epithelial changes. Of note, in a single study of epithelial dysplasias of the stomach, one half of the cases considered to be dysplastic by generalists were diagnosed as non-neoplastic by gastrointestinal pathologists. Thus, when a definitive diagnosis of dysplasia cannot be rendered, the use of the term *indefinite for dysplasia* is encouraged. As in other organs, intraobserver variation is diminished as the severity of the lesions increases.

In differentiating low-grade dysplasia from reactive and regenerative changes it is important to note both the cytologic and architectural features of these lesions. In regenerative changes the cells are frequently cuboidal and appear immature with basophilic cytoplasm secondary to reduced mucus secretion. These regenerative nuclei are often large, vesicular, and at times pleomorphic. Yet although the nuclear features show variation, the architectural features remain that of normal epithelium with basally localized nuclei, with only mild pseudostratification (Fig. 4-2). Mitotic figures, when present, are confined to the basal aspects of the glands. Finally, with transit of the epithelium from the basal portion of the glands to the luminal surface, a corresponding increase in cell maturation should be seen.

PROGNOSIS AND THERAPY

Although it is quoted that approximately 50% of low-grade GED will undergo regression, in some of these cases the "low-grade" dysplasia may in fact represent reactive or regenerative epithelial changes. Nonetheless, the importance of early detection is emphasized by the fact that more than half of gastric cancers are discovered after a diagnosis of dysplasia. Among all low-grade dysplasias identified, 20% to 30% of cases will show persistence of the lesion without progression and an additional 15% of cases will progress to high-grade dysplasia or infiltrating carcinoma. Progression of high-grade dysplasias to infiltrating carcinoma may be seen in 80% to 85% of cases, with regression observed in only 5% of cases. The time between the discovery of high-grade dysplasia and a diagnosis of adenocarcinoma varies between a few weeks to years.

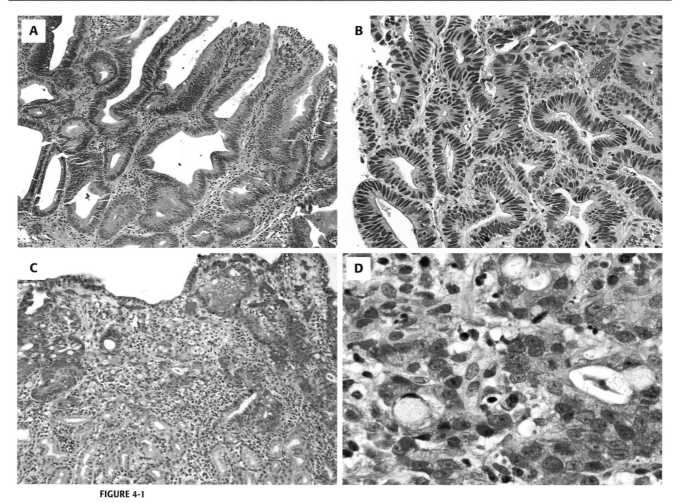

FIGURE 4-1

Gastric epithelial dysplasia. **A,** The histologic features of low-grade dysplasia include nuclear enlargement and elongation, nuclear crowding, and pseudostratification. Overall, the architecture of the surface epithelium is only moderately distorted. **B,** In high-grade dysplasia, in addition to the atypical cytologic features characterized by the complete loss of nuclear polarity and marked cellular and nuclear pleomorphism, the glands form complex structures and grow in a back-to-back formation. **C,** In this example of intramucosal carcinoma arising in high-grade dysplasia, the neoplastic cells begin to grow in a syncytial pattern. **D,** High-power view of the intramucosal carcinoma shown in C highlights the marked cytologic atypia of this early infiltrating gastric cancer. Note the single signet ring cells in the left side of the image.

Follow-up is usually recommended after a diagnosis of low-grade dysplasia; endoscopy every 3 to 12 months during the first year is advised, secondary to the risk of progression to carcinoma. Following a diagnosis of high-grade dysplasia, endoscopic mucosal resection offers a nonsurgical and potentially curative alternative for the treatment of dysplasia and intramucosal carcinoma. When there is question as to the severity of the lesion, clinical follow-up with repeat biopsy is recommended.

■ GASTRIC ADENOMAS

CLINICAL FEATURES

In contrast to flat gastric epithelial dysplasia, gastric adenomas are localized growths of dysplastic epithelium that project above the surrounding gastric mucosa. Gastric adenomatous polyps follow fundic gland and hyperplastic polyps in overall incidence, accounting for approximately 10% of gastric polyps in North America. This incidence increases with age and peaks in the seventh decade. The male-to-female ratio is approximately 2:1. Most adenomas are found incidentally at the time of endoscopy.

Unlike for the colon, gastric adenomas are not the major precursor for adenocarcinoma; most gastric adenocarcinomas are not associated with an adenoma. However, gastric adenomas are a direct precursor to some gastric carcinomas and also serve as markers for increased risk of adenocarcinoma in other areas of the stomach.

Gastric adenomas have been shown to harbor molecular alterations in the *APC, KRAS,* and *Tp53* genes, similar to that described for the colon. However, although the colon demonstrates a well-characterized adenoma-carcinoma sequence of molecular genetic events, these events are only rarely present in the stomach. For

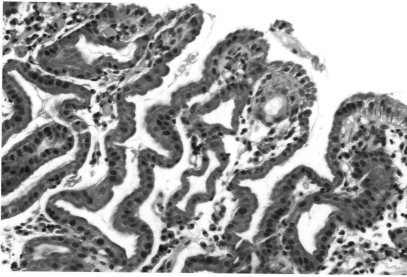

FIGURE 4-2

Reactive epithelial changes simulating gastric epithelial dysplasia. Although the reactive epithelial changes in this picture include nuclear hyperchromasia and enlargement, other features of dysplasia including prominent nuclear pseudostratification, nuclear crowding, and nuclear elongation are lacking.

example, alterations in the *APC* gene are frequently seen in gastric adenomas, but these alterations are rarely seen in gastric adenocarcinomas.

GASTRIC ADENOMA—FACT SHEET

Definition
- Localized, neoplastic growths of dysplastic epithelium that project above the surrounding gastric mucosa

Incidence
- Account for approximately 10% of gastric polyps

Morbidity and Mortality
- Related to risk for malignant progression
- Infiltrating carcinoma more common in intestinal-type adenomas > 2 cm in size
- May serve as biomarker for adenocarcinoma elsewhere in the stomach

Gender, Race and Age
- Males more than females
- Incidence increases with age, peaking in 7th decade

Clinical Features
- Often arise in the setting of intestinal metaplasia and atrophy
- Gastric-type adenomas associated with familial adenomatous polyposis

Prognosis and Therapy
- Polypectomy and complete excision are curative
- Prognosis dependent on whether infiltrating carcinoma present

PATHOLOGIC FEATURES

GROSS FINDINGS

Gastric adenomas occur throughout the stomach with the antrum being the most common location. They range in size from a few millimeters to several centimeters. They may be sessile or pedunculated.

MICROSCOPIC FINDINGS

Gastric adenomas are histologically divided into intestinal and foveolar types based on the type of glandular epithelium they display. Intestinal-type adenomas resemble those seen in the colon and are characterized by the presence of goblet or Paneth cells (Fig. 4-3A and B). Foveolar-type adenomas are lined by gastric foveolar epithelial cells containing neutral mucin (see Fig. 4-3C). Intestinal-type adenomas are more prevalent than the gastric foveolar-type adenoma and often arise in a background of intestinalized and atrophic gastric mucosa (Fig. 4-4). Compared with gastric foveolar-type adenomas, intestinal-type adenomas have a greater likelihood to show both high-grade dysplasia and to harbor adenocarcinoma.

Both types of gastric adenoma show dysplastic epithelial changes ranging from low- to high-grade, although high-grade dysplasia is rare in gastric foveolar type adenomas. Low-grade dysplastic epithelial changes include loss of polarity, nuclear enlargement, nuclear hyperchromasia, prominent nucleoli, pseudostratification, pleomorphism, and mitoses. In high-grade dysplasia, the glandular architecture becomes increasingly complex with

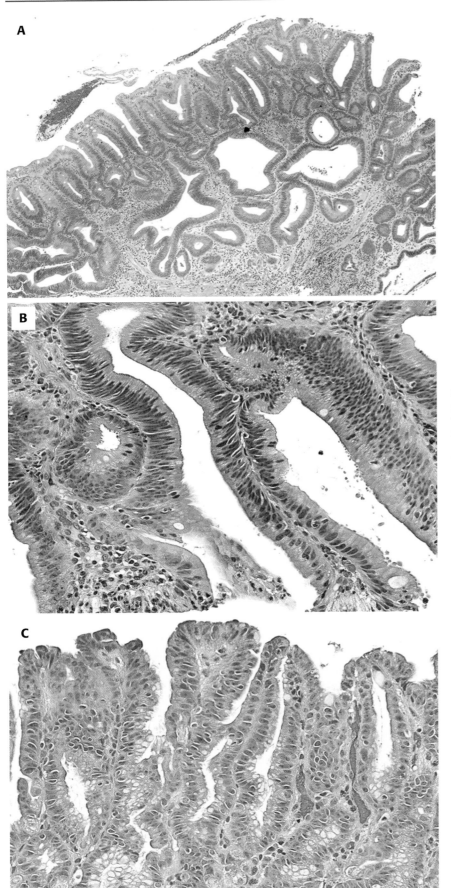

FIGURE 4-3

Intestinal-type adenoma. **A,** Low-power view of an intestinal type adenoma with enlarged hyperchromatic nuclei and several goblet cells. **B,** High-power view showing features of low-grade dysplasia including hyperchromatic nuclei, pseudostratification, and nuclear elongation. Note the presence of intestinal meta-plasia (goblet cells) scattered among the dysplastic epithelium. **C,** In foveolar-type adenomas, the adenomatous cells com-posed of dysplastic foveolar cells with loss of polarity, nuclear enlargement, nuclear hyperchromasia, and prominent nucleoli.

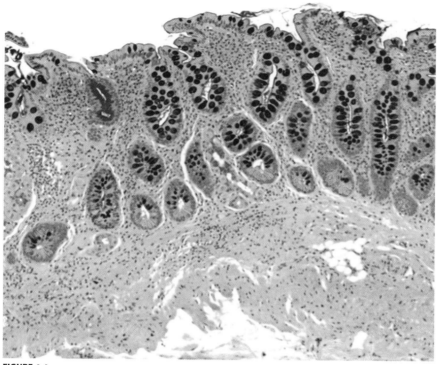

FIGURE 4-4

Background mucosa associated with an intestinal-type gastric adenoma. There is often marked intestinal metaplasia of the gastric mucosa, as seen in this PAS-AB stain highlighting the intestinal-type goblet cells (acid mucin).

GASTRIC ADENOMA—PATHOLOGIC FEATURES

Gross Features

- Pedunculated or sessile growth pattern
- Most common in the antrum
- Range in size from a few millimeters to several centimeters
- Cannot be reliably distinguished from benign gastric polyps endoscopically

Microscopic Features

- Divided into intestinal-type and gastric-type
- Intestinal-type defined by presence of goblet cells or Paneth cells
- Gastric-type composed of gastric foveolar epithelial cells
- Background mucosa often shows atrophic intestinal metaplasia
- High-grade dysplasia associated with crowding of glands, cribriform glands, full-thickness nuclear stratification, and complete loss of nuclear polarity

Genetics

- Associated with genetic alterations of *APC*, *KRAS*, *Tp53*, and microsatellite instability

Differential Diagnosis

- Pyloric gland adenoma
- Hyperplastic polyp
- Reactive epithelial change

---

irregular branching, gland budding, and cribriforming. Cytologically, the nuclei show more severe atypia with enlarged, hyperchromatic, vesicular nuclei, and prominent nucleoli. There is also complete loss of nuclear polarity with the atypical nuclei reaching the luminal surface of the epithelium.

DIFFERENTIAL DIAGNOSIS

The differential diagnosis is any pathologic entity in which the epithelium undergoes reactive changes can enter into the differential diagnosis with a gastric adenoma, including fundic gland polyps and hyperplastic polyps. In all cases, recognition of the lack of cytologic atypia and presence of surface maturation should lead to the correct diagnosis. Another neoplastic entity to be considered is a pyloric gland adenoma.

PROGNOSIS AND THERAPY

Because endoscopy cannot distinguish gastric adenomas from other benign gastric polyps, all gastric polyps should be examined histologically for evidence of neoplastic epithelium. The reported frequency of carcinoma arising within an adenoma ranges from approximately 3% up to 40%. The risk of carcinoma is greater in larger polyps (>2 cm), but even smaller adenomas can show malignant transformation. The risk of a separate gastric adenocarcinoma in the adjacent nonadenomatous mucosa may be as high as 30%. As mentioned, gastric adenomas are endoscopically indistinct from other benign gastric polyps, and, therefore, all gastric polyps should be treated with complete excision of the polyp.

■ PYLORIC GLAND ADENOMA

CLINICAL FEATURES

Pyloric gland adenoma is a rare neoplastic entity that was first reported in the 1970s but has only recently been studied and described. A retrospective study that excluded fundic gland polyps observed that pyloric gland adenomas were 2.7% of all gastric polyps. Although they are rare, they are precancerous lesions that are found frequently in association with adenocarcinoma. In separate studies, adenocarcinoma was diagnosed in 30% and 12% of each respective study of pyloric gland adenoma. There is a female predominance of disease, which has been observed in a range of 2:1 to 14:2. The mean age at diagnosis is in the seventh decade.

The genetics of pyloric gland adenoma and adenocarcinomas arising out of pyloric gland adenoma are not well characterized. In a study from the 1990s of pyloric gland adenomas of the gallbladder, no alterations were found by either APC mutational analysis, K-RAS codon 12 mutational analysis, or p53 expression. No comparable study of APC, K-RAS, or p53 has been published for gastric pyloric gland adenomas. A more recent study of changes in DNA copy numbers by microarray-based comparative genomic hybridization (CGH) revealed no significant differences between intestinal-type gastric adenomas and pyloric gland adenomas. Both intestinal-type and pyloric gland adenomas have gains in chromosomes 8, 9q, 11q, and 20 and losses in chromosomes 5q, 6, 10, and 13. The genetic basis of pyloric gland adenomas remains an area in need of further study.

PATHOLOGIC FEATURES

GROSS FINDINGS

Gastric pyloric gland adenomas are most often detected as polypoid lesions localized to the gastric body in 73% to 90% of cases. At the time of diagnosis, they have a mean size of approximately 16 mm.

PYLORIC GLAND ADENOMA—FACT SHEET

Definition
- Localized, neoplastic growths of dysplastic epithelium with pyloric gland differentiation that project above the surrounding gastric mucosa

Incidence
- Not well studied; 2.7% of all gastric polyps in a single study

Morbidity and Mortality
- Frequently identified with concurrent adenocarcinoma

Gender, Race, and Age
- Majority of patients are female
- Incidence increases with age, peaking in seventh decade
- Race is not well studied

Clinical Features
- The most common background is in autoimmune gastritis

Prognosis and Therapy
- Polypectomy and complete excision is curative, although data are limited
- Prognosis dependent on whether infiltrating carcinoma present

---

PYLORIC GLAND ADENOMA—PATHOLOGIC FEATURES

Gross Features
- Pedunculated growth pattern
- Most common in the body of the stomach
- Mean size is 16 mm
- Cannot be reliably distinguished from benign gastric polyps endoscopically

Microscopic Features
- Background mucosa often shows a gastric pattern with intestinal metaplasia
- Amphophilic to eosinophilic cytoplasm with a ground-glass quality
- Low-grade dysplasia is associated with well-organized glands of bland, nonpleomorphic, basally located nuclei
- High-grade dysplasia associated with crowding of glands, cribriform glands, nuclear stratification, and loss of nuclear polarity

Genetics
- Not characterized

Differential Diagnosis
- Gastric adenoma
- Hyperplastic polyp
- Reactive epithelial changes

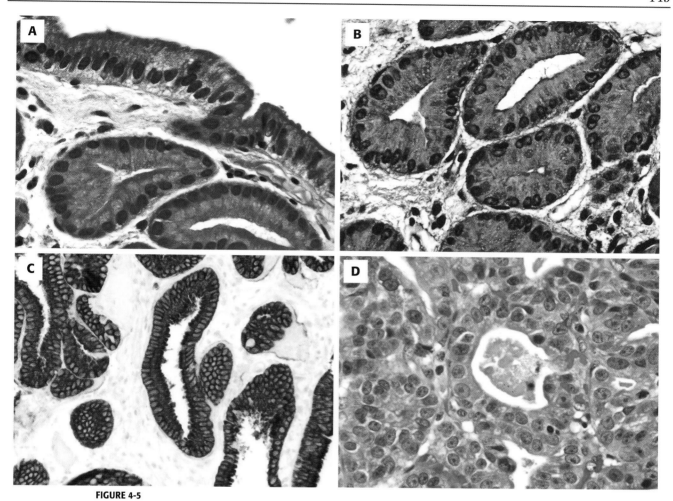

FIGURE 4-5

Pyloric gland adenoma. **A,** Pyloric gland adenoma with low-grade dysplasia. These cells are columnar with pink to basophilic cytoplasm and uniform nuclei that are basally located. **B,** PAS/Alcian Blue staining of pyloric gland adenoma emphasizes the lack of a well-defined mucin cap. **C,** MUC6 immunohistochemistry intensely labels the cytoplasm of pyloric gland adenoma including the glands of the surface epithelium. **D,** Pyloric gland adenoma with high-grade dysplasia. These glands are crowded with increased complexity and some luminal necrosis. There is an increased nuclear-to-cytoplasmic ratio with pleomorphic nuclei. The luminal necrosis is concerning for the possibility of intramucosal invasion.

MICROSCOPIC FINDINGS

Pyloric gland adenoma is comprised of tubular glands composed of cuboidal or columnar cells (Fig. 4-5). The cytoplasm is ground-glass and either eosinophilic or amphophilic. Compared with gastric foveolar type adenomas, pyloric gland adenomas do not have a well-formed mucin cap. In pyloric gland adenomas with low-grade dysplasia the cells are typically cytologically bland: there is plentiful cytoplasm; the nuclei are basally located; and there is minimal nuclear pleomorphism. Some pyloric gland adenomas display a monolayer of neoplastic cells and have been graded with "no dysplasia" akin to sessile serrated adenomas of the colon, but they are still neoplastic. In pyloric gland adenomas with high-grade dysplasia, the nuclei can be pseudostratified and hyperchromatic with marked pleomorphism.

Immunohistochemical studies have demonstrated that pyloric gland adenomas frequently express MUC6 and MUC5AC. This pattern of expression is in contrast to gastric foveolar–type gastric adenomas, which express MUC5AC, but do not express MUC6.

The background, nonlesional stomach shows gastritis, which is most frequently autoimmune in origin (33.9%). The background gastritis pattern may also be etiologically *Helicobacter pylori* (41.5%) or chemical-type gastropathy (20.8%).

DIFFERENTIAL DIAGNOSIS

The main differential diagnoses for pyloric gland adenomas include reactive epithelial changes, gastric foveolar type adenomas, and gastric intestinal–type adenomas.

Because of their bland cytologic appearance, pyloric gland adenomas are often most difficult to distinguish from gastric foveolar type adenomas. Helpful histologic features in the identification of pyloric gland adenoma are the basally located bland nuclei with amphophilic to eosinophilic ground-glass cytoplasm and lack of an apical mucin cap.

PROGNOSIS AND THERAPY

Limited follow-up clinical data are available for patients with pyloric gland adenoma. Given that there is a high incidence of invasive carcinoma present at the time of diagnosis, careful evaluation of the lesion and the surrounding nonlesional mucosa is prudent. In a recent study, three patients with deeply invasive adenocarcinoma arising from pyloric gland adenoma had long-term follow-up. One patient had survived for 10 years with local recurrence at the surgical site. The two other patients were alive at 2 and 10 months post operatively. These limited data suggest the need for complete surgical removal of adenocarcinomas arising from pyloric gland adenoma.

■ GASTRIC ADENOCARCINOMA

CLINICAL FEATURES

Gastric cancer is the second most common cancer worldwide, and despite decreasing mortality and incidence rates, it remains a leading cause of cancer-related deaths. Overall, gastric cancer rates are higher in developing countries and in lower socioeconomic groups. The lowest rates are found in North America, Northern Europe, and Africa, while the highest rates are found in Japan, Costa Rica, East Asia, and Eastern Europe. Gastric cancer peaks in the seventh decade of life and is extremely rare before the age of 40. Gastric cancer affects men twice as often as women.

Over the past several decades, gastric cancer rates have been decreasing in the United States and throughout the world. However, these trends reflect the decreasing incidence of cancers arising in the distal stomach. Proximal gastric cancers arising from the gastroesophageal junction or the gastric cardia have, in fact, been increasing in incidence at rates greater than for any other cancer, suggesting proximal cancers may have a distinct pathogenesis from their distal counterparts and are more like esophageal adenocarcinomas. In fact, because of this, the seventh edition of the TNM staging uses the following modification from prior editions: "a tumor the epicenter of which is within 5 cm of the GE junction and also extends into the esophagus, is classified and staged using the esophageal carcinoma scheme. Tumors with an epicenter in the stomach greater than 5 cm from the GE junction or those within 5 cm of the oesophagogastric junction without extension in the esophagus are classified and staged using the gastric carcinoma scheme."

Several risk factors have been associated with the development of gastric cancer. Migration studies suggest the importance of environmental factors on gastric cancer rates as immigrants from high-incidence countries retain the same rates of their original country, while future generations acquire the incidence rates of their new countries. Environmental factors such as diet and smoking have been linked to gastric cancer. Diets rich in nitrites, nitrates, salt, smoked foods, and complex carbohydrates are associated with increased gastric cancer risks, whereas diets rich in fresh fruits and vegetables are associated with reduced cancer risks through their antioxidant properties. Cigarette smoking is also associated with a twofold and threefold increased risk of gastric cancer.

Gastric carcinoma has a weak association with chronic atrophic gastritis with intestinal metaplasia, especially type III metaplasia, which shows incomplete intestinal metaplasia with sulfomucin-secreting goblet cells. However, the presence of type III metaplasia is not a reliable screening tool for gastric carcinoma. Gastric carcinomas of the intestinal type have a greater association with intestinal metaplasia than do the diffuse type of cancers.

Several studies have shown *H. pylori* infection to significantly increase the risk of both intestinal and diffuse types of gastric carcinomas, and it is now recognized as an established cause of gastric cancer. The risk of gastric cancer is significantly increased if the *H. pylori* infection is acquired in childhood or is present for greater than 10 years prior to diagnosis of cancer. *H. pylori* infection may also be associated with the increased cancer risk seen in people with blood group A because it adheres to the Lewis blood group and facilitates chronic infection in these individuals. A recent prospective study demonstrated that *H. pylori* eradication at the time of localized gastric cancer resection decreased the future risk of gastric cancer arising in other locations of the stomach.

Another infectious agent, Epstein-Barr virus (EBV), has been associated with a subset of undifferentiated gastric carcinomas with intense lymphoid infiltrates. Proximal gastric carcinomas have not been linked to *H. pylori* infection but appear closely related to Barrett's esophagus. However, the exact pathogenesis of these cancers remains unclear. Other factors that increase the risk of gastric cancer include a history of prior gastrectomy, pernicious anemia, obesity, and hypertrophic gastropathy.

Multiple genetic alterations in gastric cancers have been described; however, a definitive sequence of gastric tumorigenesis has not been defined. Although the vast majority of gastric cancers occur sporadically, some

GASTRIC ADENOCARCINOMA—FACT SHEET

Definition
- Malignant neoplasm of gastric epithelium

Incidence
- Second most common cancer worldwide
- Incidence varies considerably (lowest rates in North America, Northern Europe, and Africa and highest rates in Japan, Costa Rica, East Asia, and Eastern Europe)

Morbidity and Mortality
- Responsible for 2.5% of cancer deaths in the United States
- Leading cause of cancer deaths worldwide
- Five-year survival rate is 10% to 15%

Gender, Race, and Age
- Males more than females
- Average age at diagnosis in 7th decade

Clinical Features
- Risk factors include diets high in nitrites, low socioeconomic status, and cigarette smoking
- Associated with chronic gastritis, *Helicobacter pylori*, and partial gastrectomy
- Often presents at a late stage
- Proximal cancers may have different etiology

Prognosis and Therapy
- Prognosis related to pathologic stage and tumor differentiation
- Surgical resection most effective treatment for early stage (T1 and T2)
- Adjuvant therapy recommended for advanced-stage carcinomas

GASTRIC ADENOCARCINOMA—PATHOLOGIC FEATURES

Gross Features
- May be exophytic, flat, or ulcerated; linitis plastica corresponds to broad area of diffuse gastric wall thickening

Microscopic Features
- Classified as intestinal type or diffuse type
- Intestinal type: well-formed glands lined by columnar to cuboidal epithelial cells
- Diffuse type: individual or poorly formed nests of cells growing in an infiltrative pattern
- May have prominent desmoplastic response

Genetics
- Sporadic carcinomas associated with *APC*, *K-RAS*, and *Tp53* alterations
- 10% of carcinomas are caused by hereditary factors (E-cadherin mutations).

Immunohistochemical Findings
- Variable CK7/CK20 profile (most common CK7+/CK20−)
- CEA positive
- EMA positive

Differential Diagnosis
- Reactive processes
- Lymphoma (for diffuse type)
- Severe dysplasia
- Metastatic disease

genetic conditions have also been linked to gastric cancer. Patients with Li-Fraumeni syndrome, familial adenomatous polyposis, hereditary nonpolyposis colon cancer, and *BRCA2* mutations all have increased risk of developing gastric cancer. In addition, mutations in the adhesion molecule E-cadherin have been associated with autosomal dominant hereditary diffuse gastric cancer.

PATHOLOGIC FEATURES

GROSS FINDINGS

The majority of gastric carcinomas are located in the pylorus and antrum (50% to 60%), followed by the cardia (25%), and the body or fundus (15% to 25%). Advanced gastric cancers of the intestinal type commonly appear as polypoid, fungating masses with surface ulceration (Fig. 4-6A). In contrast, diffuse-type cancers may appear as infiltrating or depressed cancers with no obvious mass present in the mucosa. Linitis plastica is a rare lesion in which the majority of the stomach wall is infiltrated by diffuse-type cancer

conferring a thick, firm, leathery appearance to the stomach (see Fig. 4-6B).

Early gastric cancers are defined as those confined to the submucosa regardless of lymph node status and are often subtle lesions found upon periodic screening (see Fig. 4-6C). The Japanese Gastroenterological Endoscopic Society devised a complex classification scheme for the macroscopic appearance for early gastric cancers, which aids in the detection of early subtle cancers at the time of endoscopy, but this classification scheme has weak correlation with prognosis.

MICROSCOPIC FINDINGS

The overwhelming majority (95%) of malignant gastric cancers are adenocarcinomas. Although various classification schemes for gastric cancer have been proposed, the Lauren and the World Health Organization (WHO) classification systems are the most widely used. The Lauren scheme separates gastric adenocarcinomas into intestinal and diffuse subtypes. The intestinal subtype of gastric adenocarcinoma histologically resembles colorectal adenocarcinoma. It is characterized by well-formed glands lined by columnar to cuboidal epithelial cells (Fig. 4-7). Intraluminal mucin is often present, whereas intracytoplasmic mucin droplets are uncommon. Diffuse-type gastric adenocarcinoma is composed of individual

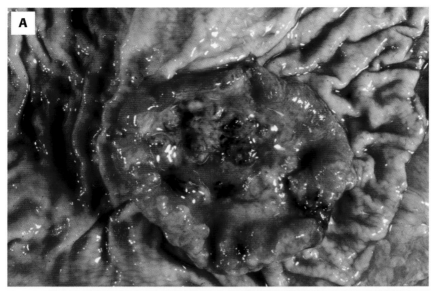

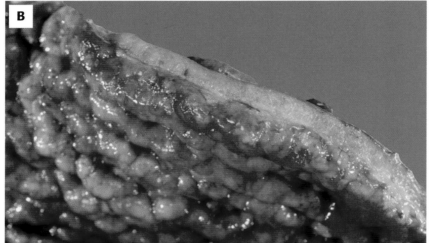

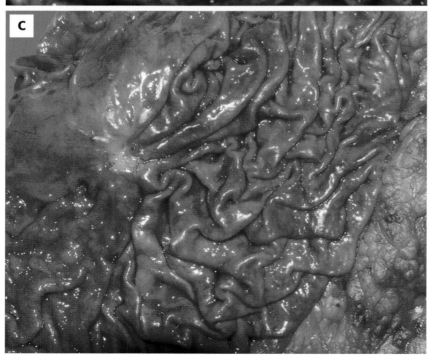

FIGURE 4-6

Gross appearances of gastric carcinoma. **A,** Intestinal-type adenocarcinoma. This advanced carcinoma presented as a large, exophytic, polypoid mass. **B,** Linitus plastica. The gastric wall is markedly thickened, firm, and fibrotic. In contrast to the intestinal-type carcinoma, the mucosa appears relatively normal. **C,** Early gastric cancer. In this example, the adenocarcinoma presents as a small area of mucosal ulceration.

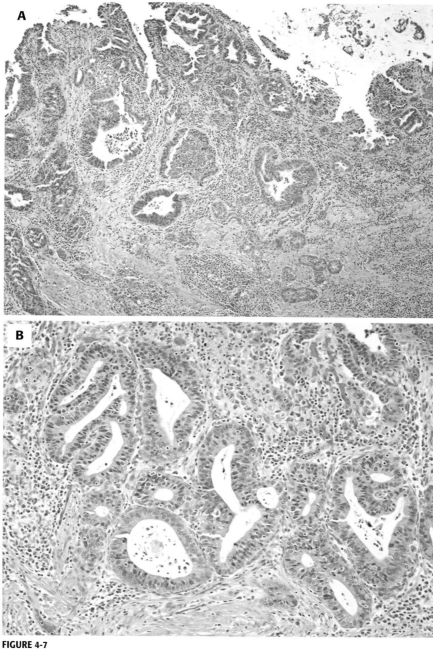

FIGURE 4-7

Intestinal-type gastric adenocarcinoma. **A,** Low-power view of intestinal type adenocarcinoma composed of infiltrating moderately differentiated neoplastic glands. **B,** Higher-power view showing the formation of complex glandular structures lined by cuboidal to columnar cells and complete loss of nuclear polarity.

or poorly formed nests of cells growing in an infiltrative pattern (Fig. 4-8). Often these cells take on a signet ring cell appearance with the intracytoplasmic mucin pushing the nucleus of the neoplastic cell to the periphery. The amount of mucin present in these cells may be highly variable and may be difficult to appreciate in poorly differentiated carcinomas. One rare presentation of diffuse-type gastric adenocarcinoma occurs in the setting of hereditary diffuse gastric cancer. In one third of families with hereditary diffuse gastric cancer there is a germline E-cadherin mutation. These patients with a germline E-cadherin mutation have a high risk of gastric cancer and may present with invasive carcinoma during their teenage years. Although this presentation is

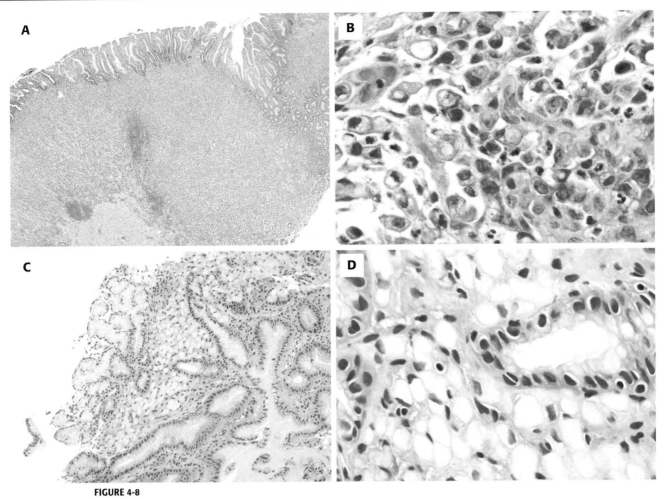

FIGURE 4-8

Diffuse-type gastric adenocarcinoma. **A,** Low-power view of diffuse type adenocarcinoma showing the complete effacement of the gastric wall by the infiltrate. In contrast to the intestinal type of adenocarcinoma, no well-formed glands are identified at this power. **B,** High-power view highlighting the individual tumor cells that diffusely infiltrate the submucosa. The cells are cytologically malignant with large, atypical nuclei, prominent nucleoli and intracytoplasmic mucin-filled vesicles that impart the "signet ring" appearance. **C,** In this example of diffuse-type adenocarcinoma, an innocuous collection of large cells with homogeneous pale cytoplasm is present beneath the surface epithelium. **D,** A higher-power view of these cells reveals the bland-appearing nuclei that are compressed to the cell periphery by the intracytoplasmic mucin.

rare, examination of the histologic precursors of this hereditary carcinoma is instructive for reviewing the various morphologic variants of signet ring cell carcinomas (Fig. 4-9).

Some gastric adenocarcinomas show features of both intestinal and diffuse types; these are classified as mixed types. It is important to note that the terms intestinal and diffuse are not synonymous with well- and poorly differentiated carcinomas. Some observers believe that when using the Lauren classification, adenocarcinomas should be further classified by their location; proximal cancers involving the cardia appear to have a different pathogenesis than their distal counterparts. A strong desmoplastic response to the tumor cells may be present, contributing to the firm, rigid stomach wall often seen in these lesions (Fig. 4-10).

The WHO scheme subtypes gastric adenocarcinomas based on the predominant morphologic component of the tumor. The subtypes include papillary, tubular, mucinous, signet ring cell, adenosquamous, and undifferentiated types. These tumors may then be further classified as well, moderately, or poorly differentiated.

Variants of gastric adenocarcinoma include medullary carcinoma in which greater than 50% of the tumor is poorly differentiated with no fibrous stroma. A subset of gastric carcinomas associated with Epstein-Barr virus (EBV) has a similar "lymphoepithelial" appearance (Fig. 4-11). Another variant of adenocarcinoma with features of typical gastric adenocarcinoma and adjacent areas resembling hepatocellular carcinoma has been reported.

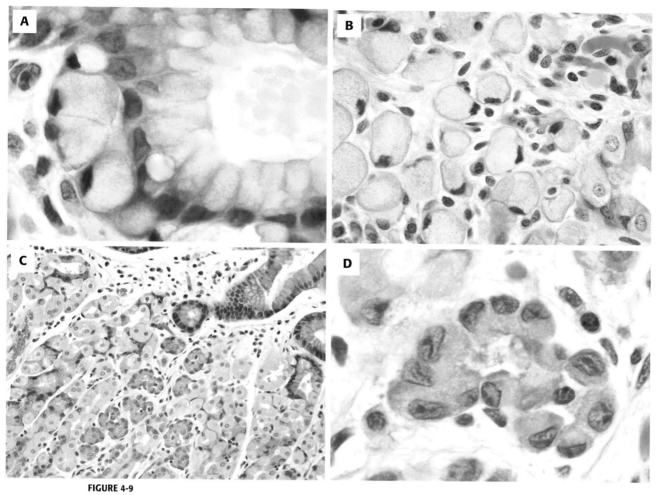

FIGURE 4-9

Signet ring cells in hereditary diffuse gastric adenocarcinoma. **A,** Pagetoid spread of signet ring cells. **B,** Intramucosal invasion of signet ring cells. **C,** Replacement of a gland with signet ring cells. **D,** Higher magnification.

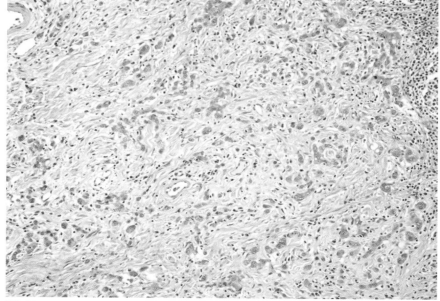

FIGURE 4-10

Desmoplastic response. There is a marked fibrotic response to the diffusely infiltrating signet ring tumor cells. This degree of desmoplasia can lead to the gross thickening of the stomach wall ("linitus plastica").

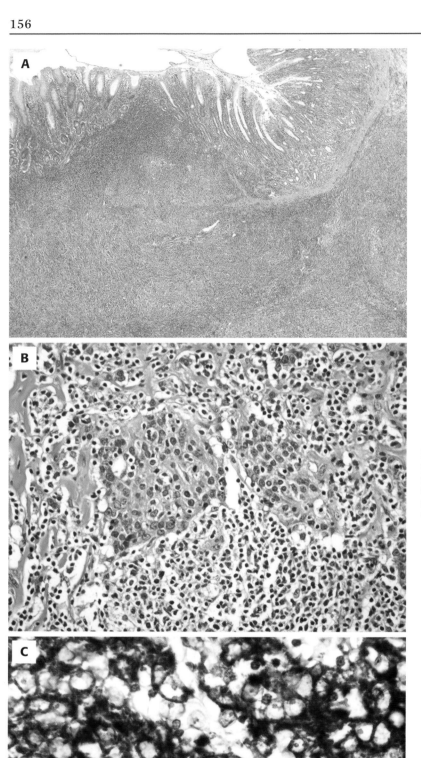

FIGURE 4-11

Epstein-Barr virus–associated gastric carcinoma. **A,** At low magnification, the lesion is ulcerated and notable for its dense lymphocytic inflammation. **B,** At high magnification, lymphocytes are intimately admixed with epithelial cells. **C,** Keratin staining highlights the neoplastic epithelial cells.

ANCILLARY STUDIES

Gastric adenocarcinomas are cytokeratin, epithelial membrane antigen, and CEA positive. CK7/CK20 profiles vary considerably with the majority being CK7 positive and CK20 negative.

Differential Diagnosis

The main difficulty encountered in the differential diagnosis of gastric carcinomas occurs with the diffuse type of gastric cancer. As the cells of this type of gastric cancer are often single and inconspicuous in a background desmoplasia and inflammation, it can often be mistaken for a variety of benign processes including gastritis or reactive endothelial cells seen in granulation tissue. Diffuse-type carcinoma may also mimic lymphoma because of its diffuse pattern of growth and round cell outlines. Therefore, pathologists should have a high degree of suspicion for diffuse-type gastric cancer when evaluating gastric biopsies. Stains for cytokeratin, EMA, and mucin should highlight the neoplastic cells. In addition, another diagnostic challenge exists in differentiating invasive intestinal-type carcinoma from severe dysplasia. Carcinoma should be characterized by a syncytial growth pattern, effacement of normal architecture with back-to-back glandular formations, or single cells percolating through the lamina propria.

PROGNOSIS AND THERAPY

Gastric adenocarcinoma has an overall poor prognosis with 5-year survival rates of 10% to 15%. Poor prognostic indicators include older age, proximal tumor location, venous or lymphatic invasion, CEA levels greater than 10 ng/mL, and CA19-9 levels greater than 37 g/mL. The best predictor of prognosis is the pathologic stage, which includes the depth of invasion, the extent of nodal involvement, and the presence or absence of distant metastasis. Surgical resection remains the standard of care. Adjuvant chemotherapy is not used routinely but does play a role in high-risk patients treated with inadequate resections. Greater than 50% of patients present with unresectable metastatic or locally advanced disease. In these cases, palliative treatments may include palliative surgery, radiation, or endoscopic procedures.

■ NEUROENDOCRINE TUMORS

CLINICAL FEATURES

Gastric neuroendocrine tumors (carcinoid tumors) are relatively rare lesions accounting for approximately 6% of all neuroendocrine tumors diagnosed. Among all stomach neoplasms, they account for less than 1% of lesions encountered. Historically, the nomenclature of neuroendocrine tumors has been inconsistent and can often be a point of confusion between pathologists and clinicians. For pathologists, the term *carcinoid* broadly applies to all low-grade or well-differentiated neuroendocrine tumors, regardless of the type of secreted hormone. In contrast, for many clinicians, neuroendocrine tumors are classified based on the hormone secreted, and the term *carcinoid* implies that the tumor secretes serotonin. In an attempt to harmonize these differences in terminology, the WHO *Classification of Tumors, Pathology, and Genetics of Tumors of Endocrine Organs* (2000) histologically classified neuroendocrine tumors on are the degree of differentiation; the categories and well-differentiated neuroendocrine tumor; well-differentiated neuroendocrine carcinoma; poorly differentiated neuroendocrine carcinoma. Based on this system, carcinoids would be considered well-differentiated neuroendocrine neoplasms and small cell carcinoma would be considered poorly differentiated neuroendocrine carcinomas. However, there has been limited consensus and reproducibility using this WHO classification, and further work needs to be done to address the classification of these tumors. Indeed, some observers would classify the diagnosis based on a combination of differentiation and invasion or spread. In this schema, the descriptive terms for diagnosis would be *carcinoid* (neuroendocrine tumor), *neuroendocrine carcinoma*, and *small cell carcinoma*. For the purpose of this chapter we will use the terms *carcinoid* and *neuroendocrine tumor* interchangeably.

WHO recognizes three types of gastric neuroendocrine tumors: type I, tumors arising in a setting of autoimmune chronic atrophic gastritis; type II, tumors associated with either multiple endocrine neoplasia type 1 (MEN-1) or Zollinger-Ellison syndrome; and type III, sporadic lesions. Type I and II tumors are typically small (<1 cm), multifocal, and associated with elevated levels of serum gastrin. Type III tumors are typically larger, solitary, and unassociated with hypergastrinemia.

Type I carcinoids comprise 65% of all carcinoid tumors. They are associated with chronic atrophic autoimmune gastritis; many such carcinoid tumors occur in patients with pernicious anemia. The pathogenesis is as follows: patients with autoimmune gastritis produce auto-antibodies to the oxyntic cells of the gastric mucosa; the inflammatory process causes chronic destruction of these oxyntic cells, resulting in decreased intrinsic factor; decreased intrinsic factor results in decreased vitamin B_{12} absorption; and decreased vitamin B_{12} leads to the development of pernicious anemia. Destruction of the oxyntic epithelium is accompanied by disappearance of the acid-producing parietal cells, an increase in the pH of the stomach, and the loss of negative feedback to the G- (gastrin-producing) cells in the antrum leading to hypergastrinemia. Thus, the constant stimulus of gastric antral gastrin is the physiologic inducer of type I gastric carcinoid. The interval between the initial diagnosis of pernicious anemia and the establishment of gastric carcinoid varies from 1 to 18 years.

Type II neuroendocrine tumors account for approximately 15% of gastric neuroendocrine tumors and are associated with the Zollinger-Ellison syndrome and MEN-I syndrome. The gastrinoma of Zollinger-Ellison syndrome causes hypergastrinemia, which leads to the hypertrophy of chief-, parietal- and ECL-cells. The pathophysiology of this lesion is similar to that of type I gastric neuroendocrine tumors, leading to primary hyperplasia of the ECL cells and secondarily to genetic susceptibility to tumorigenesis. However, unlike the generally benign nature of the type I, type II tumors can be somewhat more aggressive.

Approximately 20% of all gastric carcinoids are type III carcinoids. This group is a sporadic form of carcinoid with no identified predisposing factor. These tumors can be composed of ECL, EC, or X cells. They are more likely to be classified as carcinomas than either type I or type II carcinoids. Grossly, type III tumors tend to be solitary and large (>2 cm in diameter). Instead of gastric fundus or body locations, these tumors are located in the prepyloric region. Type III tumors show a higher propensity for invasion and/or metastases.

In general, gastric neuroendocrine tumors associated with hypergastrinemia are relatively benign, whereas sporadic lesions require aggressive surgical management. Gastric carcinoids, however, can be managed initially by endoscopic resection of accessible tumors, with biopsies surrounding flat mucosa for evaluation of the setting in which they have arisen. This initial endoscopic resection may be followed by regular endoscopic surveillance. Commonly there is a rather vast and non specific constellation of symptoms in those presenting with gastric carcinoid. The majority of patients present with epigastric pain (12% to 80%), vomiting (13% to 19%), hematemesis (24%), diarrhea (12%), weight loss (21%), and melena (13% to 31%). Despite the classic clinical teaching regarding symptoms in patients with carcinoid tumors, only 10% suffer from the "carcinoid syndrome." The carcinoid syndrome is particularly associated with patients with type III gastric carcinoid. The gastric carcinoid

syndrome results from copious production of neuroendocrine hormones including serotonin and tachykinins (substance P, histamine). These hormones clinically manifest as flushing, diarrhea, asthma (bronchoconstriction), facial edema, and headache. Thirty percent of the patients with neuroendocrine tumors show no symptoms.

PATHOLOGIC FINDINGS

GROSS AND ENDOSCOPIC FINDINGS

Generally, gastric neuroendocrine tumors are small polypoid, firm, well-circumscribed elevations of the mucosal surface. Larger tumors can show central umbilicaton with focal superficial erosion (Fig. 4-12). Hypergastrinemia-associated tumors, particularly type II

GASTRIC NEUROENDOCRINE TUMORS—FACT SHEET

Definition
- Neoplasms of the diffuse neuroendocrine system of the gastrointestinal tract

Incidence and Location
- Rare-annual incidence of 1 to 2:100,000
- 6% of all carcinoid tumors
- Account for 30% of gastrointestinal carcinoid tumors
- Occur most commonly in the fundus and body

Morbidity and Mortality
- Type I gastric carcinoid has a 5-year survival rate of > 93%; metastases are rare
- Type III tumors have the worst prognosis
- Type III lesions have a 5-year survival rate of only 50% with a large percentage of these patients developing lymph node metastases and liver metastases
- Type II carcinoids have a prognosis intermediate between types I and III

Gender, Age, and Race Distribution
- Demographics depend on whether the tumor is type I, II, or III
- Type I has a female predominance and a mean diagnosis in the sixth decade
- Type II has no gender predominance and a mean diagnosis in the fourth decade
- Type III has a slight male predominance and a mean diagnosis in the fifth decade

Clinical Features
- Symptoms often vague and nonspecific
- Carcinoid syndrome seen in 10% of cases

Prognosis
- Related to subtype of gastric carcinoid
- Tumor size > 2 cm, increased mitotic rate, nuclear anaplasia, or necrosis are all indicators of possible aggressive behavior

GASTRIC NEUROENDOCRINE TUMORS—PATHOLOGIC FEATURES

Gross Findings

- Small, well-circumscribed submucosal lesions
- Larger tumors can show central umbilicaton
- Gastrin-associated tumors, type II, are often small and have multiple foci
- Type I and II carcinoid tumors commonly located in the corpus and fundus
- Type III tumors tend to be solitary and located in the prepyloric region

Microscopic Findings

- Uniform small round cells with rare mitotic figures
- Fine, speckled chromatin pattern
- Solid, ribbon-like, trabecular or nesting growth patterns

Immunohistochemical Features

- Positive immunoreactivity with the neuroendocrine markers synaptophysin, chromogranin A, or neuron-specific enolase
- Positive immunoreactivity to pancytokeratin markers

Differential Diagnosis

- Glomus tumors

carcinoids, are often small and have multiple foci. Endoscopically, the tumors are mostly located in the corpus and fundus of the stomach and measure less than 1 cm in diameter. As mentioned earlier, type III tumors are located in the prepyloric region and tend to be solitary and larger than types I and II.

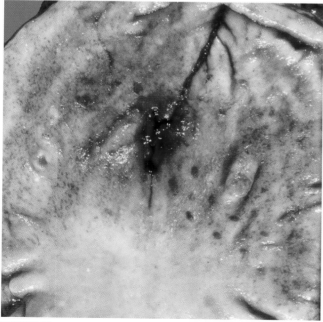

FIGURE 4-12

Gross appearance of gastric carcinoid. Gastric carcinoid presenting as polypoid, firm, well-circumscribed elevations of the mucosal surface. The larger lesions, as shown in this example, show central umbilicaton with focal superficial erosions.

MICROSCOPIC FINDINGS

The morphology of gastric neuroendocrine tumors is similar to neuroendocrine tumors primary to other anatomic sites. There are typically small round proliferating cells growing in patterns of monomorphic nest, trabeculae, festoons, or glandlike formations. Cytologically, the tumor cells have uniform, centrally located nuclei. The chromatin is fine, often displaying a "salt and pepper" pattern, with amphophilic cytoplasm. Typically these lesions are located in the mucosa, often with an overlying intact rim of superficial epithelium (Fig. 4-13A). The tumors can frequently invade the gastric wall, producing a desmoplastic reaction. Histologic features of increased mitotic rate, nuclear anaplasia, or necrosis are all indicators of possible aggressive behavior.

ANCILLARY STUDIES

The diagnosis of gastric neuroendocrine tumors can be confirmed by performing endocrine stains. The gold standard for diagnosis of all gastric neuroendocrine tumors is that they have positive immunohistochemical staining with the neuroendocrine markers synaptophysin, chromogranin A, or neuron-specific enolase (see Fig. 4-13B). Neuroendocrine tumors can also show immunoreactivity to pancytokeratin markers. The expression pattern of tissue-specific transcription factors, such as CDX2, TTF1, and PDX1, can assist in the classification of the primary site of origin in cases of neuroendocrine tumor metastasis. PDX1 expression with absence of CDX2 and TTF1 is strongly correlated with neuroendocrine tumors of gastric or duodenal origin. Immunohistochemical staining may also be performed for the determination of specific hormones expressed by the tumor; although this may be helpful in determining the subtype of gastric carcinoid, these studies are not conclusive.

DIFFERENTIAL DIAGNOSIS

The main differential diagnosis of gastric carcinoid tumors is with glomus tumors. Glomus tumors are composed of small round cells with centrally placed hyperchromatic nuclei and thus are generally similar to carcinoid tumors. However, there are distinct differences. Glomus tumor cells have lumpy, coarse chromatin instead of the finely granular chromatin of carcinoids. In addition, these cells have a pale eosinophilic to clear cytoplasm, whereas carcinoids have amphophilic cytoplasm. Ultrastructurally, glomus tumors have smooth muscle derivation and thus show immunoreactivity for smooth muscle actin. Most importantly, these tumors do not show immunoreactivity for synaptophysin or chromogranin.

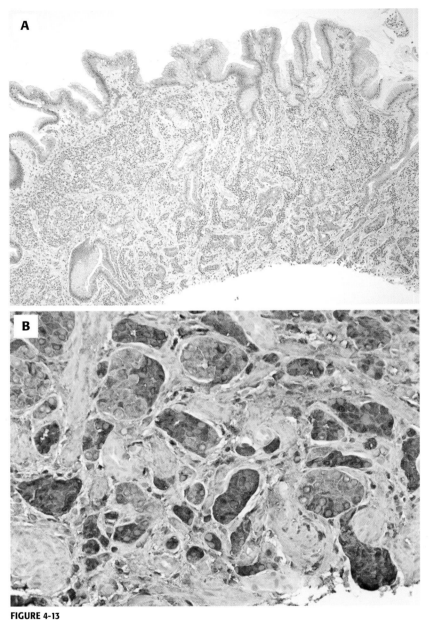

FIGURE 4-13

Histologic features of gastric carcinoid. **A,** Well-differentiated gastric carcinoid lesions are composed of small uniform cells with eosinophilic cytoplasm, centrally located round nuclei with finely dispersed chromatin, and prominent nucleoli. In this example, the tumor cells grow in a trabecular pattern. Typically these lesions are located within the gastric mucosa with an overlying intact rim of superficial epithelium. **B,** Chromogranin is expressed virtually universally in gastric carcinoid tumors. Immunostaining reveals uniform cytoplasmic labeling.

PROGNOSIS AND THERAPY

In general, gastric neuroendocrine tumors have a relatively good prognosis compared with primary epithelial gastric lesions. Gastric neuroendocrine tumors have survival rates that correlate with the extent of tumor spread at the time of diagnosis. The 5-year survival rate of localized versus regional versus distant spread is 73% versus 65% versus 25%, respectively. Among the subtypes of gastric neuroendocrine tumors, type I has the best 5-year survival rate of 93%, yet a small subset of these patients develops lymph node or liver metastases. Not surprisingly, type III tumors have the worst prognosis. It is estimated that patients with these lesions have a 5-year survival rate of 50% with a large percentage developing lymph node and liver metastases. It is important to note that although a worse prognosis may depend on the type of gastric neuroendocrine tumor, the most important and worst prognostic factor for all neuroendocrine tumors is a tumor size of greater than 2 cm. Type II carcinoids have a prognosis between types I and III.

5

Non-Neoplastic and Inflammatory Disorders of the Small Bowel

■ **Chanjuan Shi, MD, PhD** ■ **Elizabeth Montgomery, MD**
■ **Christine A. Iacobuzio-Donahue, MD, PhD**

■ PEPTIC DUODENAL DISEASES

CLINICAL FEATURES

Peptic duodenitis and peptic ulcer disease (PUD) represent a continuum of the same disease process, namely acute and chronic inflammation of the duodenal mucosa resulting from the toxic effects of excess gastric acid. It is most common in Westernized countries and estimated to affect up to 10 % of the population. Peptic disease is more common among patients who are older than 40 years and male.

Our current understanding of peptic duodenal diseases is that gastric peptic ulcers primarily result from altered mucosal defenses, whereas peptic duodenitis and peptic ulcers of the duodenum are associated with increased acid production. Chronic infection with *Helicobacter pylori* is highly correlated with peptic disease of the duodenum and is associated with greater than 80 % of peptic ulcers in this region. Peptic disease of the duodenum is also commonly seen in patients who smoke, take nonsteroidal anti-inflammatory drugs (NSAIDs) chronically for other conditions, have renal insufficiency, or have duodenal immotility, which allows prolonged contact with gastric acid. Cystic fibrosis predisposes to ulcers resulting from decreased bicarbonate secretion.

The clinical features of peptic duodenitis are essentially the same as for PUD, with the most common symptom being burning epigastric pain relieved by eating. In severe cases, the pain may be constant and accompanied by nausea and vomiting.

Patients with multiple duodenal ulcers represent the most severe form of the disease; multiple duodenal ulcers most often accompany Zollinger-Ellison syndrome (ZES). Examples of ulcer disease in ZES include ulcers in the distal duodenum or jejunum, repeated perforating ulcers, or the presence of multiple ulcers. In the absence of ZES, refractory ulcers may be seen in patients with a prior intestinal wall perforation by the ulcer, smokers, chronic NSAID users, patients with gastric outlet obstruction/duodenal stenosis, or individuals who have had a gastric bypass procedure.

PATHOLOGIC FEATURES

GROSS FINDINGS

Peptic duodenitis is most commonly seen in the duodenal bulb. The endoscopic appearance of peptic duodenitis varies from simple erythema to friability, erosions, and nodularity of the mucosa. Nodularity and frank polypoid lesions most often correspond to Brunner's gland hyperplasia. In PUD, patients have symptoms that are similar to those of peptic duodenitis but also have evidence of mucosal ulceration. Duodenal ulcers resemble ulcers in other sites and show complete breakdown of the mucosa (Fig. 5-1).

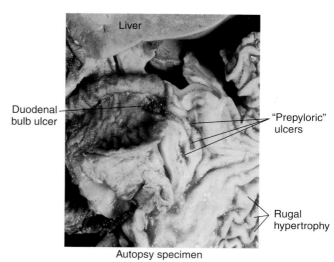

Liver

Duodenal bulb ulcer

"Prepyloric" ulcers

Rugal hypertrophy

Autopsy specimen

FIGURE 5-1

Peptic duodenal ulcer. An acute duodenal ulcer is seen in the bulb. Several small acute ulcers are also present in the prepyloric region.

The edges may show reactive and regenerative epithelial changes, acute inflammation, and granulation tissue formation. Most duodenal ulcers are circular and rarely exceed 3 cm in diameter. Ulcers located posteriorly in the duodenal bulb are more likely to bleed than those located elsewhere because of its proximity to the pancreaticoduodenal and gastroduodenal arteries. Penetration of a duodenal ulcer into one of these vessels may produce massive hemorrhage.

MICROSCOPIC FINDINGS

The microscopic findings characteristic of peptic duodenal disease include one or more of the following: inflammatory cells in the epithelium or lamina propria, damaged epithelium with or without gastric foveolar metaplasia, mucosal hemorrhage and edema, and Brunner's gland hyperplasia with prominent ingrowth above the muscularis mucosae (Figs. 5-2 through 5-4). Gastric foveolar metaplasia provides a definitive clue to the etiology of the mucosal injury and likely represents an adaptation to chronic exposure to hyperacidicity (see Fig. 5-4). In the most severe form, the villi are blunted and may be entirely lost. The superficial epithelium is damaged and shows reactive and regenerative changes, including mild nuclear atypia, as well as gastric foveolar metaplasia and erosions. Active inflammation is present within the villi and crypts (Fig. 5-5). Lymphoid aggregates, vascular dilatation, and edema may all be present. When peptic duodenitis progresses to erosive peptic duodenitis, superficial loss of the

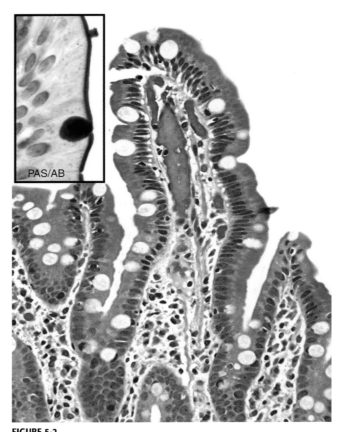

FIGURE 5-2

Normal duodenum, biopsy (H&E). The inset picture shows a combination periodic acid-Schiff and alcian blue (PAS/AB) histochemical stain. The normal brush border forms a discrete alcianophilic line; this brush border is disrupted in many pathologic processes.

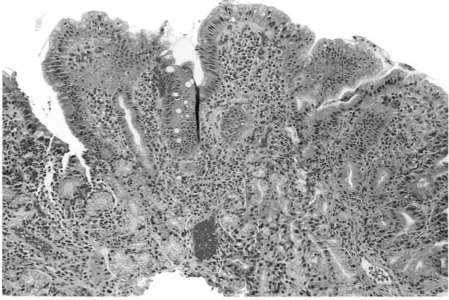

FIGURE 5-3

Chronic active peptic duodenitis, duodenal biopsy (H&E). Surface gastric foveolar metaplasia, increased lamina propria chronic inflammation with patchy active inflammation and prominent intramucosal Brunner glands.

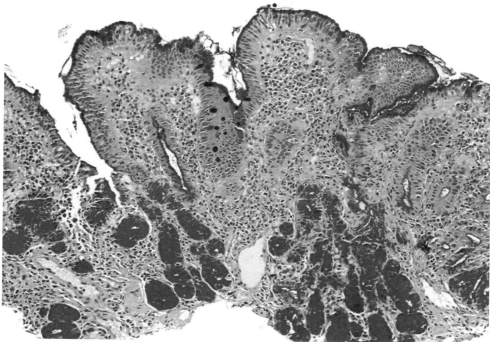

FIGURE 5-4

Chronic active peptic duodenitis, duodenal biopsy (PAS/AB). The PAS highlights the extensive surface gastric foveolar metaplasia and the intramucosal Brunner glands. The only residual alcianophilic epithelium is scattered goblet cells.

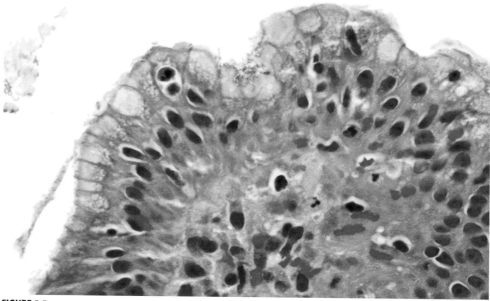

FIGURE 5-5

Chronic peptic duodenitis, duodenal biopsy (H&E). Foveolar metaplasia, with *H. pylori* organisms and neutrophilic inflammation.

duodenal mucosa occurs, leading to mucosal ulceration with associated acutely inflamed granulation tissue, necrosis, and hemorrhage. Often biopsy samples taken from the ulcer edges will show changes of peptic duodenitis (e.g., reactive epithelial changes, gastric foveolar metaplasia).

ANCILLARY STUDIES

Diff-Quik stains have utility in peptic duodenitis by demonstrating the presence of *H. pylori* organisms in association with the metaplastic gastric foveolar epithelium because these cells express the same surface receptors as

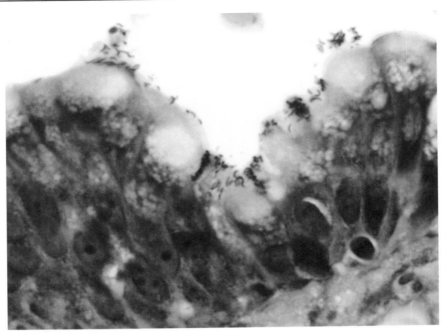

FIGURE 5-6
Chronic peptic duodenitis with *H. pylori* organisms, duodenal biopsy (Diff-Quik stain). The surface of this foveolar metaplasia is covered by *H. pylori* organisms.

normal gastric epithelium (Fig. 5-6). A combination periodic acid-Schiff and alcian blue (PAS/AB) stain highlights the presence of neutral mucin characteristic of the gastric foveolar metaplasia (see Fig. 5-4). "Lipid hang-up" is physiologically normal vacuolization of the enterocyte cytoplasm resulting from a recent fatty meal (Fig. 5-7). These vacuoles are PAS/AB negative (Fig. 5-8); a similar finding is seen in abetalipoproteinemia.

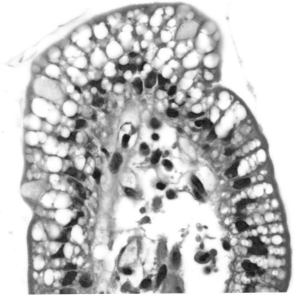

FIGURE 5-7
"Lipid hang-up," duodenal biopsy (H&E). This is physiologically normal enterocyte vacuolization resulting from a recent fatty meal.

DIFFERENTIAL DIAGNOSIS

Other inflammatory disorders that affect the small bowel can enter into the differential diagnosis with peptic changes, including upper gastrointestinal (GI) tract Crohn's disease and portal hypertensive duodenopathy. In both Crohn's disease and portal hypertension, the inflammatory changes in this region may be nonspecific and include mild to moderate villous blunting and chronic inflammation, and gastric mucin cell metaplasia. Specific features to aid in the diagnosis of Crohn's disease include granulomas, possible evidence of lower GI tract inflammatory disease, and the patchy nature of the acute and chronic changes. Gastric heterotopia may also be included in the differential diagnosis with peptic duodenitis resulting from the prominent gastric foveolar epithelium. However, unlike peptic duodenitis, gastric heterotopia can be recognized by normal-appearing oxyntic glands in association with the surface gastric mucinous epithelium.

PROGNOSIS AND THERAPY

The eradication of *H. pylori* and the use of acid-suppressive therapies improve symptoms in most patients with peptic duodenitis. Medical therapy is mainly intended to reduce gastric acid by small meals, antacids, and histamine-2 (H_2) blockers. Antibiotics may be added to the treatment regimen if *H. pylori* organisms are present. Avoidance of

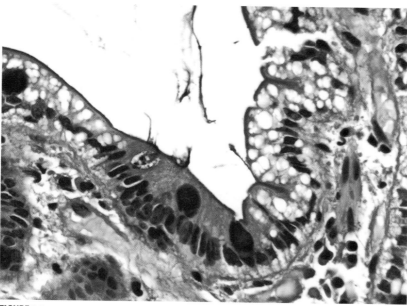

FIGURE 5-8

"Lipid hang-up," duodenal biopsy (PAS/AB). The enterocyte vacuolization in lipid hang-up is PAS/AB negative, and the overlying alcianophilic brush border is intact (compare with PAS-positive foveolar metaplasia in Fig. 5-4). The center shows a section of nonvacuolated normal enteroctyes.

substances that promote gastric acid secretion, such as ethanol or aspirin is also recommended.

Bleeding ulcers are estimated to be responsible for up to 50 % of all cases of acute hemorrhage from the upper GI tract. Up to 5 % of patients may have bleeding that is brisk enough to cause hematochezia. Even if initially controlled, re-bleeding can affect up to one third of patients, most commonly patients in the seventh decade of life or beyond, or those with a visible vessel in the ulcer base. Refractory ulcers heal slowly or follow a relapsing and remitting course. Scarring of duodenal ulcers may lead to duodenal stricturing and obstruction.

Free perforation of a duodenal ulcer into the peritoneal cavity can be a catastrophic, life-threatening event. Most patients with this complication are elderly, and the perforations are associated with NSAID use in up to half of cases. However, in patients younger than 75 years, smoking may be a stronger risk factor for perforation than NSAIDs.

■ MALABSORPTIVE DISORDERS

The term *malabsorption* is broadly used to describe any type or degree of dysfunction in the uptake of substances that are normally retained or absorbed by the small intestine. The underlying causes of malabsorption are broad and include luminal factors such as lactose deficiency and motility disorders, among others. In contrast, the malabsorption syndrome more specifically refers to the constellation of clinical findings that include

diarrhea, steatorrhea, and associated secondary changes including weight loss and vitamin deficiencies from reduced absorption of nutrients.

CELIAC DISEASE

CLINICAL FEATURES

Once considered to be a rare childhood disorder, celiac disease (CD; also known as gluten-induced enteropathy, celiac sprue, or nontropical sprue) is now understood to be a multisystem autoimmune disorder that affects 1 % of the population. In the most comprehensive U.S. study in which more than 13,000 adult and pediatric patients were screened, the overall prevalence of CD in a group with no risk factors was 1:133, while it was 1:22 in the first-degree relatives of an index case, 1:39 in second-degree relatives, and 1:56 in patients with either GI symptoms or an extragastrointestinal disorder associated with CD. The mean age of diagnosis is in middle adulthood.

According to the guidelines proposed by the European Society for Pediatric Gastroenterology and Nutrition and on recommendations from the National Institutes of Health Consensus Conference on Celiac Disease, unequivocal evidence of improvement on a gluten-free diet (GFD) is needed for definitive diagnosis of symptomatic CD. Celiac disease is present if histologic changes are found on small intestinal biopsy while the patient consumes a gluten-containing diet and unequivocal clinical improvement occurs while he or she maintains a GFD. A diagnosis of CD based solely on serologic markers (anti-transglutaminase II and anti-endomysial immunoglobulin A [IgA] is not accepted practice.

The classification and diagnosis of CD are based on GI manifestations; however, patients with extraintestinal complications are increasingly being recognized (Table 5-1). The clinical presentation of CD ranges from asymptomatic to severe malnutrition. The most common manifestations of CD include abdominal pain, increased frequency of bowel movements, weight loss, bone disease, anemia, and weakness. CD may be divided into three clinical subtypes. In the classic, symptomatic form of the disease, patients exhibit chronic diarrhea, abdominal distension, pain, weakness, and, in advanced cases, malabsorption. In contrast, in the atypical form of the disease, GI symptoms may be less pronounced to absent. Instead, extraintestinal features such as anemia, osteoporosis, short stature, infertility, and neurologic

TABLE 5-1

Extragastrointestinal Disorders Associated with Celiac Disease

Endocrine disorders
Type 1 diabetes mellitus
Autoimmune thyroid disorders
Addison's disease
Reproductive disorders (infertility, miscarriages)
Osteoporosis
Alopecia areata
Neurologic disorders
Cerebellar ataxia
Neuropathy
Epilepsy
Migraines
Cardiac disorders
Idiopathic dilated cardiomyopathy
Autoimmune myocarditis
Hepatic disorders
Primary biliary cirrhosis
Autoimmune hepatitis
Autoimmune cholangitis
Other
Dermatitis herpetiformis
Anemia
Selective IgA deficiency
Sjögren's syndrome
Juvenile chronic arthritis
Turner's syndrome
Down syndrome
Dental enamel defects

problems are predominant. Finally, some patients have asymptomatic or silent CD; they lack classic or atypical symptoms but have unequivocal villous atrophy found incidentally for other reasons or following serologic screening.

The pathogenesis of CD involves environmental, genetic, and immunologic features, and can be viewed as both luminal events and cellular events leading to the eventual activation of immune cells and ensuing tissue damage.

ENVIRONMENTAL

Enteric exposures to certain glutamine-rich proteins in the dietary grains wheat, rye, and barley are known to be essential for the development of CD. The actual proteins that can trigger the disease are the gliadins in wheat, the hordeins in barley, and the secalins in rye. Many of these peptides are poorly digested by the intestinal tract proteases and make their way intact through the epithelium into the lamina propria. Once in the lamina propria, intact peptides are deamidated by tissue transglutaminase converting the abundant glutamine residues to glutamic acid, thus rendering them negatively charged. The negative charged peptides are more efficiently bound to the specific HLA-DQ2 or HLA-DQ8 receptors on the surface of the antigen presenting cells. Intestinal DQ2- or DQ8-restricted CD4+ T cells then recognize the deamidated gliadin peptides and elaborate inflammatory cytokines.

GENETIC

The major genetic risk factors for CD are the HLA class II genes *HLA-DQ2* and *HLA-DQ8*. Approximately 95% of all patients with CD have a DQ2 heterodimer, and almost all remaining patients with CD have a DQ8 heterodimer. Gene dosage correlates with the risk for developing CD, with patients homozygous for DQ2 carrying the greatest risk. CD is concordant in 70% to 80% of monozygotic twins, 30% to 40% of HLA-identical siblings, and less than 20% of dizygotic twins, a rate similar to that for all first-degree relatives. However, recent linkage studies suggest that non-HLA disease-associated genes may also play a role.

IMMUNOLOGIC

It is well accepted that DQ2- and DQ8-restricted CD4+ T-cell populations that recognize disease-activating peptides are present in the intestinal mucosa of CD patients. When activated, these cells elaborate cytokines such as interferon-γ that promote inflammation and intestinal injury. Nonspecific upregulation of the gut immune system may also play a role, as evidenced by the frequent overt clinical GI symptoms that develop in

CELIAC DISEASE—FACT SHEET

Definition

- A multisystem autoimmune disorder caused by an immune response to dietary gluten and related proteins

Incidence

- 1% of the U.S. population
- 1 in 133 patients with no risk factors
- 1 in 29 patients with at least one first-degree relative with CD

Morbidity and Mortality

- 20-fold higher risk for enteropathy-associated T-cell lymphoma
- 30-fold higher risk for small intestinal adenocarcinomas
- 2- to 4-fold higher risk for oropharyngeal and esophageal carcinomas

Gender, Race, and Age Distribution

- Wide age range: children and adults
- Well known in Northern Europeans, rare in Southeast Asians, incidence unknown in Africans, common in pockets in the Middle East

Clinical Features

- Variable: ranges from asymptomatic to severe malnutrition
- Most common presentation is weight loss, abdominal pain, diarrhea
- Extraintestinal manifestations include type 1 diabetes, osteoporosis, dermatitis herpetiformis, and various neuropathies

Prognosis and Therapy

- Complete resolution of GI pathology with strict GFD
- Refractory CD refers to those patients on GFD without resolution of disease—up to 80% of cases associated with a clonal T-cell population.

CELIAC DISEASE—PATHOLOGIC FEATURES

Gross Findings

- Attenuated to absent villi (as seen under a dissecting microscope)

Microscopic Findings

- Variable degrees of villous atrophy
- Chronic inflammation
- Intraepithelial lymphocytes
- Epithelial damage
- Crypt hyperplasia

Differential Diagnosis

- Bacterial overgrowth
- Colchicine toxicity
- Refractory sprue
- Lymphocytic enteritis
- Radiation enteritis

patients with clinically silent CD after viral gastroenteritis, traveler's diarrhea, or GI surgery.

High-risk groups to be screened for CD are those with the presence of other autoimmune diseases such as type 1 diabetes mellitus and autoimmune thyroiditis, a family history of CD, selective IgA deficiency, or dermatitis herpetiformis. CD is also more common in certain pediatric populations, including those with Down syndrome, where the frequency of CD is as high as 10%. In this group, CD is usually not detectable on the basis of GI symptoms. Other manifestations may dominate the clinical picture, including failure to thrive, osteoporosis, refractory iron deficiency anemia, arthritis, peripheral neuropathies, cerebellar ataxia, dermatitis herpetiformis, and infertility.

PATHOLOGIC FEATURES

GROSS FINDINGS

Typically the gross specimen consists of a tiny biopsy. If the specimen is assessed under a dissecting microscope (which is seldom done), delicate villi are attenuated to absent. Endoscopically, villous flattening can be suggested.

MICROSCOPIC FINDINGS

The hallmark features of CD are intraepithelial and lamina propria chronic inflammation leading to villous atrophy and malabsorption. The earliest change in CD is the presence of increased intraepithelial lymphocytes within the villi and throughout the villous epithelium with extension to the villous tips (Fig. 5-9). With persistent disease, epithelial damage ensues with associated villous blunting, crypt hyperplasia, and increased chronic inflammation of the lamina propria (Figs. 5-10 and 5-11). In severe CD, complete loss of villous architecture is seen with the bowel mucosa appearing atrophic. The patient may or may not have active inflammation, but it is usually focal. Because the disease may be patchy, up to six different biopsy samples must be taken. Such sampling will ensure that some sections will be oriented correctly to determine the degree of villous atrophy, as well as the degree of epithelial lymphocytosis, epithelial damage, and inflammation.

Upon initiation of a GFD, patients often report a marked improvement in symptoms. Microscopically, intestinal biopsies show diminished surface epithelial injury, a reduced number of intraepithelial lymphocytes, and partial return of villous architecture. Long-term changes on a GFD include return to normal villous architecture, normal mitotic proliferative activity, and clearance of chronic inflammation. If gluten is restored to the diet, a rapid return of all lesions and malabsorption will ensue.

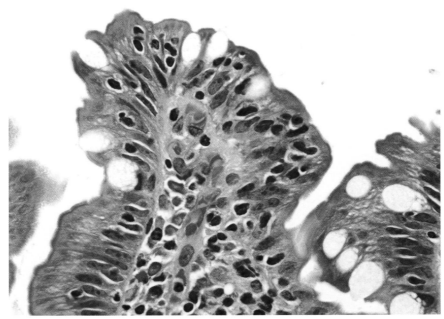

FIGURE 5-9

Latent celiac disease, duodenal biopsy (H&E). Increase in villus intraepithelial lymphocytes with normal villus architecture. The villus intraepithelial lymphocytes are more numerous at the tip of the villus, a characteristic pattern of celiac disease.

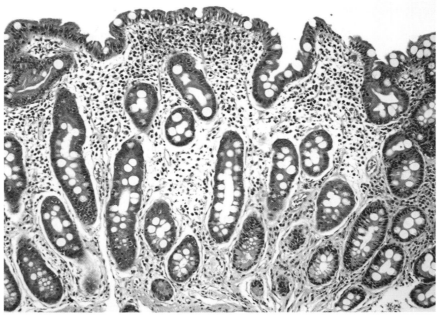

FIGURE 5-10

Celiac disease, duodenal biopsy (H&E). Fully developed celiac disease showing marked villous blunting, increased surface intraepithelial lymphocytes, and marked crypt hyperplasia.

ANCILLARY STUDIES

The histologic features of CD on routine stains are quite characteristic; thus, ancillary studies are not necessary for the diagnosis, although some observers have advocated immunophenotyping of intraepithelial lymphocytes (see Fig. 5-11).

DIFFERENTIAL DIAGNOSIS

In the absence of an appropriate clinical history, a number of additional entities can enter into the differential diagnosis of CD based on the histologic features, including tropical sprue, bacterial overgrowth, and various drug toxicities such as colchicine. In tropical sprue, the

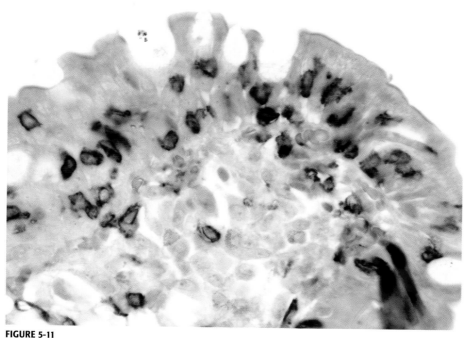

FIGURE 5-11

Celiac disease, duodenal biopsy (CD3 immunohistochemistry). CD3 highlights an increased number of intraepithelial T-lymphocytes in this blunted duodenal villus.

characteristic histologic changes are resulting from a postinfectious enteritis. A travel history and appropriate serologic studies for infectious organisms may help determine this possibility. In bacterial overgrowth syndrome, in addition to the villous atrophy, the degree of active inflammation of the villi and crypts is often in excess of that expected for CD. A prior history of abdominal surgery or bypass procedure may be found in these patients and in some cases a prior antibiotic history. Finally, in some patients taking colchicine for gout or other indication, small bowel damage simulating CD may be found. The histologic clues are numerous ring mitoses and loss of goblet cell polarity.

PROGNOSIS AND THERAPY

A lifelong adherence to a GFD is the mainstay of safe and effective treatment of CD. Commonly substituted grains in the GFD include rice, corn, quinoa, and buckwheat. Serum antiendomysial, anti-transglutaminase II, and antigliadin antibodies are used to screen and check the effectiveness of a GFD. Patients whose disease does not respond to dietary therapy should undergo a systematic evaluation including review of the patients' diet by an expert dietician and review of the original biopsy slides. Associated conditions that must be ruled out include pancreatic insufficiency, lymphocytic colitis, bacterial overgrowth, and true refractory sprue with a clonal T-cell population.

The most frequent malignant complication of CD is a high-grade T-cell non-Hodgkin's lymphoma (NHL) of the upper small intestine defined as enteropathy-associated T-cell lymphoma (EATL). This rare T-cell disorder is 20 times more common in patients with CD. The EATL immunophenotype is consistent with a derivation from a clonal proliferation of intraepithelial lymphocytes (IELs). In some cases, EATL represents the end-stage evolution of refractory CD unresponsive to a GFD. In 80% of cases of refractory CD, an abnormal clonal population of IELs can be demonstrated characterized by T-cell receptor gene rearrangement. This is the precursor lesion to EATL, and it is associated with a high risk for ulcerative jejunitis and lymphomatous transformation characterized clinically by weight loss, diarrhea, abdominal pain, fever, lymphadenopathy, hepatomegaly, and at times a palpable abdominal mass. Approximately 50% of patients require laparotomy for complications of hemorrhage, perforation, or obstruction. In previous studies, the 5-year survival rate was 10%.

Patients with CD have more than a 30-fold increased risk for small bowel adenocarcinoma as compared with the general population, and 13% of patients with a small bowel adenocarcinoma have underlying CD. Other malignancies potentially associated with CD include papillary thyroid carcinoma and malignant melanoma.

The question of whether the early diagnosis and treatment of CD reduces the risk for developing other autoimmune diseases is still under debate. There are several lines of evidence that support the notion that

CD is a causative factor in the development of other autoimmune diseases. The presence of autoimmune disease is closely related to the duration of gluten exposure and the age of initiation of a GFD, with children diagnosed and treated before 2 years of age having little subsequent increased risk. Older children diagnosed with CD have a higher than expected frequency of organ-specific autoantibodies that tend to disappear after starting a GFD.

UNCOMMON CAUSES OF MALABSORPTION

A rare but important disorder related to CD is tropical sprue (postinfective tropical malabsorption), defined as intestinal malabsorption of unknown etiology, occurring among residents in or visitors to the tropics. No single etiologic agent has been identified to account for tropical sprue. However, evidence in favor of an infectious etiology is that an infection often initiates and sustains tropical sprue; tropical sprue occurs in specific geographic areas (West Indies and the Indian subcontinent) where enteric infections are common; in some areas tropical sprue is endemic; aerobic bacteria colonize the patient's small intestine and may be toxic producing; and recovery from tropical sprue with antibiotics is usually rapid and dramatic. Protozoan infections such as with *Cyclospora* have been suggested to play a role. Other factors such as epithelial damage may also contribute to the condition because folate and vitamin B_{12} deficiencies are commonly present in these patients. In severe tropical sprue there can be resulting diminution in epithelial mitosis accompanied by nuclear enlargement, changes that are the epithelial counterpart to maturational derangements in the marrow and macrocytic anemia (megaloblastic changes). Genetic or ethnic predispositions have also been suggested.

The mucosal lesion in tropical sprue is nonspecific, with epithelial blunting, chronic inflammation, and focal neutrophil infiltrates in the epithelium and lamina propria (Fig. 5-12). A completely flat biopsy finding like that seen in CD is rare in tropical sprue, but epithelial dysfunction, as in CD, is central to its pathogenesis. Unlike CD, in which mucosal changes are greatest in the proximal small bowel, lesions in the ileum are as prominent as in the proximal small bowel in tropical sprue. This fits well with the resulting secondary vitamin B_{12} and folate deficiency states that are uncommon in CD. Intraepithelial lymphocytes are increased in tropical sprue but are often more numerous in the crypts than in the villi.

Bacterial overgrowth is another cause of malabsorption. All causes of bacterial overgrowth are related to stasis; thus, these disorders are also known as stasis syndrome. Causes of stasis in the small bowel include motor/neural disorders such as diabetic neuropathy and scleroderma, as well as structural lesions, such as diverticula and surgical anastomoses. The pathophysiology of stasis is largely caused by anaerobic bacteria that deconjugate bile salts, deplete vitamin B_{12}, and damage surface epithelium. Stasis in the small bowel, regardless of the etiology, may result in abnormal inflammatory changes in the mucosa. As with most small bowel disorders, the histologic features are nonspecific and include mild to moderate villous blunting, which may be accompanied by an increase in lamina propria mononuclear cells and focal neutrophilic infiltrates in the epithelium. At low power these changes may mimic partially developed or treated CD, although bacterial overgrowth typically lacks the intense intraepithelial lymphocytosis of CD, and the findings may be focal.

■ MICROVILLUS INCLUSION DISEASE

Microvillus inclusion disease is one of several causes of intractable diarrhea in infancy.

CLINICAL FEATURES

Babies with intractable diarrhea of infancy have a clinical presentation including the presence of diarrhea for more than 2 weeks, severe nutritional malabsorption, and negative stool cultures. Their condition is life-threatening and can require total parenteral nutrition. When a baby has such a presentation, the clinical differential diagnosis is mostly among autoimmune enteropathy and lesions displaying primary enterocyte abnormalities. These are rare conditions and are considered once causes of protracted diarrhea (which responds to bowel rest in contrast to intractable diarrhea) are excluded (Bruton's agammaglobulinemia, allergic enteropathy, and severe infection).

Microvillus inclusion disease is an uncommon congenital enteropathy, producing intractable secretory diarrhea in early infancy. It is an inherited disease in an autosomal-recessive genetic trait pattern and, not surprisingly, more common among highly inbred populations. Synonyms used for this disease include Davidson's disease, familial microvillus atrophy, congenital microvillus atrophy, and intestinal microvillus dystrophy (a variant of microvillus inclusion disease). The outcome is typically poor, with most patients requiring small bowel transplantation. Rare cases have resolved.

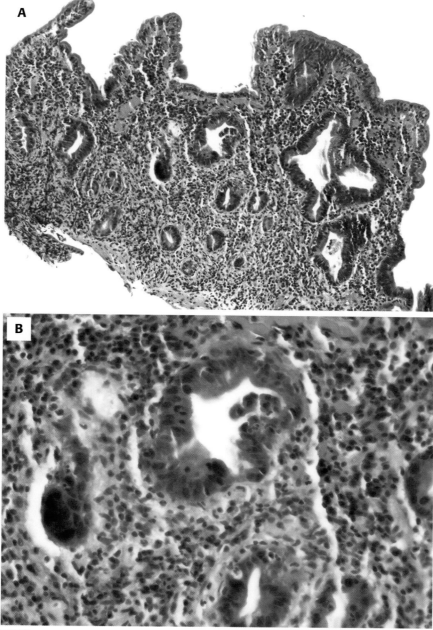

FIGURE 5-12
Tropic sprue, duodenal biopsy (H&E). **A,** There are villous attenuation and increased chronic inflammation in the lamina propria. **B,** Focal neutrophil infiltrates are seen in the epithelium and in the lamina propria.

PATHOLOGIC FEATURES

GROSS FINDINGS

Microvillus inclusion disease usually results in biopsy specimens rather than specific gross specimens.

MICROSCOPIC FINDINGS

Biopsy samples of duodenal mucosa show moderate villous blunting with no active inflammatory reaction or intraepithelial lymphocytosis. The optimal specimen is a small intestinal sample; duodenal biopsy is

MICROVILLUS INCLUSION DISEASE—FACT SHEET

Definition

- A primary enterocyte anomaly that results in intractable diarrhea of infancy

Incidence and Location

- Rare

Morbidity and Mortality

- High morbidity and mortality

Gender, Race, and Age Distribution

- No gender predominance, affects infants, autosomal recessive, common in populations prone to consanguinity (tribal Saudis, Native Americans)

Clinical Features

- Intractable diarrhea of infancy requiring total parenteral nutrition

Prognosis and Therapy

- Invariably fatal without surgical intervention (small bowel transplantation) or total parenteral nutrition

MICROVILLUS INCLUSION DISEASE—PATHOLOGIC FEATURES

Gross Findings

- Villous atrophy

Microscopic Findings

- Atrophic villi without inflammation
- Damaged brush border

Ancillary Studies

- CD10 immunohistochemistry highlights the damaged brush border
- Ultrastructural studies show intraepithelial inclusions

Differential Diagnosis

- Celiac disease
- Variant forms (e.g., tufting enteropathy)

most commonly used. Architecturally, diffuse intestinal villous atrophy without inflammation is a characteristic feature. Because of increased crypt cell apoptosis, either crypt hypoplasia or hyperplasia can be found. The characteristic histologic changes in the enterocytes are confined to the villous tips and distal villous lateral borders. Changes are difficult to discern at the base of the villus and in the crypt epithelium; the enterocytes appear normal in these regions. Cytologically, a bubbly vacuolated appearance of the apical cytoplasm with extensive or patchy absence of the brush border is a specific sign for the diagnosis (Fig. 5-13). Typical targetoid cytoplasmic inclusions are occasionally identified in the surface enterocytes. Instead of a sharp linear brush border that stains with PAS or alkaline phosphatase histochemically, a bright apical cytoplasmic blush is present and is the most easily recognized change of microvillus inclusion disease (Fig. 5-14).

ANCILLARY STUDIES

ULTRASTRUCTURAL FINDINGS

Ultrastructurally, identification of apical microvillus inclusions in surface enterocytes in intestinal tract biopsy samples makes a definitive diagnosis, and adhesion molecule defects have been implicated (Fig. 5-15). It is important to ensure that surface enterocytes are studied; villus base and crypt enterocytes may lack inclusions.

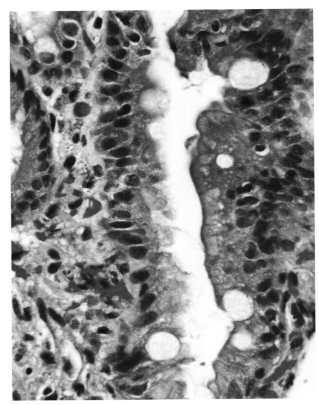

FIGURE 5-13

Microvillus inclusion disease, duodenal biopsy (H&E). The section of enterocytes on the left have complete loss of the brush border and apical vacuolization (special stains show these vacuoles to have the same staining affinities as the normal brush border [e.g., alcianophilic, CD10 positive]). The section of enterocytes on the right have an intact brush border, but do have early apical vacuolization.

IMMUNOHISTOCHEMISTRY

Brush border biomarkers, such as carcinoembryonic antigen (CEA) and particularly CD10, are also useful in the diagnosis of microvillus inclusion disease. CEA and CD10 stains demonstrate a characteristic apical cytoplasmic staining pattern in the enterocytes (Fig. 5-16).

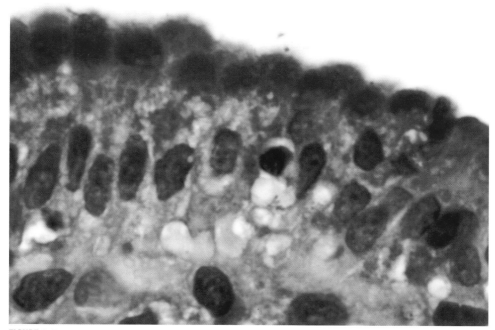

FIGURE 5-14

Microvillus inclusion disease, duodenal biopsy (PAS/AB). The apical vacuoles here are alcianophilic. Notice complete absence of normal brush border (compare with Fig. 5-1).

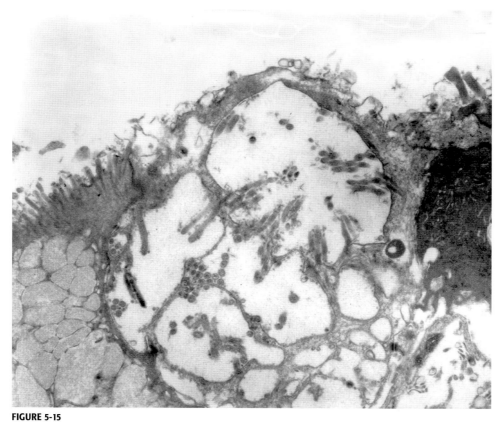

FIGURE 5-15

Microvillus inclusion disease, duodenal biopsy. The enterocyte cytoplasmic vacuoles are shown to be full of microvilli. The overlying and adjacent surface has abnormal villi.

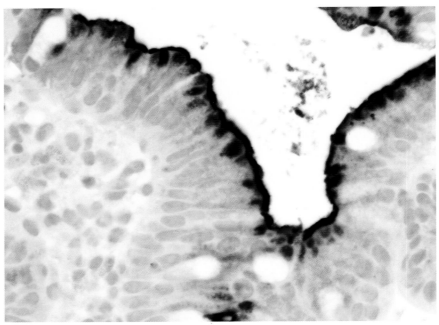

FIGURE 5-16

Microvillus inclusion disease, duodenal biopsy (MVID; CD10 immunohistochemistry). The CD10 stain mirrors other brush border markers in MVID (alkaline phosphatase, PAS/AB, carcinoembryonic antigen, etc.), which all show an apical cytoplasmic blush instead of the normal restriction of staining to a discrete brush border.

DIFFERENTIAL DIAGNOSIS

A variant of this condition (possibly an incomplete form) is called "tufting enteropathy" or "intestinal epithelial dysplasia" and features epithelial "tufts" at the tips of blunted villi (disorganized surface enterocytes with focal crowding). Because the clinical differential diagnosis is with autoimmune enteropathy, this must also be considered. It differs by featuring variable villous atrophy, a prominent lamina propria mononuclear infiltrate, intraepithelial lymphocytosis in the crypt, and depletion of goblet and Paneth cells.

PROGNOSIS AND THERAPY

The prognosis is poor. Small bowel transplantation is often attempted, but most patients do not survive to adulthood.

■ LYMPHANGIECTASIA

CLINICAL FEATURES

Primary intestinal lymphangiectasia is usually diagnosed before the age of 3 years. Most patients have growth retardation. GI complaints that vary in severity consist of diarrhea, vomiting, abdominal pain, and steatorrhea. If large segments of the gut are involved, secondary edema resulting from protein-losing enteropathy and malabsorption may occur. The edema is usually generalized, but asymmetric edema is not uncommon.

RADIOLOGIC FEATURES

Reported findings in lymphangiectasia on computed tomography (CT) include diffuse nodular thickening of the bowel wall with ascites in the absence of adenopathy or hepatosplenomegaly. Hypodense streaks of the small bowel wall secondary to markedly dilated lymphatic channels are also described. A "halo sign," or the presence of three rings on CT imaging, is also seen. A low-attenuation inner ring is pathologically correlated with dilated lacteals, focal edema, and an increased number of foamy histiocytes within the jejunal mucosa. The middle ring of very low attenuation represents dilatation of the lacteals and edema in the submucosa. The higher attenuation outer ring is imparted by the remainder of the bowel wall: the muscularis propria and serosa.

PATHOLOGIC FEATURES

GROSS FINDINGS

Resections are not performed for this condition, but the mucosa displays features of lymphangiectasia at endoscopy; white villi or spots are seen, as are white nodules and submucosal elevations with or without white mucosa.

PRIMARY INTESTINAL LYMPHANGIECTASIA (WALDMANN'S DISEASE)—FACT SHEET

Definition
- Rare digestive disorder characterized by abnormally enlarged (dilated) lymph vessels supplying the lamina propria of the small intestine

Incidence and Location
- Unknown

Morbidity and Mortality
- Growth retardation common
- Reduced life span
- Poor prognosis associated with delay in diagnosis

Gender, Race, and Age Distribution
- Presents in infancy
- No gender or racial predilection

Clinical Features
- Edema and nonbloody diarrhea
- Edema in primary intestinal lymphangiectasia is usually bilateral
- Secondary types often manifest as unilateral edema, which is caused by various neoplastic, infiltrative, and inflammatory lesions affecting one side of the body
- Steatorrhea, malabsorption, lymphocytopenia, and hypogammaglobulinemia
- Chylous ascites and chylous pleural effusions

Prognosis and Therapy
- The long-term course is variable
- Slow progression with intermittent clinical remissions
- Treatments include a high-protein, low-fat diet with added medium-chain triglycerides; octreotides have been reported to decrease intestinal protein losses

PRIMARY INTESTINAL LYMPHANGIECTASIA (WALDMANN DISEASE)—PATHOLOGIC FEATURES

Gross Findings
- Numerous white spots at endoscopy

Microscopic Findings
- Many dilated lacteals with no inflammatory process

Differential Diagnosis
- Dilated lacteals resulting from obstruction. Diagnosis requires clinicopathologic correlation

MICROSCOPIC FINDINGS

Small biopsy samples taken from these patients may be nondiagnostic, but they simply display multiple dilated lacteals, a finding easy to overlook without knowledge of an often dramatic CT appearance (Fig. 5-17).

DIFFERENTIAL DIAGNOSIS

The differential diagnosis is lymphangiectasia from extramural obstruction or from certain infections (e.g., Whipple's disease [WD], mycobacterial enteritis). The diagnosis is thus a clinicopathologic one, although the infectious etiologies are excluded by noting macrophages and performing appropriate special stains.

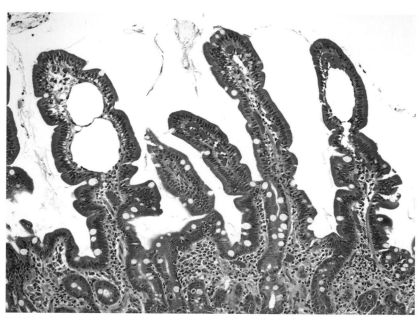

FIGURE 5-17
Primary intestinal lymphangiectasia, duodenal biopsy (H&E). Dilated lymphatics in small intestinal villi are a nonspecific finding, but in the context of endoscopic and clinical findings can be diagnostic of primary lymphangiectasia.

PROGNOSIS AND THERAPY

The long-term course is variable, but the disease is usually slow to progress, with intermittent clinical remissions. The reported medical treatments of lymphangiectasia are a high-protein, low-fat diet with added medium-chain triglycerides. Octreotides have been reported to decrease intestinal protein losses.

■ INFECTIOUS ENTERITIS

The majority of infectious agents that affect the colon can also affect the small bowel, and these are addressed in Chapter 9. In particular, *Yersinia* species, viral agents, and histoplasmosis are found in the small bowel and may mimic Crohn's disease. Somewhat unique to the small bowel is WD.

CLINICAL FEATURES

WD is a rare systemic bacterial infection caused by *Tropheryma whipplei* (an actinomycete). WD was first described by George Whipple at Johns Hopkins in 1907 as "intestinal lipodystrophy" based on accumulation of lipids in intestinal mucosa and lymph nodes. The bacterial etiology of this condition was confirmed by electron microscopy in 1961.

There is a striking male predominance (8 to 10:1); white men in the fourth to fifth decades of life are most commonly affected. Patients present with diarrhea, low-grade fever, weight loss, malabsorption, abdominal pain, arthralgia, anemia, lymphadenopathy (50%), and cardiac and central nervous system symptoms (10%). WD usually involves the postbulbar duodenum and jejunum. Thus, biopsy samples should be taken from both the proximal and distal duodenum, as well as the jejunum.

PATHOLOGIC FEATURES

GROSS FINDINGS

Endoscopically, the lesions can present as yellowish white plaques or as pale yellow shaggy mucosa, or they can have an erythematous, friable appearance.

MICROSCOPIC FINDINGS

The characteristic appearance of small intestinal biopsy consists of blunted and rounded villi with distension of the lamina propria by foamy pink macrophages

---

WHIPPLE'S DISEASE—FACT SHEET

Definition
- An infection caused by *Tropheryma whipplei* (an actinomycete) that most commonly affects the proximal small bowel (but may affect any organ, including the central nervous system)

Incidence and Location
- Rare

Morbidity and Mortality
- Low if the disease is recognized and treated

Gender, Race, and Age Distribution
- Most common in white males, usually adults

Clinical Features
- Diarrhea and malabsorption
- Low-grade fever
- Weight loss
- Abdominal pain, arthralgias, and anemia
- Lymphadenopathy (50%)
- Cardiac and central nervous system symptoms (10%)

Prognosis and Therapy
- Good with appropriate antibiotic therapy

WHIPPLE'S DISEASE—PATHOLOGIC FEATURES

Gross Findings
- Yellowish white plaques, pale yellow shaggy mucosa, or an erythematous friable appearance at endoscopy

Microscopic Findings
- Blunted and rounded villi with distention of lamina propria by foamy pink macrophages and dilated lacteals

Ancillary Studies
- PAS-D stains demonstrate macrophages containing PAS-positive, diastase-resistant rod- or sickle-shaped bacterial inclusions.

Differential Diagnosis
- Infection with *Mycobacterium avium* species

(Figs. 5-18 and 5-19). The macrophages contain PAS-positive, diastase-resistant rod- or sickle-shaped bacterial inclusions. The bacterial inclusions can also be present in the extracellular space of the lamina propria, and in epithelial cells, fibroblasts, endothelial cells, and smooth muscle. Lymphatic obstruction gives rise to dilated lacteals containing lipid deposits, a helpful feature that suggests the diagnosis of WD on hematoxylin and eosin stain. The classic histologic

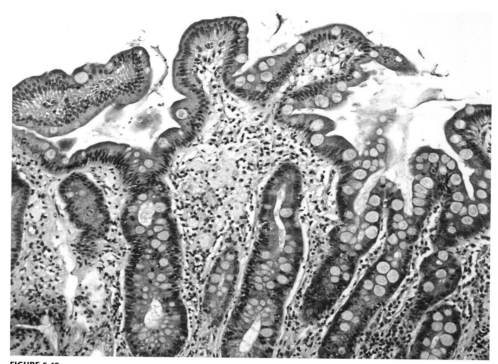

FIGURE 5-18

Whipple's disease, duodenal biopsy (H&E). There is mild villus blunting and distension of lamina propria by an infiltrate of foamy histiocytes (*center*).

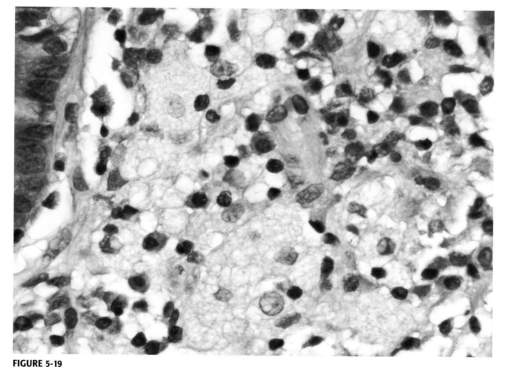

FIGURE 5-19

Whipple's disease, duodenal biopsy (H&E). Foamy histiocytes typical of Whipple's disease. Special stains are needed to exclude other causes of increased lamina propria histiocytes.

features of intensely PAS-positive foamy macrophages and dilated lacteals with large lipid droplets are characteristic of WD.

ANCILLARY STUDIES

ULTRASTRUCTURAL FINDINGS

The etiologic agent is seen as intracellular rods.

IMMUNOHISTOCHEMISTRY

The Whipple antigen can be detected by immunohistochemical analysis using a polyclonal rabbit antibody produced against a cultured strain of *T. whipplei* (Fig. 5-20). The antigen is a component of the bacterial cell wall. This is a sensitive and specific method.

OTHER STUDIES

Polymerase chain reaction (PCR) assays for 16S ribosomal RNA genes of *T. whipplei* are available. With electron microscopy, PAS stain, and Whipple immunostain, it is still possible to see retained bacterial products months and even years after initiation of therapy despite clinical improvement. Thus, PCR may be the best tool to monitor treatment response because the bacterium has been

shown to become undetectable shortly after initiation of antibiotic treatment. The bacterium of WD has also been successfully grown in a human fibroblast cell line.

DIFFERENTIAL DIAGNOSIS

The differential diagnosis includes other causes of foamy macrophages in the lamina propria, such as *Mycobacterium avium* complex infection and malacoplakia (see Chapter 9). The prominent dilatation of lacteals together with PAS-positive macrophages favors WD. Mycobacterial enteritis displays less striking dilatation of lacteals, and acid fast stains highlight the agent. The typical targetoid (Michaelis Gutmann) bodies are sought to diagnose malacoplakia, but GI tract malacoplakia more typically affects the colon.

PROGNOSIS AND THERAPY

Most patients respond dramatically to antibiotics (trimethoprim and sulfamethoxazole). However, some patients can have a chronic relapsing course, with organisms persisting in affected tissues for a long time despite extended antibiotic treatment.

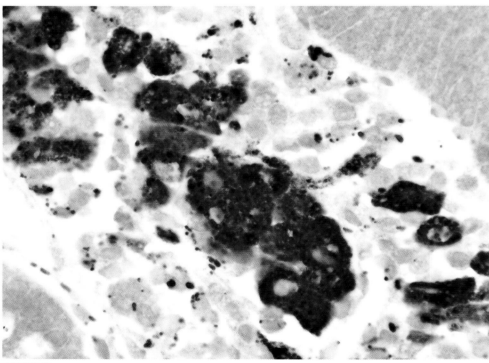

FIGURE 5-20
Whipple's disease, duodenal biopsy (Whipple immunohistochemistry). Although the organisms can be seen on PAS stain, this is not specific to *Tropheryma whipplei* (e.g., *Mycobacterium avium-intracellulare* [MAI] also stains with PAS), so an immunostain is helpful to confirm them as *T. whipplei*. Stains for acid-fast organisms are negative for *T. whipplei*.

ENTERIC ISCHEMIC DISEASE

CLINICAL FEATURES

Acute mesenteric ischemia can result from emboli, arterial and venous thrombi, or vasoconstriction secondary to low flow; in an inpatient population, this is frequently a result. Based on a 2000 review by the American Gastroenterologic Association, mortality rates reported over the past 15 years remain as high as they did more than 70 years ago and average about 70%, with a range of about 60% to 90%. Diagnosis before intestinal infarction is the key factor to improve these poor results. Relief of persistent vasoconstriction, which is the cause of nonocclusive mesenteric ischemia and occurs in association with occlusive forms of ischemia, is another important factor.

Patients have severe abdominal pain that persists for more than 2 or 3 hours. Patients at risk include those older than 50 years with congestive heart failure, cardiac arrhythmias, recent myocardial infarction, hypovolemia, hypotension, or sepsis. A history of previous arterial emboli, vasculitis, deep vein thromboses, hypercoagulable states (protein C and S deficiencies, antithrombin III deficiency, and activated protein C resistance, among others), or chronic postprandial pain also places a patient in the high-risk group. In younger patients, polyarteritis nodosa, Henoch-Schönlein purpura, and other causes of systemic vasculitis can result in mesenteric ischemia.

Chronic mesenteric ischemia ("intestinal angina") is characterized by postprandial abdominal pain and marked weight loss and is caused by repeated transient episodes of inadequate intestinal blood flow, usually provoked by the metabolic demands of digestion.

RADIOLOGIC FEATURES

The primary role of abdominal plain x-ray films is to exclude other identifiable causes of abdominal pain (e.g., perforated ulcer) in a patient suspected of having mesenteric ischemia. Duplex sonography (Doppler) is highly specific (92% to 100%) for identification of occlusions or severe stenoses of the splanchnic vessels but less sensitive (70% to 89%). Unfortunately, duplex sonography is of no value in detecting emboli beyond the proximal main vessel. Moreover, identification of significant arterial stenosis does not establish the diagnosis of intestinal ischemia because total occlusion of two or even all three splanchnic vessels can be present in asymptomatic patients.

ENTERIC ISCHEMIC DISEASE—FACT SHEET

Definition
- Injury to the bowel caused by insufficient blood flow, regardless of etiology

Incidence and Location
- Not uncommon

Morbidity and Mortality
- High mortality for acute ischemic disease (70%)

Gender, Race, and Age Distribution
- Risk factors overlap those for vascular diseases
- Age older than 50 years
- Associated with congestive heart failure, cardiac arrhythmias, recent myocardial infarction, hypovolemia, hypotension, or sepsis
- Additional associations are history of previous arterial emboli, vasculitis, deep vein thromboses, and hypercoagulable states
- Chronic postprandial pain associated with high-risk patients
- Polyarteritis nodosa, Henoch-Schönlein purpura, and other causes of systemic vasculitis in younger patients

Clinical Features
- Acute mesenteric ischemia: severe abdominal pain that persists for more than 2 or 3 hours
- Chronic mesenteric ischemia ("intestinal angina"): postprandial abdominal pain

Prognosis and Therapy
- Poor prognosis for acute ischemia (70% mortality)
- Treatment includes anticoagulation and operations to revascularize the affected segment; chronic ischemia is treated by angioplasty or revascularization procedures
- When bowel wall necrosis and peritonitis have ensued, the necrotic segment must be excised as promptly as possible

---

ENTERIC ISCHEMIC DISEASE—PATHOLOGIC FEATURES

Gross Findings
- Acute ischemic disease: varying degrees of necrosis, with or without perforation and peritonitis
- Chronic ischemia: strictures

Microscopic Findings
- Acute: necrosis of villi followed by necrosis of the bowel wall, depending on how long the process has been ongoing; sometimes the etiology is apparent (thrombus, vasculitis, intussusception, adhesions)
- Chronic: mural fibrosis, sclerotic submucosa, attenuated villi
- Hyalinized lamina propria

Differential Diagnosis
- In chronic ischemic disease with strictures, Crohn's disease, and NSAID ulcers. Crohn's disease has more abundant inflammation. NSAID injury shows overlapping features and must be correlated with history; causes of ischemia must be sought

Standard CT has been used in the detection of intestinal ischemia with varying results. As on plain radiography of the abdomen, most abnormalities on CT occur late in the course of the disease. Highly suggestive findings, including portal venous gas and pneumatosis intestinalis, are seen only after gangrene has developed. CT diagnosis of mesenteric vein thrombosis is more valuable.

Selective mesenteric angiography is considered by most authorities on vascular disorders of the bowel as the gold standard for the diagnosis of mesenteric ischemia. The sensitivity (74% to 100%) and specificity (100%) seem to justify the reliance placed on this test. Opponents of routine angiography note difficulties in performing angiography in critically ill patients. Furthermore, they point out that the large number of negative results in examinations performed to identify patients with mesenteric ischemia early in the course of the disease offsets the value of the study. The most serious potential drawback is the possible critical delay in surgical intervention.

PATHOLOGIC FEATURES

GROSS FINDINGS

In contrast to the case in the colon, small bowel ischemia is not usually diagnosed on biopsies; instead, a resected segment of small bowel is received.

Depending on the point at which the segment of ischemic small intestine is resected, it may appear dusky and overtly necrotic (acute mesenteric ischemia) or strictured from cycles of injury and repair (chronic ischemic diseases). If there is pneumatosis, the segment of small bowel may be crepitant. When disease is mild, there is mucosal ischemia but not transmural ischemia.

MICROSCOPIC FINDINGS

In early acute ischemia, the tips of the villi are affected, and they are hyperemic and display necrosis of enterocytes (Fig. 5-21). As the process develops, the submucosa and muscularis propria become necrotic (Fig. 5-22). Massive submucosal edema is accompanied by influx of neutrophils. Later, perforation and peritonitis ensue. When examining such cases, the vessels should be studied for evidence of vasculitis or thrombi (Fig. 5-23). When reporting such cases, one should always note the presence of serosal adhesions (they are almost always found) because they may have been the source of the ischemic episode if no vascular damage is detected. In cases of chronic intermittent ischemia, the lamina propria is hyalinized and the surface is atrophic with attenuated villi but minimal inflammation. There may be fibrosis of the submucosa and muscularis propria, and usually serosal adhesions can be identified.

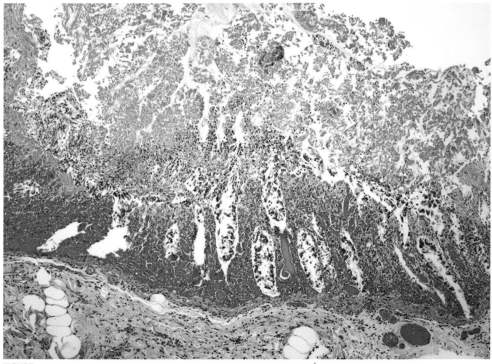

FIGURE 5-21

Ischemic enteritis, ileal resection (H&E). Early ischemia manifested by enterocyte necrosis with luminal fibrinopurulent debris *(top)* and extensive lamina propria hemorrhage.

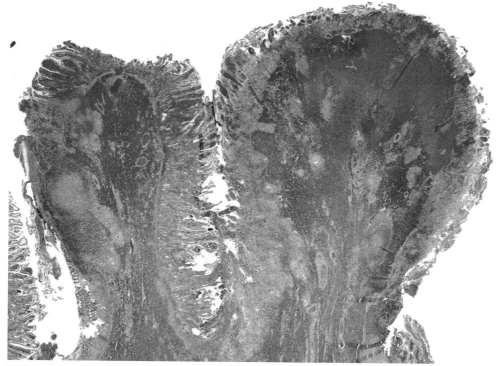

FIGURE 5-22
Ischemic enteritis secondary to vasculitis, jejunal resection (H&E).

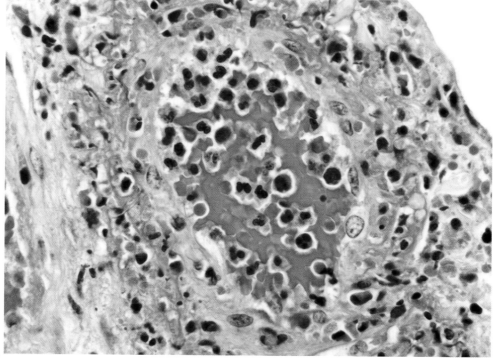

FIGURE 5-23
Ischemic enteritis secondary to vasculitis, jejunal resection (H&E). Vasculitis in a submucosal artery. The arterial wall shows fibrinoid necrosis and a marked neutrophilic infiltrate. Marked submucosal hemorrhage and mucosal necrosis.

GASTROINTESTINAL GVHD—FACT SHEET

Definition
- GI mucosal damage caused by the engraftment of donor T-lymphocytes

Incidence
- 10% to 40% of patients with allogeneic hematopoietic stem cell transplant
- Up to 13% of patients with autologous hematopoietic stem cell transplant
- <1% of patients with solid organ transplant

Morbidity and Mortality
- Responsible for approximately 50% of transplant-related deaths

Clinical Features
- Viable
- Most common symptom is secretary diarrhea

Prognosis
- <50% of patients achieved a complete resolution following treatment
- Transplant-related mortality for nonresponders is 49% to 75%

GASTROINTESTINAL GRAFT-VERSUS-HOST DISEASE—PATHOLOGIC FEATURES

Gross Findings
- Mucosal edema and erythema
- Ulcer, nodularity, friability
- Diffuse bleeding
- Mucosal sloughing

Microscopic Findings
- Epithelial cell apoptosis
- Cryptal dropout
- Cryptal abscess
- Ulcer
- Mucosal denudation

Differential Diagnosis
- CMV infection
- Cryptosporidium infection
- Toxicity from conditioning regimen
- Mycophenolate mofetil

severe cases, complete crypt loss, villous atrophy, or even extensive mucosal denudation can be seen (Fig. 5-26). In such cases, definitive apoptosis may be absent. Other morphologic findings associated with GVHD in the small bowel are variable villous blunting, pericapillary hemorrhage resulting from endothelial apoptosis, and variable mononuclear inflammatory cell infiltrates. Based on Snover's original grading criteria, intestinal

GVHD can be graded as follows: grade I, mild epithelial cell apoptosis; grade II, apoptosis with abscesses; grade III, extensive crypt dropout/individual crypt necrosis; and grade IV, total denudation of areas of the mucosa.

Diagnostic chronic GI GVHD presentations are only seen in the esophagus, including esophageal web, strictures, and submucosal fibrosis. In the small bowel, chronic GVHD results in nonspecific features of lamina propria fibrosis, mucosal atrophy, and crypt distortion without basal plasmacytosis.

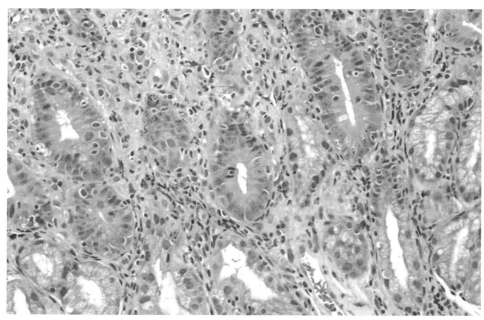

FIGURE 5-24

Graft-versus-host disease (GVHD), duodenal biopsy (H&E). Epithelial cell apoptosis is the key histologic feature for GI GVHD. In the small bowel, apoptosis is especially prominent in the neck and deep crypts, characterized by vacuoles and punctate nuclear debris.

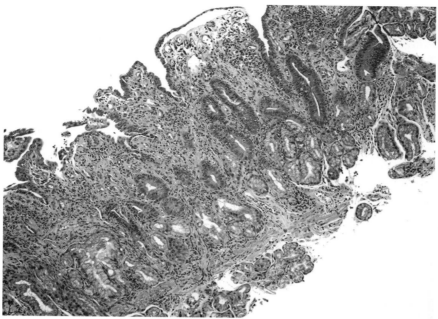

FIGURE 5-25

Grade III GVHD, duodenal biopsy (H&E). There are villous attenuation, crypt destruction/dropout, prominent intracryptal apoptosis, and increased chronic inflammation in the lamina propria. Surface epithelial injury with focal mucosal sloughing is present.

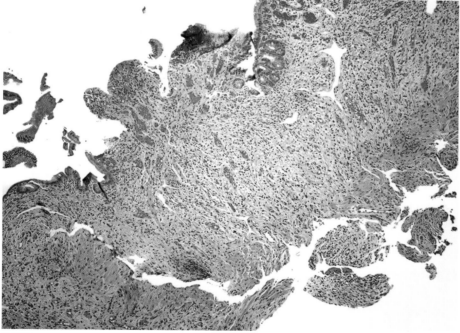

FIGURE 5-26

Grade VI GVHD, duodenal biopsy (H&E). There are extensive crypt loss, mucosal denudation and granulation tissue formation.

DIFFERENTIAL DIAGNOSIS

Other conditions such as infections and drug toxicities can mimic GI GVHD in patients who have received hematopoietic stem cell transplantation. Treatments for these conditions are, however, essentially very different from those for patients with GVHD. Therefore, differentiation of GI GVHD from its mimics is very important.

Cytomegalovirus (CMV) infection is one of the common complications following stem cell transplantation. CMV enteritis may occur concomitantly with GI GVHD. They also share similar histologies; both cause increased epithelial cell apoptosis. Sometimes, nuclear inclusions in CMV enteritis can be very sparse; an immunohistochemical study for CMV may be needed to exclude CMV infection in the GI biopsies from patients suspected with GVHD. Infection with cryptosporidium can also cause epithelial cell apoptosis in the small bowel. Careful examination of microvillous surface of the small bowel mucosa may help identify the organisms.

For patients with early onset of GI GVHD, the differential diagnosis includes toxicity from conditioning regimen given before transplantation. Patients with drug toxicity can present with nausea, vomiting, and diarrhea, similar symptoms seen in patients with GI GVHD. Epithelial cell apoptosis, increased mitotic activity, and crypt cell regeneration can be observed histologically. However, the histologic changes caused by conditioning regimen therapy usually resolve 20 days after transplantation. Mycophenolate mofetil is a common immunosuppressive drug used in transplant patients. Mycophenolate mofetil may cause entire gastrointestinal mucosal injury. In the ileum and colon, mycophenolate mofetil may cause GVHD-like changes such as mild crypt architectural disarray or villous blunting, edema, and increased crypt epithelial apoptosis.

PROGNOSIS AND THERAPY

Patients with acute GVHD are treated with low-dose corticosteroids for several weeks. If lower-dose steroids are not successful in controlling GVHD, higher dose steroids are required. For those with no response to steroids, a second-line agent can be added. Second-line agents include cyclosporine, tacrolimus, antihthymocyte globulin, and mycophenolate mofetil. Development of acute GVHD after bone marrow transplant is associated with a lower survival rate. Only 30% to 40% of patients with acute GVHD have some responses to the above treatments. Patients with no response have a mortality rate as high as 75%.

AUTOIMMUNE ENTEROPATHY

CLINICAL FEATURES

Autoimmune enteropathy (AIE) is a rare disease that occurs when the body's own immune system attacks the intestinal mucosa and leads to severe malabsorption symptoms. Patients with AIE suffer from severe and persistent inflammatory diarrhea, abdominal pain, weight loss, and malnutrition. Classically, patients present with chronic diarrhea in the first months of life. Weight loss and malnutrition can be so severe that

---

AUTOIMMUNE ENTEROPATHY—FACT SHEET

Definition
- GI mucosal damage caused by antienterocyte autoantibodies

Incidence
- 25% of infants with intractable diarrhea
- Rare in adult

Morbidity and Mortality
- Failure to thrive

Clinical Features
- Protracted hypersecretory diarrhea
- Weight loss
- Malnutrition

Prognosis
- High mortality rate for IPEX (approximately 30%)

---

parenteral nutrition is required. The symptoms are unresponsive to dietary restriction.

AIE is considered to be the most common cause of protracted diarrhea of infancy or early childhood. Although AIE generally occurs in children, adult-onset AIE has also been described. The patients usually generate a variety of autoantibodies against self-antigens in different organs including the pancreas, small intestine, and thyroid. Therefore, in addition to AIE, other autoimmune diseases such as diabetes mellitus, thyroiditis, or hemolytic anemia may also be seen in such patients.

Immunodysregulation, polyendocrinopathy, enteropathy, and X-linked inheritance (IPEX) syndrome is a particular form of AIE seen in male infants caused by mutations in *FOXP3* gene on X chromosome. AIE can also be seen in a subset of patients with common variable immunodeficiency (CVID) or IgA deficiency.

PATHOLOGIC FEATURES

GROSS FINDINGS

Endoscopic findings include loss of the normal architecture, ulceration, and hyperemic mucosa. The entire GI tract can be involved, though the most severe disease is often seen in the small bowel.

MICROSCOPIC FINDINGS

Multiple biopsies from the small bowel and colon are usually required for diagnosis. Microscopically, there are variable lymphoplasmacytic infiltrates in the lamina propria, deep cyrpt lymphocytosis, and increased crypt apoptotic bodies (Fig. 5-27). Often surface lymphocytosis is not as evident as seen in CD. In severe cases, intense neutrophilic inflammation with cryptal abscess formation or ulceration can be present. Another major histologic feature of AIE is villous blunting, which could be mild, moderate, or severe accompanied by crypt hyperplasia (Fig. 5-28). In addition, goblet cells or Paneth cells may be absent from the epithelium of the GI tract. A subset of patients can display loss of endocrine cells.

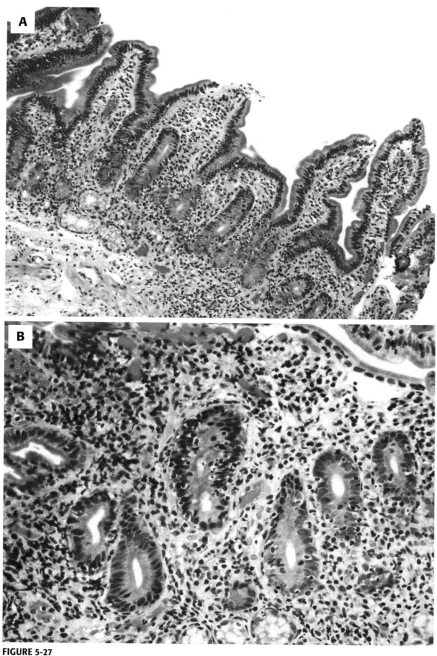

FIGURE 5-27

Autoimmune enteropathy, duodenal biopsy (H&E). **A,** Duodenal mucosa with no goblet cells and mild villous blunting. **B,** Prominent intraepithelial lymphocytes in the deep crypts and increased chronic inflammation in the lamina propria.

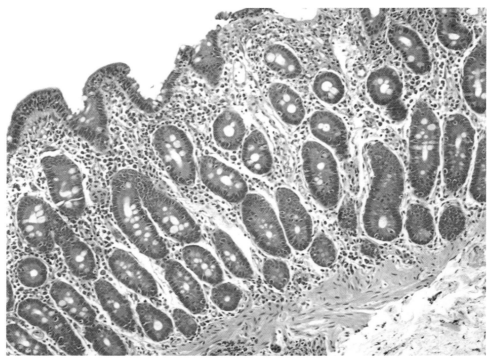

FIGURE 5-28
Autoimmune enteropathy, duodenal biopsy (H&E). There are marked villous attenuation, crypt hyperplasia, mildly prominent intraepithelial lymphocytes in the deep crypts, and complete loss of Paneth cells.

AUTOIMMUNE ENTEROPATHY—PATHOLOGIC FEATURES

Gross Findings
- Villous atrophy
- Mucosal erythema

Microscopic Findings
- Villous atrophy
- Dense lymphoplasmacytic infiltrates in the lamina propria
- Prominent intraepithelial lymphocytosis
- Increased crypt apoptotic bodies
- Absent Goblet cells or Paneth cells

Differential Diagnosis
- Celiac disease
- Common variable immunodeficiency
- Eosinophilic enteropathies
- Microvillus inclusion disease
- Enteroendocrine cell dysgenesis

DIFFERENTIAL DIAGNOSIS

Differential diagnosis with CD can be difficult. Both diseases have increased lamina propria inflammation, intraepithelial lymphocytosis, and villous blunting. However, in contrast to CD, there is a relative paucity of surface lymphocytosis in AIE. In addition, patients with CD usually respond well to a gluten-free diet. Celiac serology may also help diagnose CD. In infants with intractable diarrhea, some common illnesses such as infections and food sensitive enteropathies need to be excluded. Eosinophilic enteropathies can be differentiated from AIE by presence of abundant intraepithelial eosinophils in the absence of the other key features of AIE (loss of goblet or Paneth cells). Other rare differential diagnoses for AIE in infancy include microvillus inclusion disease, which is described in the previous section and typically lacks prominent inflammation.

Common variable immunodeficiency (CVID) is the second most common primary immunodeficiency syndrome, after selective IgA deficiency. It is caused by dysfunction of B cell differentiation, consequently resulting in hypogammaglobulinemia, diminished ability to produce antibody in response to vaccines or infections, and recurrent and chronic infections. Patients with common variable immunodeficiency (CVID) have a high incidence of chronic GI symptoms, mainly diarrhea. A small subset of CVID patients develops anti-enterocyte antibodies; their GI biopsies show changes consistent with autoimmune enteropathy. In CVID patients without anti-enterocyte antibodies, small bowel biopsies can also show histologic changes resembling AIE, including marked villous atrophy with destruction of occasional crypts, increased epithelial cell apoptosis in crypts, and prominent intraepithelial lymphocytes. Intraepithelial neutrophils also can be seen in GI biopsies from a subset of patients with CVID (Fig. 5-29). However, CVID is characterized by the paucity of plasma cells in the lamina propria and more prominent intraepithelial lymphocytosis in the surface epithelium (Fig. 5-30). In addition, in contrast to autoimmune

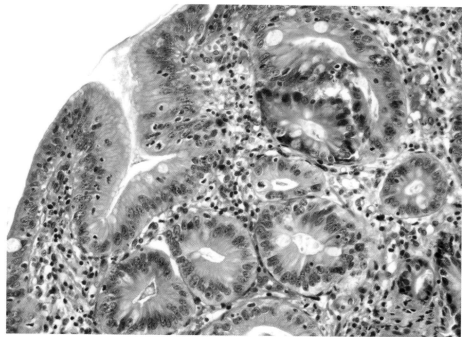

FIGURE 5-29

Common variable immunodeficiency, duodenal biopsy (H&E). The duodenal mucosa shows villous blunting, gastric mucin-cell metaplasia, and intraepithelial neutrophils. Despite the active inflammation, note that there are no plasma cells in the lamina propria.

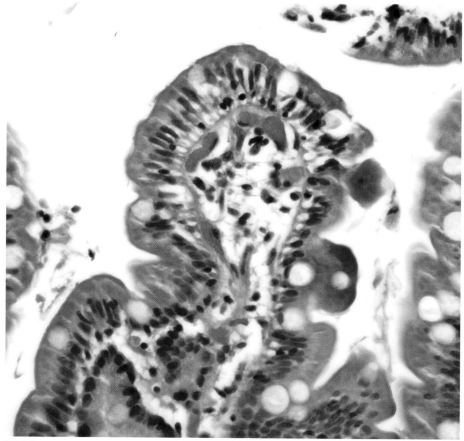

FIGURE 5-30

Common variable immunodeficiency, small bowel biopsy (H&E). An intact villus is present showing mild prominence in intraepithelial lymphocytes at the tip. The lamina propria is devoid of plasma cells.

enteropathy, goblet cells are usually present in the surface mucosa of the intestine.

PROGNOSIS AND THERAPY

The mainstay of treatment for AIE is immunosuppressive therapy. In infancy, nutritional support and adequate hydration are also needed to ensure optimal growth and development. Most of the patients respond well to the treatment with a high survival rate. Restoration of goblet cells or Paneth cells is observed in some patients after treatment (Fig. 5-31). However, IPEX patients usually have a poor response to the therapy and are associated with a high mortality rate. Currently hematopoietic cell transplantation is the only curative therapy available to IPEX patients.

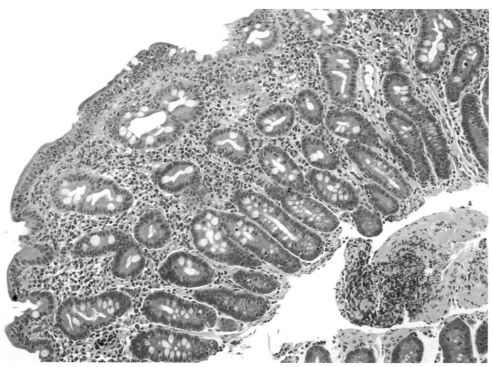

FIGURE 5-31

Autoimmune enteropathy, duodenal biopsy (H&E). This is a biopsy from the same patient shown in Figure 5-28. The biopsy was taken after treatment. Note that there are some Paneth cells in the crypts.

6

Neoplasms of the Small Intestine

■ Toby C. Cornish, MD, PhD ■ H. Parry Dilworth, MD

The small intestine represents 75% of the length and 90% of the surface area of the gastrointestinal tract, yet neoplasms of the small intestine are rare, accounting for only 1% to 2% of all gastrointestinal neoplasms and less than 1% of all cancers in the United States. Four major types of primary neoplasms arise in the small intestine. They are, in order of descending frequency, adenocarcinomas, carcinoid tumors, lymphomas, and sarcomas. The small intestine is also the most common tubular gastrointestinal site for involvement by secondary tumors, which are more than twice as common as primary small intestinal tumors. In this chapter, we discuss primary adenocarcinomas, carcinoids, and common secondary tumors of the small intestine. Lymphomas and sarcomas are discussed elsewhere.

■ ADENOCARCINOMAS OF THE SMALL INTESTINE

CLINICAL FEATURES

Adenocarcinomas are the most common primary malignancies of the small intestine, comprising from 30% to 50% of all small bowel malignancies. Primary adenocarcinomas are still rare lesions, however, and account for only 2% of gastrointestinal tract tumors and 1% of all gastrointestinal tract cancer deaths. They present in older adults (median 67 years), with a male predominance, and are more common in African-Americans than whites. Like colorectal adenocarcinomas, the vast majority of small intestinal adenocarcinomas are sporadic and arise from adenomatous polyps. Risk factors for small intestinal adenocarcinoma are similar to those for colorectal adenocarcinoma, and their incidence rates correlate highly worldwide. Risk factors for sporadic adenocarcinoma reportedly include smoking and consumption of alcohol, red meat, and fats. Increased body mass index may also be a risk factor. The remaining adenocarcinomas arise in the background of certain

predisposing conditions, including certain polyposis syndromes, Crohn's disease, gluten-sensitive enteropathy (GSE), ileostomy, and ileal conduit. Familial adenomatous polyposis (FAP) carries the greatest increase in risk for small intestinal adenocarcinoma (100- to 200-fold), followed by Crohn's disease and GSE, each of which is increased 80-fold. Other polyposis syndromes with increased risk include hereditary nonpolyposis colon cancer syndrome, Peutz-Jeghers syndrome, and juvenile polyposis syndrome.

The majority of small intestinal adenomas are located in the duodenum, and, like their colonic counterparts, exhibit three major histologic types: tubular, tubulovillous, and villous (Fig. 6-1). Most adenomas occur singly, and the presence of multiple adenomas in the small intestine is unusual in the absence of FAP. Because of their potential to undergo malignant transformation, adenomas should be removed. Endoscopic polypectomy is appropriated for pedunculated tumors, while large sessile lesions require endoscopic mucosal resection or surgical resection.

Adenocarcinomas arising sporadically and in the setting of most predisposing conditions occur most frequently in the duodenum, where 65% are periampullary. The incidence decreases progressively through the rest of the small intestine. Adenocarcinoma arising in Crohn's disease is a notable exception to this rule. In Crohn's disease, 70% of adenocarcinomas are found in the ileum, the primary site of the inflammatory process (Figs. 6-2 and 6-3).

The most common presenting symptoms of small intestinal adenocarcinoma are abdominal pain, obstruction, and occult gastrointestinal bleeding. Patients with duodenal adenocarcinomas may present with gastric outlet obstruction, while the combination of obstructive jaundice with occult gastrointestinal bleeding is characteristic of ampullary tumors. More distal lesions tend to result in severe, cramping abdominal pain. Intestinal obstruction can be caused by progression of an apple core lesion or by a large intraluminal polypoid mass. Distal adenocarcinomas tend to present with advanced disease (stage III or IV).

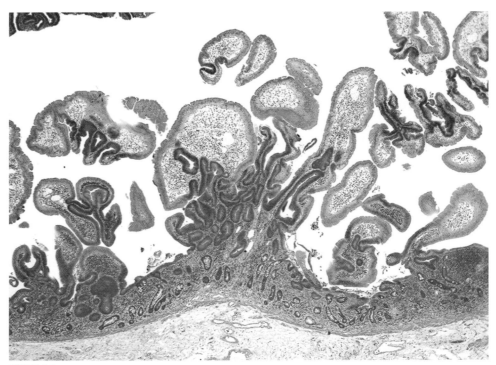

FIGURE 6-1

Duodenal adenoma. Adenomatous epithelium with pseudostratified enlarged hyperchromatic nuclei. There is no evidence of high-grade dysplasia and no lamina propria invasion.

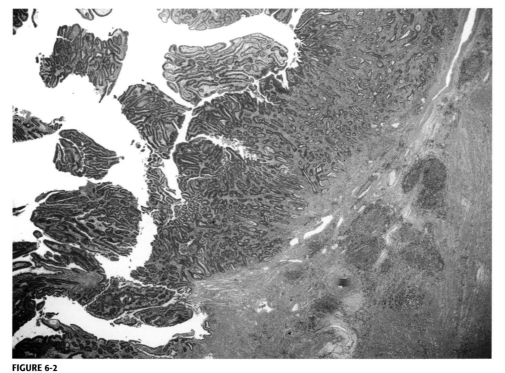

FIGURE 6-2

Terminal ileum resection in Crohn's disease. An invasive moderately differentiated adenocarcinoma fills the submucosa (*center* and *upper right*) and undermines a dysplasia-associated lesion/mass (DALM; *left*).

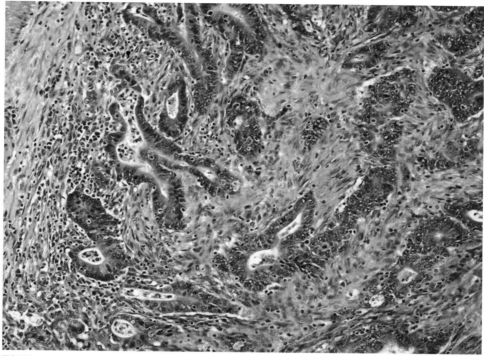

FIGURE 6-3

Terminal ileum resection in Crohn's disease. Invasive adenocarcinoma in submucosa. Irregular glands with prominent nuclear pleomorphism, luminal necrotic debris, and extensive desmoplasia.

SMALL INTESTINAL ADENOCARCINOMA—FACT SHEET

Definition

- Primary malignant epithelial tumor of the small intestine

Incidence and Location

- Most common malignancy of the small intestine (30% to 50% of small bowel malignancies)
- Overall rare lesions, 2% of GI tumors, and 1% of GI cancer deaths

Gender, Race, and Age Distribution

- Presents in older adults (median 67 years)
- Male predominance
- More common in African-Americans than whites

Clinical Features

- Vast majority of cases are sporadic
- Similar to colorectal adenocarcinomas in risk factors and development from sporadic adenomatous polyps
- Minority arise in the background of predisposing condition: most commonly FAP, GSE, and Crohn's disease
- Common symptoms: abdominal pain, obstruction, occult GI bleeding
- Combination of obstructive jaundice with occult GI bleeding characteristic of ampullary tumors
- Most patients present with advanced disease (stage III or IV)

Prognosis and Therapy

- Poor outcome in all locations
- 5-year disease-free survival rate approximately 30%
- Most deeply invasive and metastatic at time of diagnosis
- Proximal lesions: pancreaticoduodenectomy or endoscopic polypectomy or mucosectomy (polypoid or superficial tumors)
- Distal lesions: segmental resection with accompanying mesentery
- Chemotherapy and radiation appear to have little proven role

Duodenal lesions can typically be detected on routine endoscopy, whereas more distal lesions may require push or capsule enteroscopy, intraoperative endoscopy, or radiographic imaging modalities. Endoscopic ultrasound (EUS) may be of use to assess depth of invasion and local lymph node metastasis.

PATHOLOGIC FEATURES

GROSS FINDINGS

The macroscopic appearance depends largely on the site of the adenocarcinoma. The majority of the duodenal and ampullary tumors are small exophytic masses at the time of presentation. Distal tumors tend to be large, annular, constricting ("apple core") lesions with circumferential involvement of the bowel wall. Rarely, tumors can have a linitis plastica-like appearance. Macroscopic evaluation and tissue sampling should capture the data necessary for TNM staging (Table 6-1). As in the colon, depth of

TABLE 6-1

TNM Classification of Tumors of the Small Intestine

T—Primary Tumor	N—Regional Lymph Nodes	M—Distant Metastasis	Stage Grouping			
TX—Primary tumor cannot be assessed	NX—Regional lymph nodes cannot be assessed	M0—No distant metastasis	Stage 0	Tis	N0	M0
T0—No evidence of primary tumor	N0—No regional lymph node metastasis	M1—Distant metastasis	Stage I	T1, T2	N0	M0
Tis—Carcinoma in situ	N1—Metastasis in 1 to 3 regional lymph nodes		Stage IIA	T3	N0	M0
T1—Tumor invades lamina propria, muscularis mucosa or submucosa	N2—Metastasis in 4 or more regional lymph nodes		Stage IIB	T4	N0	M0
T1a—Tumor invades lamina propria or muscularis mucosa			Stage IIIA	Any T	N1	M0
T1b—Tumor invades submucosa			Stage IIIB	Any T	N2	M0
T2—Tumor invades muscularis propria			Stage IV	Any T	Any N	M1
T3—Tumor invades subserosa or nonperitonealized perimuscular tissue (mesentery or retroperitoneum*) with extension 2 cm or less						
T4—Tumor perforates visceral peritoneum or directly invades other organs or structures (includes other loops of small intestine, mesentery, or retroperitoneum more than 2 cm and abdominal wall by way of serosa; for duodenum only, invasion of pancreas)						

*The nonperitonealized perimuscular tissue is, for jejunum and ileum, part of the mesentery and, for duodenum in areas where serosa is lacking, part of the retroperitoneum.

Data from Sobin LH, Gospodarowicz MK, Wittekind CH, editors: *International Union Against Cancer (UICC): TNM classification of malignant tumors,* ed 7, Oxford, 2009, Wiley-Blackwell.

A help desk for specific questions about the TNM classification is available at http://www.uicc.org.

invasion and serosal involvement must be documented. Duodenal adenocarcinomas requires additional sampling to evaluate the depth of retroperitoneal extension and involvement of the pancreas.

MICROSCOPIC FINDINGS

Small bowel adenocarcinomas are histologically similar to colorectal adenocarcinomas (see Figs. 6-2 and 6-3). They are characterized by cellular pleomorphism, complex glandular architecture, luminal necrosis (so-called dirty necrosis), and invasion of the lamina propria and bowel wall. Most adenocarcinomas are moderately differentiated, and one third are poorly differentiated. Histologic grading and classification (e.g., mucinous, adenosquamous) have little bearing on prognosis, though, which is primarily a product of anatomic extent, resectability, and lymph node status. The majority of small bowel adenocarcinomas have invaded through the bowel wall by the time of diagnosis. Notably, intramucosal carcinomas of the small bowel are staged as T1 tumors (rather than Tis). This is caused by the rich mucosal lymphatics that confer metastatic potential to these lesions.

Residual adenomatous epithelium from a preexisting adenoma is present in the majority of proximal tumors but often cannot be demonstrated in large, distal small intestinal adenocarcinomas, presumably resulting from tumor overgrowth. Adenomatous epithelium can be mimicked by tumors metastatic to the gastrointestinal mucosa, and a sharp transition from normal to overtly malignant epithelium is highly suggestive of secondary involvement of the mucosa.

DIFFERENTIAL DIAGNOSIS

The main differential diagnostic consideration is metastatic disease, because the small intestine is the most common gastrointestinal site for metastatic disease. Immunohistochemistry is primarily used to exclude metastatic disease, specifically, metastatic adenocarcinomas (e.g., colon, breast, lung) or other mimickers of poorly differentiated carcinoma (e.g., melanoma, lymphoma). Secondary tumors of the small intestine are discussed in more detail later in this chapter.

SMALL INTESTINAL ADENOCARCINOMA—PATHOLOGIC FEATURES

Gross Findings

- Duodenum (most in the periampullary region) >> jejunum (first 30 cm) > ileum (Crohn's disease)
- Duodenal and ampullary lesions: smaller exophytic masses
- Distal tumors: large annular, constricting lesions with circumferential bowel wall involvement
- Rarely tumors can have a linitis plastica appearance
- Gross sampling should include data important for TNM staging (see Table 6-1)
- Sampling background mucosa and assessing for adenoma are important

Microscopic Findings

- Similar histologically to colorectal adenocarcinomas
- Adenocarcinoma is characterized by pleomorphism, complex glandular architecture, luminal necrosis, and invasion into the lamina propria and bowel wall
- Most are moderately differentiated, and one third are poorly differentiated
- Degree of differentiation and special histologic subsets (e.g., mucinous, adenosquamous) have little bearing on prognosis
- Majority of small bowel adenocarcinomas have invaded through the bowel wall
- Preexisting adenoma is present in the majority of proximal tumors but often cannot be demonstrated in large distal small intestinal adenocarcinomas

Immunohistochemistry

- Immunohistochemistry is primarily used to exclude metastatic disease, specifically, metastatic adenocarcinomas (e.g., colon, breast, lung) or other mimickers of poorly differentiated tumor (melanoma and lymphoma)
- Coordinate labeling for CK7/CK20 or CK7+, CK20− might be helpful to rule out metastatic colon adenocarcinomas

Differential Diagnosis

- Metastatic adenocarcinomas (e.g., colon, breast, ovary, lung)
- Poorly differentiated malignancies (e.g., lymphoma, melanoma)
- Endometriosis

PROGNOSIS AND THERAPY

Small bowel adenocarcinomas are lethal tumors, with a 5-year survival rate of approximately 30%. Survival is diminished in duodenal tumors and in patients older than 75 years of age. Surgery is the treatment of choice and the only modality with curative potential. Small polypoid or superficial tumors may be amenable to endoscopic polypectomy, mucosectomy, or, in the duodenum, a transduodenal resection. Larger proximal lesions may require pancreaticoduodenectomy, and distal tumors require segmental resection with accompanying mesentery. Chemotherapy and radiation have little role in small bowel adenocarcinomas.

■ ADENOCARCINOMAS OF THE AMPULLA OF VATER

The ampulla of Vater is the usual site for convergence of the common bile duct, main pancreatic duct (duct of Wirsung), and duodenum. The ampulla opens through the duodenal papilla and acts as a conduit for bile and pancreatic juices. This unique microenvironment may account for the disproportionate incidence of periampullary adenocarcinomas in the small intestine. Ampullary adenocarcinoma accounts for approximately 7% of carcinomas in the periampullary region and 0.2% to 0.5% of all gastrointestinal malignancies.

CLINICAL FEATURES

Adenocarcinoma of the ampulla of Vater is associated with adenomas in 80% to 90% of cases. The average age of presentation for ampullary adenomas is the middle-50s, whereas adenocarcinoma typicaly presents in the middle-60s. Adenocarcinoma is more common in whites than African-Americans and more common in men than women. Ampullary adenomas and adenocarcinomas are far more likely to become symptomatic at an earlier stage than other small intestinal adenocarcinomas. Obstruction of the ampulla frequently produces jaundice and bile duct dilatation and occasionally results in pancreatitis, cholelithiasis, or choledocholithiasis. Other findings are nonspecific and include weight loss, abdominal pain, and occult bleeding. Typical laboratory abnormalities include increased bilirubin, ALT, AST, and alkaline phosphatase. Ampullary adenomas and adenocarcinomas are visualized endoscopically or, if large enough, by CT. Endoscopic ultrasound (EUS) can also be used to evaluate for invasion.

PATHOLOGIC FEATURES

GROSS FINDINGS

Sporadic ampullary adenomas (Fig. 6-4) usually present as polypoid masses, between 1 and 3 cm. Adenomas can also be located entirely intra-ampullary, in which case the gross appearance with be of a bulging ampulla rather than an exophytic mass. Adenocarcinomas appear as an infiltrating mass invading nearby structures. Seventy-six percent of adenocarcinomas are 2 cm or larger.

MICROSCOPIC FINDINGS

The proximal portion of the ampulla is lined by pancreatobiliary epithelium contiguous with the common bile duct and main pancreatic duct, and, distally, small

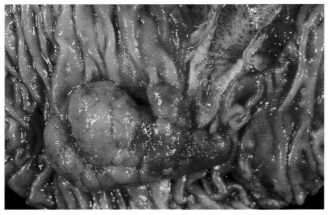

FIGURE 6-4

Ampullary adenoma. A pancreaticoduodeneectomy specimen reveals a villous adenoma at the ampulla of Vater. The common bile duct, dissected lengthwise, is grossly dilated.

intestinal epithelium contiguous with the duodenum. The vast majority of ampullary adenomas demonstrate only intestinal-type epithelium identical to other intestinal adenomas. A smaller number of adenomas show a mixture of intestinal-type and pancreatobiliary-type epithelium. Approximately 6% of adenomas are composed entirely of pancreatobiliary-type epithelium. These lesions resemble papillary tumors of the bile ducts and pancreas and have papillary projections with cuboidal epithelium and scant fibrous cores. They lack the abundant Paneth cells found in intestinal-type adenomas. In addition to typical adenomas, flat-type dysplasia can also be seen in the ampulla. When adenomatous epithelium extends into periampullary ductules in the smooth muscle of the sphincter of Oddi, care must be exercised to not misdiagnose the adenoma as an invasive carcinoma. Lack of a desmoplasia and a clear continuity with benign ductular epithelium support a noninvasive diagnosis. Likewise, caution must be exercised when evaluating an ampullary adenoma, as there is a high incidence of invasive carcinoma in these lesions.

Intestinal-type adenocarcinomas of the ampulla of Vater are identical to those found elsewhere in the small and large intestines and account for 85% of ampullary adenocarcinomas. The remaining adenocarcinomas are primarily of the pancreatobiliary-type. These are very similar to adenocarcinomas of the pancreatic duct and extrahepatic bile ducts and are composed of small nests and simple glands composed of a single layer of cuboidal or low columnar cells with rounded, pleomorphic nuclei. The glands and nests are surrounded by a desmoplastic stroma, and features of intestinal adenocarcinomas such as pseudostratification and luminal necrosis are lacking. Intestinal-type and pancreatobiliary-type neoplasms can be difficult to distinguish, especially when poorly differentiated, and immunohistochemistry can be helpful. Intestinal-type ampullary neoplasms are usually positive for cytokeratin (CK) 20, MUC2, and CDX2 and negative for CK7 (approximately 75%), MUC1, and MUC5AC. Pancreatobiliary-type ampullary neoplasms are usually positive for CK7, MUC1, and MUC5AC and negative for CK20, MUC2, and CDX2. Other types of ampullary adenocarcinomas (e.g., mucinous, adenosquamous) are infrequent.

In staging ampullary adenocarcinomas, noting the relationship to the disorganized smooth muscle of the ampulla itself is important. Lesions invading only the sphincter are T1, whereas those truly involving the muscularis propria are T2 (Table 6-2).

DIFFERENTIAL DIAGNOSIS

Pancreatobiliary neoplasms arising in the common bile duct or pancreas can colonize the ampullary epithelium or, if invasive, may directly involve the ampulla and be misdiagnosed as an ampullary adenoma or adenocarcinoma. Careful gross examination and review of clinical information is necessary when assigning the correct primary site to periampullary tumors. Metastasis from distant sites to the ampulla of Vater is exceedingly rare, but has been reported.

PROGNOSIS AND THERAPY

Pedunculated ampullary adenomas without high-grade dysplasia can be resected endoscopically if smaller than 1 cm. Adenomas that are larger than 1 cm or demonstrate high grade dysplasia are best managed by transduodenal ampullectomy or pancreaticoduodenectomy. Slightly less than half of adenomas will demonstrate invasive adenocarcinoma on resection. Pancreaticoduodenectomy is the standard of care for resectable ampullary adenocarcinomas. The 5-year survival rate for ampullary adenocarcinomas resected by pancreaticoduodenectomy is approximately 40%. Pancreatobiliary-type adenocarcinomas reportedly have a worse prognosis than intestinal-type adenocarcinomas.

TABLE 6-2

TNM Classification of Carcinoma of the Ampulla of Vater

T—Primary Tumor	N—Regional Lymph Nodes	M—Distant Metastasis	Stage Grouping			
TX—Primary tumor cannot be assessed	NX—Regional lymph nodes cannot be assessed	M0—No distant metastasis	Stage 0	Tis	N0	M0
T0—No evidence of primary tumor	N0—No regional lymph node metastasis	M1—Distant metastasis	Stage IA	T1	N0	M0
Tis—Carcinoma in situ	N1—Regional lymph node metastasis		Stage IB	T2	N0	M0
T1—Tumor limited to ampulla of Vater or sphincter of Oddi			Stage IIA	T3	N0	M0
T2—Tumor invades duodenal wall			Stage IIB	T1, T2, T3	N1	M0
T3—Tumor invades pancreas			Stage III	T4	Any N	M0
T4—Tumor invades peripancreatic soft tissues or other adjacent organs or structures			Stage IV	Any T	Any N	M1

Data from Sobin LH, Gospodarowicz MK, Wittekind CH, editors: *International Union Against Cancer (UICC): TNM classification of malignant tumors*, ed 7, Oxford, 2009, Wiley-Blackwell.
A help desk for specific questions about the TNM classification is available at http://www.uicc.org.

■ SMALL INTESTINAL CARCINOID TUMORS

Carcinoid tumors (well-differentiated neuroendocrine tumors) of the small intestine represent approximately one third of small intestine neoplasms and 2% of all gastrointestinal tumors. Small intestinal carcinoids are derived from two separate embryonic divisions of the alimentary tract: the foregut (duodenum) and the midgut (jejunum and ileum). These different embryonic origins correlate with distinct neuroendocrine differentiation and clinical behavior.

CLINICAL FEATURES

Duodenal (foregut) carcinoids are the second most common tumor in the duodenum after adenocarcinomas, and they represent approximately 20% of all gastrointestinal tract carcinoids. Overall, duodenal carcinoids are more common in men (males to females, 1.5:1) with a median age of 59 years (range, 33 to 90 years). Two thirds of duodenal carcinoids are gastrinomas (G-cell tumors), which can be sporadic or associated with multiple endocrine neoplasia-1 (MEN-1) syndrome. The remaining third are mostly somatostatinomas (D-cell tumors), and a small percentage are of an undefined type. Functional gastrinomas and somatostatinomas present in slightly younger patients than nonfunctioning tumors and are slightly more common in females. Nonfunctioning gastrinomas are usually located in the duodenal bulb, and their functional counterparts are found equally in all parts of the duodenum. Somatostatinomas have a predilection for the periampullary region. The few reported cases of poorly differentiated neuroendocrine tumors (small cell carcinomas) occurred exclusively in the periampullary region of men aged 51 to 76 years. These small cell carcinomas have a uniformly dismal prognosis.

The majority of ampullary carcinoids present with obstructive jaundice and biliary dilatation, while nonampullary duodenal carcinoids present with nonspecific symptoms, most commonly abdominal pain and upper gastrointestinal bleeding. Rarely, a duodenal carcinoid will present with obstruction. Only one third of gastrinomas are functional and cause Zollinger-Ellison syndrome (ZES). Functional duodenal gastrinomas account for half of all ZES cases, with the remainder result for pancreatic endocrine tumors. One third of somatostatinomas are associated with von Recklinghausen's disease. The somatostatinoma syndrome (i.e., diabetes mellitus, diarrhea, cholelithiasis), which can be seen with pancreatic islet cell tumors, is virtually never seen in its entirety with

CARCINOID TUMORS OF THE SMALL INTESTINE—FACT SHEET

Definition

- Carcinoid tumors are synonymous with well-differentiated neuroendocrine tumors and are neoplasms of the gastrointestinal diffuse neuroendocrine system

Incidence and Location

- Represent 30% of small bowel neoplasms and 40% of GI carcinoid tumors
- Seen primarily with roughly equal incidence in the duodenum and ileum

Gender, Race, and Age Distribution
Duodenal Carcinoids

- Median age of 59 years (range 33 to 90 years)
- More common in men (M:F, 1.5:1)

Jejunoileal Carcinoids

- Median age of diagnosis is 62 years (range 13 to 93 years)
- No particular sex predilection

Clinical Features
Duodenal Carcinoids

- One third of gastrinomas are functional and cause Zollinger-Ellison syndrome
- One third of somatostatin cell tumors are associated with von Recklinghausen's disease
- Nonampullary tumor: present with nonspecific symptoms, abdominal pain, upper GI bleeding, and rarely duodenal obstruction
- Ampullary tumor: present often with jaundice and biliary dilatation

Jejunoileal Carcinoids

- 5% to 7% have carcinoid syndrome (accounts for most cases of carcinoid syndrome)
- Abdominal pain or small bowel obstruction
- Bowel obstruction resulting from intussusception, the mechanical effect of the tumor, or mesenteric ischemia
- Often have metastases to lymph nodes or liver

Prognosis and Therapy

- Pathologic features associated with behavior that should be noted: size, invasion beyond submucosa, mitotic activity, and lymph node involvement
- Resection of the involved segment and small bowel mesentery
- Resection may be required for palliation in cases with metastatic disease

Duodenal Carcinoids

- Generally indolent (overall 4% mortality)
- Majority of somatostatinomas and gastrinomas are aggressive lesions
- Aggressive behavior best predicted by invasion beyond the submucosa and lymph node or distant metastases

Jejunoileal Carcinoids

- Worse prognosis than those of the duodenum, with a 21% mortality rate
- Survival negatively correlated with distant metastases (liver), tumor multiplicity, mitotic rate, invasion beyond submucosa, and female gender

intestinal somatostatinomas. Proximal small intestinal carcinoids virtually never produce the carcinoid syndrome.

Distal small bowel carcinoids are found primarily in the ileum and less commonly in the jejunum. Rarely they are found in association with a Meckel's diverticulum. The ileum is the single most common site for carcinoids, comprising 28% of all carcinoid tumors. Distal small bowel carcinoids account for one-fifth of gastrointestinal neuroendocrine tumors, and most are enterochromaffin cell serotonin-producing carcinoids. The median age at diagnosis is 62 years (range, 13 to 93 years) without gender predilection.

Patients with jejunoileal carcinoids often present with abdominal pain or small bowel obstruction; metastases to lymph nodes or the liver are also common. Bowel obstruction or abdominal pain may be resulting from intussusception, the mechanical effect of the tumor, or mesenteric ischemia. Ischemia can result from vascular compromise by large bulky mesenteric nodal metastasis, mesenteric vascular invasion, or microvascular metastasis. The carcinoid syndrome (e.g., watery diarrhea, flushing, endocardial fibrosis) manifests when serotonin production by the tumor exceeds the metabolic capacity of monoamine oxidase (MAO) in the liver and lungs. Carcinoid syndrome is usually, but not always, associated with metastasis to the liver and is seen in 5%

to 7% of cases. Jejunoileal carcinoids account for the majority of all carcinoid syndrome cases.

Nearly one third of patients diagnosed with a small intestinal carcinoid have a synchronous or metachronous carcinoma (e.g., colon, stomach, lung, breast).

Duodenal tumors are readily diagnosed by endoscopy. The location of jejunoileal tumors makes diagnosis more problematic because they are not amenable to colonoscopy and conventional imaging techniques (computed tomography and barium contrast studies) are not particularly sensitive. In these circumstances, scintigraphic studies with radiolabeled somatostatin analogues (octreotide and lanreotide) are a sensitive detection method of both primary and metastatic lesions.

PATHOLOGIC FEATURES

GROSS FINDINGS

Duodenal carcinoids are small polypoid lesions typically less than 2 cm in diameter. They tend to be submucosal lesions, and the overlying mucosa may be focally ulcerated (Fig. 6-5). Large, infiltrative tumors may occur but are infrequent. Gastrinomas tend to be smaller than somatostatinomas. A minority of duodenal carcinoids are multicentric (15%).

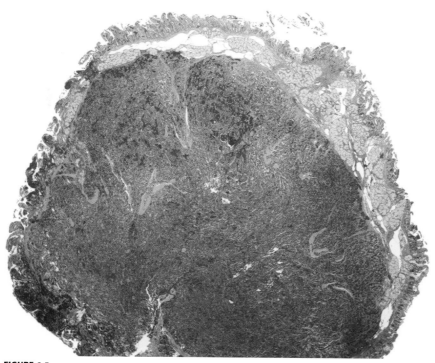

FIGURE 6-5
Polypoid duodenal carcinoid. The neoplasm is primarily located in the submucosa, with infiltration into the mucosa (left center). The mucosa is otherwise intact.

Jejunoileal carcinoids, in contrast, are twice as likely to be multicentric (30%). They tend to be large (>2 cm) and locally advanced with deep involvement of the bowel wall and mesentery. They frequently cause significant mesenteric fibrosis and obstruction, resulting in a characteristic "kinking" of the bowel that is evident grossly and radiologically. Tumor-induced angiopathy may produce frank ischemia. Like duodenal carcinoids, jejunoileal carcinoids are typically centered in the deep mucosa or submucosa, and the overlying mucosa is usually intact or slightly eroded.

MICROSCOPIC FINDINGS

A malignant carcinoid is differentiated from a benign lesion solely by the presence of metastasis. Even clinically malignant tumors show little to no cellular pleomorphism, hyperchromasia, or increase in mitotic activity. Carcinoids are characterized by a monotonous proliferation of small bland polygonal cells with a moderate amount of cytoplasm and round regular nuclei with the "salt and pepper" chromatin typical of neuroendocrine tumors (Fig. 6-6). Cytologic features do not vary by cell of origin, and immunohistochemistry is required for this distinction. Small intestinal carcinoids are typically submucosal and are not well circumscribed, with small groups of tumor cells frequently extending into the mucosa and the bowel wall (see Figs. 6-5 and 6-6).

Carcinoids demonstrate variable architectural growth patterns. Although these patterns have no prognostic significance, they can be characteristic of certain carcinoid subtypes. The main architectural patterns are insular or nested (type A), trabecular (type B), and acinar (type C) (Figs. 6-7 through 6-10). These patterns often overlap, and multiple patterns are typically seen within any single tumor. Duodenal gastrinomas can manifest any of a variety of architectural growth patterns, whereas somatostatinomas characteristically demonstrate a prominent acinar growth pattern and frequent intraluminal psammoma bodies (Figs. 6-9 and 6-11). Jejunoileal carcinoids, like gastrinomas, do not display any consistent growth patterns. They typically display prominent nested growth with more trabecular and acinar growth peripherally (see Figs. 6-7 and 6-10). These tumors are often larger and extend deeply into the bowel wall. They can be associated with significant fibrosis.

Although carcinoid tumors can show immunohistochemical evidence of multiple hormone production, this information is usually not clinically significant. The vast majority of small intestinal carcinoids are positive for chromogranin and synaptophysin, and these markers are useful in confirming the diagnosis of carcinoid. Immunohistochemical identification of specific cell types (e.g., G-cells) is of limited utility because the functional status of tumors does not correlate with immunohistochemical labeling.

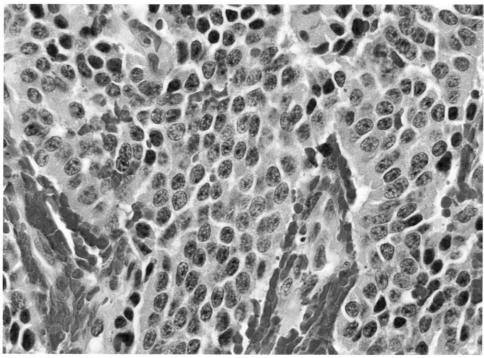

FIGURE 6-6

Duodenal carcinoid. Typical of carcinoids is striking monotony of the cellular proliferation with round nuclei and finely clumped ("salt and pepper") chromatin with small indistinct nucleoli.

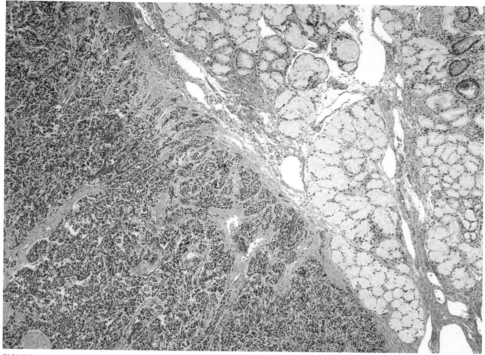

FIGURE 6-7

Duodenal carcinoid. Submucosal carcinoid extending to the base of the small intestinal mucosa. The tumor primarily has a nested growth pattern with a trabecular pattern at the edge of the mucosa.

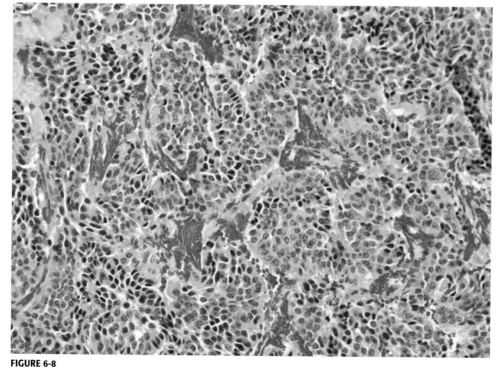

FIGURE 6-8

Duodenal carcinoid with nested (insular) growth pattern.

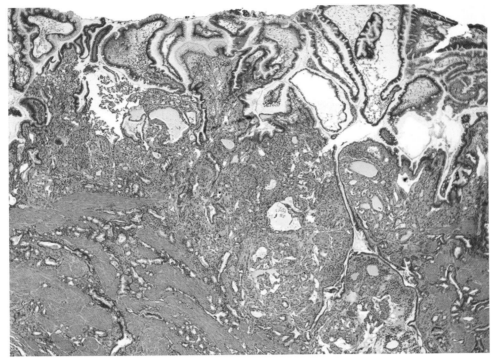

FIGURE 6-9

Periampullary somatostatinoma. The tumor extensively infiltrates the mucosa *(top)* and muscularis mucosae and submucosa *(bottom)*. The prominent acinar pattern is even apparent at this low power.

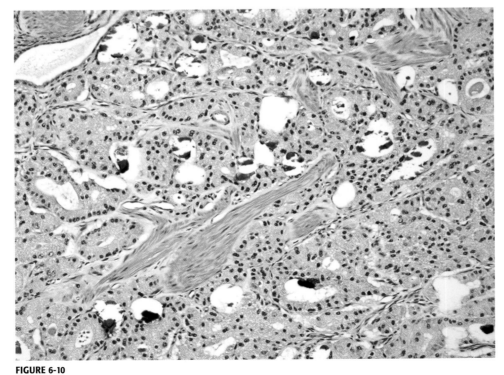

FIGURE 6-10

Periampullary somatostatinoma. The monomorphous cells have an acinar growth pattern with numerous intraluminal psammoma bodies.

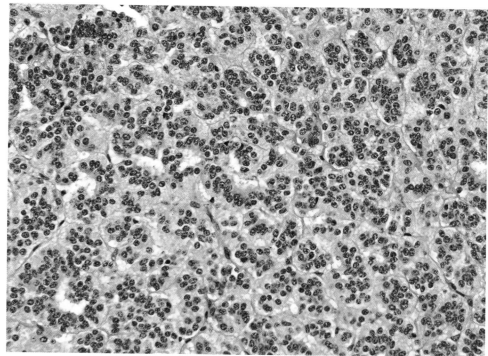

FIGURE 6-11
Jejunal carcinoid with trabecular growth pattern.

CARCINOID TUMORS OF THE SMALL INTESTINE—PATHOLOGIC FEATURES

Gross Findings

Duodenal Carcinoids

- Somatostatinomas: predilection for periampullary region
- Gastrinomas: functional type found in all parts of duodenum, nonfunctional type usually found in bulb
- Small polypoid lesions typically less than 2 cm in diameter
- Gastrinomas tend to be smaller than somatostatinomas
- Submucosal based with an overlying mucosa that may be focally ulcerated
- Infiltrative larger tumors are infrequent
- Multicentricity of tumors is seen in 15% of cases

Jejunoileal Carcinoids

- Primarily in the distal 60 cm of the ileum and less commonly the jejunum
- Twice as likely as duodenal tumors to have tumor multicentricity (30%)
- Tend to be large (> 2 cm in diameter)
- Frequently locally advanced disease, deep mural, lymph node, and mesenteric involvement
- Mesenteric tumor involvement causing significant mesenteric fibrosis and subsequent obstruction and kinking of the bowel
- Like duodenum, typically centered in the deep mucosa or submucosa; the overlying mucosa is typically intact or only slightly eroded

Microscopic Findings

- The distinction between benign and malignant carcinoid is based on the presence or absence of metastasis rather than on histology alone

- Monotonous proliferation of small bland polygonal cells with moderate amount of cytoplasm and round regular nuclei with "salt and pepper" chromatin
- Morphologic features of the cells do not differ by cell of origin (need immunohistochemistry)
- Pleomorphism and significant mitotic activity are uncommon
- Carcinoids demonstrate variable architectural growth patterns: nested (type A), trabecular (type B), and acinar (type C)
- Patterns often overlap and multiple patterns are typically seen within single tumor
- Typically poorly circumscribed, submucosal based with some mucosal extension
- Somatostatinomas often have a prominent acinar growth pattern with frequent intraluminal psammoma bodies
- Jejunoileal carcinoids and gastrinomas have variable histology and often prominent nested growth, with more trabecular and acinar growth peripherally
- Jejunoileal tumors often extend deeply into the bowel wall and can be associated with significant fibrosis

Immunohistochemistry

- Vast majority positive for chromogranin and synaptophysin (useful in confirming the diagnosis)
- Jejunoileal tumors tend to be enterochromaffin cell serotonin-producing carcinoids
- Specific cell types (e.g., G-cells) can be identified by immunohistochemical labeling—utility of this is limited because the functional status of tumors does not correlate with immunohistochemistry

Differential Diagnosis

- Primary or metastatic adenocarcinomas (particularly somatostatinomas)
- Other metastatic lesions (particularly melanoma or lobular breast cancer)

DIFFERENTIAL DIAGNOSIS

Carcinoids with a prominent acinar pattern may mimic adenocarcinomas. In such cases, the bland monotonous appearance of the carcinoid, in combination with strong labeling for neuroendocrine markers, are helpful features. The trabecular growth pattern seen at the periphery of carcinoids may be confused with metastatic lesions such as lobular breast cancer. The nested pattern can be mimicked by lamina propria and lymphatic invasion by melanoma, lymphoma, or other poorly differentiated tumors (Figs. 6-12 through 6-14). Where metastatic disease is a concern, immunohistochemistry is often definitive.

PROGNOSIS AND THERAPY

Overall behavior is difficult to predict but is dictated primarily by the stage of disease. Duodenal carcinoids are generally indolent (4% overall mortality); however, two thirds of somatostatinomas and half of functional gastrinomas behave aggressively. Poor outcome in duodenal

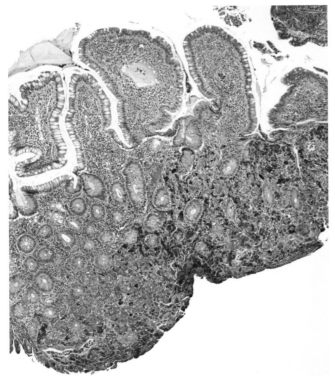

FIGURE 6-12

Metastatic melanoma to the small intestine. The bulk of the tumor is in the base of the lamina propria *(bottom)*. The tumor cells expand the lamina propria, pushing the glandular elements apart. Prominent lymphangiectasia is seen in the villi *(top)*, which is a common finding in metastatic tumors.

tumors is best predicted by invasion beyond the submucosa or by lymph node and distant metastases. Jejunoileal carcinoids have a worse prognosis than those of the duodenum, with a 21% mortality rate. Survival is negatively correlated with distant metastases, multiple tumors, mitotic rate, invasion beyond submucosa, and female gender.

Patients with small bowel carcinoid tumors should be treated with segmental resection of the bowel and associated mesentery. Even in those with metastatic disease, resection may be required for palliation, specifically to relieve obstruction.

■ SECONDARY TUMORS

Involvement of the small intestine by secondary tumors can occur by direct extension, intraperitoneal spread, or lymphohematogenous metastasis. Secondary tumors are 2.5 times more common than primary small intestinal neoplasms. Melanoma, breast, colon, and lung carcinoma are among the most common metastatic tumors involving the small intestine. Pancreatic and gastric carcinomas may also involve the small intestine by direct extension, whereas ovarian cancer is the mostly likely to involve the small intestine by serosal implantation. Secondary involvement of the small intestine may present as a thickened bowel wall or mass lesion with obstruction, intussusception, or perforation. Some tumors may even present as a mucosal polyp if exceptionally small. Features favoring a metastatic tumor include the presence of multiple lesions, the absence of a dysplastic precursor, a histologic appearance of tumor being "bottom heavy" or encroaching from below, and a lack of ulceration. When the mucosa is involved, an abrupt transition from normal epithelium to overtly malignant neoplasm supports involvement by a secondary tumor. In addition to metastatic adenocarcinomas (e.g., colon, breast, lung), mimickers of poorly differentiated carcinoma (e.g., melanoma and lymphoma) can present diagnostic challenges. Immunohistochemistry should be employed when the nature of the primary neoplasm is in doubt and is especially helpful in cases of poorly differentiated malignancies.

The most common malignancy to metastasize to the small intestine is melanoma (see Figs. 6-12 through 6-14). Melanoma can be differentiated from carcinoma, lymphoma, and carcinoid tumors using immunohistochemistry. Melanoma is positive for S-100 and melan-A and negative for leukocyte common antigen (LCA)/CD45, cytokeratins, and neuroendocrine markers. Primary melanomas of the small intestine are exceedingly rare, and melanoma in the small intestine can safely be assumed to be a secondary tumor even when a primary site is not evident.

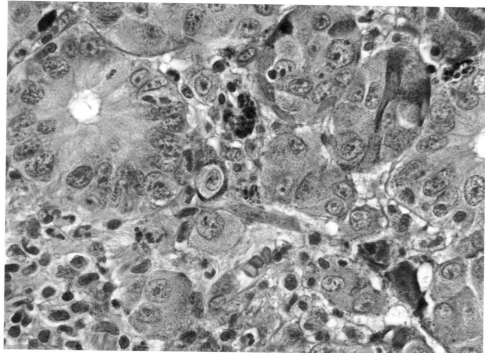

FIGURE 6-13

Metastatic melanoma to the small intestine. Tumor cells fill the lamina propria, invading as individual cells and small groups. They have abundant cytoplasm with fine brown pigment, marked nuclear pleomorphism, and prominent nucleoli.

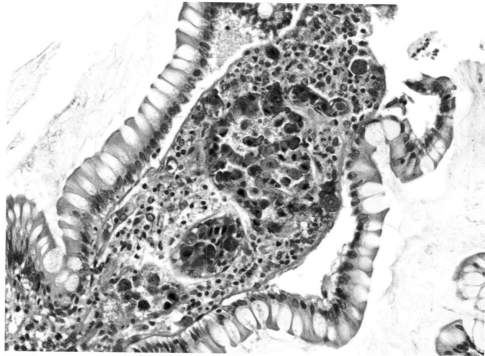

FIGURE 6-14

Metastatic melanoma filling lymphatics in a small intestinal villous mimicking nodular growth.

Metastatic colonic adenocarcinoma presents additional difficulties as it is morphologically identical to small intestinal adenocarcinoma (Figs. 6-15 and 6-16). The histologic clues discussed previously can be helpful in making a distinction, as can coordinate labeling for CK7 and CK20 (Table 6-3). Colonic adenocarcinomas are almost always positive for CK20 and negative for CK7, while small intestinal adenocarcinomas are positive for CK7 and variably positive for CK20. Both are usually CDX2 positive. Additionally, the presence of a precursor (adenoma) favors small intestinal adenocarcinoma although distinguishing "colonization" of the small bowel from a true adenoma is sometimes challenging. Interestingly, small bowel adenomas often express CK7.

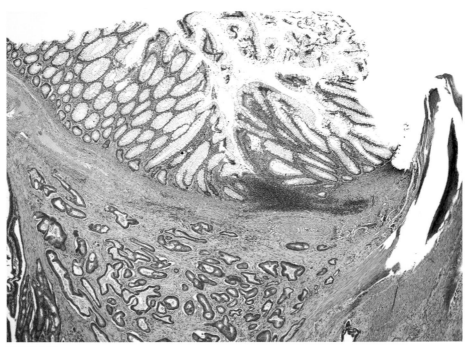

FIGURE 6-15

Ileal resection with metastatic colonic adenocarcinoma. The metastatic adenocarcinoma has a "bottom heavy" appearance because it undermines the normal small intestinal mucosa.

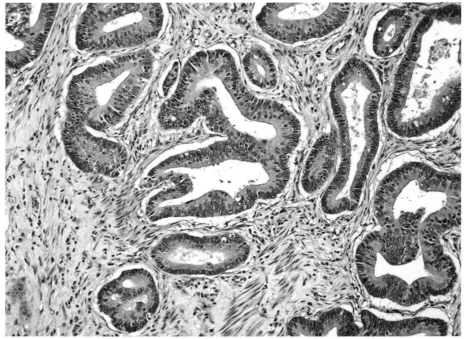

FIGURE 6-16

Ileal resection with metastatic colonic adenocarcinoma. The adenocarcinoma undermines the normal small intestinal mucosa. The adenocarcinoma has ragged glands with prominent surrounding desmoplasia.

TABLE 6-3

Cytokeratin 7 and 20 Expression in Small Intestine and Colorectal Adenocarcinomas

	Small Intestinal Adenocarcinoma	Colorectal Adenocarcinoma
CK7+/CK20+	67% (16/24)	4% (1/23)
CK7−/CK20+	0% (0/24)	91% (21/23)
CK7+/CK20−	33% (8/24)	0% (0/23)
CK7−/CK20−	0% (0/24)	4% (1/23)

Positive labeling, greater than 10% cells decorated.
Data from Chen ZM, Wang HL: Alteration of cytokeratin 7 and cytokeratin 20 expression profile is uniquely associated with tumorigenesis of primary adenocarcinoma of the small intestine. Am J Surg Pathol 2004; 28:1352-1359.

Cytokeratins 7 and 20 are insufficient for excluding other common primary carcinomas because pancreatobiliary, stomach, lung, ovarian, and endometrial tumors may share the same CK7/CK20 pattern seen in small intestinal adenocarcinomas. Immunohistochemical panels should therefore be tailored to the differential diagnoses under consideration. Lung carcinoma will be positive for thyroid transcription factor-1 (TTF-1). Ovarian carcinoma can be positive for estrogen receptor (ER) and progesterone receptor (PR). Breast carcinoma can be positive for ER, PR, and gross cytic disease fluid protein (GCDFP). Pancreatobiliary carcinomas are usually positive for MUC1 and negative for MUC2, CDX2, and DPC4. Adenocarcinoma of the prostate is positive for P504S, prostate-specific membrane antigen (PSMA), and prostate-specific antigen.

7

Gastrointestinal Mesenchymal Tumors

■ **Thong Nguyen, DO** ■ **Cyril Fisher, MD, DSc, FRCPath**
■ **Elizabeth Montgomery, MD**

■ GASTROINTESTINAL STROMAL TUMOR

Gastrointestinal stromal tumors (GISTs) are soft tissue tumors that either express C-kit/CD117 protein or have *C-KIT* or platelet-derived growth factor receptor-α *(PDGFRA)* mutations and show spindle cell or epithelioid morphology. The earlier literature attempted to classify them as smooth muscle or nerve sheath tumors. The term *stromal tumor* was introduced in 1983, after Mazur and Clark failed to find ultrastructural evidence of smooth muscle or nerve sheath differentiation in several gastric tumors.

GISTs have been shown to display differentiation toward interstitial cells of Cajal (ICC), which normally govern gut motility. The availability of specific antibodies and clarification of their immunohistochemical profile has facilitated uniform diagnosis.

CLINICAL FEATURES

GISTs comprise 5% to 10% of all sarcomas and represent about 1% of all GI malignancy. In the United States, 3300 to 4350 new GISTs are reported annually. About 20% to 25% of gastric GISTs are malignant, and the number is higher for intestinal GISTs, 40% to 50%. They are most common in adults 50 to 60 years of age. These tumors vary in differentiation and prognosis according to their location within the GI tract. GISTs are rare in the esophagus, 50% to 70% involve the stomach, 25% to 40% the small intestine (of which 10% to 20% arise in the duodenum, 27% to 37% in the jejunum, and 27% to 53% in the ileum), and less than 10% are colorectal (50% colonic, 50% rectal). GIST-type tumors arising in the omentum, peritoneum, and retroperitoneum have been identified, comprising 6.7% of the large Armed Forces Institute of Pathology (AFIP) series of 1008 GISTs.

Tumors present with primary mass, pain, hemorrhage, or metastasis, and two thirds exceed 5 cm in diameter at presentation. GISTs often metastasize to the abdominal cavity and liver, rarely to bone, soft tissue, skin, lymph nodes, and lungs. Metastasis can occur more than 10 years after surgical resection, underscoring a need for long-term follow-up.

There are three hereditary syndromes of which GIST is a component. First, GIST is found in patients with neurofibromatosis-1 (NF-1). NF-1 is an autosomal dominant genetic disorder resulting from a defect in the *NF1* gene on chromosome 17; affected patients have a deficiency of neurofibromin protein. The clinical

---

GASTROINTESTINAL STROMAL TUMORS—FACT SHEET

Definition

- Gastrointestinal stromal tumor (GIST) is a soft tissue tumor arising from the GI tract that typically expresses CD117 or has *C-KIT* or platelet-derived growth factor receptor α *(PDGFRA)* mutations and shows spindle cells or epithelioid morphology

Incidence and Location

- GIST is extremely rare in the esophagus. It is commonly found in the stomach and intestine
- Up to 5000 cases per year in the United States

Morbidity and Mortality

- Intestinal GIST is more likely to be malignant than gastric GIST

Gender, Race, and Age Distribution

- Adults with no gender predominance; may be overrepresented in African-Americans

Clinical Features

- Site-specific presentation of mural mass

Prognosis and Therapy

- Median survival for esophagus, 29 months; in stomach, 20% of patients die of disease; in the small bowel, about 40% of patients die of disease; similar for colon; appendix tumors rare
- Treatment includes imatinib and newer tyrosine kinase inhibitors
- Patients with exon 11 mutations in the *C-KIT* gene are most likely to respond to this treatment

features of NF-1 include café-au-lait spots, freckling, neurofibromas, malignant peripheral nerve sheath tumors, ganglioneuromas, and GISTs. GISTs arising in the setting of NF-1 tend to be multiple, typically involving the small intestine, and lack *PDGFRA* and *C-KIT* mutations. Instead, GISTs in NF-1 have been shown to have somatic inactivation of their wild-type *NF1* allele, leading to inactivation of neurofibromin, and causing activation of MAP-kinase pathway. Second, familial GIST, in patients with germline *C-KIT* or *PDGFRA* mutations, manifests as a syndrome of GIST, hyperpigmentation, urticaria pigmentosa, mastocytosis, dysphagia, and hyperplasia of ICC. Of the documented families, most have *C-KIT* gene alterations but the *PDGFRA* gene is occasionally affected. Third, GIST is a component of Carney's triad (gastric GIST, paraganglioma, and pulmonary chondroma). GIST in Carney's triad occurs in young individuals, has epithelioid morphology, and shows a strong female predominance. No specific genetic alteration has been identified for Carney's triad.

RADIOLOGIC FEATURES

Radiologic features are not specific, but most large mural gastric masses are GISTs. An example of a gastric epithelioid GIST is seen in Figure 7-1.

PATHOLOGIC FEATURES

GROSS FINDINGS

Tumors vary in diameter from less than 1 cm to greater than 20 cm, and can be submucosal, intramuscular, or subserosal, although most are centered in the muscularis propria. Generally GISTs are relatively well marginated. They can be solid or cystic with variable hemorrhage and necrosis, including mucosal ulceration and tumor cavitation. Figure 7-2 shows a small intestinal GIST.

MICROSCOPIC FINDINGS

There are spindle, epithelioid, and (rare) pleomorphic forms in a variety of patterns and with modifications resulting from stromal features. The two principal cell types are spindle and epithelioid (Figs. 7-3 through 7-7), which can coexist in varying proportions. About 70% of gastric GISTs and most of those in the small and large intestine are spindled. Most esophageal and rectal GISTs are malignant spindle cell tumors. The spindle cells are relatively short, are often uniform, and have tapered nuclei with amphophilic or eosinophilic slightly fibrillary cytoplasm. They form cellular sheets and

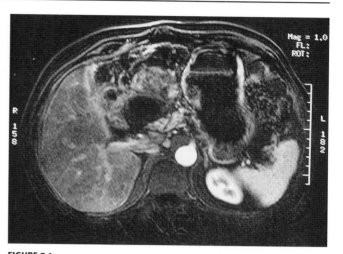

FIGURE 7-1

Imaging study from a patient with a large gastric stromal tumor. It was mistaken for a primary liver lesion by the radiologist.

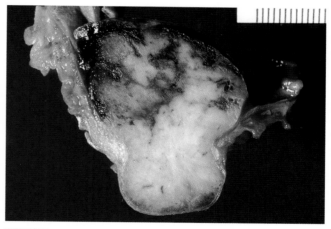

FIGURE 7-2

Small intestinal stromal tumor. This lesion is malignant with metastases to the liver.

fascicles with whorled, storiform, or palisaded patterns. The epithelioid cells have more abundant cytoplasm, with perinuclear halos and well-defined cell borders. Epithelioid GISTs have also been termed *leiomyoblastomas* or *epithelioid smooth muscle tumors*. Clear cell, signet ring, oncocytic, and plasmacytoid variants occur, but multinucleated cells are uncommon. Mitoses vary from none to many. Truly pleomorphic tumors are rare, although both pleomorphism and even unusual differentiation (e.g., skeletal muscle) can be seen in lesions that have been treated with imatinib or related tyrosine kinase inhibitors. The stroma is scanty, but fibrous septa sometimes delineate tumor nests in an organoid pattern. Myxoid or cystic change or hyalinization is sometimes seen, and there can be a variable lymphoplasmacytic inflammatory infiltrate.

GASTROINTESTINAL STROMAL TUMORS—PATHOLOGIC FEATURES

Gross Findings
- Mural mass with variable appearances, including cysts

Microscopic Findings
- Spindle cell or epithelioid, sometimes with "skeinoid" fibers in stroma (particularly in small intestine); sometimes cells have paranuclear vacuoles

Immunohistochemistry
- Positive for CD117, DOG1, CD34, variable actin, S-100 protein, and PDGFRA

Molecular Testing
- Most mutations in *C-KIT* in exon 11, and most mutations in *PDGFRA* in exon 18
- Some mutations predictive of response to targeted therapy
- Laboratories that offer testing can be found at http://www.amptestdirectory.org

Differential Diagnosis
- Smooth muscle (desmin-positive, CD117−) and neural (S-100+, CD117−) tumors
- Sometimes fibromatosis/desmoid has false-positive results for CD117/C-kit

ANCILLARY STUDIES

ULTRASTRUCTURAL FINDINGS

Early studies failed to reveal well-developed smooth muscle differentiation. A minority (about 20%) of GISTs show focally incomplete features of smooth muscle differentiation, with arrays of cytoplasmic intermediate filaments and dense bodies. Many GISTs show neuronal-like differentiation with interdigitating neurite-like cytoplasmic processes that contain microtubules, smooth endoplasmic reticulum, and intermediate filaments. Dense core neuroendocrine granules, some of which are also associated with the prominent Golgi apparatus, and synapse-like structures have been described, but these are not usual features of ICC and might represent entrapped autonomic nerve. There are numerous mitochondria and occasional cell-to-cell junctions (including with smooth muscle cells and neurons).

Skeinoid fibers, which are amorphous periodic acid–Schiff–positive foci of haphazardly arranged modified collagen fibers with a periodicity of 45 nm, are seen rarely, usually in (small) intestinal tumors, benign and malignant, including those in the duodenum. Some GISTs, including CD117/CD34-positive cases, show no ultrastructural differentiation.

IMMUNOHISTOCHEMISTRY

In the 1980s and early 1990s, immunohistochemical studies attempted to confirm supposed smooth muscle, neural, or dual differentiation in GISTs and to relate immunophenotype to behavior. Varying proportions were shown to have smooth muscle actin (SMA), muscle-specific actin (MSA), and desmin, with smaller numbers of cases displaying S-100 protein positivity. Significant numbers remained, however, with no specific markers or only vimentin. Gastrointestinal autonomic neural tumors (GANTs) were variably immunoreactive for neuron-specific enolase (NSE), neurofilaments, synaptophysin, and S-100 protein. In 1994, CD34 was shown to be a reliable marker for the majority of GISTs, and from 1998, CD117 positivity became definitional (Fig. 7-8).

CD117 (KIT), the product of the *C-KIT* gene, is expressed among normal ICCs, mast cells, melanocytes, a variety of epithelia, fetal endothelial cells, and a subset of CD34-positive hematopoietic stem cells. Staining is usually cytoplasmic, but can be membranous in mast cells, melanocytes, and germ cells.

With immunohistochemistry, CD117 is positive (diffuse cytoplasmic staining with membranous accentuation) in the vast majority of benign and malignant GISTs. GISTs with spindle cell and epithelioid morphology are both positive, although less intensely in the latter. Smooth muscle tumors (SMA and desmin positive) and schwannomas (S-100 protein positive) are negative for CD117.

A variety of commercial antibodies to CD117 are available, with varying specificity and sensitivity. For example, using the rabbit polyclonal CD117 antibody marketed by Santa Cruz Biotechnology (C-19, sc-168) positivity is essentially confined to GISTs, among the similar tumors in the differential diagnosis. The rabbit polyclonal antibody A4502, manufactured by Dako (Carpinteria, CA), however, has been reported to stain (the cytoplasm of) lesional fibroblasts and myofibroblasts, including some examples of fibromatosis, and solitary fibrous tumor; awareness of this may prevent misdiagnosis of such tumors as GISTs. These "falsely positive" tumors lack kit mutations and respond only minimally to imatinib treatment.

A small number (2% to 10%) of otherwise typical GISTs are CD117 negative. These are predominantly epithelioid in cell morphology. It has been shown that protein kinase C theta (PKCT) is constitutively activated in all GISTs, including those that are C-kit negative, although by immunoblotting, PKCT expression in these is 50% lower than in C-kit-positive GISTs. Virtually all GISTs were positive with an antibody to PKCT phospho Thr[538]. DOG1 (discovered on GIST-1) antibodies also label most GISTs and may be helpful in that they tend to label GISTS that lack CD117 expression.

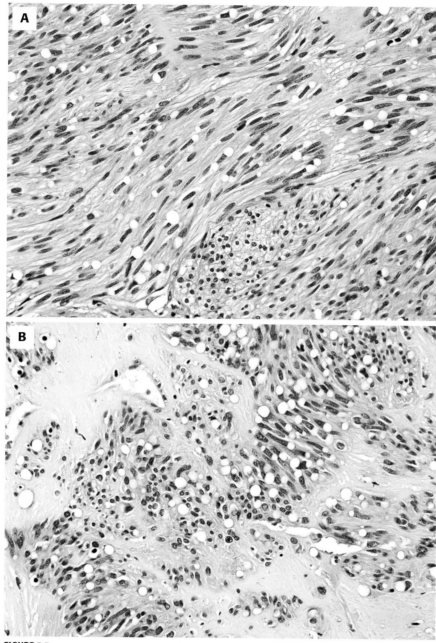

FIGURE 7-3

Gastric stromal tumors exhibiting paranuclear vacuoles. **A,** Such vacuoles are also a feature of smooth muscle tumors, but they are seldom so numerous in true smooth muscle tumors. **B,** Myxoid stroma is seen, a feature that would not be present in a smooth muscle tumor, and the nuclei have more tapered ends than smooth muscle tumor nuclei.

CD34 is positive in 47% to 100% of GISTs, and its expression varies with location within the GI tract. Miettinen and associates found, among CD117-positive tumors, 100%, 90%, 47%, 65%, 96%, and 64% of cases to be CD34-positive in esophagus, stomach, small intestine, colon, rectum, and extraintestinal locations, respectively. Among malignant gastric and small intestinal GISTs, 88% and 55% were CD34-positive. Tumors that are CD34-positive are almost always CD117-positive,

and most CD34-negative tumors are CD117 positive. CD117 is sometimes lost in metastases. It should be noted that CD34 is also positive in occasional smooth muscle tumors, including epithelioid variants.

Antibodies against platelet-derived growth factor receptors α and β (PDGFRA and PDGFRB), which are produced by Santa Cruz Biotechnology (pAb, no.sc-338 for PDGFRA and pAb, no. sc-339 for PDGFRB), are also available and label a subset of CD117-negative

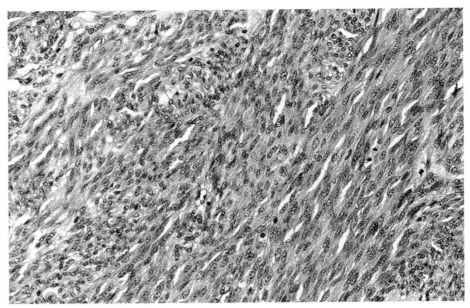

FIGURE 7-4

Small intestinal GIST. Corresponds to the gross lesion depicted in Figure 7-1 and is highly cellular and mitotically active.

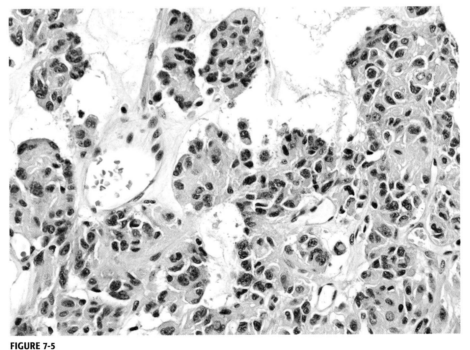

FIGURE 7-5

Epithelioid gastric GIST. Such tumors have been termed "leiomyoblastomas" in the past.

GISTs. However, some fibromatoses cases also show labeling with PDGFRA and PDGFRB antibodies.

SMA is found only focally in up to half of GISTs in an inverse frequency of expression to that of CD34 (the two sometimes showing a mosaic distribution); benign GISTs of the small intestine have the highest proportion of SMA positivity. h-Caldesmon (an actin-binding cytoskeleton-associated protein) is positive in about 80% of GISTs, supporting myoid differentiation, and calponin in about 25%. Desmin is focally positive in up

to 20% of tumors of the esophagus and omentum/peritoneum and in a small proportion of benign (but not in malignant) GISTs in the stomach and small intestine. Cytokeratins are rarely positive but are occasionally seen in malignant epithelioid GISTs.

A few have neurogenic differentiation, with positivity for S-100 protein (especially in small bowel tumors), PGP9.5, and NSE, and a few of these additionally express SMA, implying both neurogenic and myoid differentiation. Both GISTs and ICCs express

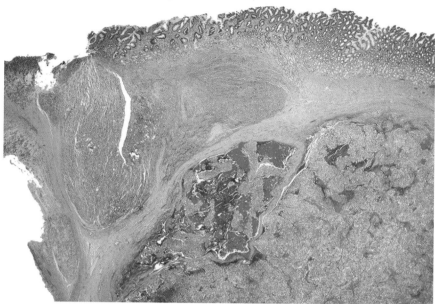

FIGURE 7-6

Epithelioid gastric GIST. On the left portion of the field, this lesion has invaded the mucosa, a feature associated with a poor prognosis. Note that the tumor is centered in the muscularis propria.

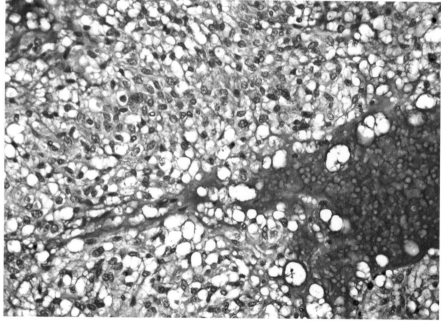

FIGURE 7-7

Epithelioid gastric GIST. Note the prominent cytoplasmic vacuoles and uniform nuclei; nuclear pleomorphism is unusual in GISTs and its presence should prompt the pathologist to consider other diagnoses.

embryonic smooth muscle myosin heavy chain messenger RNA.

FINE-NEEDLE ASPIRATION BIOPSY

Fine-needle aspiration can be used to diagnose GISTs with appropriate immunohistochemistry but cannot be used to assess malignant potential.

MOLECULAR STUDIES

Two receptors in the type III receptor tyrosine kinase subfamily have been shown to play an important role in the pathogenesis of GIST: (1) C-kit receptor and (2) platelet-derived growth factor receptor-α (*PDGFRA*). The genes encoding for these two receptors are both located in chromosome 4. The protein structure of these

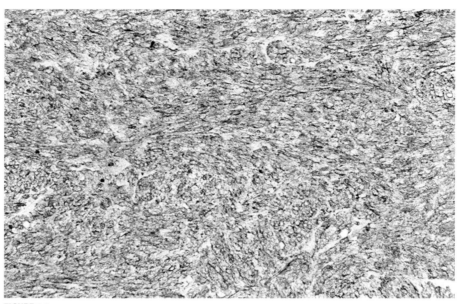

FIGURE 7-8

CD117/C-kit expression in GIST, with cytoplasmic and membranous labeling. CD117 staining is seen regardless of malignant potential in the vast majority of stromal tumors.

receptors are also similar, including an extracellular (EC) domain, transmembrane (TM) domain, juxtamembrane (JM) domain, and tyrosine kinase (TK) domains. As a result of their similarities, activating mutation in either one of these two genes will lead to activation of similar signal transduction pathways leading to GIST formation.

In sporadic GISTs, 85% to 90% of the cases have mutations in the *C-KIT* gene while 10% to 15% of the remaining cases do not. The mutations of *C-KIT* gene occur in order of decreasing frequency: exon 11, exon 9, exon 13, and exon 17. The types of mutations in exon 11 include: in-frame deletions (60% to 70%) of one to several codons at 5′ end of codon 11 and region between codons Gln^{550} to Glu^{561}; missense point mutations (20% to 30%) at Trp^{557}, Val^{559}, Val^{560}, and Leu^{576}; and internal tandem duplications of 1 to more than 20 codons at 3′ end of codon 11. The clinical significance associated with mutations in exon 11 is that they may play a role in predicting response to treatment. Most mutations of the *C-KIT* gene occur at this exon (juxtamembrane domain). The juxtamembrane domain is an intracytoplasmic domain located between the transmembrane and tyrosine kinase domains and its function, after activation, is to induce dimerization of two C-kit receptors, which leads activation of the downstream signal transduction pathways.

At exon 9, encoding the extracellular domain, most of the cases show 6-nucleotide duplications encoding Ala^{502}-Tyr^{503} and this mutation is usually encountered in intestinal GISTs. At exon 13, the most common mutation is the 1945A>G substitution leading to $Lys^{642}Glu$. At exon 17 encoding the tyrosine kinase II domain, the most common mutation is the 2487T>A

substitution leading to $Asn^{822}Lys$. Interestingly, seminoma and mastocytoma are two neoplasms that also express CD117; these both commonly have mutations in exon 17. In contrast, CD117-positive GIST rarely shows mutations at codon 17 and more commonly has exon 11 mutations.

As noted, 10% to 15% of sporadic GIST lack *C-KIT* gene mutations. About 35% to 63% of these cases have mutations in the *PDGFRA* gene. Mutations of *PDGFRA* gene occur, in order of decreasing frequency, in exon 18 (>80%), exon 12, and exon 14. In exon 18, a missense mutation leading to $Asp^{842}Val$ is commonly seen. In exon 12, a missense mutation is reported, $Val^{561}Asp$. In exon 14, a missense mutation is seen, $Asn^{659}Lys/Tyr$.

Understanding the specific mutations in *C-KIT* and *PDGFRA* genes is important because of the following five clinical implications. First, in terms of prognosis, GISTs with exon 11 mutations are associated with longer event-free and overall survival than GISTs with exon 9 mutations and GISTs with no detectable kinase mutation. Second, GISTs with exon 11 mutations have a better response to imatinib than GISTs with exon 9 mutation in C-*KIT* gene, GISTs with *PDGFRA* mutation, and wild-type GISTs. Third, in terms of dosing of imatinib, cases of metastatic/advanced GISTs with exon 9 mutation require higher doses of imatinib to achieve a response. Fourth, knowing the mutation status in the *C-KIT* and *PDGFRA* genes occasionally identifies patients who have unidentified genetic diseases. Specifically, in patients with wild-type GISTs, there is enrichment for NF-1 and Carney triad. Finally, when GISTs show resistance to first-line tyrosine kinase inhibitor such as imitanib, identification of secondary mutations can help in choosing a second-line tyrosine kinase inhibitor (e.g., sunitinib) for treatment. An excellent resource for arranging for molecular testing of GISTs, as well as other molecular tests, is found through the Association for Molecular Pathology at http://www.amptestdirectory.org/.

DIFFERENTIAL DIAGNOSIS

The differential diagnosis includes the other mesenchymal tumors discussed in this chapter, but in most cases, the differential diagnosis should include smooth muscle tumors, schwannomas, and occasionally fibromatosis.

PROGNOSIS AND THERAPY

BEHAVIOR

GENERAL

Perfect separation of benign and malignant GISTs cannot be achieved. However, the main prognostic factors identified have been mitotic count and tumor size. Both size and mitotic activity are continuous variables, and researchers have taken different cut-off points. Guidelines using combinations of maximum dimension and mitotic count for defining risk have recently been proposed as in Table 7-1, but are imperfect because they do not take site into account. Refined schemes have been developed for gastric and small bowel GISTs (Tables 7-2 through 7-4).

Site-specific analyses, including a large AFIP series of 1008 cases, have shown location, size, mitotic count, and age to be independent prognostic variables. Small intestinal tumors are the most aggressive. However, in

no site are size and mitotic count alone sufficient for long-term prediction of behavior, so no definite criteria proposed for diagnosis of malignancy are predictive of outcome. For unclear reasons, malignant examples appear to be overrepresented in African-Americans.

REGIONAL

Esophagus. GISTs account for a minority of esophageal stromal tumors (and leiomyomas for the majority), and involve the lower third or gastroesophageal junction, predominantly in males. They can be spindled or epithelioid and display the usual variety of patterns. All are CD117 and CD34 positive, and about 15% have SMA or desmin. The majority are malignant. In the series of Miettinen and coworkers, 9 of 16 patients died of disease, including all with tumors larger than 10 cm, and none with tumors smaller than 5 cm. Median

TABLE 7-1

Proposed Guidelines Using Combinations of Maximum Dimension and Mitotic Count for Defining Risk

	Size (cm)	Mitotic Count/50 hpf
Very low risk	<2	<5
Low risk	2-5	<5
Intermediate risk	<5	6-10
	5-10	<5
High risk	>5	>5
	>10	Any
	Any	>10

hpf, high-power field.

TABLE 7-2

Prognosis of Gastric versus Small Bowel GISTs

Stomach GISTs; 20% Tumor-Related Deaths		Small Intestinal GISTs; 40% Tumor-Related Deaths	
Size/mitoses/50 hpf	Outcome (with metastases)	Size/mitoses/50 hpf	Outcome (with metastases)
<10 cm, <5 mitoses/50 hpf	3%	<5 cm, <5 mitoses/50 hpf	3%
>10 cm, ≥5 mitoses/50 hpf	86%	>10 cm, ≥5 mitoses/50 hpf	86%
>10 cm, <5 mitoses/50 hpf	11%	>10 cm, <5 mitoses/50 hpf *or* <5 cm, ≥5 mitoses/50 hpf	>50%
<5 cm, ≥5 mitoses/50 hpf	15%	5-10 cm, ≥5 mitoses/50 hpf	24%

hpf, high-power field.

Data from Miettinen M, Lasota J: Gastrointestinal stromal tumors: review on morphology, molecular pathology, prognosis, and differential diagnosis. Arch Pathol Lab Med 2006; 130:1466-1478.

TABLE 7-3

Suggested Prognostic Criteria for Resected GISTs Arising in the Stomach

Category	Group	Size and Mitotic Activity	Prognostic Features
Benign	1	≤2 cm, ≤5 mitoses/50 hpf	No tumor-related mortality detected
Probably benign	2 3a	>2 cm, ≤5 cm, ≤5 mitoses/50 hpf >5 cm, ≥10 cm, ≥5 mitoses/50 hpf	Very low malignant potential, <3% progressive disease
Uncertain or low malignant potential	4	≤2 cm, >5 mitoses/50 hpf	No progressive disease (too few cases available to reliably determine prognosis)
Low to moderate malignant potential	3b 5	>10 cm, ≥5 mitoses/50 hpf >2 cm, ≤5 cm, >5 mitoses/50 hpf	12%-15% tumor-related mortality
High malignant potential	6a 6b	>5, ≤10 cm, >5 mitoses/50 hpf >10 cm, >5 mitoses/50 hpf	49%-86% tumor-related mortality

Data from Miettinen M, Lasota J: Gastrointestinal stromal tumors: review on morphology, molecular pathology, prognosis, and differential diagnosis. Arch Pathol Lab Med 2006; 130:1466-1478.

TABLE 7-4

Suggested Prognostic Criteria for Resected GISTs Arising in the Jejunum and Ileum

Category	Group	Size And Mitotic Activity	Prognostic Features
Practically benign	1	<2 cm, ≤5 mitoses/50 hpf	No evidence of progressive disease
Low malignant potential	2	>2 cm, ≤5 cm, <5 mitoses/50 hpf	<5% progressive disease
Moderate malignant potential	3a	>5 cm, ≤10 cm, ≤5 mitoses/50 hpf	10%-30% progressive disease
High malignant potential	3b	>10 cm, ≤5 mitoses/50 hpf	≥50% progressive disease/tumor-related mortality
	4	≤2 cm, >5 mitoses/50 hpf	
	5	>2 cm, <5 cm, >5 mitoses/50 hpf	
	6a	>5 cm, ≤10 cm, >5 mitoses/50 hpf	
	6b	>10 cm, >5 mitoses/50 hpf	

Data from Miettinen M, Lasota J: Gastrointestinal stromal tumors: review on morphology, molecular pathology, prognosis, and differential diagnosis. Arch Pathol Lab Med 2006; 130:1466-1478.

survival was 29 months. However, a subset of GISTs of the gastroesophageal junction is minute, multiple, and presumably does not progress, because these "seedling" GISTS are encountered commonly (approximately 10%) in autopsies and resections when the entire gastroesophageal junction is embedded (Fig. 7-9)

Stomach. About 20% are result in patient deaths. The consensus is that 5 mitoses per 50 high-power fields (hpf) and size greater than 5 cm are adverse prognostic factors. The 5-year survival rate of gastric GISTs is about 80%, with improvement in completely resected cases. There is no evidence that radical surgery improves survival, so the least extensive surgical procedure compatible with complete excision is advisable. Gastric GISTs are more frequent in males.

Epithelioid GISTs (formerly called *leiomyoblasto-mas*) comprise about 10% of gastric GISTs, of which about 80% are benign. Large tumors in the fundus or cardiac area and posterior wall are more likely to be malignant.

Duodenum. Duodenal GISTs are most common in the second part, and 35% to 50% are malignant. Miettinen and associates studied 156 duodenal GISTs, with the following results: 12 patients whose tumors were less than 2 cm with mitoses less than or equal to 5/50hpf had no recurrence, metastases, or tumor-related death during follow-up of 6 years. However, 18 of 21 patients (86%) with tumors greater than 5 cm with greater than 5 mitoses/50 hpf had metastases and disease-related death with a median survival time of 21 months.

Jejunum and Ileum. About 40% result in patient deaths. These GISTs can be spindled, epithelioid, or mixed; mixed and epithelioid tumors are associated with worse behavior than spindled tumors. The presence of

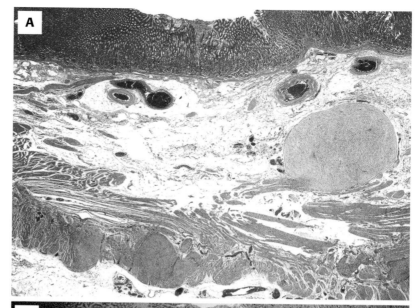

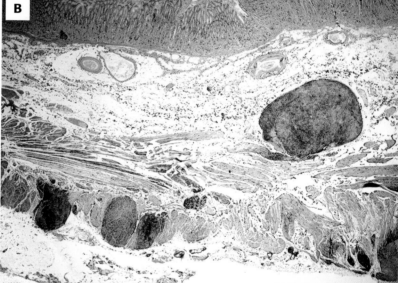

FIGURE 7-9

"Seedling" GISTs of the gastroesophageal junction are common and apparently do not progress to clinically evident lesions. Several small nodules are seen on H&E **(A),** and highlighted by CD117 **(B)** and CD34 **(C)** staining.

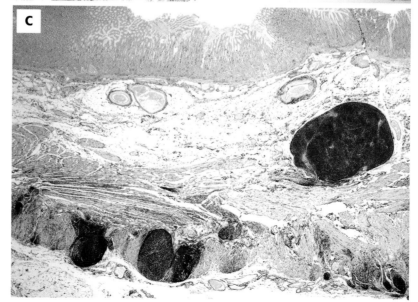

skeinoid fibers, PAS-reactive thick collagen fibers, present in about 45% of the cases, is a favorable prognostic factor. As in other sites, the most important factors determining the prognosis are tumor size and mitotic index. Small (<5 cm) with few mitoses (≤5 mitoses/50 hpf), convey an excellent prognosis. In contrast, large (>10 cm) mitotically active (>10 mitoses/50 hpf) GISTs are highly aggressive. Most small intestinal GISTs have mutation in exon 11 of *C-KIT* with few cases showing mutations in exons 9 and 17 of *C-KIT*. These mutations lack prognostic significance. *PDGFRA* mutations are rare in small bowel GISTs.

Colon. Tumors are most common in adults in the sixth decade of life in the ascending and descending portions of the colon and usually present with pain or a mass. Except for small subserosal lesions, they are typically transmural tumors with intraluminal and outward-bulging components. Morphologically they are heterogeneous, with spindle cells in fascicles, palisades or storiform arrangement, and sometimes an organoid pattern; a minority have epithelioid cells in varying proportions.

Moyana and colleagues and Tworek and associates have taken a size of 5 cm and 5 mitoses per 10 hpf as thresholds for malignancy, but Miettinen and coworkers found lower levels. In their series, tumors smaller than 1 cm did not recur, whereas in larger tumors 20% with minimal mitoses and all with more than 5 mitoses per 50 hpf metastasized or caused patient deaths. Interestingly, the few cases with skeinoid fibers had a better prognosis.

Appendix. GISTs of the appendix are rare. Miettinen and Sobin described four cases in men 56 to 72 years of age (mean 63 years). Two tumors occurred in patients who had undergone surgery for appendicitis-like symptoms: one was an incidental finding during surgery for a malignant gastric epithelioid GIST and one was an incidental autopsy finding. One was a polypoid GIST projected outward from the proximal part of the appendix. Three tumors were partially obliterating nodules, eccentrically expanding the appendiceal wall. All four were spindle cell tumors, and three of them contained extracellular collagen globules (skeinoid fibers); none had atypia or mitotic activity (< 1 mitosis per 50 hpf). Follow-up revealed death resulting from cardiovascular disease in one case (4 years after appendectomy) and liver failure because of malignant gastric epithelioid GIST metastatic to the liver in another case 15 years after the appendectomy.

Anorectum. These are rare tumors. St. Mark's Hospital in London (a specialist lower GI institution) had only 25 "leiomyosarcomas" of the rectum in a 25-year period. Thirty-two percent to 54% of rectal GISTs are malignant, the smallest being 1.6 cm, but most exceed 5 cm and have greater than 5 mitoses per 50 hpf. In the series of Miettinen and colleagues of 133 anorectal GISTs, 54% recurred or metastasized (to liver, lung, or bone), sometimes after a long interval. Seventy percent of patients whose tumors were larger than 5 cm and with greater than 5 mitoses per 50 hpf died. One tumor smaller than 2 cm and with fewer than 5 mitoses per 50 hpf recurred, but no patients died. Eighteen of 29 cases (62%) had GIST-specific *C-KIT* mutations, mainly in exon 11. Survival rates are around 60% at 5 years and 20% to 50% at 10 years (for patients with curative rather than palliative resections).

Extragastrointestinal GISTs. These GISTs have been described by a number of observers. Some data suggest that single omental GISTs unattached to the GI tract resemble gastric lesions, raising the possibility that they are gastric GISTs that have extended into the omentum. In contrast, multiple omental GISTs are more reminiscent of small bowel GISTs and thus may arise in the small bowel and metastases/extensions. Solitary examples are associated with a better prognosis than multiple ones. Kit reactive Cajal cells are absent in the omentum.

TREATMENT

Complete excision is the initial treatment. Gene product-targeted therapy, utilizing STI571, a 2-phenylaminopyrimidine derivative that is a selective inhibitor of *C-KIT*, and PDGFR tyrosine kinases has been ongoing since 2002. The first case report was published in 2001. The initial response is rapid and relatively free of side effects. Treated tumors show small pyknotic nuclei in an eosinophilic myxoid background, unusual pleomorphic cells, or even heterologous differentiation (e.g., rhabdomyosarcomatous differentiation). Tumors with *kit* exon 11 mutations are more likely to respond to therapy than those with exon 9 or exon 13 mutations. Those with PDGRA mutations typically do not respond. Additional tyrosine kinase inhibitors are available (e.g., sunitinib malate) for unresponsive lesions, some of which have acquired resistance to imatinib.

■ SMOOTH MUSCLE TUMORS OF THE GASTROINTESTINAL TRACT

CLINICAL FEATURES

Smooth muscle tumors of the GI tract consist of leiomyoma and leiomyosarcoma. Clinically, smooth muscle neoplasms of the GI tract often present as polypoid lesions extending into the gut lumen. Colonic leiomyomas classically arise in association with the muscularis mucosae and present as distal polyps on screening colonoscopy. GI smooth muscle tumors can also arise as intramural masses associated with the muscularis propria. In general, esophageal leiomyomas often present as intramural masses while leiomyomas and leiomyosarcoma of the

SMOOTH MUSCLE TUMORS OF THE GASTROINTESTINAL TRACT—FACT SHEET

Definition
- Smooth muscle tumors of the GI tract are spindle cell tumors showing differentiation along smooth muscle lines

Incidence and Location
- These are rare tumors, but leiomyomas are the most common spindle cell tumor of the esophagus
- Leiomyomas also arise in association with the muscularis mucosae of the colorectum
- In the remainder of the GI tract, true smooth muscle tumors are far outnumbered by gastrointestinal stromal tumors but tend to be malignant (leiomyosarcomas)

Morbidity and Mortality
- Leiomyomas are benign; approximately 75% of patients with leiomyosarcomas of the GI tract die of their tumors

Gender, Race, and Age Distribution
- No gender or race preference
- Occurs in adults (average 60 years)

Clinical Features
- Smooth muscle tumors of the esophagus often present as intramural mass while smooth muscle tumors of the colon usually present as polypoid lesions
- Smooth muscle tumors of small intestine can present as either intramural mass or polypoid lesions

Prognosis and Therapy
- Poor prognosis for leiomyosarcomas; leiomyomas are benign
- All lesions except small polyps of colorectum (leiomyomas) are treated surgically; there is no targeted chemotherapy as there is for GISTs and the tumors have no characteristic mutations

SMOOTH MUSCLE TUMORS OF THE GASTROINTESTINAL TRACT—PATHOLOGIC FEATURES

Gross Findings
- Not specific; esophageal leiomyomas are whorled whitish masses
- Leiomyosarcomas in other sites are mural and variably necrotic, and usually well marginated

Microscopic Findings
- Spindle cells with perpendicularly oriented fascicles of brightly eosinophilic spindle cells with blunt-ended cigar-shaped nuclei and sometimes paranuclear vacuoles
- Abundant mitosis, cytologic atypia, and necrosis

Immunohistochemistry
- Positive for desmin, SMA, calponin, caldesmon
- Negative for CD117 and S-100 protein
- Occasional focal keratin common in leiomyosarcoma
- Usually negative for CD34

Differential Diagnosis
- GIST primarily, which is CD117 positive and desmin negative, and nerve sheath tumors (positive for S-100)

RADIOLOGIC FEATURES

The radiologic features are not specific and are not distinguishable from those of GIST.

PATHOLOGIC FEATURES

GROSS FINDINGS

The gross appearance of these tumors is nonspecific. Esophageal leiomyomas form whorled masses similar to uterine leiomyomas. The occasional leiomyomas arising in the muscularis mucosae of the colorectum present as polyps. Leiomyosarcomas of the colorectum have been described as intraluminal bulging polypoid masses.

MICROSCOPIC FINDINGS

True smooth muscle tumors have the same features of smooth muscle differentiation seen elsewhere in the body, namely perpendicularly oriented fascicles of spindle cells with brightly eosinophilic cytoplasm with longitudinal striations and blunt-ended nuclei with paranuclear vacuoles (Figs. 7-10 through 7-14). Leiomyosarcoma is characterized by mitoses, cytologic atypia, and necrosis.

ANCILLARY STUDIES

ULTRASTRUCTURAL FINDINGS

The ultrastructural features are those of smooth muscle differentiation elsewhere (thin filaments, pinocytotic vesicles, attachment plaques, and interrupted external lamina).

colon often have a polypoid configuration. In the esophagus, the vast majority of spindle cell tumors are true leiomyomas—even the AFIP was only able to collect 17 GISTs from the esophagus. Leiomyoma of the esophagus is found in patients with a median age of 35 years with a male (about 70%), and has an indolent course. Leiomyosarcoma of the esophagus is truly rare and it follows an aggressive course. Smooth muscle tumors of small intestine are rare; it is estimated that one smooth muscle tumor occurs for every 36 GISTs. Both leiomyoma and leiomyosarcoma can be encountered throughout the small intestines of adults, presenting as a polypoid or intramural masses. Leiomyoma and leiomyosarcoma in the colon commonly present as polyps. Leiomyoma of the colon has male predominance of 2.4:1, occurs at a median age of 62 years old, and follows a benign course. Leiomyomas can occur extramurally adjoining the colon where they resemble uterine leiomyoma and even express hormone receptors. Leiomyosarcoma of the colon shows a slight male predominance and presents in adults. Leiomyomatosis has been described in small intestine and colon. True leiomyosarcoma is rare in the stomach.

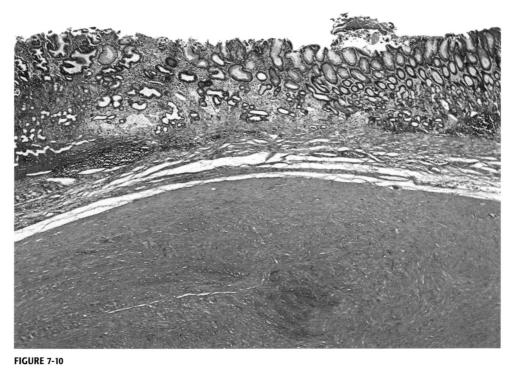

FIGURE 7-10
This gastric leiomyoma has arisen in association with the muscularis mucosae. It is brightly eosinophilic at low magnification.

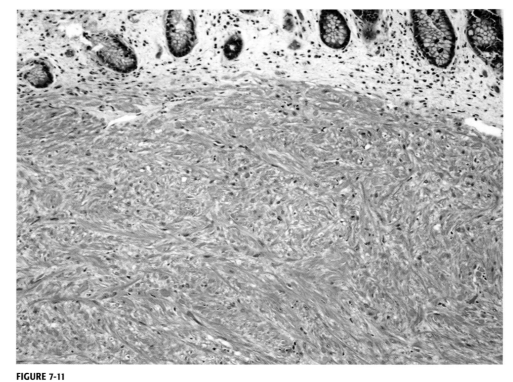

FIGURE 7-11
This distal colonic leiomyoma is hypocellular and merges with the residual muscularis mucosae. The nuclei are blunt ended.

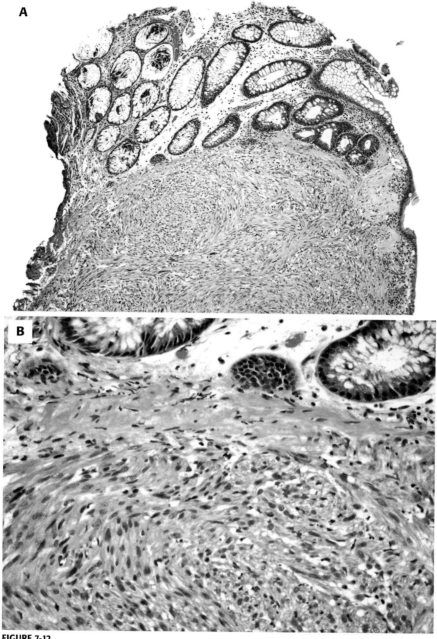

FIGURE 7-12

Leiomyosarcoma showing perpendicularly oriented fascicles of spindle cells with striking cytoplasmic eosinophilia **(A).** Compare the cellularity of this lesion **(B)** to that seen in Figure 7-11.

IMMUNOHISTOCHEMISTRY

True smooth muscle tumors are actin and desmin reactive and lack CD117/C-kit. Calponin and h-caldesmon are expressed and CD34 is typically absent. S-100 protein is absent. Some lesions display keratin expression, a feature of leiomyosarcomas in general.

DIFFERENTIAL DIAGNOSIS

The differential diagnosis is primarily with GIST and nerve sheath tumors, and the majority of lesions are readily separable based on immunohistochemistry.

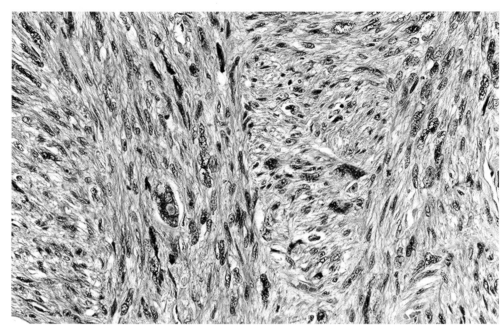

FIGURE 7-13
This leiomyosarcoma is similar to the one depicted in Figure 7-12A, but has more striking nuclear alterations.

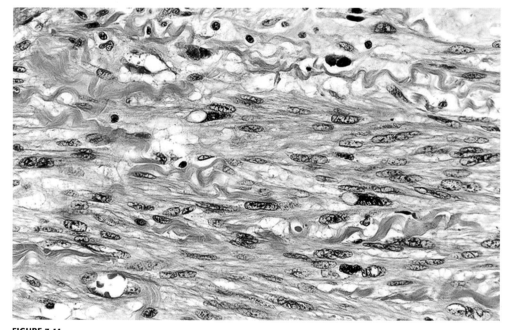

FIGURE 7-14
Leiomyosarcoma. The nuclei have blunt ends and there are scattered paranuclear vacuoles. The cytoplasm has delicate longitudinal striations.

PROGNOSIS AND THERAPY

The prognosis of leiomyomas is excellent in all sites because they are benign. In general, GI tract leiomyosarcomas have a poor prognosis, and about 75 % of patients die of their tumors.

■ SCHWANNOMAS

CLINICAL FEATURES

Most schwannomas occur in the stomach, involving the submucosa and muscularis propria. However, as a result of more widespread screening colonoscopy, colonic

SCHWANNOMAS—FACT SHEET

Definition

- Gastrointestinal schwannomas are benign nerve sheath tumors that differ from those typically found in the peripheral nervous system by lacking capsules.

Incidence and Location

- These are rare and usually affect the stomach, where they are mural
- In the colon, schwannomas often present as polypoid lesions

Morbidity and Mortality

- Gastrointestinal schwannomas are benign and typically not syndromic

Gender, Race, and Age Distribution

- No known gender/race predominance
- Present in adults

Clinical Features

- Site specific, often incidental

Prognosis and Therapy

- Benign and treated by simple excision

SCHWANNOMAS—PATHOLOGIC FEATURES

Gross Findings

- Well marginated but not encapsulated, in contrast to most schwannomas
- Generally mural in the stomach and polypoid in the colon

Microscopic Findings

- Unencapsulated infiltrative spindle cell lesion with admixed plasma cells and scattered lymphocytes
- Minimal palisading
- Striking lymphoid cuff at periphery of tumor
- Spindle and plexiform patterns seen in the colon

Immunohistochemistry

- Strong diffuse S-100 protein
- May be positive for CD34
- Negative muscle markers
- Negative for CD117

Differential Diagnosis

- Primarily GIST (usually negative for S-100, positive for CD117/C-kit), which lacks the lymphoid cuff
- Smooth muscle tumors (SMA- and desmin-positive), which have elongated blunt-ends nuclei
- Neurofibroma, which usually has wiry collagen background and can be associated with NF-1
- Benign fibroblastic polyp of the colon/perineurioma (negative for S-100, variable EMA), which has bland oval nuclei

schwannomas are encountered with increasing frequency in daily practice.

RADIOLOGIC AND ENDOSCOPIC FEATURES

Gastric tumors are not distinguishable from GISTs. Colonic schwannoma presents as a polypoid lesion ranging from 0.5 to 1.2 cm centered in the mucosa, submucosa, or muscularis propria.

PATHOLOGIC FEATURES

GROSS FINDINGS

Schwannomas are grossly similar to GISTs, having a whitish cut surface and well-circumscribed outline without a capsule.

MICROSCOPIC FINDINGS

GI tract schwannomas are not encapsulated, a feature that distinguishes them from schwannomas in the peripheral nervous system. They have a lymphoid cuff with germinal centers, and intralesional lymphocytes can be seen. They are composed of interlacing bundles of spindle cells that are only loosely palisaded (in contrast to GISTs, which, ironically, often display striking palisading). They appear similar to GISTs, but the lymphoid cuff is a tip-off that these are schwannian

(Figs. 7-15 through 7-18). In the colon, schwannomas can be classified into two types: spindle cells and plexiform. Schwannoma with spindle cell features are composed of spindle cells with wavy elongated nuclei with tapering ends, scanty eosinophilic cytoplasm, and indistinct cell borders. Schwannomas with plexiform features form nodules of spindle cells.

ANCILLARY STUDIES

IMMUNOHISTOCHEMISTRY

These benign tumors are strongly labeled with S-100 protein (Fig. 7-19) and low-affinity nerve growth factor receptor (p75). Schwannomas can show labeling with C34, glial fibrillary acidic protein (GFAP), and collagen type IV with a pericellular pattern. Calretinin is unusually negative in GI tract "schwannomas" (in contrast, schwannomas of the somatic soft tissues typically express calretinin). The tumors lack muscle markers and CD117.

ULTRASTRUCTURAL FINDINGS

Schwannoma shows characteristics of Schwann cell differentiation such as interdigitation, rudimentary cell junctions, basal lamina, and intracytoplasmic electron dense crystaloids.

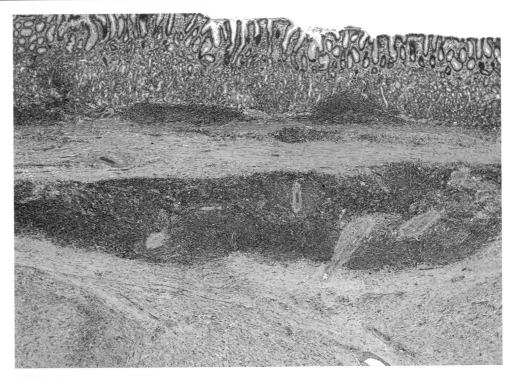

FIGURE 7-15

Gastric schwannoma. Note the striking lymphoid cuff at low magnification. This is a helpful diagnostic feature in separating these tumors (always benign) from GISTs (which may behave in a malignant fashion).

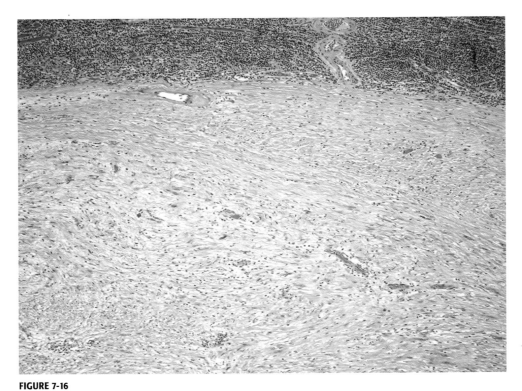

FIGURE 7-16

If this gastric schwannoma were mistaken for a GIST, the nuclear variability would result in an interpretation of a GIST of uncertain potential. The lymphoid cuff, as well as scattered intratumoral lymphocytes, are tip-offs that this is instead a benign schwannoma.

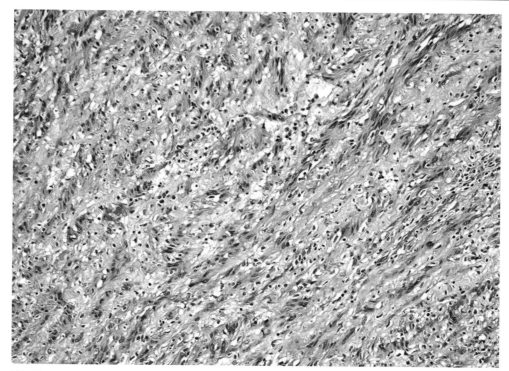

FIGURE 7-17
Gastric schwannoma. At intermediate magnification there is a mild inflammatory backdrop within the lesion.

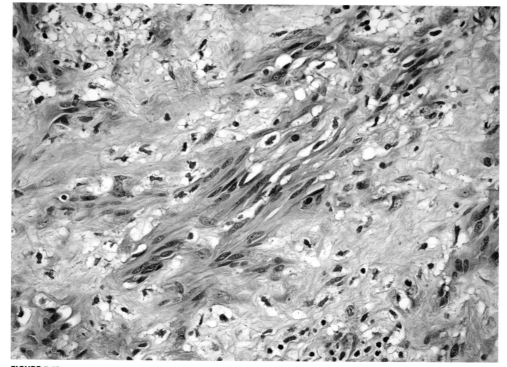

FIGURE 7-18
Gastric schwannoma. At high magnification the tapered ends of the nuclei are apparent.

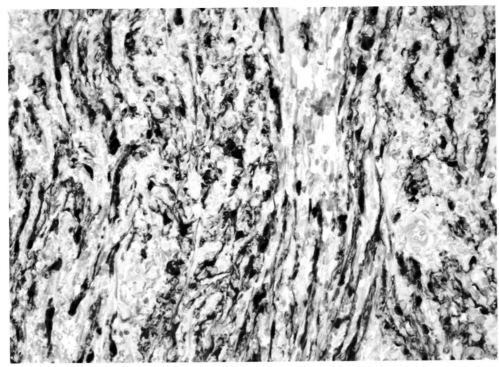

FIGURE 7-19
Gastric schwannoma. Nuclear and cytoplasmic S-100 protein expression.

MOLECULAR STUDIES

In addition to lacking calretinin labeling on immuno-histochemistry, GI "schwannomas" lack alterations in the *NF2* gene, in contrast to somatic soft tissue schwannomas.

DIFFERENTIAL DIAGNOSIS

The differential diagnoses include GIST, smooth muscle tumor, neurofibroma, and benign fibroblastic polyp (perineurioma). GISTs express CD117 and lack S-100 protein; the reverse is true for schwannoma. Smooth muscle tumors express muscle markers such as smooth muscle actin or desmin, and their nuclei are often elongated with characteristic blunt ends as compared with the wavy tapering ends of schwannoma cells. Both neurofibroma and schwannoma are labeled with S-100 protein, and the background of neurofibroma often shows collagen deposit as elongated fibers or collagenous matrix. Benign fibroblastic tumor of the colon (perineurioma) does not react with S-100. Lesions regarded as perineurioma express EMA, claudin 1 and GLUT1, but not S-100 protein.

PROGNOSIS AND THERAPY

GI schwannomas are benign.

■ NEUROFIBROMA

CLINICAL FEATURES

Neurofibroma is a rare lesion of the GI tract, accounting for about 1 in 460 colonic polyps. It commonly occurs as polyp in the colon. The tumor is also seen in the stomach and jejunum. There are three presentations of neurofibroma in the GI tract. First, about 25 % of patients with NF-I have GI tract lesions including neurofibromas, GISTs, somatostatin-producing endocrine neoplasms of the periampullary region of the duodenum, and disorders of gut motility secondary to hyperplasia of nerve plexi or ganglioneuromatosis. Second, patients with intestinal neurofibromatosis have multiple neurofibromas without clinical features of NF-1. This group is rare and there are fewer than 20 reported cases. Third, patients with nonsyndromatic (sporadic) neurofibromas manifest isolated polyps, most commonly in the colon.

Sporadic colonic neurofibromas are found in middle age patients with no gender predilection. Reported symptoms include abdominal pain, palpable masses, obstruction, intussusception, rectal prolapse, and bleeding.

ENDOSCOPIC FEATURES

In patients with NF-1 or intestinal neurofibromatosis, multiple polyps are seen. In sporadic examples, a single polyp is identified.

NEUROFIBROMA—FACT SHEET

Definition
- Neurofibroma is a benign nerve sheath tumor composed of Schwann cells, axons, fibrobasts, and perineurial-like cells

Incidence and Location
- Neurofibroma occurs in three clinical settings: neurofibroma associated with NF-1; non–NF-1–associated intestinal neurofibromatosis, and solitary nonsyndromic neurofibroma
- Neurofibroma occurs in colon, stomach, and small intestine

Morbidity and Mortality
- Benign tumor

Gender, Race, and Age Distribution
- No known gender/race predominance

Clinical Features
- Site-specific

Prognosis and Therapy
- Benign; no recurrence except those associated with syndromic disease

NEUROFIBROMA—PATHOLOGIC FEATURES

Gross Findings
- Multiple colonic polyps in neurofibromatosis 1 (NF-1) and non–NF-1–associated neurofibromatosis
- Single polyp in solitary neurofibroma

Microscopic Findings
- Neurofibroma can have solitary, plexiform, and diffuse patterns
- In solitary neurofibroma, a proliferation of spindle cells with wavy, tapered-end nuclei situation in a collagenous matrix
- Plexiform pattern characteristic of NF-1–associated lesions

Immunohistochemistry
- Spindle cells are labeled with S-100 and NSE
- Negative to focal-weak positive for calretinin

Differential Diagnosis
- Schwannoma (lymphoid cuff and intralesional inflammation)
- Ganglioneuroma (ganglion cells present)
- GIST (CD117-positive)
- Mucosal neuroma associated with MEN 2B consists of hyperplastic bundles of nerve fibers, including frequent axons reminiscent of traumatic neuroma

PATHOLOGIC FEATURES

GROSS FINDINGS

Colonic neurofibromas are usually small but range from 0.5 to 7 cm with pale gray well-demarcated cut surfaces. Multiple polyps are seen in patients with NF-1.

MICROSCOPIC FINDINGS

Neurofibroma can present in three patterns: solitary, plexiform, and diffuse. In case of solitary neurofibroma, a proliferation of spindle cells with wavy, tapered-end nuclei situation in a collagenous matrix is seen (Figs. 7-20 and 7-21). In patients with NF-1, neurofibromas can display a plexiform architecture characterized with multiple variably sized subserosal nodules. Plexiform architecture is virtually diagnostic of NF-1.

ANCILLARY STUDIES

IMMUNOHISTOCHEMISTRY

The spindle cells in neurofibroma express S-100 protein and neuron-specific enolase. They are negative or weakly positive for calretinin. A population of CD34-positive supporting cells is commonly present in neurofibromas.

DIFFERENTIAL DIAGNOSIS

The main differential diagnoses include schwannomas, ganglioneuroma (presence of ganglion cells), and GIST (positive CD117). Mucosal neuroma is also in the differential diagnosis. It is a rare entity, highly associated with multiple endocrine neoplasia type 2B (MEN 2B). In that syndrome, mucosal neuromas are found most commonly on the lips and tongue and are vanishingly rarely in the GI tract. Histologically, mucosal neuromas consist of hyperplastic bundles of nerve fibers, including frequent axons, an appearance very different from that of neurofibroma, schwannoma, and various other nerve sheath tumors.

PROGNOSIS AND THERAPY

Neurofibroma is benign. It often does not recur except in cases associated with NF-1.

■ PERINEURIOMA AND BENIGN FIBROBLASTIC POLYP OF THE COLON

CLINICAL FEATURES

Perineurioma is a rare benign nerve sheath tumor showing perineurial cell differentiation. This tumor can be seen in the colon and small intestine, although

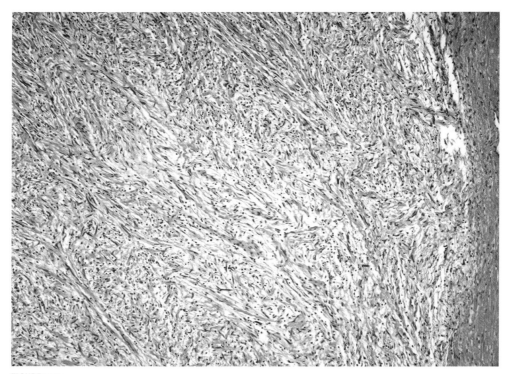

FIGURE 7-20
Neurofibroma. Note the prominent wiry collagen.

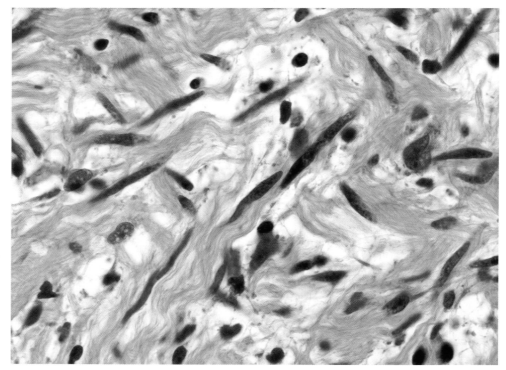

FIGURE 7-21
Neurofibroma. The nuclei appear plastered against the wiry collagen.

most examples are colonic. The tumor shows a female predominance and is typically encountered at screening colonoscopy. The patient age ranges from 35 to 77 years with a median age of 51 years. Similar lesions have been described as "benign fibroblastic polyp of the colon," and some authors believe that the two lesions are identical because the diagnosis of perineurioma is based on the detection of immunolabeling in keeping with perineurial differentiation. "Benign fibroblastic polyps of the colon" were initially described as incidental lesions detected in adult patients undergoing screening colonoscopy. All the reports describe this polyp arising from the colon, commonly in the distal colon. The incidence is about 0.2%. The patients' age ranges from 37 to 84 years with the mean age of 61.5 years. They present as small polyps at endoscopy with size ranging from 0.2 cm to 1.5 cm and the median size of 0.45 cm. About two thirds of the patients also have other polyps such as hyperplastic polyp or adenoma at the time of biopsy.

ENDOSCOPIC FEATURES

Colonic perineuriomas are small and sessile polyps. Lesions described as benign fibroblastic polyps are also small endoscopically detected polyps (size range 0.2 to 1.5 cm).

PATHOLOGIC FEATURES

GROSS FINDINGS

The tumors often present as colonic polyps in which the size ranges from 0.2 to 0.6 cm with median size measured 0.4 cm. The tumors have been also described as submucosal masses. The cut surface is described as well circumscribed with irregular borders and having a white, solid, myxoid appearance without necrosis.

MICROSCOPIC FINDINGS

The lesion is composed of a monotonous population of bland spindle cells with oval to elongated nuclei and pale eosinophilic cytoplasm (Figs. 7-22 and 7-23). The stroma is collagenous. The adjacent surface epithelium and crypts may show hyperplastic change (Fig. 7-24), a feature also reported for "benign fibroblastic polyps of the colon." No cytologic atypia is seen.

ANCILLARY STUDIES

IMMUNOHISTOCHEMISTRY

Perineuriomas are labeled with EMA and Glut-1 antibodies. They are variably labeled with Claudin-1 and CD34. They do not express S-100, GFAP, SMA, CD117, and pan-cytokeratin. Lesions initially described as

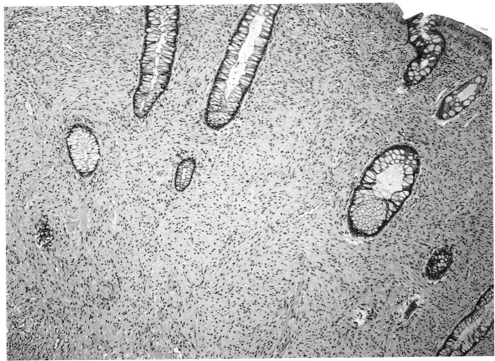

FIGURE 7-22

Perineurioma/benign fibroblastic polyp of the colon. The proliferating cells expand the lamina propria.

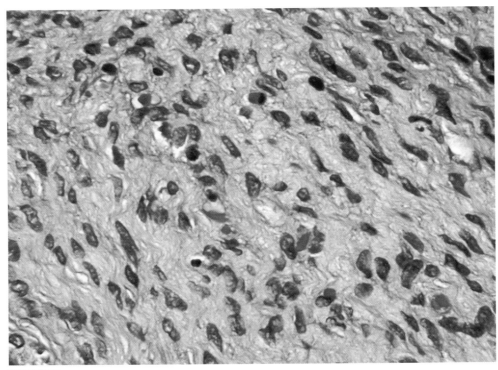

FIGURE 7-23

Higher magnification of a perineurioma/benign fibroblastic polyp of the colon. The cells are bland.

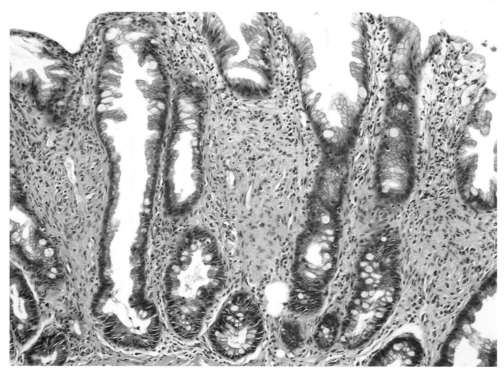

FIGURE 7-24
Perineurioma/benign fibroblastic polyps are frequently associated with serrated polyps/epithelium

"benign fibroblastic polyps of the colon" are "vimentin-only" lesions, lacking CD31, S-100, CD117/C-kit, Bcl-2, and desmin. A minority of cases were reported to display focal SMA and CD34.

ELECTRON MICROSCOPY

Perineuriomas show widely spaced spindle cells in a collagenous background with long bipolar cytoplasmic processes, pinocytotic vesicles, and sparse organelles. Wispy basal lamina may be present.

DIFFERENTIAL DIAGNOSIS

The differential diagnosis includes predominantly ganglioneuroma (presence of ganglion cells would exclude the possibility of perineurioma); neurofibroma (S-100 positive); and leiomyoma (cigar-shaped nuclei and positivity for SMA and desmin).

PROGNOSIS AND THERAPY

This is a benign tumor with no evidence of recurrence and metastasis.

■ MUCOSAL BENIGN EPITHELIOID NERVE SHEATH TUMORS

CLINICAL FEATURES

Mucosal benign epithelioid nerve sheath tumor (MBENST) is a benign tumor derived from nerve sheath that, like "Schwann cell hamartoma," cannot be classified as schwannoma or neurofibroma, but is a sporadic rather than syndromic lesion. This tumor can be seen in colonic and bladder mucosa. The mean age at presentation is 58.6 years with a slight female predominance. At endoscopy, the lesion appears as a small polyp.

PATHOLOGIC FEATURES

MICROSCOPIC FINDINGS

Most of the lesions have pushing to infiltrative borders. The epicenter of the lesion is in the lamina propria and it grows concentrically (Fig. 7-25). The tumor is composed of spindle cells and unique populations of epithelioid cells. The latter cells are round to oval shape with bland nuclei and characteristic intranuclear inclusion (Fig. 7-26).

MUCOSAL BENIGN EPITHELIOID NERVE SHEATH TUMOR (MBENST)—FACT SHEET

Definition
- Benign nerve sheath tumor that cannot be classified as schwannoma or neurofibroma

Incidence and Location
- Rare lesion seen in colonic and bladder mucosa

Morbidity and Mortality
- Benign tumor

Gender, Race, and Age Distribution
- Slight female predominance

Clinical Features
- Incidental finding

Prognosis and Therapy
- Benign

MUCOSAL BENIGN EPITHELIOID NERVE SHEATH TUMOR—PATHOLOGIC FEATURES

Microscopic Findings
- Epicenter in the lamina propria
- Spindle and epithelioid cells
- Epithelioid cells are round to oval shape containing bland nuclei with characteristic intranuclear inclusion

Immunohistochemistry
- Spindle cells labeled with S-100
- Negative for C34, CD117, calretinin, and SM31

Differential Diagnosis
- Schwannoma
- Neurofibroma (no epithelioid cells with intranuclear inclusion seen in neurofibroma)
- Similar to "Schwann cell hamartoma" except that they appear more epithelioid

ANCILLARY STUDIES

IMMUNOHISTOCHEMISTRY

MBENST expresses S-100 protein (Fig. 7-27). It is not labeled with C34, CD117, calretinin, and SM31.

DIFFERENTIAL DIAGNOSIS

MBENST should be differentiated from schwannoma and neurofibroma. Both schwannoma and MBENST are labeled with S-100 protein but GI tract schwannomas have prominent lymphocytes and spindle cells. Neurofibroma lacks epithelioid cells. Similar sporadic

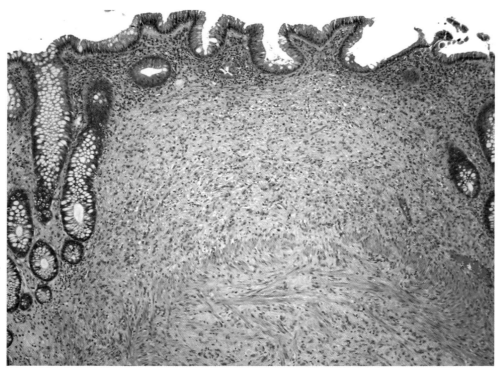

FIGURE 7-25
Benign epithelioid peripheral nerve sheath tumor. The proliferation is centered around the lamina propria and muscularis mucosae.

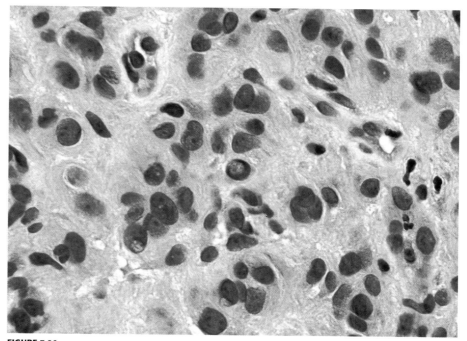

FIGURE 7-26

Benign epithelioid peripheral nerve sheath tumor. Note the striking intranuclear inclusions in the proliferating cells.

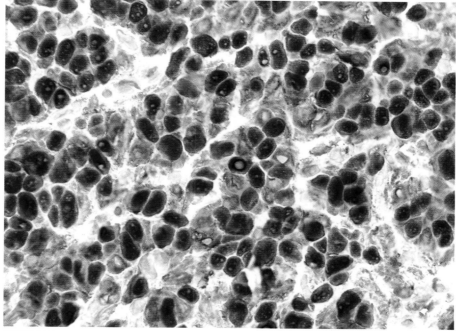

FIGURE 7-27

Benign epithelioid peripheral nerve sheath tumor. In keeping with their nerve sheath differentiation, these neoplasms are strongly S-100 protein reactive but lack expression of classic "melanoma markers," such as HMB45.

lesions that are not typical of either schwannomas, neurofibromas, or the "neuromas" of MEN 2B, but which are not so epithelioid, have been termed "Schwann cell hamartoma" and are illustrated in Figures 7-28 and 7-29.

PROGNOSIS AND THERAPY

MBENST is a benign tumor that can be managed by polypectomy.

GANGLIONEUROMA—PATHOLOGIC FEATURES

Gross Findings

- Sporadic lesions are polyps, and syndromic ones are either multiple polyps (ganglioneuromatous polyposis) or diffuse lesions that may be transmural

Microscopic Findings

- All types show a spindle cell population with interspersed ganglion cells infiltrating the lamina propria
- In diffuse ganglioneuromatosis, the lesion is centered around the myenteric plexus and typically has extensions to the lamina propria

Immunohistochemistry

- Spindle cell component is labeled with S-100 and GFAP
- Ganglion cell component is labeled with S-100, NSE, neurofilament protein (NFP), c-RET, and synaptophysin

Differential Diagnosis

- Usually easy to recognize; lesions that have sparse ganglion cells look like neurofibromas
- Synaptophysin stain may disclose scattered ganglion cells

resemble neurofibromas (differing by the presence of many ganglion cells). The ganglioneuromas in ganglioneuromatous polyposis show overlapping features with sporadic ganglioneuromas but tend to be more variable

and have more numerous ganglion cells and filiform architecture. In diffuse ganglioneuromatosis, the process is centered around the myenteric plexus and is either diffusely intramural or transmural and consists of fusiform expansions or confluent transmural ganglioneuromatous proliferations. Ganglioneuromas are depicted in Figures 7-30 through 7-33.

ANCILLARY STUDIES

IMMUNOHISTOCHEMISTRY

These lesions are easily diagnosed without immunohistochemistry, but the spindle cells react with S-100 protein, and GFAP (Fig. 7-34) and the ganglion cells mark with S-100 protein, NSE, neurofilament protein (NFP), synaptophysin, and c-RET.

DIFFERENTIAL DIAGNOSIS

The primary distinction is from neurofibroma, which is based on the presence of ganglion cells in ganglioneuromas and their lack in neurofibromas. When ganglion cells are sparse, NSE or synaptophysin staining may help detect them. Ganglioneuromas are distinguished

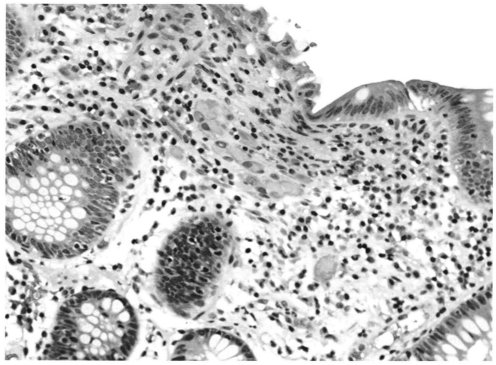

FIGURE 7-30

Ganglioneuroma. Shows a spindle cell proliferation expanding the lamina propria. This field shows a prominent collection of ganglion cells.

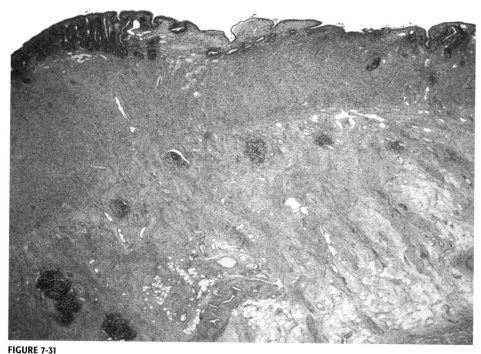

FIGURE 7-31

This ganglioneuroma, from a patient with ganglioneuromatosis (diffuse) and MEN 2B, shows transmural extension.

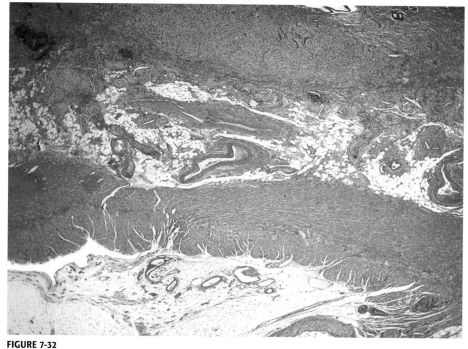

FIGURE 7-32

Another syndrome ganglioneuroma, expanding submucosal nerves.

from gangliocytic paraganglioma by the presence of epithelioid cells in gangliocytic paraganglioma; these latter cells may be positive for keratin (about half of cases), human pancreatic polypeptide, somatostatin, and chromogranin.

PROGNOSIS AND THERAPY

Sporadic ganglioneuromas are treated by polypectomy and seldom recur. These polyps are unassociated with MEN 2B and NF-1. Patients with syndromic

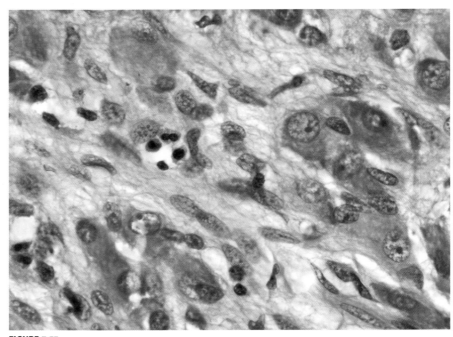

FIGURE 7-33

The ganglion cells in syndromic ganglioneuromas are often more atypical than those in sporadic examples (see Fig. 7-30), but mitotic activity is essentially absent in both forms.

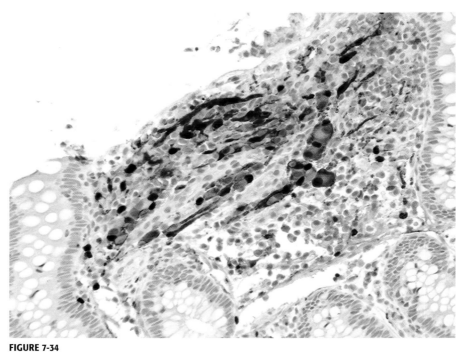

FIGURE 7-34

Ganglioneuroma. S-100 protein labels all the cells (this preparation is from the same lesion as Fig. 7-30).

ganglioneuromas must be carefully followed based on their specific syndromes. Those with NF-1 may develop other neural lesions, including malignant peripheral sheath tumors, and those with MEN 2B may develop endocrine neoplasms. Polypoid ganglioneuromas may herald Cowden's disease, tuberous sclerosis, FAP, and juvenile polyposis, whereas the diffuse type is the type most likely associated with NF-1 and MEN 2B. This type may cause strictures requiring resection, but the ganglioneuromas themselves are benign.

■ GANGLIOCYTIC PARAGANGLIOMA

CLINICAL FEATURES

These are rare and fascinating tumors, the vast majority of which are found in the duodenum in adult patients (average age about 54 years). Rare examples are found in the jejunum, pylorus, colon, and appendix. The typical presentation involves abdominal pain, gastric outlet obstruction, or bleeding. There are isolated reports of an association with neurofibromatosis, but the majority of cases are sporadic.

PATHOLOGIC FEATURES

GROSS FINDINGS

These lesions are typically centered in the submucosa, with minor extensions into the mucosa, and are 3 to 4 cm in diameter with a soft yellowish cut surface. They have infiltrative borders.

MICROSCOPIC FINDINGS

These tumors display a histologic constellation of three cell types: (1) spindle cells with the appearance of nerve sheath cells, (2) ganglion-like cells, and (3) epithelioid cells arranged in nests ("endocrine" pattern), trabeculae, or papillary structures. The proportion of the cell types is variable (Figs. 7-35 through 7-38).

ANCILLARY STUDIES

ULTRASTRUCTURAL FINDINGS

Ultrastructure shows an admixture of cells corresponding roughly to those seen by light microscopy. The epithelioid cells have cytoplasm packed with dense-core secretory granules; the ganglion-like cells have numerous secondary lysosomes, and a subset of the spindle cells produce discontinuous external lamina similar to schwannomas.

IMMUNOHISTOCHEMISTRY

On immunohistochemistry, the tumors are reactive with S-100 protein in spindle and "supporting/sustentacular" cells, synaptophysin in ganglion-like cells, and NSE staining in all three cell types. About half of cases display keratin in the epithelioid cells. A variety of hormones can be demonstrated in various fractions of gangliocytic paragangliomas, including somatostatin, human pancreatic polypeptide, serotonin, gastrin, glucagon, insulin, and vasoactive intestinal peptide.

GANGLIOCYTIC PARAGANGLIOMA—FACT SHEET

Definition
- Unusual neoplasm displaying "triphasic" differentiation

Incidence and Location
- Rare tumors that almost always occur in the duodenum

Morbidity and Mortality
- Vast majority are benign
- Morbidity is from operations aimed at their removal

Gender, Race, and Age Distribution
- No reported gender/race predilection
- Occurs in adults (average age 54 years)

Clinical Features
- Abdominal pain, gastric outlet obstruction, or bleeding
- Rare association with neurofibromatosis

Prognosis and Therapy
- Treatment is excision
- Rare reports of regional spread to lymph nodes but no disease-associated reported deaths

---

GANGLIOCYTIC PARAGANGLIOMA—PATHOLOGIC FEATURES

Gross Findings
- Centered around submucosa with infiltrative borders and yellowish surface

Microscopic Findings
- Three cell types: (1) spindle cells, (2) ganglion-like cells, and (3) epithelioid nests in variable proportions

Immunohistochemistry
- Spindle cells are positive for S-100
- Ganglion cells are synaptophysin-positive
- NSE stains all cell types
- Epithelioid component may have keratins in about 50% of samples
- Various neuroendocrine substances may be present

Differential Diagnosis
- Spindle cell–predominant lesions are distinguished from schwannomas by noting the other components
- Epithelioid-predominant lesions are distinguished from carcinoids by noting the spindle cell population

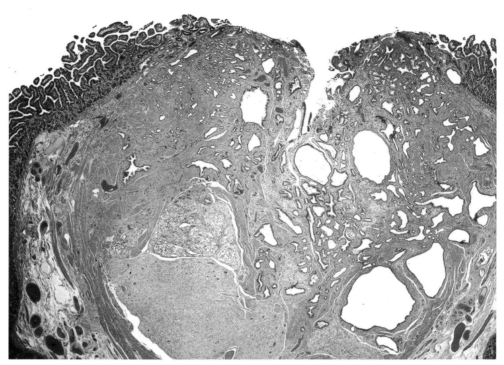

FIGURE 7-35

This gangliocytic paraganglioma arose in the ampulla. Disorganized ampullary (biliary type) glands are at the right side of the field; the lesion is at the lower left.

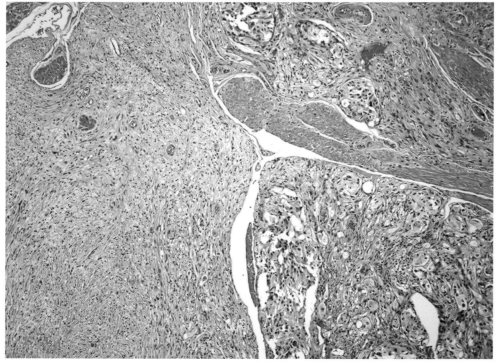

FIGURE 7-36

This gangliocytic paraganglioma shows spindle cells similar to those of a schwannoma or neurofibroma, nests of epithelioid cells, and dysmorphic ganglion cells.

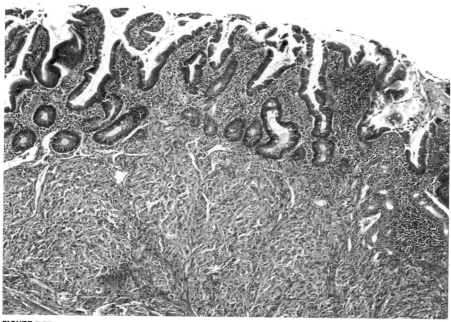

FIGURE 7-37
Epithelioid cells predominate in this gangliocytic paraganglioma; this lesion would be easily mistaken for a carcinoid tumor on a small mucosal biopsy.

DIFFERENTIAL DIAGNOSIS

In spindle cell–predominant lesions, the differential diagnosis includes GISTs and nerve sheath tumors: S-100 protein positivity excludes GISTs, and finding the admixture of other cell types excludes nerve sheath tumors. Epithelioid lesions are distinguished from carcinoid tumors and carcinomas, again by the admixture of the other cell types.

PROGNOSIS AND THERAPY

Gangliocytic paragangliomas are benign in the majority of cases. There are rare reports of regional metastases but not of tumor-associated deaths.

■ GLOMUS TUMOR

CLINICAL FEATURES

These are rare in the GI tract. The largest series (from the AFIP) had a female predominance and a median age at presentation of 55 years. The vast majority are found in the stomach, where they not infrequently present with severe bleeding producing melena. Ulcer-like pain can also be a feature. About 20% of cases in the AFIP series were detected at the time of operations for other lesions. There are also rare case reports of glomus tumor occurring in the colon.

GLOMUS TUMORS—FACT SHEET

Definition
- Gastrointestinal tract glomus tumors resemble their peripheral soft tissue counterparts

Incidence and Location
- Rare tumors usually affecting stomach and colon

Morbidity and Mortality
- Patients can present with severe GI tract bleeding, but most tumors are benign

Gender, Race, and Age Distribution
- Tumors of adults (median age 55 years) without known racial predominance
- Female predominance

Clinical Features
- About 20% are found incidentally
- Severe melena-producing gastrointestinal bleeding is common, and some are associated with ulcer-like pain

Prognosis and Therapy
- Vast majority are benign
- Treatment is surgical
- No histologic features predict the rare cases that metastasize

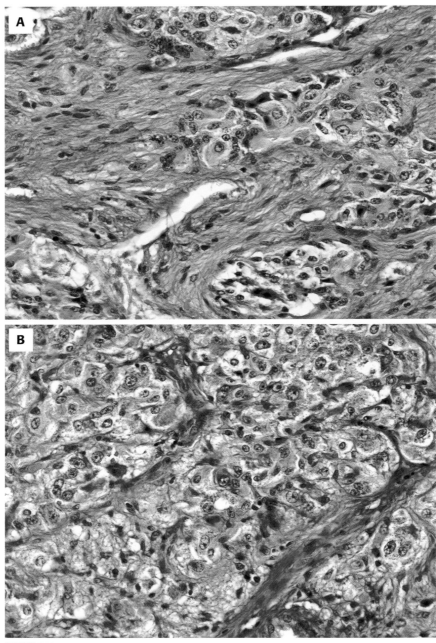

FIGURE 7-38

Gangliocytic paraganglioma. This field is from a more diagnostic area of the neoplasm depicted in Figure 7-37. **A,** Numerous spindle cells, whereas in **B,** epithelioid nests are predominant.

PATHOLOGIC FEATURES

GROSS FINDINGS

Tumors are circumscribed mural masses with a median diameter of 2.5 cm. They can bulge either into the mucosa or externally toward the serosa. They are occasionally calcified on cut surface.

MICROSCOPIC FINDINGS

Glomus tumors are multinodular at scanning magnification, the nodules separated by strands of residual muscularis propria with ulceration of the overlying mucosa. Tumor nodules are generally composed of solid sheets of cells that surround gaping capillary vessels that have a hemangiopericytoma-like pattern

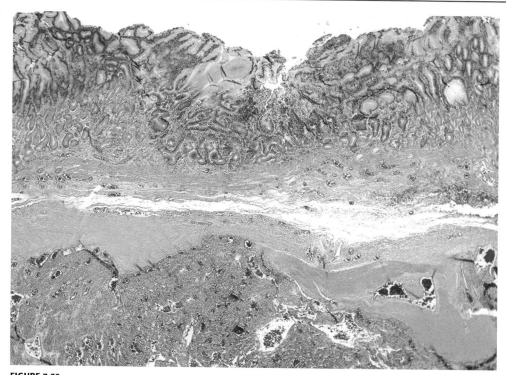

FIGURE 7-39

Gastric glomus tumors. Round cells proliferate around hemangiopericytoma-like vessels.

(Fig. 7-39). Tumor cells also tend to be present in the muscular walls of larger vessels. The individual tumor cells are round with sharply defined cell membranes, perfectly rounded nuclei, and delicate chromatin (Figs. 7-40 and 7-41). Some tumors have brightly eosinophilic cytoplasm.

GLOMUS TUMORS—PATHOLOGIC FEATURES

Gross Findings

- Tumors are usually circumscribed with a yellowish cut surface
- Some have calcifications

Microscopic Findings

- Round cells with sharply defined cell membranes and uniform nuclei
- Cells congregate around vessels displaying a hemangiopericytoma-like pattern

Immunohistochemistry

- Positive for actin and calponin
- Negative for desmin, endocrine markers, keratin, CD117/C-kit

Differential Diagnosis

- GIST (positive for CD117/C-kit, variable actin)
- Endocrine tumors (carcinoids) are keratin positive and have endocrine markers (e.g., synaptophysin, chromogranin)

ANCILLARY STUDIES

ULTRASTRUCTURAL FINDINGS

Glomus tumors are composed of modified smooth muscle cells.

IMMUNOHISTOCHEMISTRY

These tumors express SMA (Fig. 7-42), calponin, and h-caldesmon, but lack desmin. Pericellular netlike positivity is seen with basement membrane proteins (laminin and collagen type IV; Fig. 7-43). Some cases have focal CD34. Glomus tumors are negative for CD117/C-kit. Occasional cases have focal synaptophysin but these tumors lack chromogranin and keratin.

OTHER STUDIES

These tumors have been shown to lack C-KIT mutations.

DIFFERENTIAL DIAGNOSIS

The differential diagnosis includes endocrine tumors (carcinoids) and GISTs. Their occasional synaptophysin expression may lead to confusion, but a panel

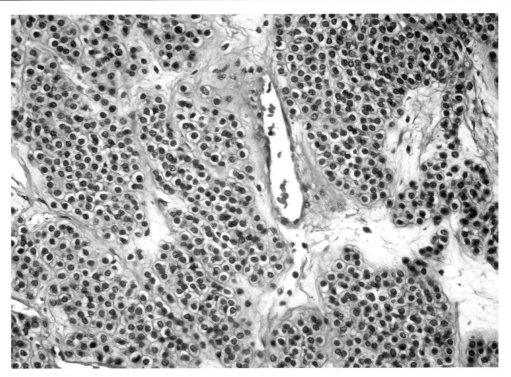

FIGURE 7-40

Gastric glomus tumors. Note the prominent cell borders.

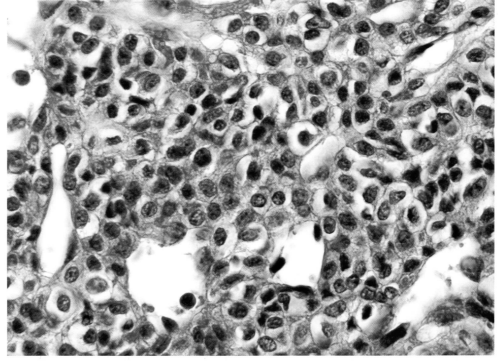

FIGURE 7-41

Gastric glomus tumors. This lesion has somewhat clear cells but also has prominent cell borders.

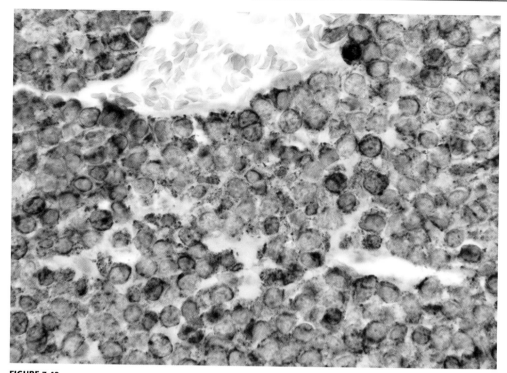

FIGURE 7-42

This is an actin stain; gastric glomus tumors consistently express actin but not desmin.

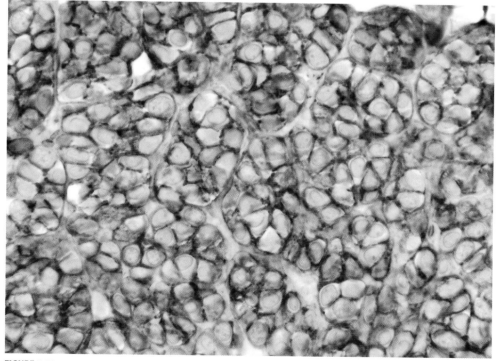

FIGURE 7-43

Gastric glomus tumors. A collagen type 4 stain highlights striking basement membranes.

approach should exclude this possibility because these tumors lack keratin and express smooth muscle markers (other than desmin).

PROGNOSIS AND THERAPY

Most glomus tumors behave in a benign fashion. However, rare examples are lethal with metastases. It is difficult to predict which will have an unfavorable outcome.

◼ INTRA-ABDOMINAL FIBROMATOSIS

CLINICAL FEATURES

This includes several entities that have similar morphologic findings but distinct clinical presentations. Pelvic fibromatosis typically involves the lower portion of the pelvis, where it presents as a slowly growing mass in young females but has no relationship to gestation. Mesenteric fibromatosis is probably the most common among the intra-abdominal fibromatosis group. It usually presents as a slowly growing mass that involves small bowel mesentery or retroperitoneum, where distinction may become extremely difficult from retroperitoneal fibrosis. Some cases are associated with pregnancy and Crohn's disease, even though the majority are considered to be secondary to trauma in individuals with the appropriate predisposition. Mesenteric fibromatosis in patients with Gardner's syndrome appears to have a substantially higher recurrence rate than in patients without this syndrome. Gardner's syndrome is an autosomal dominant familial disease with a female predilection and consists of numerous colorectal adenomatous polyps, osteomas, cutaneous cysts, soft tissue masses, and other manifestations. Gardner's syndrome is related to FAP, a disorder caused by germline adenomatous polyposis coli (APC) gene mutations. It is associated with a 7% to 12% incidence of developing fibromatosis.

RADIOLOGIC FEATURES

Although not specific, imaging studies show a mass lesion with a mesenteric epicenter, an infiltrative pattern, and a low signal on all magnetic resonance imaging sequences.

PATHOLOGIC FEATURES

GROSS FINDINGS

Grossly the tumor is firm with coarse white trabeculation resembling a scar and a gritty sensation is detected when the tumor is cut.

INTRA-ABDOMINAL FIBROMATOSIS—FACT SHEET

Definition
- Fibromatoses are myofibroblastic proliferations prone to locally aggressive behavior but do not metastasize

Incidence and Location
- Usually in the musculoaponeurotic soft tissue, but a subset is found intra-abdominally or in the mesentery

Morbidity and Mortality
- Extensive morbidity relates to local recurrences, and there are occasional lesion-related deaths from local recurrence

Gender, Race, and Age Distribution
- No gender predominance in childhood; female predominance during young adulthood; no gender predominance in older adults
- No report of racial predilection
- Occurs at all ages

Clinical Features
- Mass lesions; syndromic examples are a component of familial adenomatous polyposis/Gardner's syndrome

Prognosis and Therapy
- Treatment is primarily surgical
- Mesenteric fibromatoses in Gardner's syndrome more likely to recur

---

INTRA-ABDOMINAL FIBROMATOSIS—PATHOLOGIC FEATURES

Gross Findings
- Large infiltrative masses with firm white cut surface

Microscopic Findings
- Sweeping fascicles of myofibroblasts separated by collagen and prominent gaping thin-walled vessels

Immunohistochemistry
- May be positive for actin
- Most lack desmin
- 90% positive for nuclear β-catenin
- Many examples have spurious CD117/C-kit (cytoplasmic not membranous)
- Often express estrogen receptor-β

Differential Diagnosis
- Smooth muscle tumors that are positive for desmin and caldesmon, as well as actin
- GISTs, because fibromatoses often display cytoplasmic (not membranous) CD117/C-kit; GISTs lack nuclear β-catenin

---

MICROSCOPIC FINDINGS

Microscopically, the lesion is poorly defined with infiltrative margins consisting of spindled fibroblasts separated by abundant collagen (Fig. 7-44). Cells and

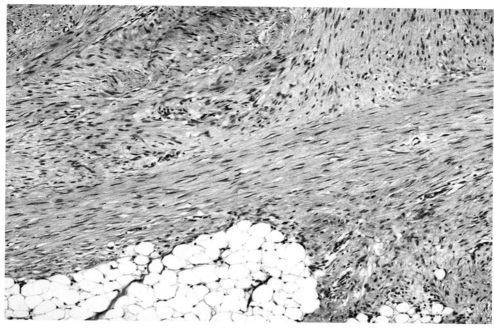

FIGURE 7-44
Fibromatosis. Shows sweeping fascicles of myofibroblasts with abundant collagen deposition.

collagen are organized in parallel arrays. Keloid-like collagen and hyalinization may be so extensive as to obscure the original pattern of the tumor. Scattered thin-walled (Fig. 7-45), elongated, and compressed vessels are usually seen with focal areas of hemorrhage, lymphoid aggregates, and, rarely, calcification or chondro-osseous metaplasia. Typically the vessels, although thin-walled, appear conspicuous at scanning magnification. The nuclei of the proliferating lesion are typically tinctorially lighter than those of the endothelial cells, and the smooth muscle cytoplasm in vessel walls is pinker than the surrounding myofibroblastic cytoplasm of the tumor cells. They have delicate nucleoli and smooth nuclear membranes (Fig. 7-46). Mitotic figures are infrequent.

ANCILLARY STUDIES

ULTRASTRUCTURAL FINDINGS

Fibromatoses display myofibroblastic ultrastructural characteristics.

IMMUNOHISTOCHEMISTRY

Because mesenteric fibromatoses are myofibroblastic lesions, they sometimes express SMA and (less frequently) desmin. They typically lack CD34.

With the observation that STI571 (imatinib) is effective against GI stromal tumors based on their expression of CD117 (KIT), pathologists are increasingly called

upon to perform immunohistochemical staining for CD117 in every spindle cell lesion in the abdomen. When mesenteric fibromatoses are evaluated using one commercially available CD117 antibody (Dako), up to 80% of cases can be reactive. In contrast, there were no reactive cases using another antibody (Santa Cruz Biotechnology, Santa Cruz, CA). This problem issue has become less problematic since about 2003; presumably the antibodies have been refined. However, because CD117 reactivity is a criterion by which GI stromal tumors are diagnosed, the lack of specificity using some antibodies can result in diagnostic confusion between fibromatoses and stromal tumors, a clinically relevant separation. Although these entities are usually readily distinguished on morphologic grounds, they sometimes pose diagnostic problems. Nuclear β-catenin is typically detected in mesenteric fibromatosis (Fig. 7-47) and not in GISTs, a finding that occasionally may be of diagnostic value in separating these entities.

Because fibromatoses can respond to antiestrogen treatments, analysis of hormone receptors has been explored using immunolabeling. Desmoid tumors are estrogen receptor-α negative but are known to express estrogen receptor-β. They have occasional androgen receptor expression.

FINE-NEEDLE ASPIRATION BIOPSY

These tumors are well collagenized, so diagnosing them by fine-needle aspiration cytology can be frustrating owing to difficulty in sampling. However, loosely cohesive

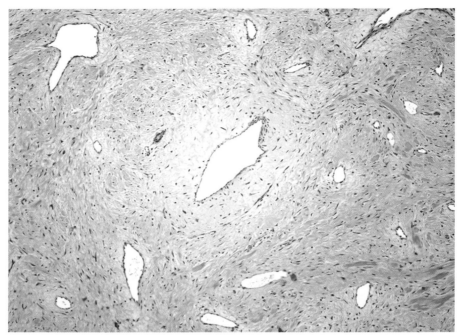

FIGURE 7-45
Mesenteric fibromatosis tends to display thin-walled vessels that appear to be "pulled open" by the proliferating myofibroblasts.

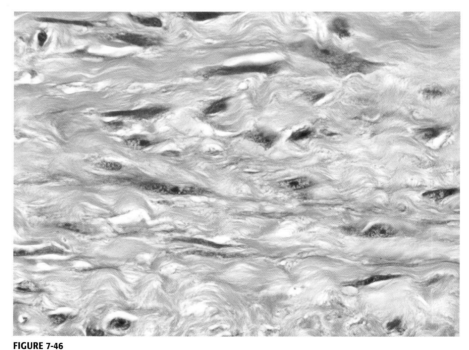

FIGURE 7-46
Mesenteric fibromatoses typically have bland cytologic features at high magnification.

and single bland spindle cells are found if there is suffi-cient fine-needle aspiration material.

OTHER STUDIES

Among patients with FAP, intestinal and extraintestinal neoplasms typically arise through bi-allelic (germline then somatic) inactivation of the APC gene, whereas the corresponding tumors in non-FAP patients occur either through somatic bi-allelic APC inactivation or somatic mutation of a single β-catenin allele. As the various FAP-associated tumors have been studied, somatic alterations of the APC/β-catenin pathway have been initially de-tected in familial examples and then subsequently demon-strated in the sporadic counterparts. It has been estimated that FAP patients in general have an 852-fold increased

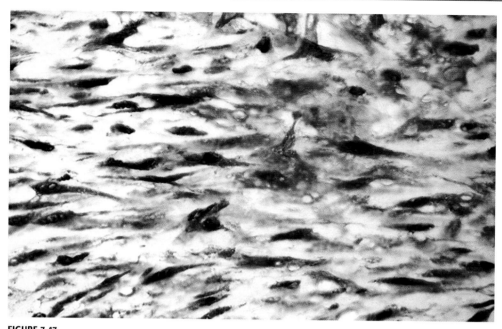

FIGURE 7-47

Nuclear b-catenin staining in fibromatoses. Cytoplasmic staining is not specific; only nuclear staining is assessed to support an interpretation of fibromatosis.

risk for developing desmoids, typically intra-abdominal lesions. In fact, there is a unique French-Canadian kindred harboring a germline mutation of codon 2643-2644 of the APC gene. These patients have a penetrance of desmoid tumors approaching 100 % and have cutaneous cysts, but few manifest colon polyposis.

DIFFERENTIAL DIAGNOSIS

The differential diagnosis includes low-grade dedifferentiation in liposarcoma/low-grade fibrosarcoma and benign fibroblastic proliferative lesions. Low-grade fibrosarcomas and low-grade dedifferentiation in liposarcomas are distinguished from fibromatoses by having scattered hyperchromatic nuclei in contrast to the bland ones in fibromatoses. Dedifferentiated liposarcoma (including the low-grade form) often shows MDM-2 gene amplification or MDM-2 and CDK4 nuclear labeling, which can be helpful in distinguishing it from fibromatosis. Sclerosing mesenteritis is also in the differential diagnosis and is discussed in the following section.

PROGNOSIS AND THERAPY

Mesenteric fibromatoses, particularly familial ones, are prone to local persistence/recurrence, doing so in 90 % of Gardner's syndrome cases and in 10 % to 15 % of sporadic ones. Fibromatoses do not metastasize. Surgical excision is the mainstay of therapy.

■ SCLEROSING MESENTERITIS

Sclerosing mesenteritis is also known as mesenteric panniculitis, retractile mesenteritis, liposclerotic mesenteritis, mesenteric Weber-Christian disease, xanthogranulomatous mesenteritis, mesenteric lipogranuloma, systemic nodular panniculitis, inflammatory pseudotumor, and mesenteric lipodystrophy.

CLINICAL FEATURES

Sclerosing mesenteritis most commonly affects the small bowel mesentery, presenting as an isolated large mass, although about 20 % of patients have multiple lesions. The cause of these lesions remains unknown, and they are assumed to reflect a reparative response, although the stimulus is not clear; prior trauma/surgery was recorded in only 4 of 84 patients in the series by Emory and associates. A portion of patients with sclerosing mesenteritis has elevated serum IgG4 level; therefore, it has been suggested that sclerosing mesenteritis is member of a group of sclerosing disorders of various organs unified by increased IgG4 production from lesional plasma cells. The prototypic disease in this group is lymphoplasmacytic sclerosing pancreatitis (autoimmune pancreatitis), which manifests vasculitis, duct-centric lymphoplasmacytic inflammation, increased serum and plasma cell IgG4. However, whereas most patients with classic IgG4-related sclerosing disorders respond to steroids, patients with sclerosing mesenteritis do not.

SCLEROSING MESENTERITIS—FACT SHEET

Definition
- Sclerosing mesenteritis is a fibroinflammatory condition of obscure etiology affecting the mesentery
- A subset of cases may be under the umbrella of a group of sclerosing diseases characterized by increased serum IgG4 level

Incidence and Location
- Rare and usually found in the small bowel mesentery

Morbidity and Mortality
- Generally indolent without recurrences
- Morbidity is from the treating surgery

Gender, Race, and Age Distribution
- No gender or racial predominance
- Adults affected (average age 60 years)

Clinical Features
- Patients present with abdominal pain, abdominal mass, or obstruction
- Typically no history of trauma or prior surgery

Radiologic Features
- Soft tissue mass in mesentery, sometimes with preservation of fat around mesenteric vessels (fat ring sign)

Prognosis and Therapy
- Treatment can be surgical or medical using steroids and tamoxifen
- Recurrence is uncommon, but occasional cases are associated with significant morbidity and even mortality

SCLEROSING MESENTERITIS—PATHOLOGIC FEATURES

Gross Findings
- Infiltrative solitary (80%) or multifocal whitish mass lesion with extensions into surrounding tissue

Microscopic Findings
- Bands of sclerotic infiltrative tissue peppered with lymphocytes and plasma cells in a background of fat necrosis
- Neutrophils not a component
- Lymphocytic phlebitis or venulitis common

Immunohistochemistry
- Focal actin and calponin
- Negative for desmin, keratin, S-100 protein
- May have "false-positive" CD117/C-kit, but lacks nuclear β-catenin
- May display IgG4-labeled plasma cells

Differential Diagnosis
- Primarily mesenteric fibromatosis, which differs by lacking the inflammatory backdrop, having less incorporated fat and fat necrosis, and by having nuclear β-catenin on immunohistochemical evaluation

lymphoma, carcinoid tumor, or carcinomatosis. A tumoral pseudocapsule may be present in half of patients with mesenteric panniculitis.

PATHOLOGIC FEATURES

GROSS FINDINGS

Lesions typically consist of a dominant, whitish, firm mass with extensions of firm, whitish tissue encasing adjacent tissues.

MICROSCOPIC FINDINGS

Typically, lesions consist of fibrous bands infiltrating and encasing fat lobules (Figs.7-48 through 7-50), with an associated admixture of inflammatory cells, typically lymphocytes, plasma cells, and eosinophils. Areas of fat necrosis are common. Lymphocytic phlebitis or venulitis (see Fig. 7-50), an overlapping feature with IgG4-related sclerosing disorders is often encountered.

ANCILLARY STUDIES

IMMUNOHISTOCHEMISTRY

There is no specific immunolabeling pattern, although the proliferating cells are often myofibroblastic by immunolabeling, displaying actin and calponin expression but not

In one large study, the patient age ranges from 23 to 87 years (mean, 60 years) without gender predilection. Most patients presented with nonspecific symptoms such as abdominal pain, palpable mass, and symptoms related to bowel obstruction.

RADIOLOGIC FEATURES

The CT appearance of sclerosing mesenteritis can vary from subtle increased attenuation in the mesentery to a solid soft tissue mass. Sclerosing mesenteritis most commonly appears as a soft tissue mass in the small bowel mesentery, although infiltration of the region of the pancreas or porta hepatis is also possible. The mass may envelop the mesenteric vessels, and, over time, collateral vessels may develop. There may be preservation of fat around the mesenteric vessels, a phenomenon that is referred to as the *fat ring sign*. This finding may help distinguish sclerosing mesenteritis from other mesenteric processes such as

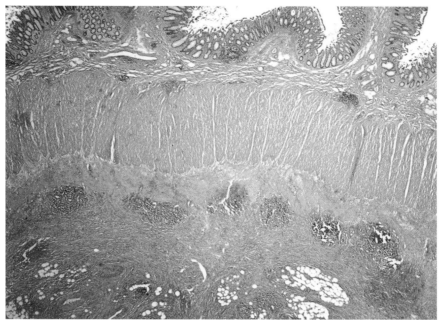

FIGURE 7-48

Sclerosing mesenteritis. A disorganized sclerotic process infiltrates mesenteric fat, usually accompanied by a lymphoplasmacytic inflammatory response but not by neutrophils.

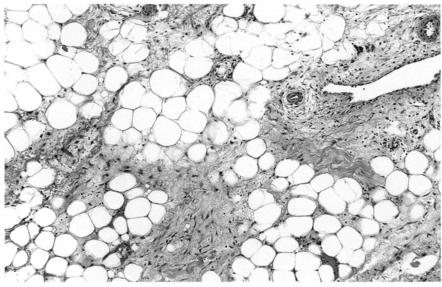

FIGURE 7-49

Sclerosing mesenteritis. Note the bland cytologic features in a sclerotic area.

desmin or caldesmon. Some cases display prominent IgG4 labeling in plasma cells (Fig. 7-51), and some examples show nonspecific CD117 expression. These lesions do not express anaplastic lymphoma kinase (ALK).

DIFFERENTIAL DIAGNOSIS

Sclerosing mesenteritis is distinguished from mesenteric fibromatosis by its abundance of inflammation and fat entrapment with fat necrosis. Fibromatosis,

while infiltrative at its periphery, grows as a solid mass composed of homogeneous sweeping fascicles of fibroblasts with minimal inflammation. Inflammatory well-differentiated liposarcoma can appear similar but differ by displaying enlarged hyperchromatic cells. Unfortunately MDM2 immunolabeling can display nonspecific nuclear staining in about 20% of sclerosing mesenteritis cases and thus cannot consistently be used to separate the two; FISH for *MDM-2* amplification is more reliable.

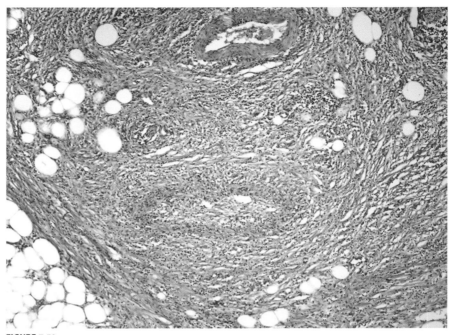

FIGURE 7-50

Many examples of sclerosing mesenteritis display a lymphocytic phlebitis pattern. Note the damaged inflamed vein beneath the uninvolved artery in this field.

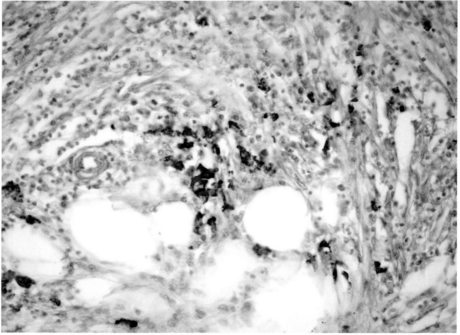

FIGURE 7-51

Sclerosing mesenteritis. Prominent IgG4 immunolabeling can be encountered in these lesions, although its significance remains unclear.

PROGNOSIS AND THERAPY

Treatment has included medical therapy alone in, surgery alone, and surgery followed by medical therapy but about half of patients seem to require no treatment. Tamoxifen in combination with prednisone has resulted in improvement in 60% of patients. Occasional patients die as a result of the lesion or complications of treatment. Sclerosing mesenteritis can have a prolonged debilitating course in a subset of patients, but the overall prognosis is favorable.

■ INFLAMMATORY FIBROSARCOMA/ INFLAMMATORY MYOFIBROBLASTIC TUMOR

Although these lesions were originally described as separate entities, they are now recognized as ends of a spectrum of tumors unified by a common molecular profile. They are grouped together by the World Health Organization.

CLINICAL FEATURES

INFLAMMATORY FIBROSARCOMA

This is most common in childhood, at a mean age of 8 years (range 2 months to 74 years). As described in the AFIP series, this tumor arises within the abdomen, involving mesentery, omentum, and retroperitoneum (more than 80% of cases), with occasional cases in the mediastinum, abdominal wall, and liver. Sometimes there are associated systemic symptoms. The tumor can be solitary or multinodular (30%) and up to 20 cm in diameter.

INFLAMMATORY MYOFIBROBLASTIC TUMOR

Also known as inflammatory pseudotumor, this entity was first well described in the lungs and later became recognized in extrapulmonary locations. Recent cytogenetic and molecular evidence in both inflammatory myofibroblastic tumor and inflammatory fibrosarcoma supports a clonal origin, implying that this process is neoplastic. It is found in soft tissue, in omentum and retroperitoneum, and involving viscera. Inflammatory myofibroblastic tumor has been reported in patients 3 months to 46 years of age, but mostly in childhood (mean age 9 years), with a slight male predominance, and some cases are associated with systemic symptoms. A small number recur, especially when multinodular.

RADIOLOGIC FEATURES

Imaging studies show poorly marginated mass lesions that are calcified in a minority of cases (nonspecific mass lesions).

PATHOLOGIC FEATURES

GROSS FINDINGS

These tumors form firm white infiltrative masses.

INFLAMMATORY FIBROSARCOMA/INFLAMMATORY MYOFIBROBLASTIC TUMOR—FACT SHEET

Definition
- Clonal proliferation composed of cells with myofibroblastic differentiation that may be multicentric and classically occurs in children with constitutional symptoms

Incidence and Location
- Rare, affecting mesentery, omentum, and retroperitoneum (more than 80% of cases), with occasional cases in the mediastinum, abdominal wall, and liver

Morbidity and Mortality
- Metastases are rare but do occur
- Multicentricity may be a feature
- Patients may die of local disease rather than systemic spread

Gender, Race, and Age Distribution
- Mean age is 7 to 9 years, but adults have been affected
- No gender or race predominance

Clinical Features
- Patients present with mass lesions and/or constitutional symptoms (anemia, weight loss, malaise)

Prognosis and Therapy
- Most examples are indolent; treatment is surgical and should not be overly aggressive

---

INFLAMMATORY FIBROSARCOMA/INFLAMMATORY MYOFIBROBLASTIC TUMOR—PATHOLOGIC FEATURES

Gross Findings
- Firm white infiltrative mass or masses

Microscopic Findings
- Three forms of spindle cell lesions: (1) fasciitis-like, with vascular, myxoid, and inflamed stroma, including plasma cells; (2) fascicular MFH or leiomyosarcoma-like spindle cell areas with inflammation; (3) sclerosed desmoid-like areas with calcification
- Lesions with more cytologic atypia are "inflammatory fibrosarcoma," but these are ends of a morphologic spectrum

Immunohistochemistry
- Reactive for actin and calponin
- Negative for desmin and caldesmon
- Keratin may be present in submesothelial areas of the tumor
- ALK may be expressed, which roughly correlates with *ALK* gene alterations

Differential Diagnosis
- Fibromatosis and sclerosing mesenteritis
- More inflamed than fibromatosis; more of a solid mass lesion than sclerosing mesenteritis; typically occurs in younger patients

MICROSCOPIC FINDINGS

Histologically there are three patterns: (1) fasciitis-like, with vascular, myxoid, and inflamed stroma, including plasma cells (Figs. 7-52 and 7-53); (2) fascicular malignant fibrous histiocytoma (MFH; Fig. 7-54) or leiomyosarcoma-like spindle cell areas with inflammation (see Fig. 7-28); and (3) sclerosed desmoid-like areas with calcification.

The tumors are composed of myofibroblasts and fibroblasts in fascicles or whorls, as well as histiocytoid cells. Pleomorphism is moderate, but mitoses are infrequently seen. There is a variable but often marked inflammatory infiltrate, predominantly plasmacytic but with some lymphocytes, and occasionally neutrophils or eosinophils as well. Fibrosis and calcification can be seen in the stroma.

ANCILLARY STUDIES

ULTRASTRUCTURAL FINDINGS

Ultrastructurally these tumors have fibroblastic and myofibroblastic features.

IMMUNOHISTOCHEMISTRY

Immunostaining is positive for SMA, and some examples express cytokeratin, especially where there is submesothelial extension. By immunohistochemistry, ALK has been detected in about 60% of cases, a finding that can sometimes be exploited for diagnosis (Fig. 7-55).

OTHER STUDIES

Gene fusions involving the *ALK* gene at chromosome 2p23 have been described in these lesions. The fusion partners have included *ATIC, CARS, TPM3, TPM4, CLTC, RANB2,* and *SEC31L.*

DIFFERENTIAL DIAGNOSIS

The differential diagnosis between inflammatory fibrosarcoma and inflammatory myofibroblastic tumor is subjective because these conditions are ends of a spectrum (one case was included in both the original papers describing these two conditions). Essentially, it depends

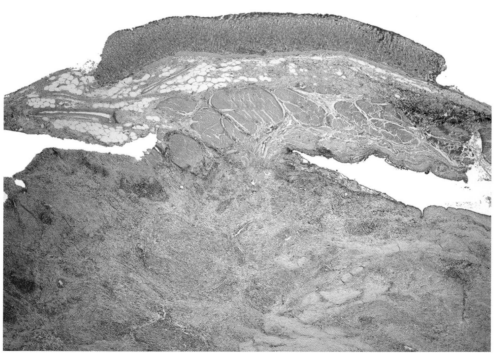

FIGURE 7-52

This inflammatory myofibroblastic tumor is centered in the adipose tissue outside the gastric muscularis propria (although it has focally extended into the smooth muscle). In contrast to the gastric schwannoma seen in Figure 7-15, the inflammation is a uniform integral part of the process rather than forming a rind that encases the lesion.

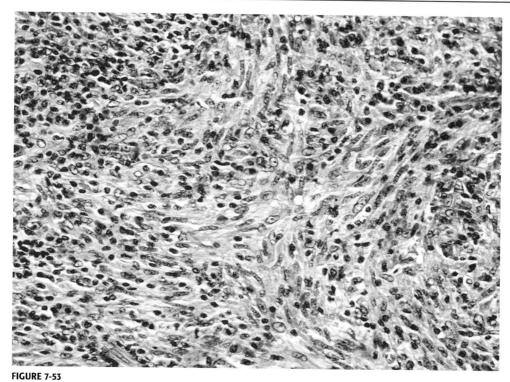

FIGURE 7-53

This inflammatory myofibroblastic tumor consists of a storiform proliferation of spindle cells with abundant plasma cells.

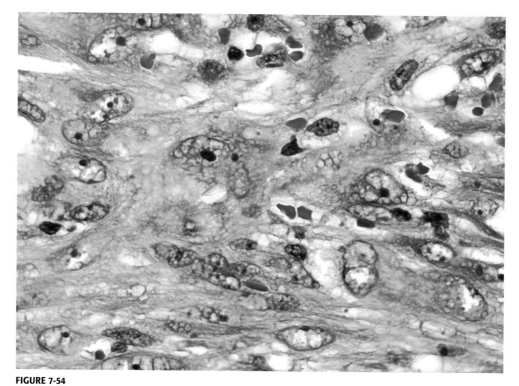

FIGURE 7-54

Inflammatory myofibroblastic tumor and inflammatory fibrosarcoma are ends of a spectrum. Lesions with cytologic alterations such as this one may be classified as inflammatory fibrosarcoma.

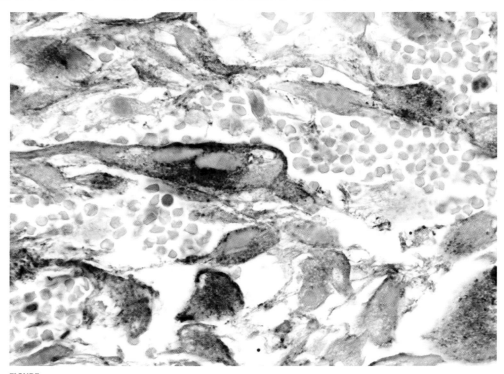

FIGURE 7-55
ALK staining in an inflammatory myofibroblastic tumor.

on the presence of pleomorphism in cases designated as "fibrosarcoma" (see Fig. 7-28). Retroperitoneal fibrosis is clinically distinctive, being more inflammatory than spindled and lacking pleomorphism. Lesions termed inflammatory MFH in the past (now known to be dedifferentiated liposarcomas) have atypical xanthomatous cells, and inflammatory leiomyosarcoma is more myoid. Solitary fibrous tumor has CD34 positivity, and sarcomatoid mesothelioma displays diffuse epithelial marker positivity.

PROGNOSIS AND THERAPY

The tumors invade adjacent viscera; in the original series, 37% recurred and three cases (11%) metastasized. One fourth of the patients died of disease.

8

Non-Neoplastic and Neoplastic Disorders of the Appendix

■ **Dora Lam-Himlin, MD** ■ **Elizabeth Montgomery, MD**
■ **Michael Torbenson, MD**

■ FIBROUS OBLITERATION OF THE APPENDICEAL LUMEN (NEURAL HYPERPLASIA)

CLINICAL FEATURES

There are no specific features as this is typically an incidental finding in about one third of appendices excised for a variety of reasons.

PATHOLOGIC FEATURES

GROSS FINDINGS

The tip of the appendix is usually affected and appears whitish on cut surface. The appendix is not enlarged and the serosa is normal.

MICROSCOPIC FINDINGS

Obliteration of the appendiceal lumen is by spindle cells in a collagenous and myxoid backdrop. The process may be confined to the mucosa ("intramucosal variant") or may replace the entire lumen and underlying crypts. These phenomena are believed to be overall proliferative, with attendant phases of growth, involution, and finally fibrosis.

ANCILLARY STUDIES

IMMUNOHISTOCHEMISTRY

Immunohistochemical staining discloses S-100 protein and neuron-specific enolase-reactive spindle cells (intermingled Schwann cells and axons, respectively), and scattered endocrine cells (if neuroendocrine stains are performed).

FIBROUS OBLITERATION OF THE APPENDICEAL LUMEN (NEURAL HYPERPLASIA)—FACT SHEET

Definition
- A spindle cell proliferation that fills and "obliterates" the appendix lumen, usually at the tip

Incidence and Location
- Found in about one third of excised appendices

Morbidity and Mortality
- None

Gender, Race, and Age Distribution
- All ages, without race or gender predisposition

Clinical Features
- Incidental finding in appendices excised for all reasons

FIBROUS OBLITERATION OF THE APPENDICEAL LUMEN (NEURAL HYPERPLASIA)—PATHOLOGIC FEATURES

Gross Findings
- Normal appendix diameter with firm white process involving lumen

Microscopic Findings
- Bland spindle cell population effacing appendix lumen with no residual mucosa

Immunohistochemistry
- S-100-positive and NSE-positive cells with scattered endocrine cells

Differential Diagnosis
- With benign mesenchymal tumors, the luminal location is the key

DIFFERENTIAL DIAGNOSIS

The differential diagnosis is with the host of spindle cell tumors of the gastrointestinal tract that are discussed in Chapter 7. However, it is the pattern that is specific here—namely, a process with its epicenter in the lumen of the appendix.

PROGNOSIS AND THERAPY

Fibrous obliteration is a benign and incidental lesion.

■ ANATOMIC ANOMALIES OF THE APPENDIX

CLINICAL FEATURES

The appendix can have a host of anatomic abnormalities including atypical location, duplication, and congenital absence. There can be complete or incomplete septa, which are seen principally in children and young adults and associated with acute appendicitis. An abnormally long appendix (normal is 7 to 10 cm) has been linked to primary acute torsion, although torsion has also been reported in appendices of normal length. Diverticula of the appendix can be congenital, in which case the muscularis propria is part of the diverticular wall, or acquired, in which case the diverticulum results from increased intraluminal pressure and mucosal herniation through a defect of the muscularis propria, often at the site of a penetrating artery. Acquired diverticula are more common than congenital diverticula and are seen in 1% to 2% of the population. However, acquired diverticula are greatly increased in patients with cystic fibrosis, in whom they are found in up to 22% of appendectomy specimens (Fig. 8-1).

■ ACUTE AND CHRONIC APPENDICITIS

CLINICAL FEATURES

Acute appendicitis is a disease of the young, most typically presenting in children and adolescents (5-15 years), but even the elderly can be affected. Perforation is most likely in the very young and in older adults. An approximate incidence of acute appendicitis is 7% to 10%. The pathogenesis of appendicitis is believed by some clinicians to reflect an initial insult to the mucosa resulting from luminal obstruction by a fecalith, fragment of undigested food, or lymphoid hyperplasia, followed by bacterial infection that progressively spreads from the

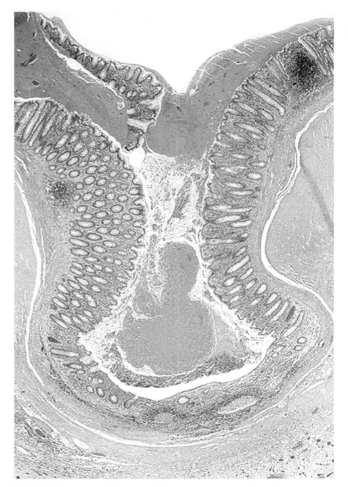

FIGURE 8-1
Acquired diverticulum in a patient with cystic fibrosis (CF).

mucosa into the wall. Approximately 70% of patients suspected to have appendicitis on clinical and imaging grounds have it on resection. Some observers believe that all appendices should be removed during surgery for suspected acute appendicitis, even when grossly normal, because nearly 20% of normal-appearing appendices may have acute inflammation on microscopic examination. A possible exception is those patients who might require urologic surgery in the future, because their appendices may later serve as urinary conduits. Patients with appendicitis in the setting of human immunodeficiency virus (HIV) infection have similar clinical presentations, although sometimes with a less striking elevation in the peripheral white blood cell count. In one surgical series of appendicitis and HIV infection, delays before operation increased the likelihood of perforation.

RADIOLOGIC FEATURES

Both ultrasound and computed tomography (CT) are useful in diagnosing acute appendicitis.

or pelvic fluid collections, or a complex mass representing intraperitoneal abscess.

The reported sensitivity of CT using rectal contrast medium has ranged from 97% to 100%, and the specificity has ranged from 94% to 98%. The normal appendix can be identified with CT as a tubular structure arising from the posteromedial aspect of the cecum, approximately 1 to 4 cm below the ileocecal junction. The normal appendix is identified on CT in approximately one half of children. The appendix is usually curved and may be tortuous. The free end of the appendix is mobile and can be directed medially, caudally, laterally, or retrocecally. A segment of the appendix is commonly noted at a level higher than the ileocecal valve. The maximal normal appendiceal diameter is typically 7 mm or less. The lumen of the normal appendix may fill with contrast material and may contain intraluminal air or fluid.

CT signs of acute appendicitis include a distended appendix greater than 7 mm in maximal diameter, appendiceal wall thickening and enhancement, an appendicolith, circumferential or focal cecal apical thickening, pericecal fat stranding, adjacent bowel-wall thickening, focal or free peritoneal fluid, mesenteric lymphadenopathy, and intraperitoneal phlegmon or abscess. The identification of cecal apical thickening is particularly useful in allowing a confident diagnosis of acute appendicitis if there is difficulty in identifying an enlarged appendix. Cecal apical thickening can result in a triangular-shaped space that becomes filled with contrast medium. This has been labeled the *arrowhead sign* and is a useful indicator of disease.

PATHOLOGIC FEATURES

GROSS FINDINGS

The appendix may appear grossly normal when inflammation is limited to the mucosa and submucosa. However, when inflammation extends into the muscularis propria, the appendix frequently becomes swollen and erythematous. When the serosa is affected, the peritoneum is initially dull and gray, followed by a purulent exudate. Perforation secondary to mural necrosis (gangrenous appendicitis) can follow, which may lead to abscess formation. At times, an appendix resected in the clinical setting of acute appendicitis is grossly and histologically normal, even after submission of the complete specimen for histologic examination. In these cases, an etiology is rarely found.

MICROSCOPIC FINDINGS

On microscopic examination, early lesions display mucosal erosions and scattered crypt abscesses (Figs. 8-2 and 8-3). Later, the inflammation extends into

Overall sensitivity of 85% and specificity of 92% have been reported for sonography. The normal appendix is usually not visualized at graded-compression sonography. The inflamed appendix appears as a fluid-filled, noncompressible blind-ending structure measuring greater than 6 mm in maximal diameter. In early nonperforated appendicitis, an inner echogenic lining representing submucosa can be identified. If fluid is present within the appendiceal lumen, a target appearance, characterized by a fluid-filled center, surrounded by echogenic mucosa and submucosa and hypoechoic muscularis, may be seen when imaging in the axial plane. Other findings of appendicitis include an appendicolith, which appears as echogenic foci with acoustic shadowing, pericecal or periappendiceal fluid, and increased periappendiceal echogenicity representing fat infiltration. The only sonographic sign that is specific for appendicitis is an enlarged, noncompressible appendix measuring greater than 6 mm in maximal diameter. The appendix may not be visible following perforation. The characteristic sonographic findings associated with perforated appendicitis are nonspecific, but, in the proper clinical situation, still suggest the diagnosis. The findings include focal periappendiceal

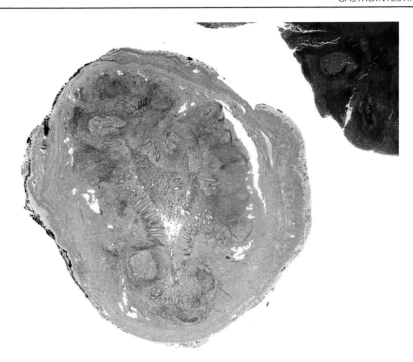

FIGURE 8-2
Acute appendicitis. At low magnification, in this example, the inflammation is confined to the mucosa and lumen.

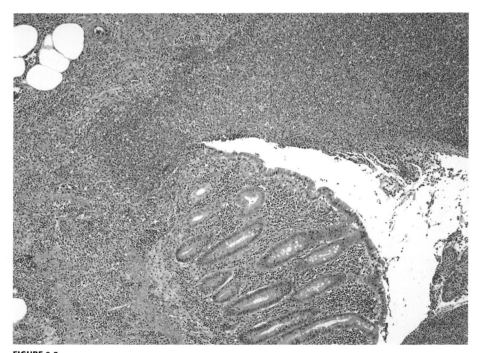

FIGURE 8-3
Acute appendicitis. The mucosa has a zone or erosion, but note that the crypt architecture is essentially preserved.

the lamina propria, and collections of neutrophils are also seen in the lumen. When the inflammation damages the muscularis propria extensively, mural necrosis can lead to perforation.

As appendices heal, two basic patterns may be seen. In the first, more typical pattern, there are mixed inflammatory infiltrates ranging from patchy and mild

to diffuse and transmural (Figs. 8-4 and 8-5). In some appendices, there may be intramural or serosal foreign body–type giant cells surrounded by granulation tissue suggestive of prior rupture. Serositis and fibrous adhesions can be present, as well as prominent submucosal fibrosis. Mucin extravasation is often seen. A second pattern, which has been termed *xanthogranulomatous*

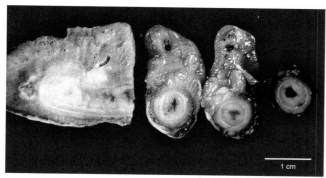

FIGURE 8-4

Gross specimen prepared from an "interval appendix." Antibiotic treatment was carried out for 4 weeks prior to appendectomy. Note the fibrous thickened wall, which suggests the possibility of Crohn's disease.

appendicitis, features a xanthogranulomatous infiltrate composed of foam cells, scattered multinucleated histiocytes, abundant hemosiderin, and luminal obliteration with spared lymphoid follicles. These latter cases share features with Crohn's disease but differ by lacking epithelioid granulomas, having fewer lymphoid aggregates, and having less profound subserosal fibrosis. However, occasional patients having features similar to those described previously are found to have Crohn's disease on follow-up, so careful clinical correlation is always important in such cases.

More recently, patients who present with a ruptured acute appendicitis are treated with antibiotic

ACUTE APPENDICITIS—PATHOLOGIC FEATURES

Gross Findings

- Thickened diameter, depending on severity of process. There may be perforation. Serosa may be dulled (from periappendicitis).

Microscopic Findings

- Early lesions display mucosal erosions and scattered crypt abscesses; later, the inflammation extends into the lamina propria and collections of neutrophils are also seen in the lumen
- When the inflammation extensively damages the muscularis propria, mural necrosis can lead to perforation
- In appendectomies performed in patients with prior appendicitis, there are mixed inflammatory infiltrates ranging from patchy and mild to diffuse and transmural
- In some appendices, there may be intramural or serosal foreign body–type giant cells surrounded by granulation tissue suggestive of prior rupture
- Serositis and fibrous adhesions, as well as prominent submucosal fibrosis, may be present
- Mucin extravasation is often seen
- A second pattern, *xanthogranulomatous appendicitis*, features a xanthogranulomatous infiltrate composed of foam cells, scattered multinucleated histiocytes, abundant hemosiderin, and luminal obliteration with spared lymphoid follicles

Differential Diagnosis

- *Interval appendices* share features with Crohn's disease but differ by lacking epithelioid granulomas, having fewer lymphoid aggregates and having less profound subserosal fibrosis.

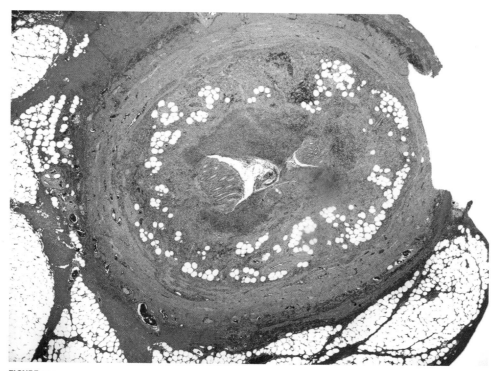

FIGURE 8-5

"Interval appendix." Note the mural chronic inflammatory cell aggregates in a concentric pattern. This pattern has been likened to a "string of pearls." See Guo G, Greenson JK: Histopathology of interval (delayed) appendectomy specimens: strong association with granulomatous and xanthogranulomatous appendicitis, *Am J Surg Pathol* 27:1147–1151, 2003.

therapy and drainage followed by a delayed or "interval appendectomy." In this setting, about two thirds of cases contain granulomas compared with less than 10% of acute appendicitis controls. About one third of interval appendectomy cases have xanthogranulomatous inflammation (cases with acute appendicitis do not display this pattern). A Crohn's-like appearance is found about half the time in interval appendices. Without the appropriate clinical history, these changes may be misinterpreted as Crohn's disease.

DIFFERENTIAL DIAGNOSIS

The differential diagnosis is with inflammatory bowel disease, which is described in subsequent text, and with infections. The diagnosis is often one of exclusion.

PROGNOSIS AND THERAPY

Treatment is appendectomy. Complications include wound infection, urinary retention, bowel obstruction, intra-abdominal abscesses, urinary tract infections, and pneumonia, all more likely if the appendix has perforated. Rarer complications include fistula formation, pylephlebitis, and liver abscesses. The overall mortality for appendectomy is about 0.3%. In individuals older than 65 years, this figure is closer to 5%.

■ PERIAPPENDICITIS

CLINICAL FEATURES

Preoperative mechanical manipulation of the appendix alone may result in mild diffuse granulocytic infiltration of the serosa, but when inflammation is accompanied by fibrin deposition and/or adhesions in the absence of luminal active inflammation, this is a potentially clinically significant finding. Periappendicitis alone is found in 1% to 5% of appendices resected for clinically acute appendicitis, the majority of which are attributable to salpingitis. In two large series, periappendicitis was attributable to a variety of processes: gonococcal and chlamydial salpingitis; yersiniosis, Meckel's diverticulitis, and associated intraperitoneal abscess; urologic disorders; colon neoplasms; infectious colitis; abdominal aortic aneurysm; bacterial peritonitis; and gastrointestinal perforation.

RADIOLOGIC FEATURES

These vary with the etiology of the periappendicitis.

PATHOLOGIC FEATURES

GROSS FINDINGS

The appendix is not enlarged, and the serosa is dulled or whitish depending on the severity of the periappendicitis. The lumen and mucosa appear normal.

MICROSCOPIC FINDINGS

Depending on the stage of the lesion, there is a serosa-confined (or possibly with extension into muscularis propria) lesion (Fig. 8-6) consisting of neutrophils and fibrin if the process is acute or with adhesions (scarring) and chronic inflammation if the process is chronic. The lumen is unaffected.

ANCILLARY STUDIES

The pathologist's finding of periappendicitis on an appendectomy specimen in the absence of luminal disease should alert the surgeon to take measures to identify the source of the serosal injury. If the patient is a woman, the female genital tract is a likely source, but as noted previously, any abdominal process may result in periappendicitis.

PROGNOSIS AND THERAPY

The treatment and prognosis depend on the inciting extra-appendiceal lesion.

PERIAPPENDICITIS—PATHOLOGIC FEATURES

Gross Findings
- Serosal thickening or exudates with normal muscularis and lumen

Microscopic Findings
- Serosal fibroinflammatory process and normal lumen

Differential Diagnosis
- With appendicitis
- Diagnosing periappendicitis as appendicitis is misleading to the clinician, who needs to find the true source of the inflammatory process; appendicitis has luminal involvement

---

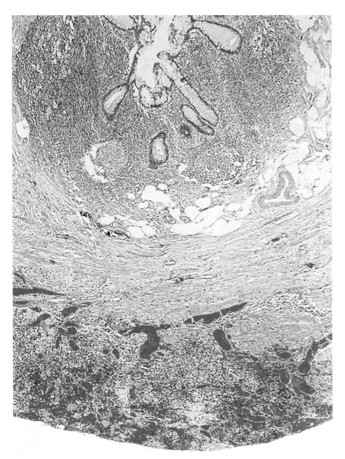

FIGURE 8-6
Periappendicitis with acute and chronic serositis with fibrosis and adhesions. The mucosa is free of acute inflammation.

■ INFECTIOUS CAUSES OF ACUTE APPENDICITIS

CLINICAL FEATURES

Infections of the appendix can be caused by bacteria, viruses, fungi, or parasites. In most cases of acute appendicitis, no organisms are identified by histology. Although specific infectious causes of acute appendicitis are only rarely identified, certain agents can occasionally be implicated. A few specific infections are noted in the following sections.

BACTERIAL INFECTIONS

Cultures reveal mixed aerobic and anaerobic isolates in almost all cases. In one study of 41 children with acute appendicitis, an average of 14.1 isolates per specimen was detected. Bacterial isolates are almost always limited to normal flora and believed to play a secondary role following mucosal injury. Bacteria belonging to the *Bacteroides fragilis* group are the most frequently isolated anaerobes, whereas *Escherichia coli* is the most frequently isolated aerobe. Bacteria belonging to the *Streptococcus milleri* group are also common aerobes, but may be of greater significance because they have been linked to a markedly increased (seven-fold) risk of abscess formation.

ACTINOMYCES

Actinomyces israelii is a rare cause of appendicitis. *A. israelii* can rarely lead to infections of the small intestine, appendix, or colon. Histologically, the long filamentous organisms stain dark blue on routine hematoxylin and eosin preparations and are particularly easy to recognize when associated with characteristic sulfur granules. Active inflammation in the mucosal wall is typically present, and fistula formation, rupture of the appendix, and abscess formation may complicate the clinical course. *Actinomyces turicensis* has also been implicated in appendicitis and is frequently accompanied by aerobic bacterial isolates of the *Streptococcus anginosus* group.

CAMPYLOBACTER

Campylobacter jejuni is an uncommon cause of bacterial appendicitis (approximately 2%). The patients are generally young children with grossly normal appendices. Histologically, the active inflammatory changes are limited to the mucosa, consisting of cryptitis and surface erosions with focal accumulations of histiocytes that occasionally result in a granulomatous appearance.

CLOSTRIDIUM DIFFICILE AND SHIGELLA

Clostridium difficile infections and shigellosis involving the appendix are almost always associated with more general colonic disease, although appendicitis can be a rare clinical presentation. Overall, the histologic findings are identical to those seen in the colon (see Chapter 9).

MALAKOPLAKIA

Malakoplakia is most commonly seen in the urinary tract but can occasionally be found in the appendix (Figs. 8-7 and 8-8). In general malakoplakia results from

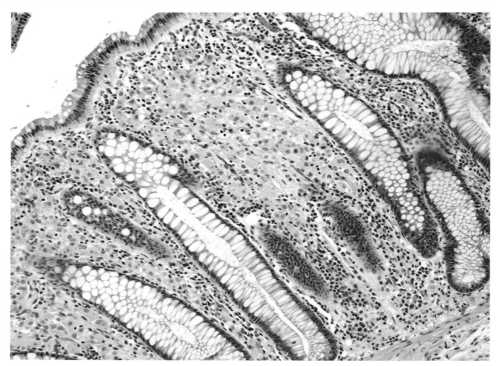

FIGURE 8-7

Malakoplakia showing sheets of histiocytes infiltrating the laminae propria.

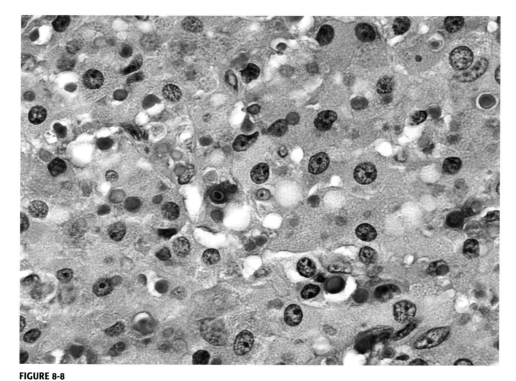

FIGURE 8-8

Malakoplakia. Note the admixed Michaelis-Gutmann bodies in this example of malakoplakia (round, laminated structures with a targetoid appearance).

INFECTIOUS CAUSES OF ACUTE APPENDICITIS—FACT SHEET

Definition
- Cases of acute appendicitis in which a specific infectious etiology is identified

an abnormal immune response in which bacteria are incompletely digested and accumulate in histiocytes. The histologic findings typically consist of a diffuse or nodular thickening of the mucosal wall resulting from the accumulation of numerous macrophages, including many that are eosinophilic, with scattered lymphocytes and plasma cells. Most characteristic are the admixed Michaelis-Gutmann bodies, which are round, laminated structures with a targetoid appearance that can be highlighted with iron or calcium stains.

SPIROCHETOSIS

Spirochetosis is caused by *Brachyspira aalborgi* and can occasionally be seen in the appendix. In one study, spirochetosis was detected in 1.9 % of incidentally removed appendices, 0.7 % of appendices in patients with clinical acute appendicitis plus histologic acute appendicitis, and 12.3 % of patients with clinical acute appendicitis but no histologic changes. Therefore, spirochetosis may contribute to clinical symptoms in patients with otherwise normal appendices. Spirochetosis of the small intestine and colon is more commonly found in HIV-infected patients than in non-HIV-infected patients, but little information is available on whether this is also true for the appendix. Overall, adults appear to be more commonly infected than children. From a histologic standpoint, spirochetosis is characterized by a hazy hematoxylin-positive band of about 3 μm in thickness that lies along the epithelial brush border (Fig. 8-9). Silver stains highlight the organisms (Fig. 8-10). Typically, there is no inflammatory response, even though organisms can be seen by electron microscopy within epithelial cells and macrophages.

TUBERCULOSIS

Tuberculosis of the appendix is almost always accompanied by gastrointestinal or pulmonary tuberculosis, although isolated infections have been reported. The histologic findings are identical to those seen elsewhere in the body.

YERSINIA

When *Yersinia enterocolitica* is specifically sought, infections are found in approximately 4 % of cases of acute appendicitis. In general, *Yersinia* tends to cause acute enteritis in young children and terminal ileitis and mesenteric adenitis in older children and young adults. *Y. enterocolitica* and *Y. pseudotuberculosis* infection can cause granulomatous

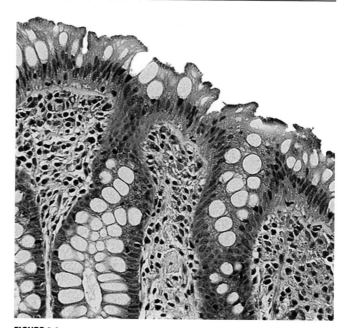

FIGURE 8-9
Appendiceal spirochetosis. Note the "haze" present on the surface of the epithelial cells.

inflammation with large epithelioid noncaseating granulomas surrounded by prominent lymphoid cuffs. In these cases of granulomatous inflammation, prominent acute inflammation is common and lymphoid hyperplasia is essentially always present (Figs. 8-11 and 8-12).

FUNGAL INFECTIONS

Fungal infections such as aspergillosis and mucormycosis can involve the appendix, typically as a component of systemic infection. Patients are typically immunosuppressed owing to organ transplantation or chemotherapy.

PARASITE INFECTIONS

Enterobius vermicularis is one of the most common parasites seen in the appendix. However, at our hospital, only 4 of 1584 appendices removed over a 17-year period from patients 15 years of age or younger had *Enterobius* infections. Individuals in late childhood and early adolescence have the highest frequency of infection (ages 5 to 15 years), which can reach as high as 24 % in some studies. The organism is most commonly found in the lumen with no mucosal inflammatory response (Figs. 8-13 and 8-14). In one study in which close to 22,000 appendices were evaluated, granulomatous inflammation and increased eosinophils in the lamina propria were quite rare and were both noted in less than 2 % of infections. It is of interest to note that an inverse relationship between active mucosal inflammation and pinworm infection has been noted in several studies. Mucosal inflammation, when present, has been more strongly linked to the presence of parasite ova.

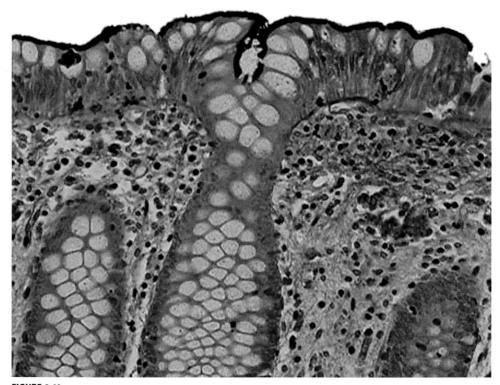

FIGURE 8-10

Warthin-Starry staining in spirochetosis.

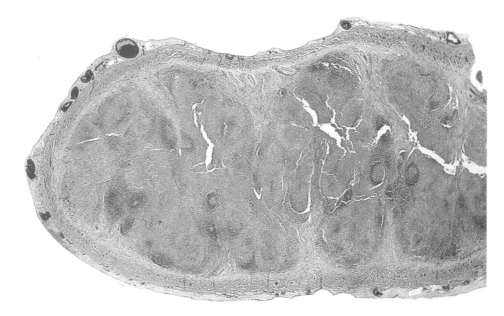

FIGURE 8-11

Yersinia appendicitis. Note the necrotizing lymphoid hyperplasia.

VIRAL INFECTIONS

Viral gastroenteritis does not typically result in appendectomy, although some examples of appendicitis are, no doubt, caused by viral agents. Viral enteritis classically results in surgical excision of the appendix when it leads to ileocecal intussusception and ileocolectomy. Intussusception is most often attributable to lymphoid hyperplasia in the terminal ileum, which can form a "leading edge," classically in infants and young children. The viral agents most commonly implicated in this setting are rotavirus, echovirus, and adenovirus.

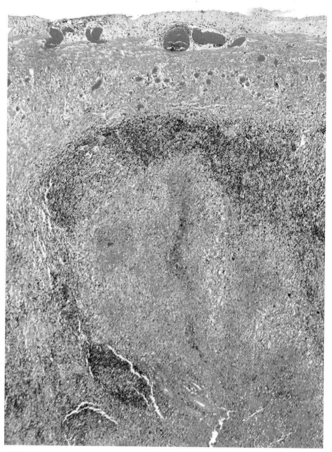

FIGURE 8-12

Yersinia appendicitis. Acute necrotizing inflammation appears within the center of lymphoid aggregates.

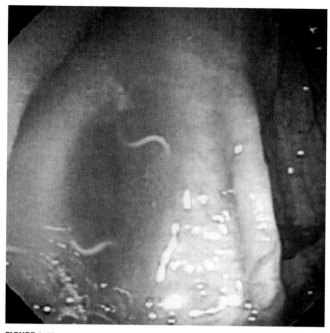

FIGURE 8-13

Enterobius vermicularis. Endoscopic photo taken from within the cecum in a patient with appendiceal disease.

The latter is detected most frequently and is so named based on its isolation from adenoids. In appendices infected with adenovirus, lymphoid hyperplasia is prominent. Erosions may be identified, but viral inclusions are found in intact mucosal epithelial cells. Zones in which inclusions may be found are selected by scanning at low magnification for areas with

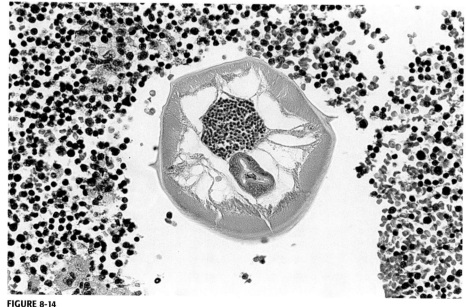

FIGURE 8-14

Enterobius vermicularis in the appendiceal lumen. Note the characteristic cuticular crests.

frayed-appearing epithelium showing loss of nuclear polarity and an eosinophilic appearance imparted by loss of goblet cell mucin. Such zones are frequently in close association with lymphoid follicles. Intranuclear adenovirus inclusions are typically of the Cowdry B type, consisting of nuclear smudging, although Cowdry A inclusions, featuring sharply demarcated globules surrounded by a clear zone, are found in a minority of cases (Figs. 8-15 and 8-16).

Cytomegalovirus may also be found in the appendices of immunocompromised hosts, where it displays the features found in other sites with endothelial cells, rather than epithelial cells, tending to be infected. It is occasionally responsible for clinical acute appendicitis.

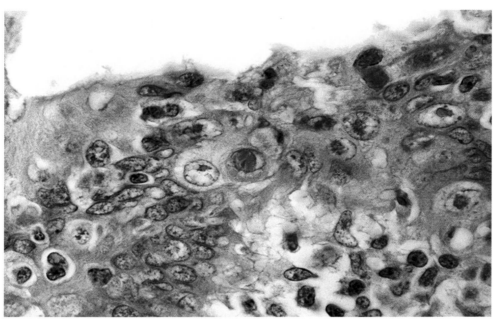

FIGURE 8-15

Adenovirus infection with epithelial cells containing both Cowdry A and Cowdry B inclusions.

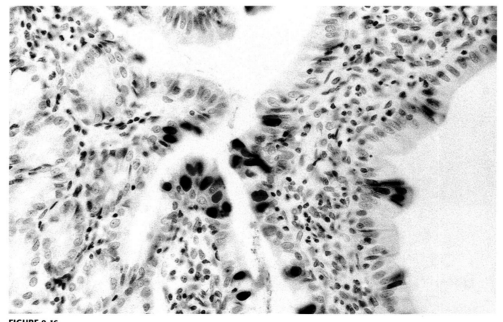

FIGURE 8-16

Note the strong nuclear expression of adenovirus on immunohistochemical staining.

INFECTIOUS CAUSES OF ACUTE APPENDICITIS—PATHOLOGIC FEATURES

- *Actinomyces*
- *Campylobacter*
- *Clostridium difficile*
- *Shigella sp.*
- Malakoplakia
- Spirochetosis
- Tuberculosis
- Yersiniosis
- Fungal infections
- Parasitic infections (usually *Enterobius vermicularis*)
- Viral agents (adenovirus)

■ ULCERATIVE COLITIS INVOLVING THE APPENDIX

CLINICAL FEATURES

The appendix may play an interesting role in inflammatory bowel disease because an appendectomy has been touted as a protective factor in ulcerative colitis in more than one study, although some evidence suggests that it is the appendicitis rather than the appendectomy that is protective. The prevalence of prior appendectomy is far lower in patients with ulcerative colitis than in control groups, although this observation does not necessarily indicate causation. Similar findings have also been observed in a murine model.

Ulcerative appendicitis, the appendiceal counterpart of ulcerative colitis, is typically present in patients with pancolitis but is also common as a "skip lesion" in patients who have left-sided or rectal disease, occurring in 20% to more than 80% of cases. In some cases, the active inflammatory disease in the appendix may be prominent, whereas that in the nearby cecum is mild.

ULCERATIVE COLITIS INVOLVING THE APPENDIX—FACT SHEET

Definition
- Appendiceal inflammatory disease (usually active chronic) in patient with ulcerative colitis

Incidence and Location
- Common in patients with ulcerative colitis and more predominantly involving the orifice than the tip

Morbidity and Mortality
- Same as for ulcerative colitis

Gender, Race, and Age Distribution
- Same as that for ulcerative colitis

PATHOLOGIC FEATURES

GROSS FINDINGS

In patients with pancolitis, the appendix may appear swollen in contiguity with the cecum and displays a smooth serosa. Like a "skip lesion" in ulcerative colitis, the appendiceal opening will display a red edematous surface in contrast to the unaffected cecal mucosa.

MICROSCOPIC FINDINGS

Ulcerative appendicitis shows the same histologic features as ulcerative colitis. There is mucosal-based active inflammation with crypt abscesses, panmucosal plasmacytosis, suppurative luminal exudate, and crypt distortion. Ulcerative appendicitis is distinguished from early acute appendicitis partly on clinical grounds, although early acute appendicitis features less crypt distortion and minimal plasmacytosis.

ANCILLARY STUDIES

IMMUNOHISTOCHEMISTRY

In ulcerative colitis, but not in acute appendicitis, immunostains can show prominent S-100 protein-reactive dendritic cells, MAC387-positive dendritic cells, as well as upregulated HLA class II antigens.

DIFFERENTIAL DIAGNOSIS

The differential diagnosis is with acute appendicitis, which often has serosal involvement. Crypt distortion is more typical of ulcerative colitis, but the separation of these entities is made by clinicopathologic correlation.

ULCERATIVE COLITIS INVOLVING THE APPENDIX—PATHOLOGIC FEATURES

Gross Findings
- Found either in continuity with pancolitis in ulcerative colitis or as a "skip" lesion in left-sided disease

Microscopic Findings
- Like those of ulcerative colitis elsewhere, featuring cryptitis, crypt distortion, basal plasmacytosis

Differential Diagnosis
- With acute appendicitis. Differs by having more crypt distortion

PROGNOSIS AND THERAPY

Prognosis and therapy is related to the patient's underlying ulcerative colitis.

■ CROHN'S DISEASE INVOLVING THE APPENDIX

CLINICAL FEATURES

The appendix is often examined in terminal ileal resections from patients with Crohn's disease, and involvement is found affected in anywhere from 0% to 60% of cases. Such operations are usually performed in adults. The majority of appendices resected from patients with typical Crohn's disease elsewhere in the gastrointestinal tract are normal, and most patients who present with isolated granulomatous appendiceal disease do not later manifest typical Crohn's disease elsewhere in the gastrointestinal tract, so many observers believe that there are two diseases: true Crohn's disease of the appendix and idiopathic granulomatous appendicitis. In contrast to the case with ulcerative colitis, prior appendectomy is thought to be a risk factor for the subsequent development of Crohn's disease.

RADIOLOGIC FEATURES

Both CT and ultrasound display mural thickening when Crohn's disease involves the appendix. However, in contrast to the typical pattern of acute appendicitis, this thickening usually extends into the ileum and or cecum.

PATHOLOGIC FEATURES

GROSS FINDINGS

The appendiceal wall is thick and fibrotic in Crohn's disease and involvement may be patchy.

MICROSCOPIC FINDINGS

In cases with clinical Crohn's disease, the appendices have the typical histologic features of Crohn's seen elsewhere in the gastrointestinal tract, with fissures, ulcers, active inflammation, and occasional granulomas (Figs. 8-17 and 8-18). The numbers of granulomas per cross-section of the appendix were studied by Dudley and Dean in appendices resected from patients with typical Crohn's disease and compared with cases of isolated "idiopathic granulomatous appendicitis." They found that cases with clinical Crohn's disease

---

CROHN'S DISEASE INVOLVING THE APPENDIX—FACT SHEET

Definition
- Appendiceal inflammatory disease in a patient known to have Crohn's disease

Incidence and Location
- Uncommon, and may be found in any part of the appendix

Morbidity and Mortality
- Same as for patient's Crohn's disease

Gender, Race, and Age Distribution
- Same as for Crohn's disease

CROHN'S DISEASE INVOLVING THE APPENDIX— PATHOLOGIC FEATURES

Gross Findings
- Thickened appendix, usually with mucosal lesions visible grossly

Microscopic Findings
- Those of Crohn's disease elsewhere, including fissures, ulcers, active inflammation, and occasional granulomas

Differential Diagnosis
- If disease is limited to the appendix, caution is advised in labeling a de novo patient with Crohn's disease and "interval" appendicitis should be considered
- Sarcoidosis is also excluded by clinicopathologic correlation

---

had 0.3 granulomas per tissue section in contrast to about 20 granulomas per tissue section in patients with "idiopathic granulomatous appendicitis." Furthermore, none of the "idiopathic granulomatous appendicitis" had recurrent disease in a mean follow-up period of 4.5 years. In another series, none of nine patients (identified among 1133 consecutive appendectomy specimens) with idiopathic granulomatous appendicitis developed Crohn's disease in a mean follow-up period of just longer than 7 years. In contrast, one patient reported in a series by Huang and Appelman with 21 granulomas per cross-section later developed Crohn's disease elsewhere in the gut, so the number of granulomas per cross-section is not entirely reliable in separating these entities (Table 8-1).

ANCILLARY STUDIES

OTHER STUDIES

Newer microbiologic techniques may provide some clues to the etiologies of granulomatous appendicitis. For example, in a 2001 study by Lamps and her

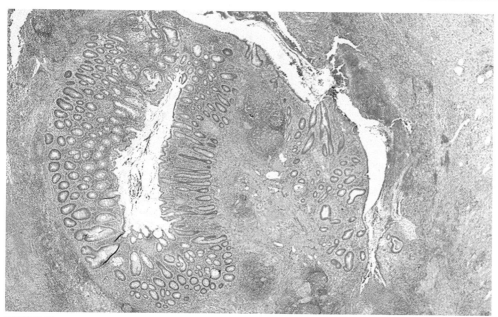

FIGURE 8-17

Crohn's disease involving the appendix displaying a fissure.

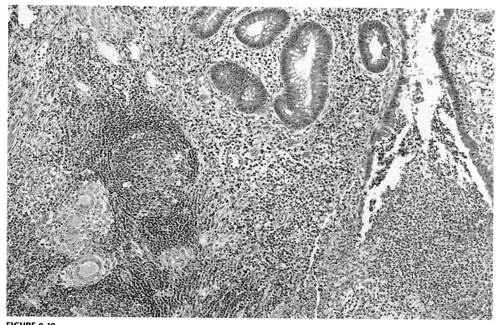

FIGURE 8-18

Appendiceal Crohn's disease showing granulomatous inflammation.

colleagues, 10 of 40 (25%) cases of granulomatous appendicitis were found to have evidence of pathogenic *Yersinia* species by polymerase chain reaction (PCR). However, now that some of the features of Crohn's disease are believed to reflect an immunologic defect in processing organisms that do not affect normal individuals, the search for a unifying infectious cause of Crohn's disease may be misleading.

DIFFERENTIAL DIAGNOSIS

Diagnosing Crohn's disease of the appendix requires a clinicopathologic correlation. If disease is limited to the appendix, caution is advised in labeling a de novo patient with Crohn's disease and a history in keeping with "interval" appendicitis should be

TABLE 8-1

Chronic Inflammatory Disorders of the Appendix

Finding	Idiopathic Granulomatous Appendicitis	Crohn's Disease	Healing Acute Appendicitis
Neutrophilic cryptitis/crypt abscesses	+	+	+
Fissures or fistulae	Occasional fissures	+	−
Transmural lymphoid aggregates	Often	Often	Occasionally
Fibrosis	Often	Often	Often
Granulomas	Numerous	Occasional	No, but may have numerous foam cells

sought. Another consideration is sarcoidosis, which is a rare event and, again, excluded by clinicopathologic correlation.

PROGNOSIS AND THERAPY

The prognosis of Crohn's disease of the appendix is that of Crohn's disease in general (see Chapter 10), because those with appendiceal involvement often have extensive ileocolic involvement.

■ CYSTIC FIBROSIS

CLINICAL FEATURES

Cystic fibrosis (CF) occurs in approximately one of every 3200 live white births (in one of every 3900 live births of all Americans). Approximately 1000 new cases of CF are diagnosed each year. More than 80% of patients are diagnosed by age 3 years; however, nearly 10% of newly diagnosed cases are age 18 or older. People with CF have a variety of symptoms including very salty-tasting skin; persistent coughing, at times with phlegm; wheezing or shortness of breath; an excessive appetite but poor weight gain; and greasy, bulky stools. Symptoms vary from person to person owing, in part, to the more than 1000 mutations of the CF gene. The sweat chloride test is the standard diagnostic test for CF.

Although recurrent pulmonary infections and pulmonary insufficiency are the hallmarks, gastrointestinal symptoms commonly antedate the pulmonary findings and may suggest the diagnosis in infants and young children. The protean gastrointestinal manifestations of CF result primarily from abnormally viscous luminal secretions within hollow viscera and the ducts of solid organs. Bowel obstruction may be present at birth because of meconium ileus or meconium plug syndrome. Complications of meconium ileus include volvulus, small bowel atresia,

perforation, and meconium peritonitis with abdominal calcifications. Older children with CF may present with bowel obstruction because of distal intestinal obstruction syndrome or colonic stricture, and tenacious intestinal residue may serve as a lead point for intussusception or cause recurrent rectal prolapse. Overall, patients with CF have a lower frequency of acute appendicitis (1.5%) than the general population (approximately 7%). In some cases, the engorged appendix itself can cause clinical symptoms of appendicitis, even though histologic examination reveals no inflammation. The incidence of acquired appendiceal diverticula is also markedly increased in cystic fibrosis patients.

RADIOLOGIC FEATURES

Radiologic studies often demonstrate thickened intestinal mucosal folds in older children and uncommonly show colonic pneumatosis, peptic esophageal stricture owing to gastroesophageal reflux, and duodenal ulcer.

Appendicitis resulting from inspissated secretions is uncommon. Of note, the mean diameter of the appendix in CF patients who do not have appendicitis is about 8 mm, and in most patients the appendix measures more than 6 mm. Therefore, the diameter of the appendix alone may not be a parameter for diagnosing appendicitis in patients with cystic fibrosis. Mucoid material is found in the appendix lumen in the majority of patients.

PATHOLOGIC FEATURES

GROSS FINDINGS

On gross examination, all hollow viscera, including the appendix, contain thick viscous tenacious mucus filling the lumina, and in the appendix it may form a plug. This abnormal mucin can cause marked engorgement of the appendix and can lead to a "sausage-like" appendix.

CYSTIC FIBROSIS INVOLVING THE APPENDIX—FACT SHEET

Definition
- Involvement of the appendix in a patient known or subsequently found to have CF
- Gastrointestinal tract involvement may be the first presentation

Incidence and Location
- CF occurs in approximately 1 in every 3200 live white births (1 in every 3900 live births of all Americans).

Morbidity and Mortality
- Same as for CF in general
- Patients typically live into their 30s with numerous respiratory infections and gastrointestinal tract complications
- Adults are prone to diabetes, osteoporosis, and gastrointestinal tract malignancies

Gender, Race, and Age Distribution
- Most cases of CF are diagnosed in early childhood
- No gender prevalence
- Most common in whites

Clinical Features
- Patients with CF have a variety of symptoms including very salty-tasting skin; persistent coughing, at times with phlegm; wheezing or shortness of breath; excessive appetite but poor weight gain; and greasy, bulky stools
- Symptoms vary owing in part to the more than 1000 mutations of the *CFTR* gene. Many patients present with gastrointestinal tract symptoms, but the incidence of appendicitis is lower in these people than in control subjects (1% to 2% vs. 7% to 10%)

Prognosis and Treatment
- Same as for CF
- Treatment of the underlying disease is directed at reducing pulmonary infections
- Most patients with CF live into their 30s

CYSTIC FIBROSIS INVOLVING THE APPENDIX—PATHOLOGIC FEATURES

Gross Findings
- The appendix, even when unaffected by appendicitis, is enlarged and distended with mucus

Microscopic Findings
- Enlarged and distended goblet cells containing normal-appearing mucin and thick inspissated eosinophilic mucin in the lumen

Differential Diagnosis
- Evaluation of the epithelium excludes neoplasms (sometimes multiple sections are required), and correlation with the clinical history is best in establishing a diagnosis of CF

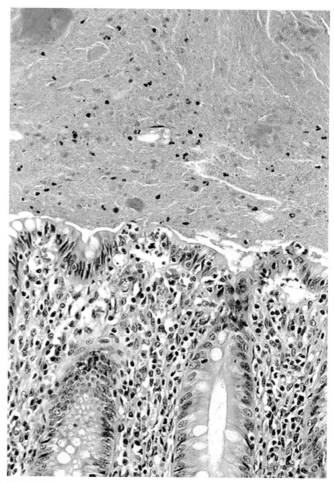

FIGURE 8-19

Cystic fibrosis. The goblet cells are more prominent than usual, and the lumen contains the thick inspissated mucin characteristic of cystic fibrosis.

MICROSCOPIC FINDINGS

In CF, the most common histologic finding is enlarged and distended goblet cells containing normal-appearing mucin, although this can be a subtle finding in many cases. Inspissated eosinophilic mucin in dilated glands can also be seen, but is a nonspecific finding. The most readily identifiable abnormality is usually the thick inspissated eosinophilic mucin in the lumen (Figs. 8-1 and 8-19).

DIFFERENTIAL DIAGNOSIS

Patients without CF sometimes have prominent inspissated mucus in their appendices, and mucinous neoplasms are also accompanied by abundant mucin. Evaluation of the epithelium excludes neoplasms (sometimes multiple sections are required), and correlation with the clinical history is best in establishing a diagnosis of CF.

PROGNOSIS AND THERAPY

The prognosis is that of CF itself. The treatment of CF depends upon the stage of the disease and the organs involved. Clearing mucus from the lungs by chest physical therapy is a cornerstone of CF treatment. Other types of treatments include TOBI (tobramycin solution for inhalation), an aerosolized antibiotic used to treat lung infections; dornase alfa (Pulmozyme), a mucus-thinning drug shown to reduce the number of lung infections and improve lung function; and azithromycin, an antibiotic recently proven to be effective in patients with CF whose lungs are chronically infected with the common *Pseudomonas aeruginosa* bacteria.

According to the Cystic Fibrosis Foundation's national patient registry, the median age of survival for people with CF extends into the early 30s. As more advances have been made in the treatment of CF, the number of adults with CF has steadily grown. Today, more than 40% of the CF population is age 18 and older. Complications for these individuals include male infertility, osteoporosis, diabetes, and gastrointestinal tract malignancies.

ENDOMETRIOSIS, DECIDUOSIS, GLIOMATOSIS

CLINICAL FEATURES

Endometriosis is well known to present in a variety of anatomic sites and affects the gastrointestinal tract in up to 40% of patients with pelvic endometriosis. The sigmoid colon is the most common site, but the appendix may be involved in about 15% of the cases. Although appendiceal endometriosis can masquerade clinically as acute appendicitis, it more typically has a nonspecific presentation, although pain may wax and wane with the menstrual cycle.

A similar phenomenon, termed *deciduosis* (ectopic decidua), has been found in the appendices of pregnant women. Deciduosis, in contrast to endometriosis, typically presents with signs and symptoms of acute appendicitis.

When present, pelvic gliomatosis can also affect the serosal aspect of the appendix. Gliomatosis peritonei is found in patients with ovarian teratomas and manifests as foci of mature glial tissue deposited ubiquitously over the serosal surfaces. It has also been reported as a rare complication of ventricular shunts, and cases of malignant transformation are recorded.

PATHOLOGIC FEATURES

GROSS FINDINGS

On gross examination, endometriosis appears as it does in other sites, as firm areas that may contain cysts filled with brown fluid. The appearances of deciduosis and gliomatosis are less specific—both appear as whitish plaques.

ENDOMETRIOSIS, DECIDUOSIS, GLIOMATOSIS—FACT SHEET

Definition
- Deposition of endometrial-type glands and stroma, decidualized endometrial-type tissue, or glial tissue in the appendix

Incidence and Location
- Affects the gastrointestinal tract in about 40% of patients with endometriosis; appendix in 15%
- Deciduosis and gliomatosis are rare

Morbidity and Mortality
- Benign processes that can result in adhesions and obstruction

Gender, Race, and Age Distribution
- Affect women in their reproductive years

Clinical Features
- Patients have nonspecific symptoms that may wax and wane with the menstrual cycle
- Deciduosis presents with symptoms and signs of acute appendicitis
- Gliomatosis presents nonspecifically

Prognosis and Treatment
- Benign overall—rarely carcinomas arise in association with endometriosis and rare malignant degeneration in gliomatosis
- Treatment is same as that for endometriosis (hormonal manipulation, lysis of adhesions that form)

ENDOMETRIOSIS, DECIDUOSIS, GLIOMATOSIS—PATHOLOGIC FEATURES

Gross Findings
- Endometriosis—firm with cysts containing brown fluid
- Deciduosis and gliomatosis—white plaques

Microscopic Findings
- Endometriosis—endometrial glands and stroma with associated fibrosis and adhesions (usually serosal)
- Deciduosis—large polyhedral cells arranged in sheets in the serosa
- Gliomatosis—nodules of glial tissue coating the serosa

Differential Diagnosis
- Endometriosis—adenocarcinoma (lacks stroma)
- Deciduosis—epithelioid malignant neoplasms (lacks mitoses)
- Gliomatosis—spindle cell neoplasms

MICROSCOPIC FINDINGS

Most examples of endometriosis affect the serosa or muscularis propria and are accompanied by abundant fibrosis and adhesions, although submucosal examples are also reported. Endometriosis of the appendix resembles examples found elsewhere, consisting of endometrial-type glands and stroma associated with hemosiderin deposition and a fibroblastic response (Figs. 8-20 through 8-22). The endometrial-type epithelium changes with the menstrual cycle. A stromal decidual reaction may be found in endometriotic foci in pregnant patients.

Deciduosis differs from endometriosis by lacking glands and consists only of large polyhedral cells arranged in sheets in the serosa or outer muscularis propria, although deciduosis has rarely been reported in the mucosa of the gastrointestinal tract. Such cells can sometimes be mistaken for malignant (often epithelial) lesions.

IMMUNOHISTOCHEMISTRY

If deciduosis raises a concern for carcinoma based on its large pink polyhedral cells, immunohistochemical stains for keratin, carcinoembryonic antigen (CEA), epithelial membrane antigen (EMA), and S-100 protein are negative. The large decidualized cells typically express vimentin, and may show desmin or muscle

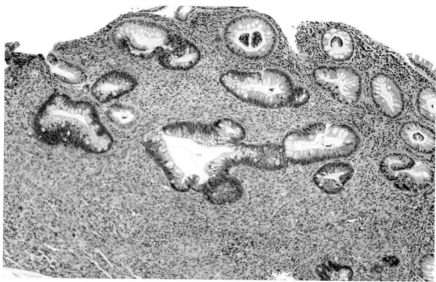

FIGURE 8-20

Endometriosis is not uncommon in the gastrointestinal tract. In this example, the condition resulted in a spindle cell lamina propria lesion that raised the possibility of a sarcoma (Kaposi's sarcoma) in the stroma, and the reactive epithelial changes suggested an epithelial lesion.

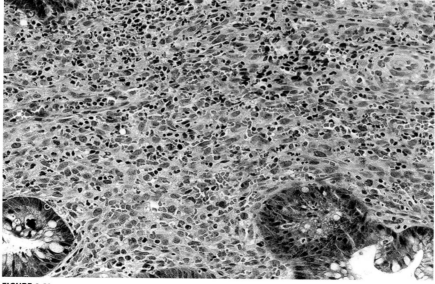

FIGURE 8-21

Higher magnification of the lesion depicted in Figure 8-20.

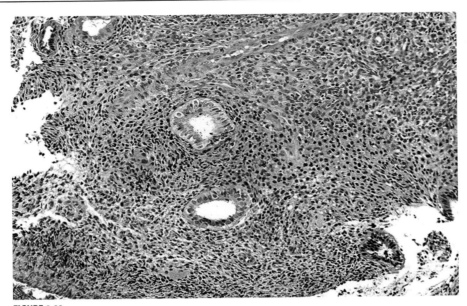

FIGURE 8-22
Appendiceal endometriosis. Additional sections of the lesion in Figure 8-20 revealed typical endometrial-type glands.

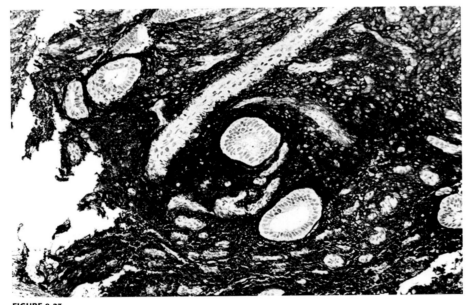

FIGURE 8-23
CD10 staining in endometriosis.

actin positivity. When the stroma of endometriosis is unaccompanied by glands, it can raise the concern that the lesion is Kaposi's sarcoma. A positive CD10 stain can be reassuring (Fig. 8-23).

DIFFERENTIAL DIAGNOSIS

The appearances of endometriosis, deciduosis, and gliomatosis are characteristic if one considers these entities.

PROGNOSIS AND THERAPY

These processes are benign, but endometriosis of the appendix is associated with adhesions (just as endometriosis in general).

■ COLONIC-TYPE (NONMUCINOUS) EPITHELIAL NEOPLASMS OF THE APPENDIX: ADENOMAS AND ADENOCARCINOMA

Colonic-type adenomas and adenocarcinomas of the appendix are nonmucinous neoplasms histologically comparable to those found in the colon.

CLINICAL FEATURES

The nonmucinous adenomas and adenocarcinomas that are characteristic of colorectal neoplasia rarely occur in the appendix. The frequency of colonic-type neoplasms in the appendix is about 2% and 7% of all adenomas and adenocarcinomas, respectively, with the remainder being mucinous neoplasms. Colonic-type neoplasms do not tend to form mucoceles and are frequently incidental findings. Most manifest clinically with appendicitis related to neoplastic luminal obstruction.

RADIOLOGIC FEATURES

Relatively little information exists on the imaging appearance of colonic type neoplasms of the appendix. The majority of cases detected on imaging are in the setting of suspected appendicitis in an older individual. A focal soft tissue mass can be seen on CT that involves the appendix but rarely demonstrates mucocele formation.

PATHOLOGIC FEATURES

GROSS FINDINGS

Gross examination may show features similar to those found in the colon, including a mass lesion and mucosal, submucosal, and serosal thickening. In comparison to mucinous lesions and carcinoids, which are frequently found at the tip of the appendix, colonic-type adenomas and adenocarcinomas reside at the appendiceal orifice. Mucocele formation (cystic dilatation of the appendix) is more likely in mucinous neoplasms, but may rarely be found in the setting of colonic-type adenomas and adenocarcinomas. The term *mucocele* does not describe a histologic entity, but rather a gross finding and should be reserved for clinicians, radiologists, and gross descriptions. Involvement by secondary appendicitis may cause a suppurative exudate. The finding of a polypoid luminal mass is exceptionally rare.

MICROSCOPIC FINDINGS

Precursor lesions of tubular adenomas, traditional serrated adenomas, and sessile serrated adenomas may all be encountered (Fig. 8-24). The histologic criteria

for these lesions in the appendix are identical to those of their colonic counterparts (see Chapter 13). The finding of adenomatous change should prompt submission of the entire appendix to exclude a higher-grade lesion.

The descriptive term *cystadenoma* is used when adenomatous lesions grow and cause cystic dilatation of the appendix (mucocele) with the histologic finding of a low-grade neoplastic lining. The lining can become flattened and attenuated as the appendix dilates. As discussed in the next section on low-grade mucinous neoplasms, the term adenoma should be reserved for lesions that are completely confined to the appendix and have no risk for intra-abdominal or peritoneal spread (pseudomyxoma peritonei).

Colonic-type (nonmucinous) adenocarcinomas of the appendix are defined as malignant tumors in which less than 50% of the lesion is composed of mucin. These lesions are rare within the appendix and appear as cuboidal or columnar neoplastic cells that form infiltrating glands resembling typical adenocarcinomas of the colon and rectum. There are high-grade nuclear alterations with full-thickness nuclear stratification, vesicular nuclei, irregular membranes, prominent nucleoli, and frequent mitoses with destructive invasion of the appendiceal wall.

ANCILLARY STUDIES

IMMUNOHISTOCHEMISTRY

Appendiceal colonic-type neoplasms express immunohistochemical markers similar to those of the colon, including reactivity for CK20 and CDX-2. They are almost universally CK-7 negative.

DIFFERENTIAL DIAGNOSIS

Sessile serrated adenomas occurring in the appendix should be separated from hyperplastic changes resulting from their potential to progress to carcinomas. The criteria remain the same as those for their colonic counterparts, including widened crypt bases and lateral branching crypts. Some examples may prove difficult to differentiate because of the overlapping hyperplastic features seen in sessile serrated adenomas.

Adenomas that produce a mucocele need to be distinguished from non-neoplastic retention cysts. Retention cysts also form a dilatation of the appendix that can be referred to as a *mucocele* by gross appearance. However, although the epithelial lining of a retention cyst may be attenuated, it is not dysplastic like that seen in the mucocele produced by an adenoma or adenocarcinoma. Simple retention cysts rarely exceed 2 cm in diameter. Mucoceles larger than 2 cm that are initially diagnosed

COLONIC-TYPE ADENOMA AND ADENOCARCINOMA OF THE APPENDIX—FACT SHEET

Definition
- Nonmucinous epithelial neoplasm

Incidence and Location
- 0.2/100,000 population
- Comprises 2% and 7% of all adenomas and adenocarcinomas of appendix
- Far less common than mucinous neoplasms

Morbidity and Mortality
- Causes acute appendicitis
- Metastasis occurs via lymphatics and hematogenous routes, sometimes involving ovaries

Gender, Race, and Age Distribution
- Males more than females
- No clear racial difference
- Disease of adulthood, average age of diagnosis is 62 years

Clinical Features
- Most are incidental findings
- Patients may present with acute appendicitis

Prognosis and Treatment
- Complete excision is curative for adenomas
- Right hemicolectomy is recommended for invasive tumors
- Metastasis occurs in 20% of patients with adenocarcinoma
- Adjuvant therapy and prognosis are comparable to colonic adenocarcinoma

COLONIC-TYPE ADENOMA AND ADENOCARCINOMA OF THE APPENDIX—PATHOLOGIC FEATURES

Gross Findings
- Mucosal thickening or ulceration
- Rarely has mucocele formation
- Rarely has a polypoid lesion

Microscopic Findings
- Identical to adenomas and adenocarcinomas found in colon

Differential Diagnosis
- Sessile serrated adenomas should be differentiated from hyperplasia
- Cystadenomas should be differentiated from simple mucoceles/retention cysts
- Adenocarcinomas should be differentiated from metastatic adenocarcinomas

as simple mucoceles are more likely to represent true neoplasms that have been undersampled.

PROGNOSIS AND THERAPY

Colonic type adenocarcinoma of the appendix develops from a tubular or tubulovillous adenoma. It is comparable to adenocarcinoma of the colon, with a malignant potential between that of appendiceal carcinoid and

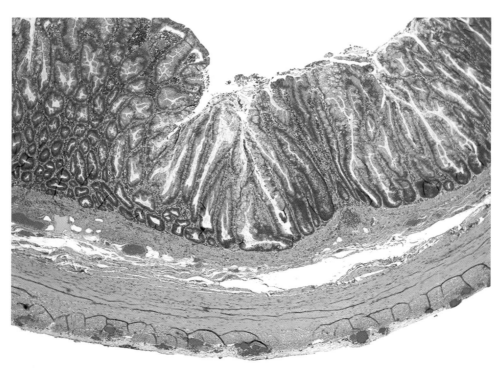

FIGURE 8-24
Sessile serrated adenoma arising in appendix. Histologic features are identical to those seen in colon.

colonic carcinoma spreading both within lymphatics and blood vessels—often to the ovaries. Metastases will subsequently develop in 20% of patients with colonic type appendiceal adenocarcinoma.

Adenomatous lesions and early colonic-type adenocarcinoma of the appendix, although uncommon, may be treated with appendectomy alone. However, as a result of the high rate of invasion and presence of nodal metastases, a right hemicolectomy is recommended. Histologic staging and adjuvant therapy are similar to those for colonic adenocarcinomas.

◾ APPENDICEAL MUCINOUS NEOPLASM

Appendiceal mucinous neoplasm is an epithelial neoplasm demonstrating a low-grade mucinous morphology that lacks overtly malignant features, but is associated with extra-appendiceal spread. The bland cytology conflicts with its biologic behavior, which often pursues an indolent, but progressive, clinical course with a relatively high mortality rate. A multitude of potentially confusing terms and competing classification schemes have been used to characterize these lesions, including terms such as *pseudomyxoma peritonei, disseminated peritoneal adenomucinosis, low-grade appendiceal mucinous neoplasm, mucinous borderline tumor of the appendix, mucinous tumor of uncertain malignant potential,* and *low-grade mucinous carcinoma.*

CLINICAL FEATURES

Mucinous neoplasms are detected in only 0.3% of surgically removed appendices, but account for nearly one third of all appendiceal epithelial tumors. Mucinous neoplasms are far more frequent than colonic-type neoplasms, comprising nearly 90% of carcinomas that arise in the appendix. Patients present with acute appendicitis symptoms, obstruction, or a palpable mass. Intussusception into the colon is a rare, but recognized, complication of appendiceal mucoceles. Patients late in the disease process may present with *pseudomyxoma peritonei* (meaning false mucinous tumor of the peritoneum), a term that should be reserved for the clinical syndrome in which patients experience slowly increasing abdominal girth caused by mucinous ascites resulting from prior mucocele rupture or transmural extension; the abdominal cavity relentlessly fills with mucin produced by the neoplastic cells.

RADIOLOGIC FEATURES

The imaging diagnosis of mucinous neoplasms hinges primarily on detection of the resulting mucocele. Abdominal radiography may suggest a soft tissue mass

MUCINOUS NEOPLASM OF THE APPENDIX—FACT SHEET

Definition
- Epithelial neoplasm usually demonstrating low-grade mucinous morphology, but associated with extra-appendiceal spread

Incidence and Location
- Rare neoplasm (0.3% of appendectomies)
- Outnumbers colonic-type epithelial neoplasms in appendix by 9:1

Morbidity and Mortality
- Peritoneal spread leads to clinical syndrome of pseudomyxoma peritonei
- Spread to ovaries can cause confusion regarding primary site of peritoneal disease
- Spread is usually via direct extension, infrequently by lymphatic or hematogenous routes

Gender, Race, and Age Distribution
- Females more than males
- No clear racial difference
- Mean age sixth decade

Clinical Features
- Patients present with acute appendicitis, obstruction, palpable mass, intussusception
- Mucinous ascites (psuedomyxoma peritonei) is a late, uncommon finding

Prognosis and Treatment
- Periappendiceal spread of acellular mucin has excellent prognosis (<4% progress to mucinous ascites)
- Periappendiceal spread of mucin with neoplastic cells (even if paucicellular) is more likely to develop mucinous ascites (33%)
- Peritoneal disease with low-grade histology has a 75% 5-year survival rate; high-grade histology is 15%
- Complete excision of a confined appendiceal neoplasm is curative
- Following peritoneal spread, aggressive surgical debulking (cytoreduction) and hyperthermic chemotherapy are treatments of choice

in the right lower quadrant, but specificity is increased when calcification is identified. Curvilinear mural calcification is highly suggestive of the diagnosis, but is seen in less than 50% of cases. Contrast enema examination will show a smooth impression on the medial aspect of the cecum, a finding that suggests an extramucosal or extrinsic process. The typical location of the filling defect will usually favor an appendiceal process.

At ultrasound, an ovoid cystic mass with or without acoustic shadowing from dystrophic mural calcification is characteristic of mucoceles from mucinous neoplasms. CT scan is more sensitive in detecting mural calcification. Identification of a separate right ovary in women is crucial for excluding processes such as a cystic ovarian neoplasm or tubo-ovarian abscess. The differential diagnosis includes periappendiceal abscess, enteric duplication cyst, mesenteric cyst, and hydrosalpinx.

PATHOLOGIC FEATURES

GROSS FINDINGS

On gross examination, the appendix is often dilated or cystic with tenacious mucin in the lumen. The wall is thick and fibrotic, sometimes with mural calcification ("porcelain appendix"). The term *mucocele* is used to describe the gross and clinical appearance of a dilated, mucin-filled appendix, but does not implicate whether the histologic appearance is benign or malignant.

When a mucocele is encountered, it is extremely important to determine whether the wall of that structure is intact or has been breached (Fig. 8-25). A gross assessment of the appendix at the time of surgery and at the grossing bench is essential. Proper surgical management of the mucocele is essential, as rupture of a neoplastic mucocele by traumatic appendectomy could be an iatrogenic catastrophe for the patient. Low-grade mucinous tumors that are completely confined to the appendix behave in a benign fashion, whereas the same tumors can behave in a malignant fashion if the mucinous contents have access to the free peritoneal cavity.

TERMINOLOGY AND MICROSCOPIC FINDINGS

The terminology of appendiceal mucinous neoplasms has been confounded by multiple classifications over the years. Some authors propose the phrase *mucinous adenoma* because of its frequently low-grade histology and indolent behavior, while others argue that peritoneal spread leads to biologic behavior similar to adenocarcinoma, and support use of that term. However, many of the appendiceal neoplasms do not have frankly invasive histology characteristic of usual adenocarcinomas.

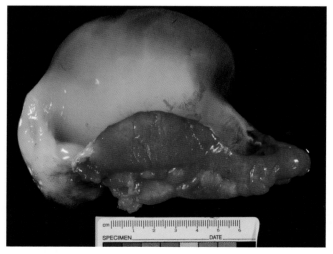

FIGURE 8-25

Low-grade appendiceal mucinous neoplasm. Gross photo showing glistening mucin confined to the lumen (the appendix has been opened longitudinally). The peritoneal surface is uninvolved, and thus the risk of pseudomyxoma peritonei would be negligible.

MUCINOUS NEOPLASM OF THE APPENDIX—PATHOLOGIC FEATURES

Gross Findings

- Dilated, cystic appendix filled with mucin
- Thickened wall, sometimes with mural calcification (porcelain appendix)
- Status of intact vs. ruptured appendix is critical to patient outcome

Microscopic Findings

- Villous or flat mucinous epithelial lining, usually of low-grade cytologic atypia: hyperchromasia, pseudostratification of nuclei, no architectural complexity, sometimes appears exceptionally bland
- High-grade lesions can also occur with severe cytologic abnormalities: loss of nuclear polarity, mucin depletion, prominent nucleoli, complex cribriform and papillary architecture
- Extension of mucin outside of appendix may be acellular or have strips, clusters, or single epithelial cells
- Involvement of peritoneum may be acellular or show low-grade or high-grade morphology

Differential Diagnosis

- Cystadenoma of colonic-type epithelium origin (tubular adenoma, sessile serrated adenoma)
- Endometriosis

In view of this, the nomenclature *low-grade appendiceal mucinous neoplasm* or *mucinous neoplasm of low malignant potential* have come into favor. These terms do not carry the same implications as the terms *adenoma* or *carcinoma*.

Appendiceal mucinous neoplasms can be classified as low grade or high grade. Low-grade mucinous tumors are a villous or flat proliferation of mucinous epithelium with mild to moderate cytologic atypia, sometimes appearing quite bland. There is mild nuclear enlargement, pseudostratification and hyperchromasia in the absence of complex architectural features (Figs. 8-26). High-grade tumors have severe cytologic abnormalities, including loss of nuclear polarity, mucin depletion, round or ovoid nuclei with conspicuous nucleoli, and cribriform or micropapillary architectural growth patterns. These lesions may also be frankly invasive (Fig. 8-27).

As the lesion grows in the appendix, the lumen may dilate with mucin and produce a cystadenoma. The term *cystadenoma* is not a specific pathologic diagnosis but rather describes a cystically dilated appendix with an adenomatous lining, which can be either colonic-type or mucinous in nature.

The dilatation of the appendix causes weakness the muscular wall with prolapse of the epithelium or dissection of mucin through the muscularis mucosae (Fig. 8-28). Care should be taken not to interpret these diverticular-like changes as invasive carcinoma.

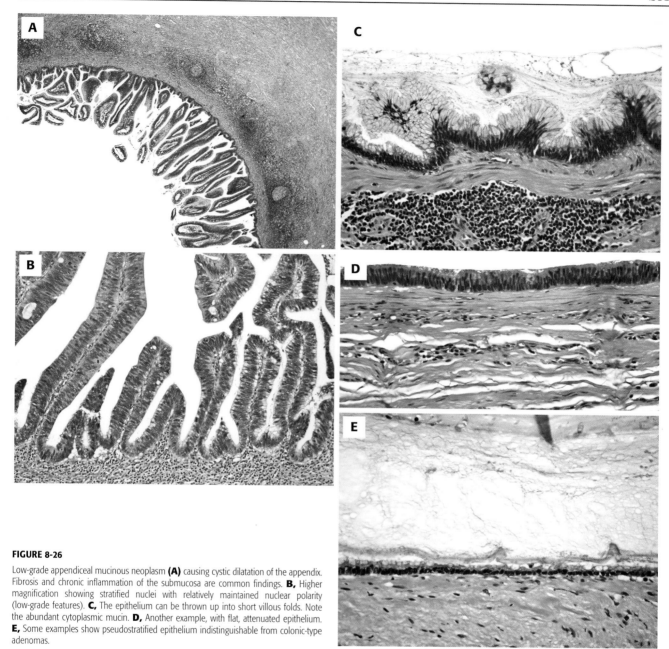

FIGURE 8-26

Low-grade appendiceal mucinous neoplasm **(A)** causing cystic dilatation of the appendix. Fibrosis and chronic inflammation of the submucosa are common findings. **B,** Higher magnification showing stratified nuclei with relatively maintained nuclear polarity (low-grade features). **C,** The epithelium can be thrown up into short villous folds. Note the abundant cytoplasmic mucin. **D,** Another example, with flat, attenuated epithelium. **E,** Some examples show pseudostratified epithelium indistinguishable from colonic-type adenomas.

Rupture or extra-appendiceal spread of mucin may be localized to the periappendiceal area. This periappendiceal spread may contain mucin that is acellular (Fig. 8-29) or cellular, harboring strips or clusters of neoplastic epithelium. As patients with acellular mucin have an excellent prognosis, it is critical to accurately assess the presence or absence of epithelial elements. Microscopic examination of the entire appendix is necessary, as lesions with extra-appendiceal tumor cells are more likely to progress to disseminated disease and result in death of the patient, even if the mucin is paucicellular and confined to the periappendiceal region.

PSEUDOMYXOMA PERITONEI

As discussed earlier, the term *pseudomyxoma peritonei* should be reserved for the clinical finding of mucinous ascites; it is not a histologic diagnosis. Underlying this phenomenon is invariably a ruptured appendiceal mucinous neoplasm with peritoneal spread, hence the discussion within this section. The histologic findings include neoplastic mucinous epithelial cells present in the peritoneal cavity with independent growth.

Histologically, the malignant cells may be extremely scant within abundant mucinous material (Figs. 8-30 and 31). Extensive sampling may be required to demonstrate

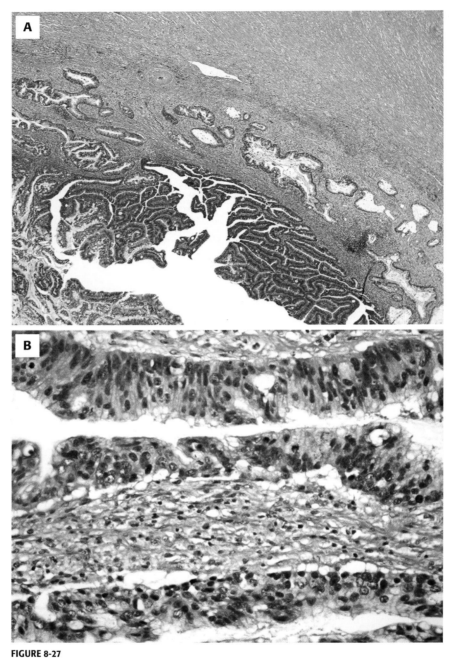

FIGURE 8-27

Adenocarcinoma arising from appendiceal mucinous neoplasm. **A,** Infiltration into the submucosa with desmoplastic stromal response. **B,** Cytologic features are high grade with loss of nuclear polarity, nuclear irregularity, and frequent mitotic figures.

them. A better prognosis is implied in the event that adequate sampling has been performed and epithelial cells cannot be demonstrated.

As with its parent neoplasm from the appendix, the classification of pseudomyxoma peritonei is plagued with a number of competing nomenclatures. Some

authors prefer the term *disseminated peritoneal adeno-mucinosis* (DPAM) to indicate histologically bland to low-grade adenomatous mucinous epithelium associated with abundant extracellular mucin and fibrosis. For high-grade lesions characterized by cytologic and architectural features of mucinous carcinoma associated

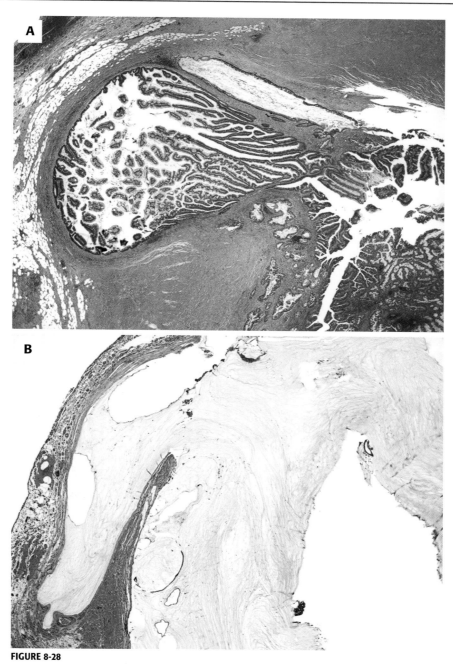

FIGURE 8-28

Prolapse of the low-grade mucinous neoplasm may occur through a weakening in the muscular wall (diverticulum). **A,** Epithelial components lining the diverticulum should not be interpreted as invasion. **B,** Acellular mucin may dissect through muscle layers, eventually rupturing through.

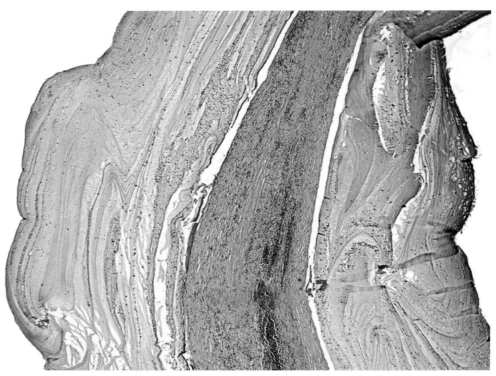

FIGURE 8-29
Pools of mucin outside of the appendix may be acellular, as in this example. Patients with acellular mucin (following extensive sampling) have a significantly better outcome than patients with mucin harboring even a few neoplastic cells.

with extracellular mucin, the compatible term *peritoneal mucinous carcinomatosis* (PMCA) is used. Lesions with histologic features of both DPAM and PMCA are identified as "peritoneal mucinous carcinomatosis with intermediate or discordant features" (PMCA-I/D). These authors have demonstrated that the high-grade histology seen in PMCA correlates with a much more aggressive clinical course as compared with DPAM. The 5-year survival rate for patients with DPAM is 75% compared to 14% for patients with PMCA.

Other observers, however, argue that the term *adenomucinosis* implies a benign adenoma-like lesion that can be misleading to patients and clinicians because this low grade lesion does progress to a significant rate of mortality. These observers prefer the analogous terms *low-grade mucinous adenocarcinoma* and *high-grade mucinous adenocarcinoma* to indicate malignancy in these lesions. Yet other authors prefer to imply the same concepts by using the terms *nonaggressive histology* and *aggressive histology* after identifying the neoplasm as "appendiceal mucinous neoplasm with extra-appendiceal spread."

Regardless of terminology used, it is prudent for the pathologist to indicate whether the lesional cells have histology that correlates with an aggressive or an indolent clinical course, and whether the mucin is acellular or cellular, following extensive sampling, because of the prognostic implications.

ANCILLARY STUDIES

IMMUNOHISTOCHEMISTRY

Mucinous neoplasms of the appendix stain in a similar pattern as adenocarcinoma elsewhere in the colon. The cells are reactive for cytokeratin (CK) 20, CDX2, carcinoembryonic antigen (CEA), and MUC2. Many neoplasms also co-express CK7.

The corresponding peritoneal disease stains in an identical manner, as would be expected.

DIFFERENTIAL DIAGNOSIS

The distinction between low-grade mucinous neoplasm of the appendix that has malignant potential from an adenoma (e.g., colonic-type tubular adenoma, sessile serrated adenoma) that has attenuated epithelium as a result of cystic dilatation can occasionally be unfeasible. Features that can be helpful include frank invasion or periappendiceal mucin characteristic of a mucinous neoplasm.

Some authors have suggested an intermediate term, *mucinous tumor of uncertain malignant potential,* when it is impossible to determine whether the

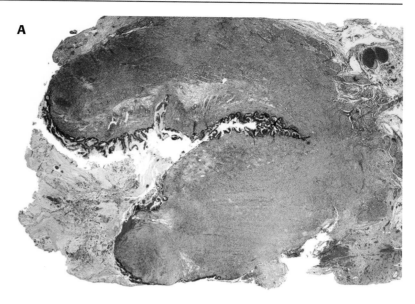

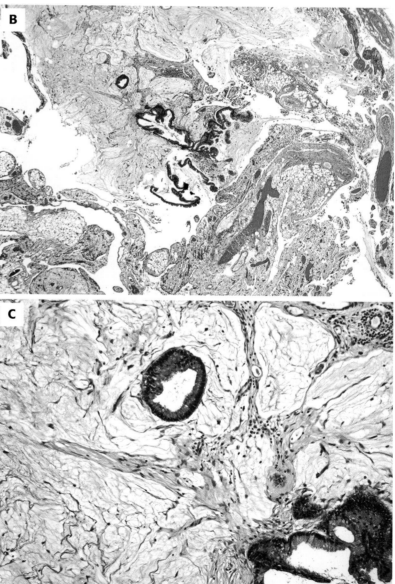

FIGURE 8-30

A patient with clinical pseudomyxoma peritonei syndrome. **A,** Examination of the appendix reveals the culprit—a low-grade appendiceal mucinous neoplasm with rupture and extra-appendiceal spread of tumor cells. **B,** A sample from the peritoneum shows abundant mucin with free-floating clusters of epithelial cells, which can be called *diffuse peritoneal adenomucinosis* (DPAM) or low-grade mucinous adenocarcinoma. **C,** On high power, the epithelial cells have low-grade cytology and are identical to the mucinous neoplasm found in the appendix. This is considered favorable histology.

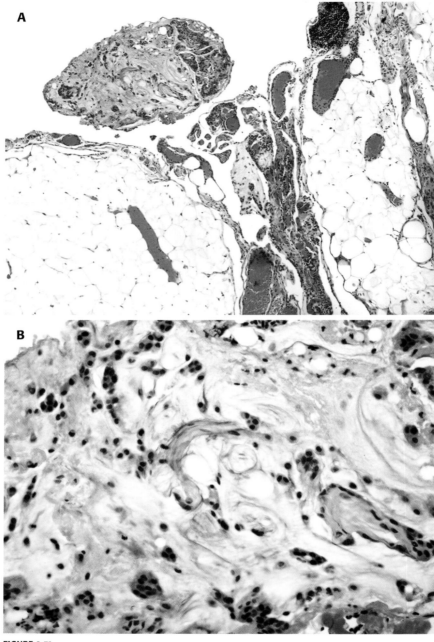

FIGURE 8-31

Another patient with pseudomyxoma peritonei. **A,** Sampling of the peritoneal cavity shows clusters of epithelial cells in abundant mucin. **B,** A high-power view of sample in **A** shows high-grade cytology with loss of polarity, high nuclear-to-cytoplasmic ratio, pleomorphism, and discohesion. Patients with this unfavorable histology have a significantly worse prognosis. These lesions are referred to as *peritoneal mucinous carcinomatosis* (PMCA) or high-grade mucinous adenocarcinoma.

appendiceal tumor is an adenoma or a mucinous neoplasm. While this additional term captures the difficulty in histologic diagnosis, other authors argue that the distinction is arbitrary and prefer to include these lesions in the category of mucinous neoplasms.

PROGNOSIS AND THERAPY

Gross examination of the appendix at the time of appendectomy and an assessment of the size of the mucocele cannot determine whether the mucocele is benign or malignant. The prudent surgical approach is to regard every mucocele of the appendix as potentially malignant. This means that special care in the resection of an appendiceal mucocele must occur to avoid trauma and possible rupture of the appendix as it is removed. Often, this means conversion of a laparoscopic appendectomy to an open laparotomy.

Appendiceal mucinous neoplasms confined to the mucosa behave in a benign fashion and complete excision is curative. Mucinous neoplasms with disseminated peritoneal mucin deposits often follow an indolent, but malignant, course. Not infrequently, appendiceal mucinous neoplasms are associated with localized periappendiceal mucin deposits, but lack diffuse peritoneal involvement. Mucin deposits in these cases may be acellular or contain neoplastic epithelium (cellular mucin). In patients with acellular periappendiceal mucin, only 4% develop diffuse peritoneal disease. In contrast, 33% of patients with cellular periappendiceal mucin develop mucinous ascites. Patients with appendiceal mucinous neoplasms and acellular periappendiceal mucin are unlikely to develop recurrent disease. Microscopic examination of the entire appendix is necessary to determine the presence of absence of cells in pools or extra-appendiceal mucin. Lesions with extra-appendiceal tumor cells are more likely to progress to disseminated disease and result in death of the patient, even if the mucin is paucicellular and confined to the periappendiceal region.

Recent evidence suggests that right hemicolectomy is not always the treatment of choice in patients with a mucinous neoplasm of the appendix. Some observers recommend a sentinel lymph node approach; if intraoperative frozen sections of appendiceal lymph nodes are negative for tumor, a right hemicolectomy is not indicated. Additionally, a cecectomy may be adequate treatment for a positive appendiceal margin.

Aggressive surgical debulking for mucinous-type tumors improves survival rate and reduces recurrence rates in patients with generalized pseudomyxoma peritonei compared with simple appendectomy. Intraperitoneal hyperthermic chemotherapy following cytoreduction of tumor bulk is the current standard of treatment for peritoneal spread.

◼ NEUROENDOCRINE TUMORS OF THE APPENDIX

Carcinoid tumors are well-differentiated neuroendocrine neoplasms arising from cells of the diffuse endocrine system. Appendiceal carcinoids arise from enterochromaffin cells and enteroglucagon cells found in the lamina propria and submucosa.

CLINICAL FEATURES

Carcinoid tumors can be found throughout the gastrointestinal tract, with the appendix being the third most common site, comprising 24.1% of gastrointestinal neuroendocrine neoplasms; the appendix follows small intestine (41.8%) and rectum (27.4%) in frequency. Carcinoid tumors comprise 75% of all neoplasms found in the appendix.

Whereas appendiceal carcinoids can occur at any age, patients tend to be much younger compared with patients diagnosed with other appendiceal neoplasms or carcinoids at other sites, approximately 20 years younger than for neuroendocrine neoplasms from other sites. These tumors occur more often in women, with a male-to-female ratio of 1:2. Appendiceal neuroendocrine neoplasms are also the most common gastrointestinal neoplasm in childhood. It is unclear whether this demographic represents the actual distribution of tumor or the age range of the population that typically undergoes appendectomy for inflammatory appendicitis or incidental appendectomy during pelvic surgery for other reasons.

CARCINOID TUMOR OF THE APPENDIX—FACT SHEET

Definition
- A well-differentiated neuroendocrine tumor of enterochromaffin cell or enteroglucagon cell origin

Incidence and Location
- Most frequent tumor of the appendix, occurring in 0.2% to 0.9% of all appendectomy specimens

Morbidity and Mortality
- Metastasis is rare, usually to regional nodes
- Hematogenous spread is exceptional

Gender, Race, and Age Distribution
- Females more than males (2:1)
- No clear racial difference
- Can occur at any age; peak incidence in young adults; mean age 42

Clinical Features
- Most are incidental findings
- Carcinoid syndrome is very rare, and is associated with metastatic liver disease

Prognosis and Treatment
- Complete excision is curative
- Right hemicolectomy is suggested for tumors larger than 2 cm, presence of regional lymph node metastasis, high mitotic count, mesoappendiceal invasion, and angioinvasion
- If only the proximal resection margin is involved, conservative local reexcision may be considered

---

CARCINOID TUMOR OF THE APPENDIX—PATHOLOGIC FEATURES

Gross Findings

- Round or oval lesion usually found at the tip of the appendix
- Most are less than 1 cm in diameter
- Cut surface is gray or yellow

Microscopic Findings

- Nested and insular pattern, sometimes with acinar or tubular structures
- Cells are uniform, round to polygonal
- Nuclei are round with inconspicuous nucleoli and speckled chromatin
- Eosinophilic or amphophilic cytoplasm may contain small granules
- Mitoses are rare

Differential Diagnosis

- Most examples are not a problem
- Can be differentiated from adenocarcinoma and goblet cell carcinoid by the absence of mucin and by neuroendocrine markers chromogranin and synaptophysin

---

The most common clinical presentation is that of an incidental nodule detected at the time of appendectomy for presumed appendicitis. Others may be found incidentally during laparotomy for other reasons. Still others may be found at autopsy. Rarely, they present with an abdominal mass, pain, or the carcinoid syndrome.

RADIOLOGIC FEATURES

Because of their small size, tendency to be confined to the appendix, and benign behavior, very few imaging features have been reported. They can be occasionally seen as a soft tissue mass or circumferential thickening on CT.

PATHOLOGIC FEATURES

GROSS FINDINGS

The majority of appendiceal neuroendocrine neoplasms are localized to the appendix at the time of diagnosis. Eighty percent are smaller than 1 cm in diameter. They are round or oval and sometimes palpable. The cut surface is gray to yellow.

MICROSCOPIC FINDINGS

Carcinoids of the appendix are morphologically similar to their small intestinal and rectal counterparts (Fig. 8-32). They are characterized by an exquisitely monotonous

proliferation of small, bland polygonal cells with a moderate amount of eosinophilic to amphophilic cytoplasm. Nuclei are round with features of neuroendocrine differentiation, including inconspicuous nucleoli and finely stippled chromatin of a "salt and pepper" quality. Pleomorphism and mitoses are rare. Morphologic features of the cells do not differ by cell of origin (immunohistochemistry is required for this distinction). Carcinoids demonstrate variable architectural growth patterns including nested (insular), trabecular, acinar, and tubular (Fig. 8-33). These patterns do not have prognostic significance and often overlap with multiple patterns seen within any single tumor. The stroma can range from delicate and vascular to dense and fibrous.

ANCILLARY STUDIES

IMMUNOHISTOCHEMISTRY

The vast majority of carcinoid tumors are diffusely reactive for immunohistochemical stains chromogranin and synaptophysin, as well as CD56 (Fig. 8-34). Some tumors express synaptophysin without expression of chromogranin. Other generic neuroendocrine markers may also be reactive (neuron specific enolase and protein gene product 9.5). Historically, silver impregnation techniques were used to identify and differentiate enterochromaffin (EC) and enteroglucagon (L) cells, as they appear morphologically identical. Argentaffin marks the serotonin-containing granules of EC cells, and argyrophil is generally positive in all endocrine cells. Specific peptide hormone markers serotonin, substance P, and occasionally somatostatin are reactive in EC cells. Glucagon, glucagon-like peptides, pancreatic polypeptide, and peptide YY are expressed in L cells. Use of ancillary studies to differentiate EC and L cell carcinoids may be useful in confirming the diagnosis but are not necessary as the tumors do not differ in prognosis.

ELECTRON MICROSCOPY

Electron microscopy reveals irregular, dense-core, membrane-bound neuroendocrine granules.

DIFFERENTIAL DIAGNOSIS

Most examples are not a diagnostic problem. Some examples of acinar pattern neuroendocrine neoplasms may mimic an adenocarcinoma, but strong diffuse staining with neuroendocrine markers such as chromogranin or synaptophysin confirms a carcinoid tumor. Goblet cell carcinoid (GCC) remains in the

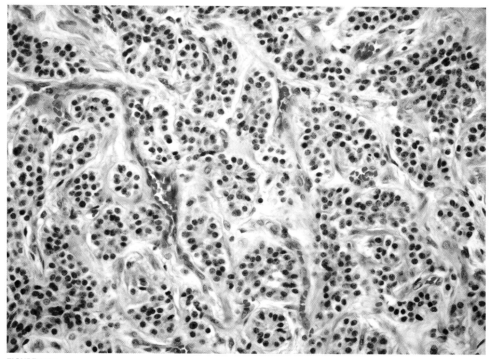

FIGURE 8-32

Carcinoid tumor of the appendix, showing a nested arrangement with uniform round cells. Nuclei lack nucleoli and the chromatin is stippled in a "salt and pepper" pattern.

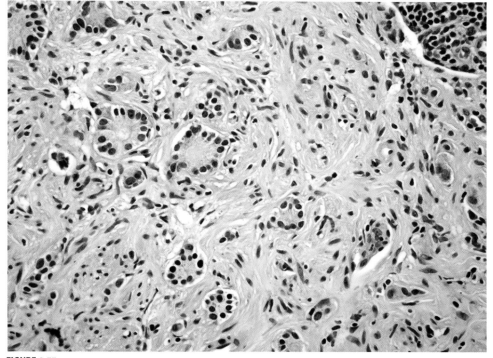

FIGURE 8-33

Tubular pattern of carcinoid tumor. In the past, carcinoid tumors of this pattern may have been referred to as "adenocarcinoid"—a now-retired term that was also used for goblet cell carcinoid and adenocarcinoma (e.g., goblet cell carcinoid). The tubular carcinoid tumor is prognostically identical to the typical carcinoid tumor and behaves in an essentially benign manner.

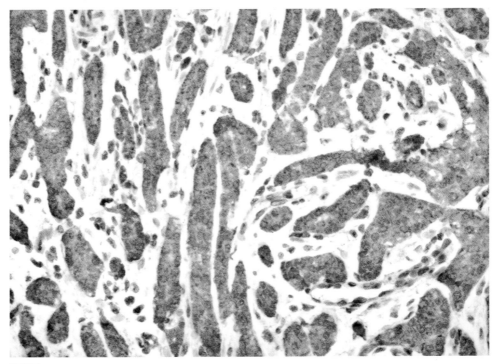

FIGURE 8-34
Typical carcinoid tumor with strong, diffuse chromogranin immunoreactivity.

differential diagnosis because of its appendiceal origin and reactivity to synaptophysin and chromogranin. However, GCCs have well-defined goblet cells with eccentric nuclei that are displaced and compressed by cytoplasmic mucin, which is not present in appendiceal neuroendocrine neoplasms. The cytoplasmic mucin can be demonstrated with a mucicarmine or alcian blue stain.

PROGNOSIS AND THERAPY

The prognosis for patients with conventional appendiceal neuroendocrine neoplasms is better than that for all other anatomic sites, and demonstrates a 5-year survival rate greater than 95%. Lymph node metastasis to regional nodes occurs in approximately 4% of all appendiceal neuroendocrine neoplasms, and this is usually in tumors larger than 2 cm. Distant metastasis occurs in about 1% of cases, once again usually only in tumors larger than 2 cm. In these rare cases, the carcinoid syndrome has been reported.

Treatment by appendectomy is curative in most cases, particularly for that less than 1 cm in greatest dimension. For cases with lymph node metastasis, tumor size larger than 2 cm, presence of regional lymph node metastasis, high mitotic count, mesoappendiceal invasion, peritoneal studding, or angioinvasion, a right hemicolectomy is advised. Cases that lack these features, but involve the proximal margin

may receive a limited reexcision. In tumors of uncertain malignancy, those between 1 and 2 cm in size, the presence of deep serosal and mesoappendiceal spread and a significant mitotic rate may predict more aggressive behavior.

■ GOBLET CELL CARCINOID AND ADENOCARCINOMA EX GOBLET CELL CARCINOID

Appendiceal GCC tumor was first recognized as a distinct entity in 1969 and remains a rare appendiceal neoplasm with uncertain histogenesis. These infiltrative tumors have a mixed phenotype, with partial neuroendocrine differentiation and intestinal-type goblet cell morphology. As such, they have been classified in the past with other neoplasms that show both neuroendocrine and glandular differentiation as *adenocarcinoid tumors,* a term that encompasses biologically diverse neoplasms such as tubular pattern carcinoid tumor and a collision tumor of typical carcinoid with a *de novo* adenocarcinoma. It is best to avoid using this term to avoid confusion; the term *adenocarcinoid* is no longer used by the World Health Organization (WHO). Distinguishing GCC from these other entities is important because the clinical characteristics and prognoses are distinct. In the past, GCC has also been proposed as crypt cell carcinoma, mucinous carcinoid, microglandular carcinoid, or amphicrine carcinoma to distinguish the entity from classical carcinoid tumor of the appendix.

CLINICAL FEATURES

GCCs occur in adults, with a mean age of 50 years. There is a female predominance with a male-to-female ratio of about 1:2. The most common clinical presentation is abdominal pain and a palpable mass (50%). Other patients present with symptoms related to acute appendicitis, and only 3% of patients are diagnosed as an incidental finding. Patients with advanced disease most frequently present with abdominal masses. In female patients with stage IV disease, 83% present with ovarian masses and a presumptive diagnosis of a primary ovarian neoplasm. Overall, less than 1% of patients have a preoperative diagnosis of a primary appendiceal tumor.

RADIOLOGIC FEATURES

Cross-sectional imaging will typically reflect the infiltrative nature of the tumor, with mild but diffuse mural thickening.

PATHOLOGIC FEATURES

GROSS FINDINGS

At gross examination, GCC tumors rarely present a discrete nodule or mass, and may present with a grossly normal appendix. As a result of their infiltrative nature, they most commonly grow in a circumferential pattern with longitudinal extension along the length of the appendix. Most tumors are greater than 2 cm in size (representing length of tumor extension rather than diameter) and have transmural infiltration of the appendiceal wall.

GOBLET CELL CARCINOID—FACT SHEET

Definition
- Appendiceal tumor with mixed phenotype: partial neuroendocrine differentiation and intestinal-type goblet cell morphology of uncertain histogenesis

Incidence and Location
- Rare, essentially exclusive to the appendix

Morbidity and Mortality
- Metastatic spread is present in more than half of patients at time of presentation (peritoneum, omentum, ovaries)
- Commonly has direct extension into the right colon
- Lymph node metastasis is present in more than a third of cases

Gender, Race, and Age Distribution
- Females more than males (2:1)
- Occurs in adults, mean age 50 years

Clinical Features
- Half present with abdominal pain and palpable mass
- Forty percent present with acute appendicitis symptoms
- Less than 5% are incidental

Prognosis and Treatment
- Prognosis is related to tumor stage at presentation and histologic grade
- Ninety-seven percent of patients have transmural invasion at the time of diagnosis
- 5-year survival:
  - Group A 100%
  - Group B 36%
  - Group C 0%
- Surgical resection most effective treatment for early stage
- Advanced disease and peritoneal spread may require additional debulking, oophorectomy, and intraperitoneal chemotherapy

---

GOBLET CELL CARCINOID—PATHOLOGIC FEATURES

Gross Findings
- Does not produce a discrete mass lesion; appendix may look normal
- Circumferential thickening with longitudinal infiltration
- Most are greater than 2 cm (tumor involvement along length of appendix)

Microscopic Findings
- Arise in mucosa or submucosa without a precursor lesion
- Concentric, infiltrative growth pattern of goblet-shaped or signet-ring cells and neuroendocrine cells

Morphologic Subtypes
- Goblet cell carcinoid, typical (group A)
  - Cohesive goblet cell clusters or linear groups
  - Minimal cytologic atypia
  - Minimal desmoplasia or distortion of appendiceal wall
- Adenocarcinoma ex GCC, signet ring type (group B)
  - Irregular and clusters of signet ring cells or goblet cells
  - Discohesive single file or single infiltrating cells
  - Significant cytologic atypia
  - Desmoplasia and destruction of appendiceal wall
- Adenocarcinoma ex GCC, poorly differentiated adenocarcinoma type (group C)
  - At least focal goblet cell morphology
  - At least greater than 1 HPF poorly differentiated carcinoma

Immunohistochemistry
- CK20+ (with coexpression of CK7 in 70%)
- Patchy, focal reactivity with endocrine markers (chromogranin, synaptophysin)
- Group A+B have MUC2+/MUC1−; group C has MUC1+/MUC2−
- Goblet cells are CEA+ and mucicarmine+

Differential Diagnosis
- Tubular pattern classical carcinoid
- Collision tumor of adenocarcinoma and carcinoid
- Classical carcinoid tumor with entrapped benign epithelium
- Metastatic adenocarcinoma with signet ring features

MICROSCOPIC FINDINGS

GCCs arise without a recognizable precursor lesion. These tumors infiltrate in a concentric manner with small clusters, linear rows, or single cells that can be difficult to appreciate on low-power examination (Fig. 8-35). They display a wide range of histologic patterns. Fundamental morphologic features common to all GCCs include:

1. The presence, at least focally, of mucin-containing goblet-shaped or signet-ring epithelial cells arranged in round or oval clusters at the primary site.
2. Neoplastic cells demonstrating at least focal immunoreactivity for neuroendocrine markers (chromogranin or synaptophysin).

Among tumors that demonstrate these characteristics, Tang and colleagues have proposed a classification based on the morphology of the tumor at the primary site. The schema divides the tumors into three groups (groups A, B, and C), which show distinct morphologic and prognostic characteristics.

Typical GCCs (group A) demonstrate well-defined goblet cells arranged in tight clusters or a cohesive linear pattern with minimal cytologic atypia and no desmoplasia (Fig. 8-36). There is minimal architectural distortion of the appendiceal wall and continued cohesiveness of tumor cells despite invasion. As tumor cells infiltrate through the muscular layers, the clusters often exhibit a compressed linear configuration aligned along the axis of the muscle fibers. This compression of groups can give rise to a single-file pattern, reminiscent of a poorly differentiated signet ring carcinoma, but the cells exhibit minimal atypia and remain cohesive (Fig. 8-37). Extracellular mucin may be seen as a result of degenerative changes.

Adenocarcinoma ex goblet cell carcinoid, signet ring type (group B) is composed of goblet cells or signet ring cells arranged in irregular, large, disorganized clusters that have lost cohesion. There is significant cytologic atypia (hyperchromatic and irregular nuclei), and a discohesive single file or single cell infiltrating pattern may be present along with desmoplasia and associated destruction of the appendiceal wall. However, despite the complete near loss of the goblet cell clustered architecture, there is at least a focal component with histologic features of typical GCC.

Adenocarcinoma ex goblet cell carcinoid, poorly differentiated carcinoma type (group C) is the least common subtype, comprising about 10% of GCCs. It has at least focal evidence of goblet cell morphology and a component of poorly differentiated adenocarcinoma defined as greater than 1 low power field (or 1 mm^2) of tumor cells, which are not otherwise distinguishable from a poorly differentiated adenocarcinoma (Fig. 8-38). The tumor cells may appear as either gland-forming, confluent sheets of signet ring cells, malignant epithelial cells with or without signet ring features, or simply an undifferentiated carcinoma.

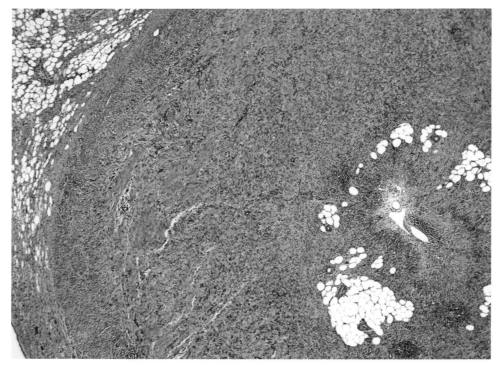

FIGURE 8-35

Goblet cell carcinoid tumor. Low-power view of the appendix emphasizes the subtle, concentric infiltrating pattern of this tumor.

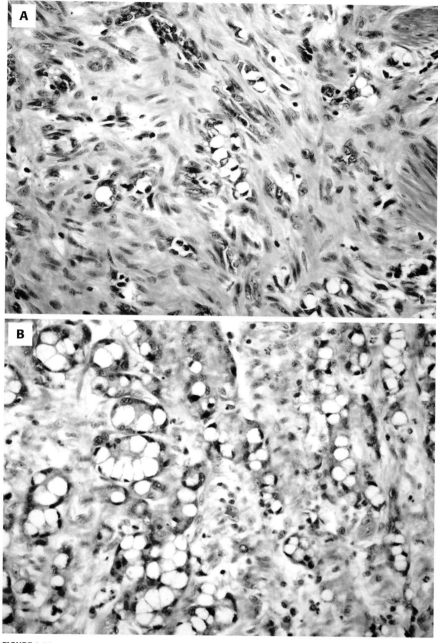

FIGURE 8-36

Typical goblet cell carcinoid (group A). **A,** Well-defined goblet cells are arranged in tight clusters or a cohesive linear pattern with minimal atypia and no desmoplasia. **B,** A more cellular example demonstrating well-formed goblet cells in tight clusters.

ANCILLARY STUDIES

IMMUNOHISTOCHEMISTRY

Nearly all goblet cell carcinoids stain for cytokeratin (CK) 20 and up to 70% coexpress CK7. The goblet cells are reactive with carcinoembryonic antigen (CEA) and the endocrine cells react at least focally with endocrine markers chromogranin and synaptophysin (Fig. 8-39). Intracytoplasmic mucin can be demonstrated with mucicarmine.

The immunoprofile for the subtypes of GCC show some variability. Group A and B both show negative immunoreactivity for MUC1 and preserved MUC2

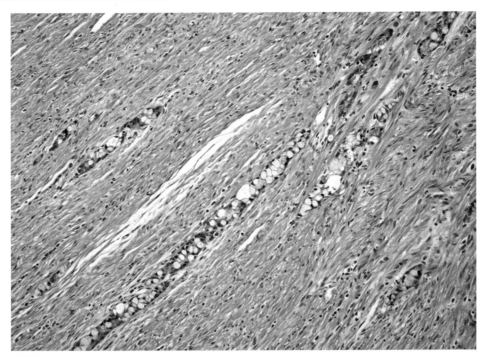

FIGURE 8-37
Typical goblet cell carcinoid (group A). A characteristic finding, the cells display a compressed, linear pattern aligned along the axis of the muscle fibers. Note how the cells are cohesive rather than infiltrating singly.

immunostaining, similar to the pattern seen in normal colonic epithelial cells. By comparison, group C tumors show MUC2 loss and MUC1 expression, a pattern similar to that seen in colorectal adenocarcinoma. The proliferative index assessed by Ki-67 is relatively low in groups A and B tumors (10% to 15%), but particularly high in the invasive component of group C tumors (80%).

ELECTRON MICROSCOPY

Dense core neuroendocrine granules can be seen, as well as intracytoplasmic globules of mucin. Occasionally, these findings occur within the same cell.

DIFFERENTIAL DIAGNOSIS

Diagnosis of GCC tumors can be perplexing as a result of unfortunate taxonomy and it is further complicated by shared histologic features with other tumors.

Classic carcinoid tumors with glandular differentiation (tubular pattern) were previously regarded as "adenocarcinoid" tumors. These tubular carcinoids can be distinguished from GCCs by their formation of glandular structures, lack of goblet or signet-ring cells, strong diffuse staining with endocrine markers, and lack of mucin.

GCCs, by comparison, have a patchy or focal staining pattern with endocrine markers. Tubular carcinoids behave indolently like classical carcinoids and should not be confused with the more aggressive GCC.

Other entities previously regarded as "adenocarcinoid" include tumors with mixed carcinoid-adenocarcinoma histology, which may represent a true collision tumor of adenocarcinoma and a separate de novo carcinoid. Alternatively, tumors with mixed morphology may represent a carcinoid tumor with entrapped non-neoplastic epithelial cells. Differentiating these tumors from GCCs can be aided by the infiltrative and concentric pattern of growth that is typical of GCC.

PROGNOSIS AND THERAPY

Compared with classic carcinoid tumors of the appendix, GCCs behave more aggressively.

Most patients (97%) have transmural extension of the tumor at the time of diagnosis and more than half present with metastatic (stage IV-type) disease. Tumor stage is related to the histologic grade of the primary tumor. Thirty-three percent of group A, 88% of group B, and 100% of group C have metastases at the time of initial presentation. Metastatic disease to other

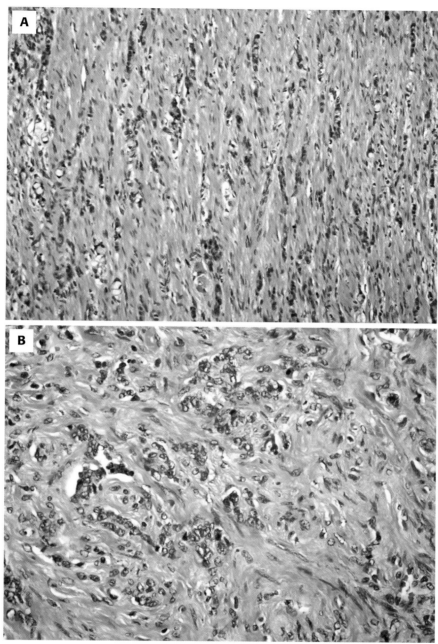

FIGURE 8-38

Adenocarcinoma (e.g., goblet cell carcinoid) (group C). **A,** The poorly differentiated tumor cells infiltrate in a somewhat discohesive manner. A few well-formed goblet cells on the left side reveal the nature of the tumor. **B,** Another example of an undifferentiated carcinoma arising from a goblet cell carcinoid. While this area does not demonstrate signet ring or goblet cell features, other areas of the same tumor have focal goblet cell morphology.

solid organs (e.g., lung, liver, bone) is exceptionally rare. The most commonly involved extra-appendiceal sites include direct extension into the right colon and ileum followed by spread to the peritoneum and omentum. The ovary is the most common site of metastasis in women (88%), usually presenting as Krukenberg tumors. Lymph node metastases are detected in more than one third of patients, dependent on the histologic subtype. Of patients with group A tumors, 20% of patients have lymph node metastasis, compared with 75% of group B and 100% of group C patients.

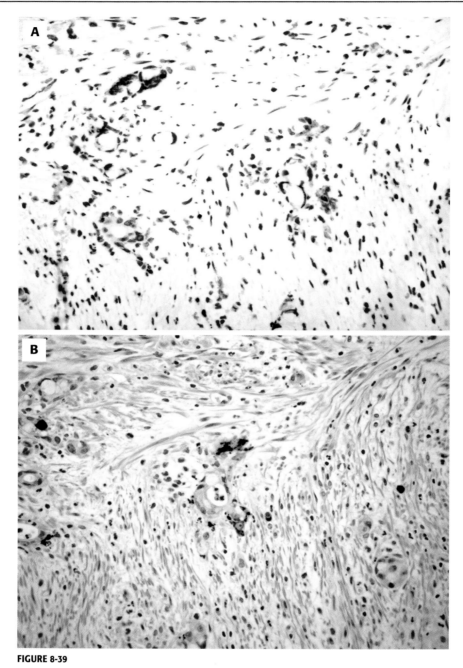

FIGURE 8-39

Positive neuroendocrine markers. **A,** An adenocarcinoma (e.g., goblet cell carcinoid tumor) shows focal reactivity to synaptophysin. **B,** Chromogranin has a similar pattern of reactivity. In comparison, typical carcinoid tumors express strong, diffuse staining of these endocrine markers.

Surgical management with right hemicolectomy is recommended after appendectomy for most cases, particularly those with an adenocarcinoma component (groups B and C). Additional debulking procedures may be needed followed by chemotherapy. Chemotherapy regimens are similar to those used for colonic adenocarcinomas. Intraperitoneal spread may warrant oophorectomy and intraperitoneal chemotherapy.

The disease-specific five-year survival for group A tumors is 100%, while groups B and C are 36% and 0%, respectively.

9

Infectious Diseases of the Colon

■ Laura W. Lamps, MD

When evaluating a colonic biopsy for possible infectious processes, the surgical pathologist must first attempt to differentiate histologic changes suggesting infectious colitis from other inflammatory processes, especially chronic idiopathic inflammatory bowel disease (ulcerative colitis or Crohn's disease). Following this determination, dedicated attempts must be made to diagnose the specific infectious organism or organisms. The surgical pathologist's ability to detect infectious processes in tissue sections has grown exponentially with the advent of new histochemical and immunohistochemical stains, in situ hybridization, and polymerase chain reaction (PCR) analysis. As these techniques have developed and become more widely available for diagnostic use, our knowledge of the pathologic spectrum that specific infectious organisms can cause has also grown, including our knowledge of those infectious processes that can closely mimic Crohn's disease, ulcerative colitis, and ischemic colitis.

Most enteric infections are self-limited. Patients who undergo endoscopic evaluation and biopsy generally have unusual clinical features such as chronic or debilitating diarrhea, evidence of systemic disease, or a history of immunocompromise. One of the most valuable (and least expensive) diagnostic aids for the surgical pathologist is a discussion with the gastroenterologist regarding specific symptoms, colonoscopic findings, travel history, food intake history (e.g., sushi, poorly cooked beef), sexual practices, and immune status.

Despite the large number of infectious agents that may affect the colon, the histologic features that they produce may be generally categorized as follows:

1. Organisms producing very mild or no histologic changes (e.g., enteroadherent *Escherichia coli*)
2. Organisms producing the histologic features of acute infectious/self-limited colitis (ASLC) or focal active colitis (FAC), such as *Campylobacter* species
3. Organisms producing suggestive or diagnostic histologic features, such as pseudomembranes, granulomas, or viral inclusions

The pattern of ASLC or FAC is one of the most common seen in infectious colitis. Typical histologic features include focal cryptitis, with or without increased neutrophils in the lamina propria and crypt abscesses; preservation of crypt architecture; and lack of basal plasmacytosis. The acute inflammatory component may be most prominent in the mid to upper crypts. The lack of crypt distortion and basal lymphoplasmacytosis helps distinguish ASLC from early ulcerative colitis. Details of specific viral, bacterial, fungal, and parasitic infections of the colon are given in the following sections.

■ VIRAL INFECTIONS OF THE COLON

A wide variety of viruses affect the colon. Manifestations of disease vary with the type of virus, specific site of infection, and immune status of the patient.

CYTOMEGALOVIRUS

Cytomegalovirus (CMV) infection occurs in both immunocompromised and immunocompetent persons, and may be found anywhere in the large bowel. The pathogenesis in truly healthy patients is poorly understood. Underlying immunocompromise should be considered when CMV infection is diagnosed, because it is an opportunistic pathogen in patients with many types of immune compromise, including those with acquired immunodeficiency syndrome (AIDS) and those who have undergone solid organ or bone marrow transplantation.

CLINICAL FEATURES

Symptoms vary with the immune status of the patient and the specific site of infection. The most common clinical symptoms are diarrhea (either bloody or watery), abdominal pain, fever, and weight loss; however, primary infections in healthy, immunocompetent persons are often self-limited. CMV is well known as a secondary pathogen superimposed on other chronic gastrointestinal (GI) diseases, such as ulcerative colitis and Crohn's disease; in such cases, CMV superinfection

CYTOMEGALOVIRUS—FACT SHEET

Definition
- Viral infection

Incidence and Location
- Anywhere in GI tract

Clinical Features
- Most common in, but not limited to, immunocompromised patients
- Frequent symptoms are diarrhea (with or without blood), abdominal pain, fever, weight loss
- May cause an ischemic picture, both clinically and pathologically
- May superinfect Crohn's disease or ulcerative colitis

Prognosis and Therapy
- Infections in healthy persons are usually self-limiting
- Ganciclovir is first line of medical therapy, but now is often used in combination with newer drugs

CYTOMEGALOVIRUS—PATHOLOGIC FEATURES

Gross Findings
- Most commonly ulcers, single or multiple, shallow or deep
- May also manifest as colitis (hemorrhagic or pseudomembranous) or obstructive mass
- Segmental or linear ulceration may mimic Crohn's disease grossly

Microscopic Findings
- Colitis featuring cryptitis, mixed inflammatory infiltrate in the lamina propria with numerous neutrophils, mucosal ulceration, crypt abscesses, crypt atrophy, and numerous apoptotic enterocytes
- Characteristic inclusions: "Owl's eye" inclusions are visible on routine hematoxylin and eosin preparations and are present in both cytoplasm and nucleus
- Inclusions are within mesenchymal and endothelial cells, often deep within ulcer bases
- No associated inflammatory reaction may be seen, particularly in severely immunocompromised patients
- Severe endothelial infection may cause ischemia

Differential Diagnosis
- Other viral infections, particularly adenovirus
- Crohn's disease
- Graft-versus-host disease
- Ischemic colitis

has been associated with high mortality, toxic megacolon, and exacerbations of the underlying GI disease.

PATHOLOGIC FEATURES

GROSS FINDINGS

CMV causes a wide variety of gross lesions in the colon. Ulcers are the most common finding (Fig. 9-1); they may be single or multiple, and either superficial or deep. The ulcers often have a well-demarcated, "punched out" appearance. Other gross findings include hemorrhagic colitis, pseudomembranous colitis (PMC), and obstructive mass lesions.

Segmental ulcerative lesions and linear ulcers mimicking Crohn's disease have been well documented in colonic CMV infection. Complications of severe ulcerative CMV infection include toxic megacolon and perforation.

MICROSCOPIC FINDINGS

The histologic spectrum of CMV infection also varies widely, ranging from a minimal inflammatory reaction to deep ulcers with prominent granulation tissue and necrosis at the base (Fig. 9-2). Typical histologic features include cryptitis, a mixed inflammatory infiltrate in the lamina propria with numerous neutrophils, and mucosal ulceration. Crypt abscesses, crypt atrophy and loss, and numerous apoptotic enterocytes may be seen as well. Characteristic inclusions with virtually no associated inflammatory reaction may be seen, particularly in severely immunocompromised patients. Inclusions are preferentially found in endothelial cells and stromal cells, and only rarely in epithelial cells. The characteristic "owl's eye" inclusions are visible on routine hematoxylin and eosin (H&E) preparations, and may be present within both the cytoplasm and the nucleus of the cell. Unlike adenovirus and herpes infections, CMV inclusions are characteristically found deep within ulcer bases, rather than at the edges of ulcers or in superficial mucosa (Fig. 9-3).

A more recently described sequel of CMV infection is segmental bowel ischemia. Mucosal changes are identical to those seen in ischemia of other causes (hemorrhagic necrosis and crypt withering). Numerous endothelial cells containing CMV inclusions are seen in the vessels of the mucosa and submucosa; vessel walls are inflamed and necrotic, and microthrombi are present within the lumen (Fig. 9-4). Presumably,

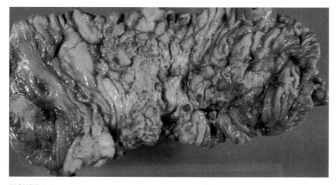

FIGURE 9-1

Colon resected from renal transplant patient with cytomegalovirus colitis. Note sharply demarcated area of coalescing ulcers.

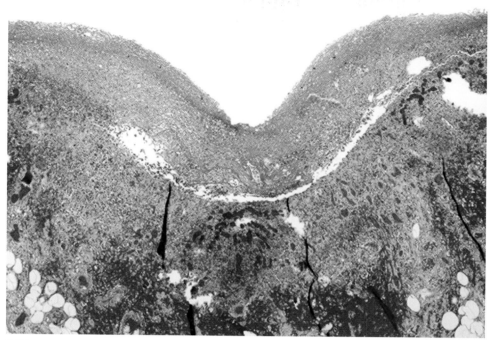

FIGURE 9-2
Colonic ulcer secondary to cytomegalovirus. Note granulation tissue and necrosis at the base (H&E).

viral infection of numerous endothelial cells initiates inflammatory mediators, leading to thrombosis and subsequent bowel ischemia.

ANCILLARY STUDIES

Examination of multiple levels and use of immunohistochemical stains is recommended when evaluating colonic biopsy specimens for CMV infection, for the diagnosis may be easily missed when only rare inclusions are present. Other useful diagnostic aids include viral culture, PCR assays, in situ hybridization, and serologic studies. Isolation of CMV in culture, however, does not imply active infection, because virus may be excreted for months to years after a primary infection.

DIFFERENTIAL DIAGNOSIS

The differential diagnosis is primarily that of other viral infections, particularly adenovirus. CMV inclusions have the characteristic owl's eye morphology, are generally located within endothelial or stromal cells, and exist within both nucleus and cytoplasm. Adenovirus inclusions, by comparison, are crescent shaped or have irregular outlines, are generally within surface epithelium, and are only intranuclear in location. As mentioned previously, CMV may mimic Crohn's disease both grossly and microscopically, and a careful search for inclusions should confirm the diagnosis of CMV infection (although

the two may coincide; Fig. 9-5). The distinction between CMV infection and graft-versus-host disease (GVHD) in bone marrow transplant patients may be particularly difficult, because both clinical and histologic features are similar. Immunohistochemistry or in situ hybridization studies should be employed to rule out CMV infection in this setting, because failure to identify CMV infection could result in delay of antiviral therapy.

PROGNOSIS AND THERAPY

The vast majority of infections in healthy persons are self-limiting. Ganciclovir has historically been the mainstay of medical therapy, but this drug has problems with toxicity and poor oral bioavailability, and resistant strains are evolving. Newer drugs such as foscarnet are now often used in combination with ganciclovir.

HERPESVIRUS

Herpetic infection of the large bowel is most commonly seen in the anorectum. Although colonic herpes infections are often seen in immunocompromised patients, they are by no means limited to this group. The symptoms and pathologic features of herpes simplex virus type 1 (HSV-1) versus HSV-2 are indistinguishable. In immunocompetent patients, herpetic infection is often self-limiting; immunocompromised persons may be at risk for dissemination and life-threatening illness.

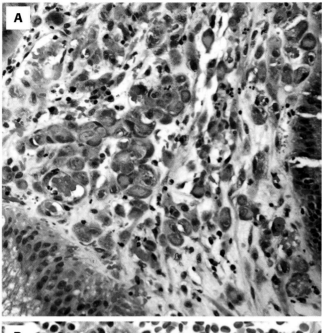

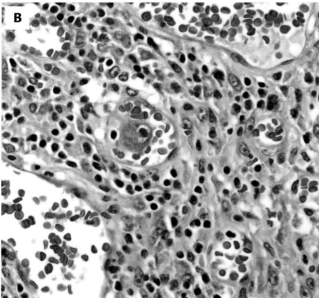

FIGURE 9-3

Characteristic "owl's eye" inclusions are seen within endothelial and mesenchymal cells in the lamina propria (H&E).

diarrhea, fever, abdominal pain, and lower GI bleeding. Fulminant, life-threatening colitis with perforation may occur rapidly in immunocompromised patients. Similar to CMV, HSV may superinfect and complicate preexisting Crohn's disease or ulcerative colitis.

PATHOLOGIC FEATURES

GROSS FINDINGS

In herpetic colitis, the most typical finding is ulceration. Ulcers are often multiple and confluent. Surrounding mucosa is often hemorrhagic and friable, and "cobblestoning" of the mucosa may be seen. In herpetic proctitis, perianal vesicles are common, and they may extend up into the anal canal and rectum. Associated proctoscopic findings include anorectal ulceration and mucosal friability.

MICROSCOPIC FINDINGS

Ulceration is the most frequent finding, accompanied by increased neutrophils in the lamina propria, and an inflammatory exudate that often contains sloughed epithelial cells. Perivascular lymphocytic cuffing and crypt abscesses may also be seen. Two types of characteristic nuclear inclusions may be found: (1) the more common smudged, ground-glass nuclear inclusion with peripheral darker, marginated chromatin (Fig. 9-6), and (2) the acidophilic inclusions with a surrounding clear halo and peripheral chromatin margination (Cowdry type A inclusion). Inclusions are detectable in less than half of biopsy specimens, and ancillary studies may be required if HSV

CLINICAL FEATURES

Herpetic proctitis is the most common cause of nongonococcal proctitis in homosexual men. Herpes infection in this area generally presents with severe anorectal pain, bloody discharge or frank bleeding, tenesmus, constipation, and fever. Concomitant neurologic symptoms (difficulty in urination and paresthesias of the buttocks and upper thighs) are well described, as is inguinal lymphadenopathy. Herpes colitis is most often seen in immunocompromised patients. Patients present with

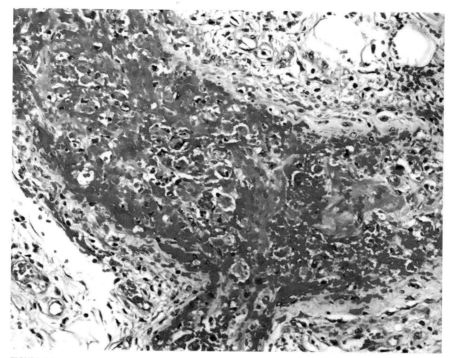

FIGURE 9-4
Thrombosed submucosal vessel with numerous cytomegalovirus inclusions within endothelial cells (H&E).

is suspected. The best place to search for the atypical cells of herpetic infection is within the mucosa at the edges of ulcers (Fig. 9-7) and in sloughed cells within the exudate. If present, inclusions are often multiple.

ANCILLARY STUDIES

Viral culture is the most valuable diagnostic aid to diagnosis; immunohistochemistry, in situ hybridization, and PCR assays may also be of use.

HERPES SIMPLEX VIRUS—PATHOLOGIC FEATURES

Gross Findings
- Anorectal or colonic ulcers, often multiple
- Associated mucosal friability and hemorrhage, sometimes "cobblestoned" mucosa

Microscopic Findings
- Ulceration, accompanied by increased neutrophils in lamina propria, and inflammatory exudate with sloughed epithelial cells
- Characteristic viral inclusions, consisting of a smudged, ground-glass nucleus with peripheral darker, marginated chromatin
- Often found in epithelium of mucosa at the edges of ulcers and in sloughed cells in exudate

Differential Diagnosis
- Other viral infections, particularly varicella
- Crohn's disease

DIFFERENTIAL DIAGNOSIS

The differential diagnosis predominantly includes other viral infections, such as CMV and varicella zoster. Morphology and location of the inclusions usually resolve the differential diagnosis, but ancillary studies may be required. Herpetic inclusions are most often in the epithelial cells of the mucosa, whereas CMV preferentially involves the endothelial and mesenchymal cells. It is also important to remember that mixed infections are common in many situations in which herpetic infection is found. Rarely, segmental ulceration and cobblestoning of mucosa may mimic Crohn's disease, and as in the case of CMV infection, HSV infection should be considered when patients with idiopathic inflammatory bowel disease experience disease flare-ups and relapses.

PROGNOSIS AND THERAPY

Acyclovir is the mainstay of medical therapy. Segmental resection to control bleeding and prevent perforation may be required in severe cases of herpetic colitis.

ADENOVIRUS

Adenovirus infection is second only to rotavirus as a cause of generally self-limiting childhood diarrhea. However, it has recently gained much attention as a

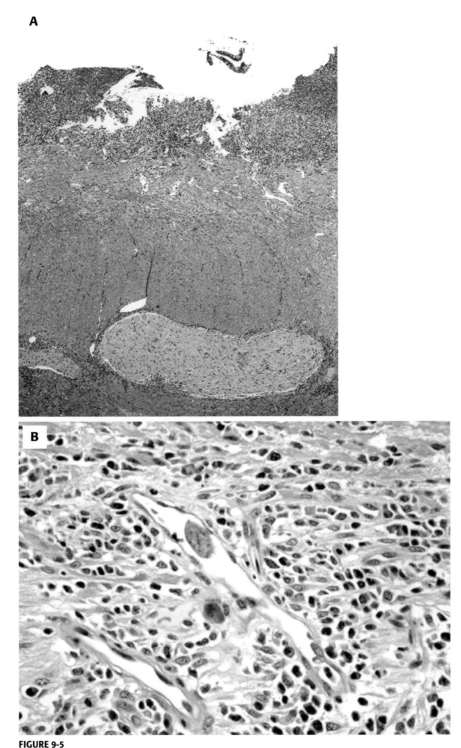

FIGURE 9-5

Cytomegalovirus (CMV) infection superimposed on chronic Crohn's disease. **A,** Note active ulcer overlying thickened colon wall with marked neural hyperplasia (H&E). **B,** CMV inclusions are seen within endothelial cells at the base of the ulcer (H&E). *(Case courtesy of Dr. Brian Quinn.)*

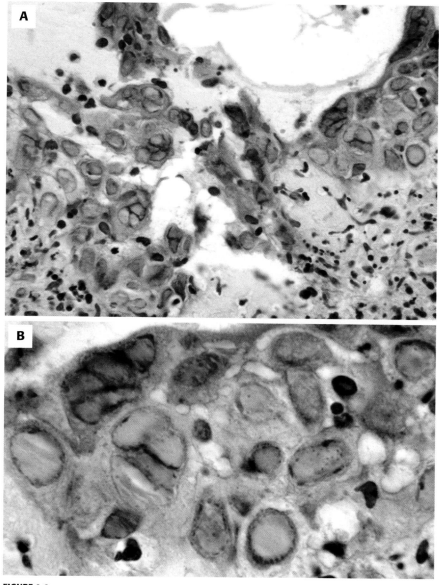

FIGURE 9-6

Typical herpes simplex virus inclusions. Note smudged, ground-glass nuclei with peripheral darker, marginated chromatin (H&E).

cause of diarrhea in immunocompromised patients, especially those with AIDS and patients who have undergone transplantation (particularly bone marrow transplantation). Adenovirus infection of the GI tract is strongly associated with concomitant acute GVHD.

CLINICAL FEATURES

Virtually all patients present with diarrhea, sometimes accompanied by fever, weight loss, lower GI bleeding, and abdominal pain.

PATHOLOGIC FEATURES

GROSS FINDINGS

Endoscopic findings typically include evidence of colitis, such as erythematous, friable, and granular mucosa.

MICROSCOPIC FINDINGS

Histologic features of adenovirus infection include epithelial changes such as superficial cellular degeneration, apoptosis of epithelial cells, and focal acute

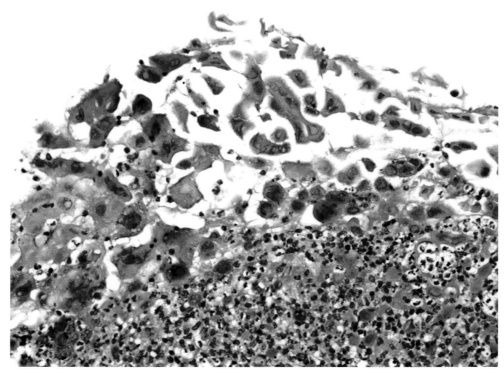

FIGURE 9-7
Ulcerated squamous mucosa in a patient with a herpetic ulcer contains typical inclusions admixed with sloughing epithelial cells and a neutrophilic infiltrate (H&E).

inflammation. Severe cases may show ulceration and exudate. Characteristic homogeneous, smudgy, eosinophilic inclusions may be seen filling the nucleus. Adenovirus inclusions are, except in rare circumstances, limited to epithelial cells; inclusions are most common within surface epithelium (Fig. 9-8) but are also seen in the colonic crypts. Inclusions are particularly common in surface goblet cells, in which they are often crescent shaped (Fig. 9-9). Cowdry type A inclusions are rarely seen, but the owl's eye morphology of CMV inclusions is absent in adenovirus infection.

ANCILLARY STUDIES

Useful aids to diagnosis of adenovirus infection include immunohistochemistry, stool examination by electron microscopy, and viral culture.

ADENOVIRUS—FACT SHEET

Definition
- Viral infection, often in immunocompromised or transplant patients

Incidence and Location
- Colon

Clinical Features
- Diarrhea in virtually all cases, sometimes accompanied by fever, weight loss, abdominal pain, or GI bleeding

Prognosis and Therapy
- Ribavirin

ADENOVIRUS—PATHOLOGIC FEATURES

Gross Findings
- Evidence of colitis including erythematous, friable, and granular mucosa

Microscopic Findings
- Superficial cellular degeneration, apoptosis of epithelial cells, and focal acute inflammation; severe cases may show ulceration and exudate
- Inclusions
  - Characteristic homogeneous, smudgy, eosinophilic inclusions fill the nucleus
  - Inclusions can be crescent shaped or targetoid
  - Most common within surface epithelium, particularly goblet cells, but can be seen in crypt epithelial cells; almost never in endothelial and mesenchymal cells

Differential Diagnosis
- Other viral infections, particularly CMV

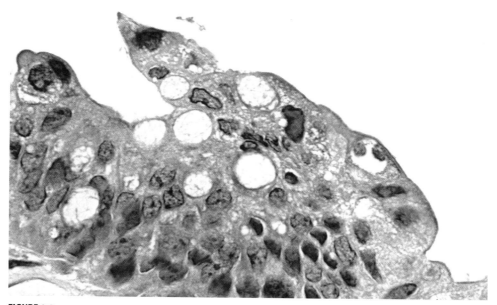

FIGURE 9-8

Homogeneous, smudgy, eosinophilic inclusions fill the nuclei of the surface enterocytes (H&E). *(Courtesy of Dr. Joel Greenson.)*

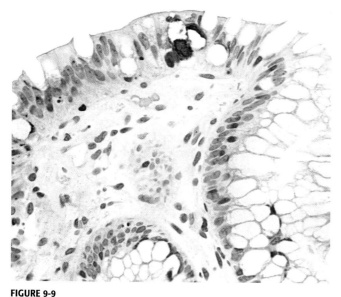

FIGURE 9-9

Crescent-shaped adenovirus inclusions within surface goblet cells (adenovirus immunostain). *(Courtesy of Dr. Joel Greenson.)*

DIFFERENTIAL DIAGNOSIS

The differential diagnosis primarily includes other viral infections, especially CMV. Morphologic differences between the two viruses, as well as differences in location within the gut (epithelium versus endothelium/mesenchymal cells) usually help resolve the differential diagnosis. Because adenovirus often coexists with GVHD, it may be overlooked if a careful search for inclusions is not undertaken.

PROGNOSIS AND THERAPY

The antiviral drug ribavirin is the mainstay of therapy.

AIDS ENTEROCOLOPATHY

AIDS enterocolopathy has been loosely defined as the morphologic changes seen in the gut of patients with HIV/AIDS and chronic diarrhea, for which no other infectious cause has been identified. Some workers believe that these changes represent either primary infection of gut epithelial cells with HIV or a secondary autoimmune reaction to viral infection. Others believe that this is a poorly understood term that does not clearly represent a specific disease entity, and thus should not be used at all. The controversy arises because asymptomatic patients may have similar morphologic findings on biopsy, and conversely severely symptomatic patients may have normal biopsy findings. In addition, there is always the added concern that a causative pathogen simply has been missed. Because patients with HIV/AIDS do have severe impairments of GI function including diarrhea, malabsorption, and weight loss, even in the absence of any demonstrable pathogen, some authors support using the term *AIDS enterocolopathy* to describe the morphologic findings, provided that the bowel has been adequately sampled and all other infectious causes have been excluded.

CLINICAL FEATURES

Patients with these abnormalities often have chronic diarrhea, but some are asymptomatic. Colonoscopy is usually normal.

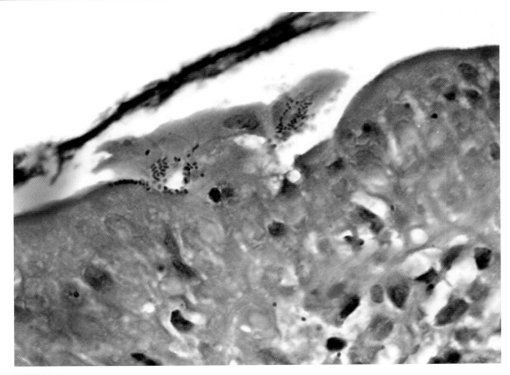

FIGURE 9-11

Enteroadherent *Escherichia coli* in an AIDS patient. A coating of gram-negative rods with little inflammatory reaction is noted at the surface of the colonic mucosa (Twort Gram with oil immersion).

important cause of traveler's diarrhea and pediatric diarrhea worldwide. Both EPEC and EAEC have been increasingly recognized as causes of chronic diarrhea and wasting in AIDS patients. Endoscopic findings are usually unremarkable, but histologic examination shows a coating of adherent bacteria at the surface epithelium, which may stain gram negative (Fig. 9-11). Degenerated surface epithelial cells with associated intraepithelial inflammatory cells may also be present. Enteroinvasive *E. coli* (EIEC) is similar to *Shigella* both genetically and in its clinical presentation and pathogenesis. Given its capacity for invasion, EIEC produces a severe dysentery-like diarrheal illness that can be a particular problem in patients with AIDS. The gross and microscopic pathology of EIEC has not been well described.

ENTEROHEMORRHAGIC ESCHERICHIA COLI

The most common strain of EHEC is 0157:H7. This infectious disease is probably markedly underdiagnosed. EHEC gained national attention in 1993 when a massive outbreak in the Western United States was linked to contaminated hamburger patties served at a fast-food restaurant. This organism adheres to intestinal epithelial cells and produces a cytotoxin similar to that produced by *Shigella* dysenteriae; however, there is no invasion. Although contaminated meat is the most frequent mode of transmission, infection may also occur through contaminated water, milk, produce, and person-to-person contact.

CLINICAL FEATURES

GI symptoms usually consist of bloody diarrhea with severe abdominal cramps and mild or no fever. Nonbloody, watery diarrhea may occur, however. Only one third of patients have fecal leukocytes. Rarely, this infection leads to frank lower GI bleeding. Affected persons may develop hemolytic-uremic syndrome or thrombotic thrombocytopenic purpura, and children and the elderly are at particular risk for serious, systemic illness.

PATHOLOGIC FEATURES

GROSS FINDINGS

Endoscopically, patients have colonic edema, erosions, ulcers, and hemorrhage, and the right colon is usually more severely affected. The edema may be so marked as to cause obstruction.

MICROSCOPIC FINDINGS

The histopathologic features are those of ischemic colitis, because the toxin is believed to induce an ischemic insult. These features include marked edema and hemorrhage in

ENTEROHEMORRHAGIC *ESCHERICHIA COLI*—FACT SHEET

Definition
- Diarrheagenic *E. coli* strain producing hemorrhagic colitis

Incidence and Location
- Preferentially involves right colon

Clinical Features
- Bloody diarrhea (rarely nonbloody) with severe abdominal cramps
- Mild or no fever
- One third of patients have fecal leukocytes
- Sometimes leads to obstructive edema or massive bleeding
- Patients at risk for hemolytic-uremic syndrome and thrombotic thrombocytopenic purpura

Prognosis and Therapy
- Mainly supportive care
- Role of antibiotics controversial
- Surgery may be required to relieve obstruction or control bleeding

ENTEROHEMORRHAGIC *ESCHERICHIA COLI*—PATHOLOGIC FEATURES

Gross Findings
- Colonic edema, erosions, ulcers, and hemorrhage

Microscopic Findings
- Mimics ischemic colitis of other causes
- Marked edema and hemorrhage in the lamina propria and submucosa
- Mucosal acute inflammation, crypt withering, and necrosis
- Microthrombi may be seen within small vessels
- Pseudomembranes may be present

Differential Diagnosis
- Ischemic colitis of other causes
- *C. difficile*—related PMC
- Rarely, idiopathic inflammatory bowel disease

the lamina propria and submucosa (Fig. 9-12), with associated mucosal acute inflammation, crypt withering, and necrosis (Fig. 9-13). Microthrombi may be seen within small vessels, and pseudomembranes may occasionally be present.

ANCILLARY STUDIES

Routine stool cultures will not distinguish 0157:H7 from normal intestinal flora, and successful culture may be impossible more than 4 days after onset of symptoms. Microbiologic diagnosis requires screening on special agar. An immunohistochemical stain for this organism has recently been described, and molecular assays for use on routinely processed tissue are being developed. If this organism is suspected, the microbiology lab should be notified so that special media and serotyping assays may be employed in a timely manner.

DIFFERENTIAL DIAGNOSIS

The differential diagnosis includes *Clostridium difficile*–related colitis, idiopathic inflammatory bowel disease, and especially ischemic colitis. Histologic features of ischemia in the right colon, particularly in patients who are not at risk for atherosclerotic disease, should prompt

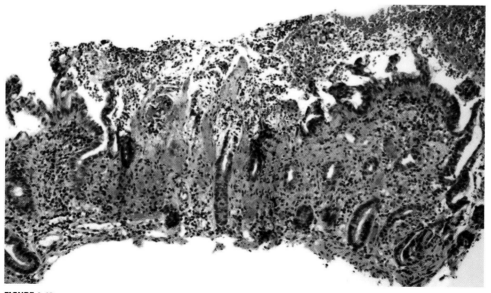

FIGURE 9-12

Enterohemorrhagic *Escherichia coli* infection. Hemorrhagic mucosal necrosis of the upper epithelium, crypt withering, lamina propria hyalinization, and microthrombi (H&E).

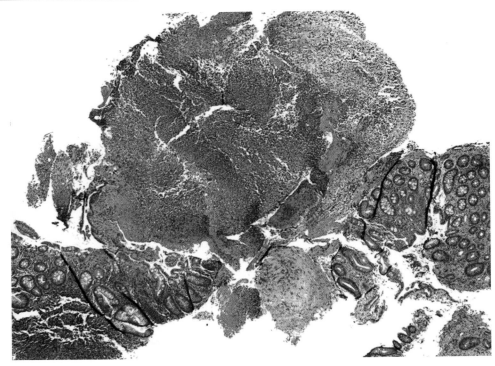

FIGURE 9-13
Enterohemorrhagic *E. coli* can have prominent necroinflammatory exudates that resemble pseudomembranes (H&E).

consideration of EHEC and the appropriate cultures. If pseudomembranes are present, differentiation from *C. difficile*–related colitis may be difficult, and cultures or the *C. difficile* toxin assay may be required. The histologic features of ischemia generally serve to distinguish EHEC from idiopathic inflammatory bowel disease.

PROGNOSIS AND THERAPY

There is no proven therapy for EHEC, and the role of antibiotic treatment is controversial, although most strains are susceptible. Surgical resection of the affected colon may be required to relieve obstruction from edema or to control bleeding.

SALMONELLOSIS

Salmonella, which are gram-negative bacilli, are transmitted through food and water and are particularly prevalent where sanitation is poor. They are an important cause of both food poisoning and traveler's diarrhea. The discussion of *Salmonella* species may be generally divided into typhoid and nontyphoid species. Enteric (typhoid) fever is usually caused by *S. typhi*; the most common nontyphoid species include *S. enteritidis*, *S. typhimurium*, *S. muenchen*, *S. anatum*, *S. paratyphi*, and *S. give*. Although historically enteric fever was considered a much more severe disease, and nontyphoid

salmonellosis a milder one, more recent literature suggests a greater degree of overlap (both clinically and pathologically) than was previously thought. The infective dose is relatively low (approximately 10^3 organisms may cause human disease). Patients with low gastric acidity are at increased risk for salmonellosis, and patients with AIDS have a greater risk for *Salmonella* infection as well as a greater likelihood of severe infection and septicemia.

CLINICAL FEATURES

There are numerous manifestations of *Salmonella* infection, including an asymptomatic carrier state (often the organism is harbored in the gallbladder), a self-limited gastroenteritis, typhoid fever, and septicemia. Patients with typhoid (enteric) fever typically present with fever (which generally rises over several days), abdominal pain, headache, and occasionally initial constipation. Abdominal rash ("rose spots"), delirium, hepatosplenomegaly, and leukopenia are fairly common. The diarrhea, which begins in the second or third week of infection, is first watery but may progress to severe GI bleeding and perforation. Nontyphoid *Salmonella* species generally causes a milder, self-limited gastroenteritis with vomiting, nausea, fever, and watery diarrhea. Occasionally these species cause bloody diarrhea or toxic megacolon.

SALMONELLOSIS—FACT SHEET

Definition

- Gram-negative enteric bacterium causing typhoid (enteric) fever or milder gastroenteritis; may mimic idiopathic inflammatory bowel disease

Incidence and Location

- Any level of colon; typhoidal form typically involves ileum, right colon, and appendix most dramatically

Clinical Features

- Typhoidal form
- Fever (rising over several days), abdominal pain, headache, and occasionally constipation
- Abdominal rash (rose spots) and leukopenia
- Diarrhea begins in the second or third week
- Diarrhea is initially watery but may progress to severe GI bleeding
- Nontyphoidal form
- Milder, self-limited gastroenteritis with vomiting, nausea, fever, and watery diarrhea
- More clinical and pathologic overlap between the typhoidal and nontyphoidal forms than previously thought

Prognosis and Therapy

- Antibiotics, supportive care

SALMONELLOSIS—PATHOLOGIC FEATURES

Gross Findings

- Typhoid
- Characteristic pathology most prominent in ileum, appendix, and colon
- Markedly thickened bowel, raised nodules correspond to hyperplastic Peyer's patches
- Aphthoid ulcers overlying Peyer's patches, linear ulcers, discoid ulcers, or full-thickness ulceration and necrosis are common
- Perforation and toxic megacolon rarely seen
- Suppurative mesenteric lymphadenitis may be present
- Nontyphoid
- Generally milder findings including mucosal redness, ulceration, and exudates

Microscopic Findings

- Typhoid
- Histiocyte is the predominant inflammatory cell
- Hyperplastic Peyer's patches with overlying acute inflammation; eventually frank ulceration begins in Peyer's patch and spreads to surrounding mucosa
- Lymphoid follicles are infiltrated and obliterated by macrophages
- Neutrophils are not prominent
- Ulcers are typically very deep, with the base at the muscularis propria
- Rare granulomas
- Occasionally significant crypt distortion
- Nontyphoid
- Features of acute self-limited colitis, variable exudate

Differential Diagnosis

- Other bacterial infections (*Yersinia, Shigella*)
- Crohn's disease
- Ulcerative colitis

PATHOLOGIC FEATURES

GROSS FINDINGS

In enteric fever, any level of the alimentary tract may be involved, but the characteristic pathology is most prominent in the ileum, appendix, and colon and is associated with Peyer's patches. Grossly, the bowel wall is thickened, and raised nodules may be seen corresponding to hyperplastic Peyer's patches. Aphthoid ulcers overlying Peyer's patches, linear ulcers, discoid ulcers, or full-thickness ulceration and necrosis are common as disease progresses. Perforation and toxic megacolon may also be seen, as may suppurative mesenteric lymphadenitis. Occasionally, the mucosa is grossly normal or only mildly inflamed and edematous. Endoscopic findings in nontyphoid salmonellosis include mucosal redness, ulceration, and exudates, but the characteristic nodularity and marked edema are not generally seen.

MICROSCOPIC FINDINGS

The histiocyte is the predominant inflammatory cell in typhoid fever (Fig. 9-14). Peyer's patches become hyperplastic, and then acute inflammation of the overlying epithelium is seen (Fig. 9-15). Eventually the lymphoid follicles are infiltrated and obliterated by macrophages. Occasional lymphocytes and plasma cells are seen, but neutrophils are not prominent. Necrosis begins in the Peyer's patch and spreads to

surrounding mucosa, which eventually ulcerates. The ulcers are typically deep, with the base at the muscularis propria. Typhoid fever may also show features more consistent with acute self-limited colitis, including prominent neutrophils, cryptitis, crypt abscesses, and overlying fibrinous exudate. Granulomas are occasionally seen. In nontyphoid salmonellosis, the pathologic features are those of acute self-limited colitis of any infectious cause. Occasionally, significant crypt distortion may be seen (Fig. 9-16).

ANCILLARY STUDIES

Stool cultures are the most helpful ancillary study, and blood cultures may also be of use if the patient is septic.

DIFFERENTIAL DIAGNOSIS

The differential diagnosis of typhoid fever includes yersiniosis and other infectious processes, as well as Crohn's disease, and there may be significant histologic overlap.

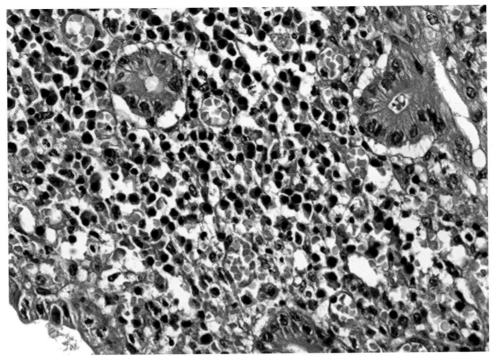

FIGURE 9-14
Mononuclear cells comprise the inflammatory infiltrate in enteric fever, with a dearth of neutrophils (H&E). *(Case courtesy of Dr. A. Brian West.)*

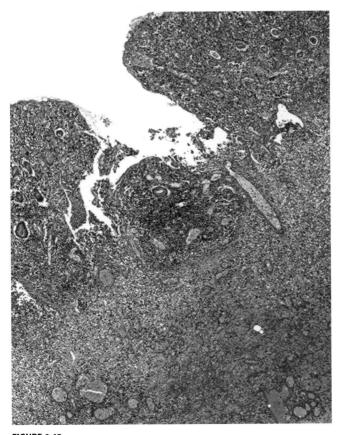

FIGURE 9-15
Ulcer overlying a Peyer's patch in typhoid fever (H&E). *(Case courtesy of Dr. A. Brian West.)*

Prominence of neutrophils and granulomas are often more prominent in the latter two diseases. The differential diagnosis of nontyphoid *Salmonella* infection also includes other causes of acute self-limited infectious colitis, as well as ulcerative colitis. In addition, *Salmonella* infection may complicate preexisting idiopathic inflammatory bowel disease. Although significant crypt distortion has been reported in some cases of salmonellosis, it is more likely to be more pronounced in ulcerative colitis. Clinical presentation and stool culture may be helpful in resolving the differential diagnosis.

PROGNOSIS AND THERAPY

Although the vast majority of *Salmonella* infections in developed countries resolve with antibiotics and supportive care, illness may progress to septicemia and death, particularly in the elderly and the very young, or in patients who are ill for other reasons. Delayed treatment is associated with higher mortality, and antibiotics are particularly important for neonates, older patients, immunocompromised persons, and patients with cardiac valve abnormalities or indwelling prostheses. *Salmonella* is sensitive to several antibiotics, including ciprofloxacin, penicillins, and quinolones. Follow-up stool cultures should be obtained to exclude chronic carrier states.

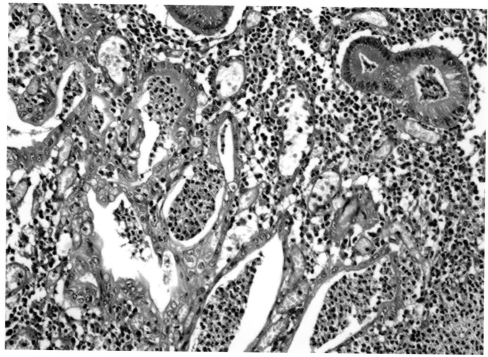

FIGURE 9-16

The architectural distortion in salmonellosis can mimic chronic idiopathic inflammatory bowel disease (H&E). *(Case courtesy of Dr. A. Brian West.)*

SHIGELLOSIS

Shigella species are virulent, invasive, gram-negative bacilli that cause severe bloody diarrhea. They are a major cause of infectious diarrhea worldwide. *Shigella dysenteriae* is the most common species isolated, although *S. sonnei* and *S. flexneri* are increasingly reported in the United States. The infective dose is low (as few as 10 to 100 species in *S. dysenteriae* type 1). *Shigella* is generally ingested from water contaminated with feces, but person-to-person transmission is also possible through the fecal-oral route. Infants, young children, and malnourished, immunocompromised, or debilitated patients are most commonly affected in developed countries. Like salmonellosis, the gross and microscopic features of shigellosis may closely mimic idiopathic inflammatory bowel disease.

CLINICAL FEATURES

Symptoms include abdominal pain, fever, and watery diarrhea, followed by bloody diarrhea. Chronic disease is rare. Perforation and hemolytic-uremic syndrome associated with *Shigella* have been rarely described. Most studies of mortality in shigellosis were performed in underdeveloped nations, and figures range from 2% to 10%. The mortality rate is significantly higher (exceeding 20%) if patients become septic.

PATHOLOGIC FEATURES

GROSS FINDINGS

The large bowel is typically affected, with the left colon more severely involved. The mucosa is hemorrhagic, with exudates that may form pseudomembranes. Ulcerations may be present as well.

SHIGELLOSIS—PATHOLOGIC FEATURES

Gross Findings

- Hemorrhagic mucosa, with exudates that may form pseudomembranes
- Ulcerations may be present as well

Microscopic Findings

- Early infection
- Acute self-limited colitis with cryptitis, crypt abscesses, ulceration
- Pseudomembranes or aphthoid ulcers may be seen
- Later infection
- Increased mucosal destruction with a predominantly neutrophilic inflammatory infiltrate
- Marked architectural distortion to an extent that mimics idiopathic inflammatory bowel disease

Differential Diagnosis

- Other infections, especially *C. difficile* and enteroinvasive *E. coli*
- Ulcerative colitis
- Crohn's disease

MICROSCOPIC FINDINGS

Early infection features acute self-limited colitis with cryptitis, crypt abscesses (often superficial), and ulceration. Pseudomembranes similar to *C. difficile* infection may be seen, as may aphthoid ulcers similar to those of Crohn's disease. As disease progresses, there is increased mucosal destruction with a mixed inflammatory infiltrate containing many neutrophils in the lamina propria. Marked architectural distortion to an extent that mimics idiopathic inflammatory bowel disease is commonly seen.

ANCILLARY STUDIES

Stool culture is essential to diagnosis. Specimens should be rapidly inoculated onto appropriate culture plates, because *Shigella* organisms are fastidious and die quickly. Multiple cultures may be necessary. Stool cultures are more sensitive than rectal swabs. PCR, DNA probes, and serologic studies are also available.

DIFFERENTIAL DIAGNOSIS

The differential diagnosis of early shigellosis is primarily that of other infections, particularly enteroinvasive *E. coli* and *C. difficile*. As disease progresses, it may be extremely difficult to distinguish shigellosis from Crohn's disease or ulcerative colitis both endoscopically and

histologically. Stool cultures and clinical presentation may be helpful in this instance.

PROGNOSIS AND THERAPY

Treatment includes supportive care with fluid and electrolyte replacement, and antibiotics, particularly in children, people who are severely ill, and HIV-positive patients. Antibiotics lessen the mortality rate and shorten the duration of the illness. Most *Shigella* species have at least some degree of antibiotic resistance; trimethoprim-sulfamethoxazole, third-generation cephalosporins, and some fluoroquinolones are drugs of choice.

CAMPYLOBACTER

Campylobacter species, particularly *C. jejuni*, are major causes of diarrhea worldwide. *Campylobacter* is the most common stool isolate identified in the United States. It is transmitted by the fecal-oral route; is found in contaminated meat, water, and milk; and is a common animal pathogen. *C. jejuni* is most commonly associated with gastroenteritis; *C. fetus* and the other less common species are more often seen in immunosuppressed patients and homosexual men. The importance of *C. fetus* may be underrecognized as a result of the difficulty of culturing it under conditions used for other *Campylobacter* strains. The infective dose is low (ingestion of as few as 500 organisms may cause disease), and invasion may occur.

CLINICAL FEATURES

Patients typically have fever, malaise, abdominal pain (often severe), and watery diarrhea, often bloody and with fecal leukocytes. Symptoms generally present within 1 to 5 days of exposure, and last for 4 to 10 days. Relapse is common, although usually less severe than the original attack. Immunosuppressed patients have a higher incidence of symptomatic infection, and symptoms are more severe. Most infections are self-limited, especially in healthy patients. Of note, Guillain-Barré syndrome and reactive arthropathy are associated with *Campylobacter* infection.

PATHOLOGIC FEATURES

GROSS FINDINGS

Endoscopic findings include friable colonic mucosa with associated erythema and hemorrhage.

MICROSCOPIC FINDINGS

Histologic examination most frequently shows features of acute infectious or self-limited colitis, including cryptitis (Figs. 9-17 and 9-18), crypt abscesses, surface epithelial damage, and a neutrophilic infiltrate in the lamina propria. Marked edema and superficial mucosal erosion with associated hemorrhage may be seen as well. Findings may be patchy or focal. Mild crypt distortion, crypt epithelial damage, and crypt loss are occasionally present, although crypt architecture is usually well preserved overall.

ANCILLARY STUDIES

The mainstay of laboratory diagnosis is culture of *Campylobacter* from stool or blood. Preliminary diagnosis may be made by detection of organisms in fresh stool smears by dark-field microscopy. Stool agglutination tests are less sensitive, and serologies are only useful late in the course of disease. Molecular techniques are under development and available for research purposes but are not widely available for clinical use.

DIFFERENTIAL DIAGNOSIS

The differential diagnosis primarily includes other forms of infectious enterocolitis that produce the acute self-limited colitis pattern; stool culture may be essential to resolving the differential.

PROGNOSIS AND THERAPY

In most uncomplicated cases of *Campylobacter* infection, fluid and electrolyte replacement is the principal therapy. Antibiotics are not generally indicated unless there is high fever, severe or bloody diarrhea, symptoms of more than 1 week, or the patient is immunocompromised or septic. Erythromycin is the antibiotic of choice.

YERSINIA

Yersinia enterocolitica and *Y. pseudotuberculosis* are the two *Yersinia* species pertinent to human GI disease. *Yersinia* is one of the most common causes of bacterial

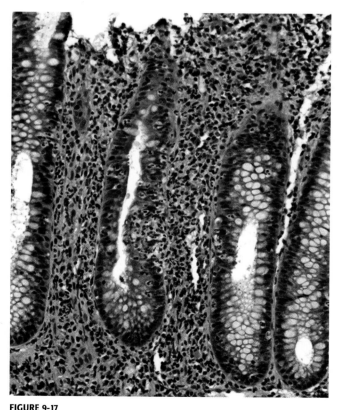

FIGURE 9-17

Campylobacter jejuni infection showing cryptitis, surface epithelial injury, and preservation of crypt architecture (H&E).

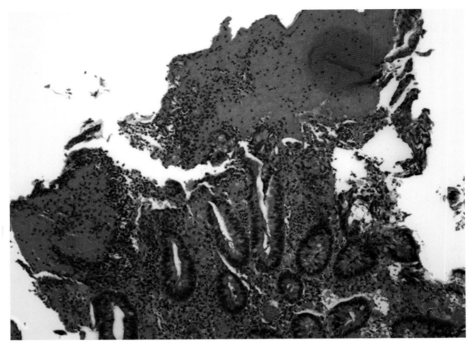

FIGURE 9-18
Campylobacter jejuni infection. Superficial ulceration, neutrophilic infiltrate, and hemorrhage are seen. (H&E).

enteritis in Western and Northern Europe, and numerous cases have been documented in North America and Australia. *Yersinia* may be found in many food products, including meats (particularly undercooked pork), dairy products, and water.

CLINICAL FEATURES

These gram-negative coccobacilli are causative agents in appendicitis, ileitis, colitis, and mesenteric lymphadenitis. In addition, they are responsible for many cases of isolated granulomatous appendicitis. Infection with either species may cause symptoms and signs of an acute abdomen, chronic abdominal pain, and diarrhea. Although yersiniosis is usually a self-limited process, chronic infections (including chronic colitis) and persistent abdominal pain have been well documented. Immunocompromised and debilitated patients, as well as patients on deferoxamine or with iron overload resulting from other causes, are at particular risk for serious disease.

PATHOLOGIC FEATURES

GROSS FINDINGS

Grossly, involved bowel has a thickened, edematous wall with nodular inflammatory masses centered around Peyer's patches. Aphthoid and linear ulcers may be seen.

YERSINIA—FACT SHEET

Definition
- Common cause of granulomatous appendicitis, enterocolitis in the United States and Europe
- Found in many food products, including meats, dairy products, and water
- May be clinicopathologic mimic of Crohn's disease

Incidence and Location
- Ileum, appendix, and colon

Clinical Features
- Signs and symptoms of enterocolitis, acute appendicitis
- Usually self-limiting, occasionally cause chronic disease
- May have mesenteric adenopathy

Prognosis and Therapy
- Usually self-limiting
- Severe cases or debilitated patients require antibiotics

Involved appendices are enlarged and mimic suppurative granulomatous appendicitis; perforation is often seen. Involved lymph nodes may show gross foci of necrosis.

MICROSCOPIC FINDINGS

Both suppurative and granulomatous patterns of inflammation may be seen, and a mixture of the two is common. GI infection with *Y. pseudotuberculosis*

DIFFERENTIAL DIAGNOSIS

The major differential diagnoses of *Yersinia* infection include other similar infectious processes, particularly mycobacterial infection and salmonellosis. Acid-fast stains and culture results should help to distinguish mycobacterial infection; clinical features and the presence of greater numbers of neutrophils, microabscesses, and granulomas may help to distinguish yersiniosis from salmonellosis.

Crohn's disease and yersiniosis may be difficult to distinguish from one another, and, in fact, have a long and complicated relationship. Both may show similar histologic features, and, in fact, isolated granulomatous appendicitis has in the past frequently been interpreted as primary Crohn's disease of the appendix. However, patients with granulomatous inflammation confined to the appendix rarely develop generalized inflammatory bowel disease. Features that may favor Crohn's disease include cobblestoning of mucosa and creeping fat grossly, and changes of chronicity microscopically, including crypt distortion, thickening of the muscularis mucosa, and prominent neural hyperplasia. However, some cases are indistinguishable on histologic grounds alone.

PROGNOSIS AND THERAPY

Most cases of yersiniosis resolve spontaneously. Yersinia is susceptible to many antibiotics, and therapy is recommended in patients with severe infections, bacteremia, or in the context of immunocompromise or debilitation.

AEROMONAS

Aeromonas, initially thought to be nonpathogenic gram-negative bacteria, are increasingly recognized as causes of gastroenteritis in both children and adults. The motile *A. hydrophila* and *A. sobria* most often cause GI disease in humans.

has characteristically been described as a granulomatous process with central microabscesses, almost always accompanied by mesenteric adenopathy. Infection with *Y. enterocolitica* has not typically been associated with discrete granulomas but has been characterized by hyperplastic Peyer's patches with overlying ulceration and accompanying acute inflammation, hemorrhagic necrosis, and palisading histiocytes. Recent studies have shown that there is significant overlap between the histologic features of *Y. enterocolitica* and *Y. pseudotuberculosis* infection and that either species may show lymphoid hyperplasia, epithelioid granulomas with prominent lymphoid cuffing, transmural lymphoid aggregates, giant cells, mucosal ulceration, cryptitis, and concomitant lymph node involvement (Figs. 9-19 through 9-21). Some cases show only nonspecific features of acute self-limited colitis.

ANCILLARY STUDIES

Special stains are not helpful in the diagnosis of *Yersinia*, for the organisms are small, may be present in low numbers, and are difficult to distinguish from normal nonpathogenic colonic flora. Cultures, serologic studies, and particularly PCR assays are the most useful diagnostic aids.

CLINICAL FEATURES

The typical presentation is bloody diarrhea, sometimes chronic, accompanied by nausea, vomiting, and cramping pain. The diarrhea may contain mucus as well as blood. The duration of illness varies widely, ranging from a few days to several years, indicating that *Aeromonas* infection can cause a chronic colitis.

AEROMONAS—FACT SHEET

Definition

- Gram-negative bacterium initially believed nonpathogenic; now increasingly recognized as cause of infectious enterocolitis; may be clinicopathologic mimic of Crohn's disease

Incidence and Location

- Colon, often segmental distribution

Clinical Features

- Bloody diarrhea, can be chronic; nausea, vomiting, cramping pain

Prognosis and Therapy

- Most cases resolve spontaneously; susceptible to multiple antibiotics if needed

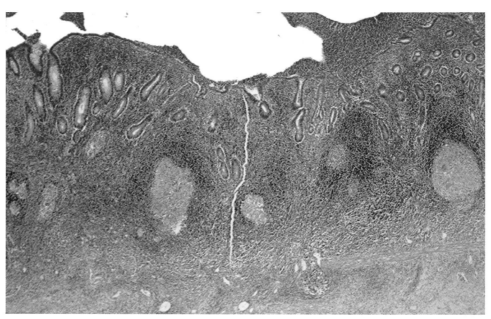

FIGURE 9-19

Yersinia enterocolitica infection. Mucosal ulceration, lymphoid hyperplasia, and epithelioid granulomas are seen. (H&E).

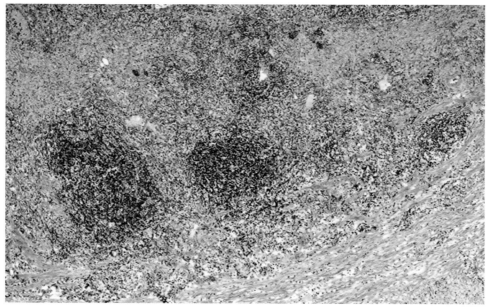

FIGURE 9-20

Linear arrangement of mural and serosal lymphoid aggregates in *Yersinia* infection can mimic Crohn's disease (H&E).

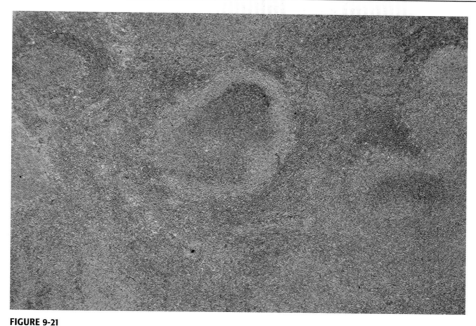

FIGURE 9-21

Yersina pseudotuberculosis infection. Granulomatous inflammation with central microabscess formation (H&E).

PATHOLOGIC FEATURES

GROSS FINDINGS

Endoscopically, signs of colitis may be seen, including edema, friability, erosions, exudates, and loss of vascular pattern; the features are often segmental and may mimic ischemic colitis or Crohn's disease. A pancolitis mimicking ulcerative colitis has also been described.

MICROSCOPIC FINDINGS

The histologic features are usually those of acute self-limited colitis. However, ulceration and focal architectural distortion may be seen (Fig. 9-22).

AEROMONAS—PATHOLOGIC FEATURES

Gross Findings
- Edema, friability, erosions, exudates, and loss of vascular pattern
- Often segmental
- Pancolitis mimicking ulcerative colitis has been seen

Microscopic Findings
- Usually those of acute self-limited colitis
- Ulceration and focal architectural distortion may be seen

Differential Diagnosis
- Crohn's disease
- Ischemic colitis (particularly grossly)
- Ulcerative colitis (grossly, if pancolitis present)

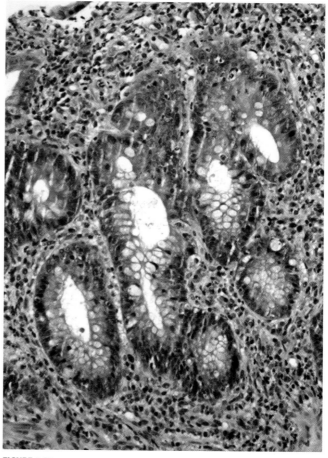

FIGURE 9-22

Cryptitis, mucosal ulceration, and architectural distortion in culture-proven *Aeromonas* infection (H&E).

ANCILLARY STUDIES

Stool cultures are critical to diagnosis.

DIFFERENTIAL DIAGNOSIS

The differential diagnosis includes other infectious processes, ischemic colitis, and chronic idiopathic inflammatory bowel disease. Culture should help exclude other infections, and typical features of ischemia (crypt withering, mucosal necrosis) are not present with *Aeromonas*. When architectural distortion is present in a patient with chronic symptoms, it may be very difficult to resolve the issue of *Aeromonas* infection versus Crohn's disease or ulcerative colitis. Some authorities recommend culturing for *Aeromonas* in all patients with refractory chronic inflammatory bowel disease.

PROGNOSIS AND THERAPY

Most cases resolve spontaneously. *Aeromonas* is susceptible to many antibiotics, which can be used in severe or chronic infections.

CLOSTRIDIAL DISEASES OF THE GUT

Clostridial organisms are responsible for pseudomembranous/antibiotic-associated colitis (usually *C. difficile*); necrotizing jejunitis or pig-bel (usually *C. perfringens*); neutropenic enterocolitis (NEC; usually *C. septicum*); and botulism (*C. botulinum*). Clostridial organisms are some of the most potent collections of toxigenic bacteria in existence, and many species are important gut pathogens.

The two species most pertinent to diagnostic colonic pathology are *C. difficile* and *C. septicum*, causative agents in PMC and NEC, respectively. *C. perfringens* (welchii) causes necrotizing enterocolitis or pig-bel; the colon is rarely affected by this process, and the jejunum is the most commonly involved site in *C. perfringens* infection.

CLINICAL FEATURES

C. difficile is the most common nosocomial GI pathogen. Infection is usually related to prior antibiotic exposure (especially orally administered antibiotics), because the organisms cannot infect in the presence of normal colonic flora.

The majority of patients are older, although infection is certainly not limited to this group. In addition, the incidence of *C. difficile* infection has increased in patients with chronic idiopathic inflammatory bowel disease, and negatively affects clinical outcome in terms of both hospitalization and need for colectomy.

Recurrent disease is common despite successful treatment and is seen in up to 50% of cases; the incidence of recurrent disease appears to be increasing. Furthermore, the incidence of severe or life-threatening *C. difficile* colitis in North America has increased recently. This increase has been linked to an epidemic strain of *C. difficile* known as strain BI/NAP1; this strain is hypervirulent, with increased production of both toxins A and B, and is resistant to fluoroquinolones.

Some patients are asymptomatic despite the presence of toxigenic strains in stool. Presentation in symptomatic patients is highly variable, ranging from mild diarrhea to PMC to fulminant colitis with perforation or toxic megacolon. Watery diarrhea is most common initially, and may be accompanied by abdominal pain, cramping, fever, and leukocytosis (sometimes marked). Bloody diarrhea is variably seen. Symptoms can occur up to several weeks after discontinuation of antibiotic therapy. Patients with more severe disease may not have diarrhea, and the only clues to diagnosis may be fever, marked leukocytosis, and a markedly tender, distended abdomen. Complications of severe infection include toxic megacolon, perforation, and death. An associated reactive polyarthritis also has been described.

NEC (typhlitis) is a serious complication of neutropenia as a result of chemotherapy in patients with marrow-based and solid tumors, as well as in patients with neutropenia of primary causes. Most patients have received chemotherapy within the previous month before the onset of colitis, and the incidence of typhlitis is believed to be related to the intensity of chemotherapy and degree of immunosuppression. *C. septicum* has been frequently reported as a causative organism, especially in adults. *C. septicum* infection is also associated with malignancies (particularly adenocarcinoma) in the colon and distal ileum, and clostridial infection may be the first indication of such a tumor. Patients usually present with the abrupt onset of GI hemorrhage, fever, abdominal pain and distention, and diarrhea. The pain often initially localizes to the right lower quadrant, but quickly progresses to peritonitis, shock, and sepsis. Perforation is a well-described complication, and infection is often fatal.

PATHOLOGIC FEATURES

GROSS FINDINGS

Endoscopically, classic PMC shows yellow-white pseudomembranes, most commonly in the left colon. The plaques bleed when scraped. The distribution

CLOSTRIDIUM DIFFICILE–RELATED PSEUDOMEMBRANOUS COLITIS—FACT SHEET

Definition

- Colitis caused by overgrowth of *C. difficile*, usually following antibiotic administration and destruction of normal gut flora
- Most common nosocomial gut pathogen

Incidence and Location

- Anywhere in colon, often patchy distribution; rectum may be spared

Clinical Features

- Usually prior, orally administered antibiotic exposure; diarrhea can happen weeks after antibiotic therapy
- Usually older patients
- Variable range of clinical disease, from mild diarrhea to fulminant colitis with toxic megacolon
- Watery diarrhea initially; may be accompanied by abdominal pain, cramping, fever, and leukocytosis
- Bloody diarrhea sometimes seen

Prognosis and Therapy

- Remove offending drug
- Supportive measures
- Oral vancomycin or Flagyl

CLOSTRIDIUM DIFFICILE–RELATED PSEUDOMEMBRANOUS COLITIS—PATHOLOGIC FEATURES

Gross Findings

- Yellow-white pseudomembranes, most commonly in the left colon; distribution may be patchy
- Plaques bleed when scraped
- Erythema and friability of the mucosa may be present, without pseudomembranes

Microscopic Findings

- Classic features
  - "Volcano" lesions with intercrypt necrosis and ballooned crypts giving rise to laminated pseudomembrane composed of fibrin, mucin, and neutrophils
  - Ballooned glands are filled with neutrophils and mucin
- Exceptions
  - Severe and prolonged PMC may lead to full-thickness mucosal necrosis
  - Some cases show only focal active colitis with occasional crypt abscesses but lacking pseudomembranous features.

Differential Diagnosis

- Ischemia
- Other infections, including *Shigella* and enterohemorrhagic *E. coli*

CLOSTRIDIUM-RELATED NECROTIZING ENTEROCOLITIS—FACT SHEET

Definition

- Neutropenic enterocolitis
- Usually in the context of previous chemotherapy
- *C. septicum* commonly implicated

Incidence and Location

- Right colon preferentially involved

Clinical Features

- Neutropenia, either resulting from chemotherapy or primary causes
- GI hemorrhage, with fever, abdominal pain and distention, diarrhea
- Perforation a frequent complication

Prognosis and Therapy

- Controversial
- Antibiotics and supportive measures, versus segmental resection of the involved bowel
- Surgery may be required to prevent or treat perforation

CLOSTRIDIUM-RELATED NECROTIZING ENTEROCOLITIS—PATHOLOGIC FEATURES

Gross Findings

- Right colon is preferentially involved
- Diffuse dilatation and edema of bowel, varying severity of ulceration and hemorrhage
- Exudates and pseudomembranes common

Microscopic Findings

- Range from mild hemorrhage to prominent submucosal edema, ulceration, marked hemorrhage, and focal necrosis
- Often with a striking absence of inflammatory cells
- Neutrophils sometimes found despite peripheral neutropenia
- Pseudomembranous exudate resembling *C. difficile*–related colitis may be seen
- Sometimes organisms seen in bowel wall with Gram stain

Differential Diagnosis

- Ischemic colitis
- PMC

may be patchy, and the rectum may be spared. Less striking findings may also be seen, including erythema and friability of the mucosa without pseudomembranes. Typical histologic findings may be seen, however, even in the absence of grossly visible pseudomembranes.

The right colon is preferentially involved in NEC, although the ileum and other sites in the colon may be affected. Gross findings include diffuse dilatation and edema of the bowel, with varying severity of ulceration and hemorrhage. Exudates and pseudomembranes resembling *C. difficile* colitis may be seen in NEC as well.

MICROSCOPIC FINDINGS

Histologically, classic PMC features "volcano" lesions with intercrypt necrosis and ballooned crypts giving rise to the typical laminated pseudomembrane composed of fibrin, mucin, and neutrophils (Fig. 9-23). The ballooned glands are filled with neutrophils and mucin, and often lose the superficial epithelial cells. More severe and prolonged PMC may lead to full-thickness mucosal necrosis. Less characteristic lesions, usually focal active colitis with occasional crypt abscesses but lacking pseudomembranous features, have been well described in association with a positive *C. difficile* toxin assay.

In NEC, microscopic changes range from mild hemorrhage to prominent submucosal edema, ulceration, marked hemorrhage, and focal necrosis, often with a striking absence of neutrophils and other inflammatory cells (Figs. 9-24 and 9-25). However, neutrophils are sometimes present despite peripheral neutropenia. A pseudomembranous exudate resembling *C. difficile*–related colitis may be seen. Sometimes organisms can be detected in the wall of the bowel on Gram stain.

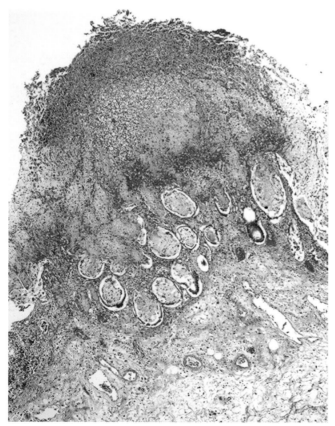

FIGURE 9-23

"Volcano" lesion of *Clostridium difficile*–related pseudomembranous colitis. Note ballooned crypts containing neutrophils, intercrypt necrosis, and laminated pseudomembrane composed of fibrin, mucus, and neutrophils (H&E).

ANCILLARY STUDIES

The *C. difficile* toxin assays are the most helpful diagnostic aid in PMC. Culture is the most helpful technique for confirming the diagnosis of *C. septicum* infection.

DIFFERENTIAL DIAGNOSIS

The term *pseudomembranous colitis* is a description of an inflammatory pattern, not a specific diagnosis. Although most cases of PMC are related to *C. difficile* infection, other infectious entities as well as ischemic colitis may have similar appearances. A hyalinized lamina propria favors the diagnosis of ischemia; other features, such as crypt withering, pseudomembranes, and mucosal necrosis, may be seen in either entity. Endoscopically, pseudomembrane formation is also seen more often in PMC, although this finding may be present in ischemia as well. History of antibiotic use and stool assay for *C. difficile* toxin may be invaluable in sorting out this differential diagnosis.

The differential diagnosis for NEC includes ischemic colitis and PMC. The appropriate clinical setting and dearth of inflammatory cells favor NEC.

PROGNOSIS AND THERAPY

Treatment of PMC includes a combination of removal of the offending drug, supportive measures, and antibiotics (oral vancomycin or metronidazole). Treatment of NEC is controversial; some recommend antibiotics and supportive measures, whereas others recommend segmental resection of the involved bowel. Surgery may be required to prevent or treat perforation in severe cases.

MYCOBACTERIAL INFECTIONS OF THE COLON

Although common in developing countries and immigrant populations, there has been a remarkable resurgence of tuberculosis in Western countries due in large part to AIDS but also to institutional overcrowding and immigrant populations. Although many cases present with pulmonary symptoms, GI symptoms may be the initial presenting findings in these patients, and primary GI tuberculosis has been well documented. The ileocecal and jejunoileal areas are the most commonly involved areas of the gut in *M. tuberculosis* infection, followed by the appendix and ascending colon. This distribution is probably caused by the organism's

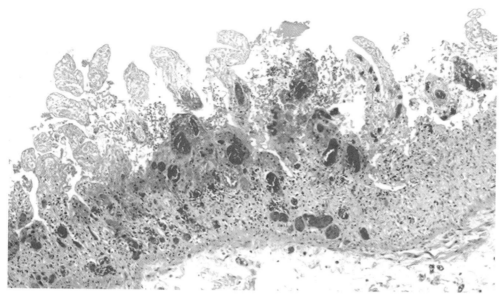

FIGURE 9-24

Necrotizing enterocolitis in chemotherapy patient. Note sections of ileum and cecum with ulceration, hemorrhagic necrosis, and a coating of surface bacteria (H&E).

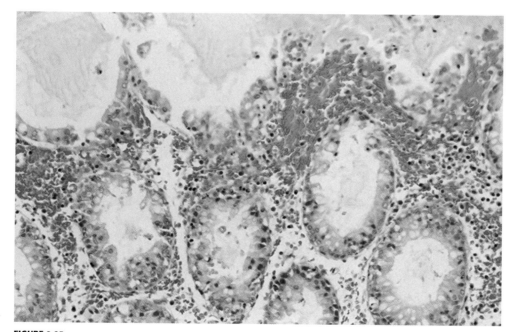

FIGURE 9-25

Necrotizing enterocolitis. Note lack of neutrophils (H&E).

affinity for lymphoid tissue. Anorectal involvement is much less common but has been well described.

Atypical mycobacteria may also involve the gut, and *Mycobacterium avium-intracellulare* (MAI) complex is the most common atypical *Mycobacterium* isolated from the GI tract. The small bowel is preferentially involved, but colonic involvement may also be present, as may mesenteric adenopathy.

CLINICAL FEATURES

Symptoms of colonic tuberculosis are nonspecific and include weight loss, fever, abdominal pain, diarrhea, or a palpable abdominal mass. Complications include hemorrhage, perforation, obstruction, or malabsorption. Mesenteric adenopathy is common. Symptoms in MAI infection are similar, and often reflect systemic disease.

Location
- *Mycobacterium tuberculosis*: anywhere in colon, but ileocecum preferentially involved
- *Mycobacterium avium-intracellulare* complex: anywhere in colon, more often small bowel involved

Clinical Features
- *Mycobacterium tuberculosis*: weight loss, fever, abdominal pain, diarrhea, or a palpable abdominal mass
- Complications include hemorrhage, perforation, obstruction, malabsorption
- Mesenteric adenopathy is common
- *Mycobacterium avium-intracellulare* complex: similar to *M. tuberculosis*; often reflects systemic disease

Prognosis and Therapy
- Medical therapy same as that for other organ systems (multidrug antimycobacterial regimens)
- Surgery required for obstruction, perforation, bleeding

PATHOLOGIC FEATURES

GROSS FINDINGS

The ileocecal valve is often deformed and gaping in cases of ileocecal *M. tuberculosis* infection. Multiple and segmental lesions with skip areas are common. Strictures and ulcers are the most common endoscopic findings, along with thickened mucosal folds and inflammatory nodules. Different gross lesions, such as strictures and ulcers, often occur together. The ulcers are often circumferential and transverse. Large inflammatory masses, usually involving the ileocecum, may be seen. Endoscopic findings with MAI infection are usually unremarkable, except for occasional white nodules, small ulcers, or hemorrhages.

MICROSCOPIC FINDINGS

In *M. tuberculosis* infection, the characteristic histologic lesion is caseating granulomas, which may be present at any level of the wall of the gut (Fig. 9-26). Granulomas are often confluent, with a rim of lymphocytes at the periphery of the granulomas. Granulomas may be hyalinized and calcified. Aphthoid ulcers or frank ulceration, as well as inflammation of submucosal vessels, may be seen as well. Acid-fast stains may demonstrate organisms, but culture may be required; in addition, excellent PCR assays are available. Purified protein derivative (PPD) tests are unreliable in immunocompromised or debilitated patients.

In MAI infection, histology varies with immune status. Immunocompetent patients show a granulomatous response (Fig. 9-27), either necrotizing or non-necrotizing. Immunocompromised patients generally have a diffuse

Gross Findings
- *Mycobacterium tuberculosis*
  - Deformed and gaping ileocecal valve
  - Multiple and segmental lesions with skip areas, thickened mucosal folds and raised nodules, ulcers
  - Strictures and ulcers are the most common endoscopic findings; ulcers are often circumferential and transverse
  - Large inflammatory masses may obstruct
- *Mycobacterium avium-intracellulare* complex
  - Usually normal colonoscopy; rare findings include white nodules, small ulcers, or hemorrhages

Microscopic Findings
- *Mycobacterium tuberculosis*
  - Characteristic histologic lesion is caseating granulomas in any part of gut wall
  - Often confluent, with a rim of lymphocytes at the periphery
  - May be rare, or hyalinized and calcified
  - With or without ulceration, inflammation of submucosal vessels
  - Acid-fast stains may demonstrate organisms
- *Mycobacterium avium-intracellulare* complex
  - Histology varies with immune status
  - Immunocompetent patients show a granulomatous response, either necrotizing or non-necrotizing
  - Immunocompromised patients have a diffuse infiltration of histiocytes containing the bacilli, with little inflammatory response

Differential Diagnosis
- Other infectious processes causing granulomas, histiocytic infiltrate
- Crohn's disease

infiltration of histiocytes containing the bacilli, with little inflammatory response (Fig. 9-28). Rarely, poorly formed granulomas occur in immunocompromised patients with MAI infection.

ANCILLARY STUDIES

Bacilli stain with acid-fast stains, as well as periodic acid-Schiff (PAS) and Gomori methenamine silver (GMS) stains. Organisms are generally abundant in immunocompromised patients, but may be hard to detect in healthy patients. Culture and PCR assays may also be helpful.

DIFFERENTIAL DIAGNOSIS

The differential diagnosis of *M. tuberculosis* infection includes other infectious processes, especially yersiniosis and other granulomatous processes such as fungal diseases. The granulomas of yersiniosis are typically noncaseating, but there may be considerable histologic overlap. Crohn's disease may be difficult to distinguish

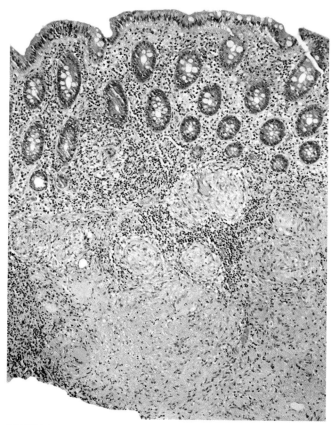

FIGURE 9-26

Colonic *Mycobacterium tuberculosis* with confluent caseating granulomas in the mucosa (H&E).

from tuberculosis; features favoring Crohn's disease are linear rather than circumferential ulcers, transmural lymphoid aggregates, and deep fistulas and fissures. Tuberculosis also commonly lacks mucosal cobblestoning. Atypical mycobacteria, such as *M. kansasii* and *M. bovis,* may yield a similar histologic picture. The differential diagnosis of MAI includes other infectious processes causing a histiocytic infiltrate, such as infection with *Rhodococcus equi.*

PROGNOSIS AND THERAPY

GI tuberculosis responds to the same medication regimen as pulmonary tuberculosis. Surgical therapy may be required for obstructive disease, perforation, or hemorrhage. MAI of the GI tract is also treated similarly to MAI infection of other organ systems, with combination therapy using antimycobacterial agents with activity against MAI.

■ SYPHILIS (*TREPONEMA PALLIDUM*)

GI syphilis commonly involves the anorectum. Homosexual males are at particularly high risk of infection, and many authorities believe that syphilis, particularly anorectal syphilis, is markedly underdiagnosed as a

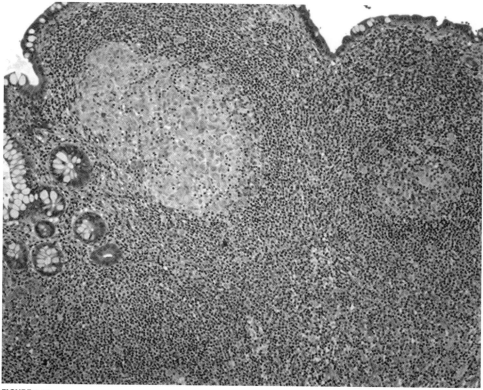

FIGURE 9-27

Mycobacterium avium-intracellulare complex infection. Note the epithelioid, noncaseating granulomas in the ileocecum of an immunocompetent person (H&E).

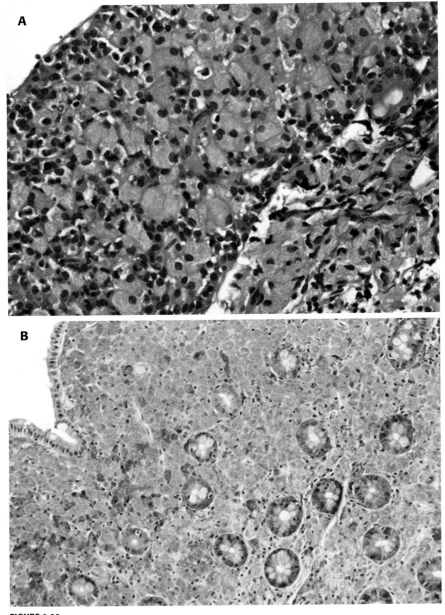

FIGURE 9-28

Gastrointestinal MAI complex infection. **A,** Infiltrate of foamy macrophages in an AIDS patient (H&E). **B,** Numerous acid-fast bacilli within foamy macrophages (Ziehl-Neelsen).

result of the variability of the clinical findings and a low index of suspicion.

CLINICAL FEATURES

Patients are often asymptomatic, but common presenting symptoms in syphilitic proctitis include pain, often with defecation; tenesmus; constipation; bleeding; and anal discharge, which may be mucoid or bloody (Fig. 9-29).

PATHOLOGIC FEATURES

GROSS FINDINGS

Gross findings in primary anorectal syphilis include anal chancres (indurated, circular lesions, single or multiple, with variable tenderness) or a mild proctitis. Signs of secondary syphilis typically present 6 to 8 weeks later, and include masses, mucocutaneous rash, or condyloma lata (raised, moist, smooth warts that secrete mucus and are associated with itching and a foul odor). Inguinal adenopathy is typical. The gross features of primary and secondary infection sometimes coexist. The mass lesions of secondary syphilis may mimic malignancy, and surgical removal without a prior biopsy should be avoided.

MICROSCOPIC FINDINGS

Histologically, syphilitic proctitis features a dense plasmacytic cell infiltrate. Cryptitis and crypt abscesses are often present as well, along with gland destruction and reactive epithelial changes. Granulomas have been reported rarely, and occasionally prominent, proliferative capillary endothelial cells may be noted (proliferative endarteriolitis). Syphilitic proctitis may be nonspecific, showing only features of acute infectious-type colitis without a significant increase in plasma cells.

ANCILLARY STUDIES

Dark-field examination, Warthin-Starry stains, serologic studies, and immunohistochemistry may be helpful diagnostic aids.

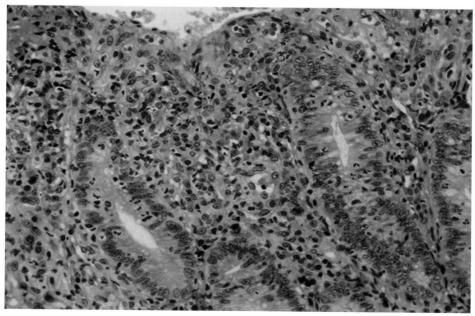

FIGURE 9-29

Syphilitic proctitis. Note cryptitis with increased plasma cells in the lamina propria (H&E). (*Courtesy of Drs. Rodger C. Haggitt and Mary P. Bronner.*)

DIFFERENTIAL DIAGNOSIS

The gross differential diagnosis of chancre includes anal fissures, fistulas, and traumatic lesions. Condyloma acuminata are more dry and keratinized than condyloma lata. The differential diagnosis histologically primarily includes other infectious processes that cause a focal active colitis.

PROGNOSIS AND THERAPY

Penicillin is the treatment of choice in most cases of syphilis. HIV-positive patients should be monitored particularly closely, because the infection may have a more aggressive course in this population.

Several other types of infectious proctocolitis are common among homosexual men and should be considered in the differential diagnosis of sexually acquired infectious proctocolitis. Patients generally present with similar symptoms regardless of infectious agent, including anal discharge, pain, diarrhea, constipation, bloody stools, and tenesmus. Proctoscopic findings range from normal to mucosal friability, erosions, and erythema.

CHLAMYDIA TRACHOMATIS

Chlamydia trachomatis (serotypes L1, L2, and L3) is the causative agent of lymphogranuloma venereum (LGV). Although the anorectum is the most common site, LGV has been described in the ileum and colon as well. Most patients have a lymphoplasmacytic infiltrate in the mucosa and submucosa, but neutrophils may also be prominent. Granulomatous inflammation is sometimes present. Crypt distortion, crypt abscesses, ulceration, fissuring ulcers, neural hyperplasia, and fibrosis have also been described. In addition, LGV may produce a striking follicular proctitis. Because of these latter features, LGV may be difficult to distinguish from Crohn's disease or ulcerative colitis, and culture, direct immunofluorescence studies, and immunohistochemistry may provide valuable diagnostic aids. Granuloma inguinale (*Calymmobacterium granulomatis*) may cause anal and perianal disease that can be clinically and histologically similar to LGV, although rectal involvement favors LGV. Warthin-Starry or Giemsa stains may aid in visualizing the Donovan bodies typical of granuloma inguinale.

NEISSERIA GONORRHEA

Gonorrhea has been reported in up to 20% of homosexual men and is frequently asymptomatic. The anorectum (alone or in combination with pharyngitis and urethritis) is a common site of gonorrheal infection. *Neisseria meningitidis* has also been isolated from the anorectums of homosexual men. Proctoscopic examination is usually unremarkable. Most histologic biopsy results in rectal gonorrhea are normal; some contain a mild increase in neutrophils and mononuclear cells or focal cryptitis. Gram-negative cocci can occasionally be seen on Gram stain of anal discharge, and culture can also be a valuable diagnostic aid.

INTESTINAL SPIROCHETOSIS

Intestinal spirochetosis is primarily seen in homosexual men, although it has been described in a wide variety of other conditions, including diverticular disease, ulcerative colitis, and adenomas. Spirochetosis represents infection by a heterogeneous group of related organisms, most importantly *Brachyspira aalborgi* and *Brachyspira pilosicoli*, which are genetically unrelated to *T. pallidum*. Patients with spirochetosis may harbor one or both of these species.

CLINICAL FEATURES

Although patients with this histologic finding often have symptoms such as diarrhea or anal pain and discharge, it is not clear that spirochetosis causes these symptoms. Many patients have concomitant infections (especially gonorrhea), thus complicating the clinical picture.

PATHOLOGIC FEATURES

GROSS FINDINGS

Any level of the colon may be involved, as may the appendix. Typically, endoscopic abnormalities are mild or absent.

MICROSCOPIC FINDINGS

On H&E, spirochetosis resembles a fuzzy, "fringed" blue line at the luminal border of the colonic mucosa (Fig. 9-30). Invasion is not seen. The changes can be very focal. Most show no associated inflammatory infiltrate, although occasionally an associated cryptitis may be seen. Warthin-Starry or similar silver stains stain the organisms intensely (Fig. 9-31). The organisms will also stain with Alcian blue (pH 2.5) and PAS.

DIFFERENTIAL DIAGNOSIS

The differential diagnosis primarily consists of a prominent glycocalyx, which should not stain with Warthin-Starry stains. Occasionally enteroadherent

INTESTINAL SPIROCHETOSIS—FACT SHEET

Definition

- Coating of the colonic luminal surface with spirilla bacteria, primarily in homosexual men

Incidence and Location

- Colon and appendix

Clinical Features

- Usually asymptomatic; some patients have diarrhea, but often coinfections complicate the clinical picture

Prognosis and Therapy

- Metronidazole or other antimicrobials; treatment of asymptomatic persons is controversial

INTESTINAL SPIROCHETOSIS—PATHOLOGIC FEATURES

Gross Findings

- Usually normal colonoscopy

Microscopic Findings

- Fuzzy, "fringed" blue line at the luminal border of the colonic mucosa
- Invasion is not seen
- May be focal
- Most have little or no associated inflammatory infiltrate
- Warthin-Starry or similar silver stains stain the organisms intensely

Differential Diagnosis

- Enteroadherent *E. coli*
- Prominent glycocalyx of colonic mucosa

E. coli can give a similar appearance, but *E. coli* should stain gram negative and not have spirillar morphology.

PROGNOSIS AND THERAPY

Treatment is somewhat controversial. Some authorities do not advocate treating asymptomatic patients. Others advocate treatment with metronidazole or other antimicrobials. There are little long-term follow-up data on treatment effects.

ACTINOMYCOSIS

Actinomycosis is caused by *Actinomyces,* filamentous anaerobic gram-positive bacteria that are normal inhabitants of the oral cavity and upper GI tract. They rarely cause disease of the alimentary tract, usually as a chronic, nonopportunistic infection, particularly *Actinomyces israelii.*

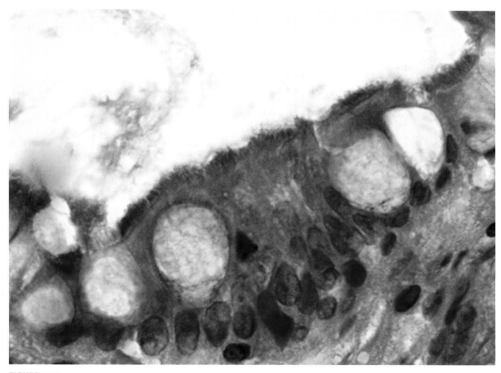

FIGURE 9-30

"Fringe" of bacteria along luminal surface in spirochetosis. No attendant inflammation (H&E with oil immersion).

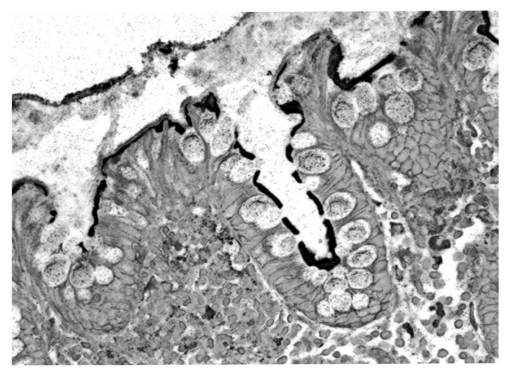

FIGURE 9-31
Spirochetes are intensely positive with silver impregnation staining (Warthin-Starry).

CLINICAL FEATURES

Infection may be at any level of the GI tract, but is usually in a solitary site. Sometimes this infection is associated with diverticular disease. Symptoms include fever, weight loss, abdominal pain, and sometimes a palpable mass. Perianal fistulas and chronic (often granulomatous) appendicitis resulting from actinomycosis have also been described.

ACTINOMYCOSIS—FACT SHEET

Definition
- Filamentous anaerobic gram-positive bacterium, a normal inhabitant of the oral cavity and upper GI tract, which rarely causes a chronic, nonopportunistic GI infection

Incidence and Location
- Any level of the GI tract, usually a solitary site

Clinical Features
- Fever, weight loss, abdominal pain, sometimes a palpable mass
- May be associated with diverticular disease
- Rare manifestations: perianal fistulas, chronic (often granulomatous) appendicitis
- May mimic carcinoma

Prognosis and Therapy
- Surgical resection or incision and drainage
- Prolonged antibiotic therapy, often intravenous
- Follow-up CT scan is recommended to assess therapy

PATHOLOGIC FEATURES

GROSS FINDINGS

Grossly, *Actinomyces* often produces a large, solitary mass, with or without ulceration, often with significant mural infiltration that may extend into surrounding structures and grossly mimic carcinoma.

ACTINOMYCOSIS—PATHOLOGIC FEATURES

Gross Findings
- Large, solitary mass, with or without ulceration
- Significant mural infiltration that may extend into surrounding structures and grossly mimic carcinoma

Microscopic Findings
- Actinomycotic ("sulfur") granules consisting of irregularly rounded clusters of bacteria bordered by eosinophilic, clublike projections (Splendore-Hoeppli material)
- Inflammatory reaction is predominantly neutrophilic, with abscess formation
- Palisading histiocytes and giant cells, as well as frank granulomas, often surround the neutrophilic inflammation
- May be a marked associated fibrotic response

Differential Diagnosis
- Gross differential: abscess of other infectious causes, lymphoma and carcinoma
- Histologic differential: other infectious processes, particularly *Nocardia*

MICROSCOPIC FINDINGS

The organism typically produces actinomycotic ("sulfur") granules consisting of irregularly rounded clusters of bacteria bordered by eosinophilic, clublike projections (Splendore-Hoeppli material). The inflammatory reaction is predominantly neutrophilic, with abscess formation (Fig. 9-32). Palisading histiocytes and giant cells, as well as frank granulomas, often surround the neutrophilic inflammation. There may be a marked associated fibrotic response.

ANCILLARY STUDIES

Gram stains will reveal the filamentous, gram-positive organisms (Fig. 9-33). GMS and Warthin-Starry stains will also stain actinomycosis. Immunofluorescence studies are also available.

DIFFERENTIAL DIAGNOSIS

The gross differential diagnosis includes abscess of other infectious causes, lymphoma, and carcinoma. The histologic differential primarily includes other infectious processes, particularly *Nocardia*. Unlike *Nocardia*, this organism is not at all acid-fast. Care should also be taken not to confuse actinomycosis with fungi or other bacteria that may form clusters and chains but are not truly filamentous, such as *Pseudomonas* and *E. coli.*

PROGNOSIS AND THERAPY

Most cases require surgical removal of the affected area, or at least drainage of any abscess. Prolonged antibiotic therapy, often intravenous in route and for several months to a year, is recommended following surgical therapy. Actinomyces is susceptible to many antimicrobial agents. Follow-up computed tomography (CT) scan is recommended to assess therapy.

■ FUNGAL INFECTIONS OF THE GASTROINTESTINAL TRACT

The importance of fungal infections of the GI tract has increased in parallel with the numbers of patients with organ transplants, AIDS, and other immunodeficiency states. Signs and symptoms of GI fungal infections are generally similar regardless of type of fungus, and include diarrhea, vomiting, melena, frank GI bleeding, abdominal pain, and fever. Although fungal infections of the GI tract are often a part of a disseminated disease process, GI symptoms and signs may well be the presenting manifestations of disease.

Fungi can often be appreciated in routine H&E sections in fulminant infections, but GMS and PAS stains remain invaluable diagnostic aids. Fungi can also be correctly classified in tissue sections based on morphologic criteria. It should be stressed, however, that if there is any doubt as to classification, fungal culture should be relied upon as the gold standard of speciation; antifungal therapy may vary according to the type of fungus identified. The differential diagnosis of the various

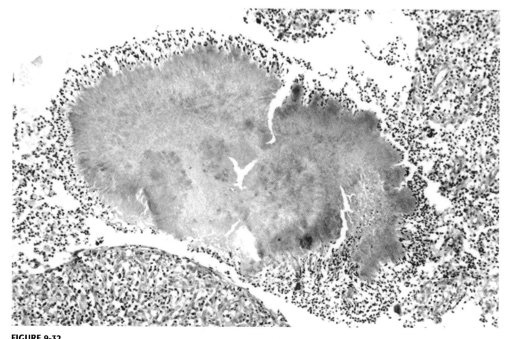

FIGURE 9-32

Clusters of Actinomyces with associated Splendore-Hoeppli material and acute inflammation (H&E). *(Courtesy of Dr. George F. Gray Jr.)*

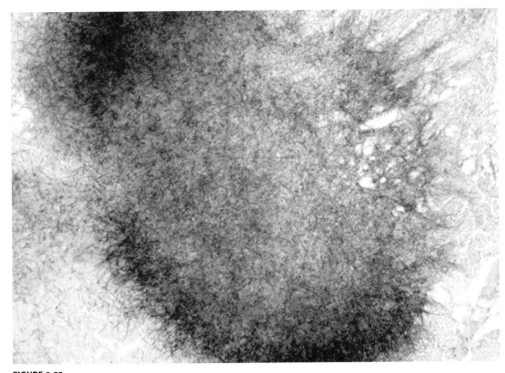

FIGURE 9-33
Filamentous gram-positive bacteria characteristic of actinomycosis are seen on Gram stain (Twort Gram).

types of fungal infection (Table 9-2) as well as helpful ancillary studies are discussed at the end of this section.

CANDIDA

Candida species may be seen at any level of the GI tract, and the GI tract is a major entryway for disseminated candidiasis. Although immunocompromised patients are most frequently affected, immunocompetent

patients can rarely contract GI candidiasis. Infection with *C. albicans* is most common, but *C. tropicalis* and *C. (Torulopsis) glabrata* may produce similar infections. It is unclear whether *Candida* produce a true primary infection, or rather secondarily superinfect preexisting ulcerative lesions of any cause.

PATHOLOGIC FEATURES

GROSS FINDINGS

Gross features of colonic candidiasis include ulceration, enterocolitis that may feature pseudomembranes, and inflammatory masses. If vascular invasion is prominent, the gross appearance of infarcted bowel may be seen. Involvement may be diffuse or segmental; some workers believe that *C. tropicalis* is more likely to be diffuse, more extensively invasive, and involve the entire alimentary tract.

MICROSCOPIC FINDINGS

The associated inflammatory response ranges from minimal if any tissue reaction to organisms (especially in immunocompromised patients) to prominent neutrophilic infiltrates, erosion/ulceration, abscess formation, and necrosis. Granulomas are not usually seen. Fungi may invade to any level of the gut wall, from submucosa to transmural invasion and perforation.

COLONIC FUNGAL INFECTIONS—FACT SHEET

Location
- Anywhere in colon

Clinical Features
- Usually occurs in immunocompromised patients
- Signs and symptoms of GI fungal infections are similar regardless of type of fungus: diarrhea, vomiting, melena, frank GI bleeding, abdominal pain, and fever
- Occasionally mass lesions may form, obstructing the bowel
- Often a part of a disseminated disease process
- GI symptoms and signs may be the presenting manifestations of disease

Prognosis and Therapy
- Most commonly intravenous amphotericin B

TABLE 9-2

Morphologic Features of Fungi Involving the Colon

Organism	Morphologic Features	Histologic Response	Major Differential Diagnoses
Aspergillus species	Hypha-septate uniform width Branching-regular acute angles Conidial head formation in cavitary lesions	Ischemic necrosis with angioinvasion Acute inflammation Occasionally granulomatous	Zygomycetes *Fusarium* *Pseudallescheria boydii*
Zygomycetes	Hypha-pauciseptate ribbon-like thin walls Branching-haphazard Optically clear on cut-section	Similar to *Aspergillus*	Similar to *Aspergillus*
Candida albicans *Candida tropicalis*	Mixture of budding yeast and pseudohyphae; occasional septate hypha	Usually suppurative May be necrotic and ulcerative Occasionally granulomatous	*Trichosporon*
Candida glabrata	Budding yeast; no true hyphae; no "halo" effect	Similar to other *Candida* species	Histoplasmosis *Cryptococcus*
Cryptococcus neoformans	Pleomorphic Narrow-based buds Usually mucicarmine positive Variable in size	Usually suppurative May have extensive necrosis Sometimes granulomatous	Histoplasmosis Blastomycosis *C. glabrata*
Histoplasma capsulatum	Ovoid, narrow-based buds Intracellular "Halo" effect around organism on H&E	Lymphohistiocytic infiltrate with parasitized histiocytes Occasional granulomas	*Cryptococcus* *P. marneffei* *C. glabrata* Intracellular parasites *P. carinii*

H&E, hematoxylin and eosin staining.

Invasion of mucosal and submucosal blood vessels is also a prominent feature of invasive candidal infection. *C. albicans* and *C. tropicalis* produce a mixture of budding yeast forms, hyphae, and pseudohyphae. *C. (Torulopsis) glabrata* features tiny budding yeast forms similar to *Histoplasma*, and does not produce hyphae or pseudohyphae.

CANDIDIASIS—PATHOLOGIC FEATURES

Gross Findings

- Ulceration, enterocolitis that may feature pseudomembranes, or inflammatory masses
- Involvement may be diffuse or segmental
- Appearance of infarction if vascular invasion is prominent

Microscopic Findings

- Prominent neutrophilic infiltrates, erosion/ulceration, abscess formation, and necrosis
- Granulomas rare
- Minimal tissue reaction in many immunocompromised patients
- Fungi may invade to any level of the gut wall, from submucosa to transmural invasion and perforation; may also invade vessels

Differential Diagnosis

- Other fungi (see Table 9-2)

PROGNOSIS AND THERAPY

Intravenous amphotericin B is the treatment of choice for invasive colonic candidiasis.

ASPERGILLUS

Aspergillus species infection of the GI tract occurs almost exclusively in immunocompromised patients. The majority of patients with GI *Aspergillus* infection have coexistent lung lesions. GI signs and symptoms and gross pathologic findings are similar to infection with *Candida* species.

PATHOLOGIC FEATURES

GROSS FINDINGS

The gross findings are similar to those of *Candida* species. Invasion of vessels often produces the classic "target lesion," consisting of a necrotic central area surrounded by hemorrhage. The bowel may appear grossly infarcted, and transmural infarction is common.

ASPERGILLUS—PATHOLOGIC FEATURES

Gross Findings
- Similar to *Candida*
- Target lesions resulting from vascular invasion
- Bowel appears grossly infarcted

Microscopic Findings
- Characteristic nodular infarction consisting of a zone of ischemic necrosis centered on a blood vessel containing fungal organisms
- Fungal hyphae extend outward from the infarct in parallel or radial arrays
- Inflammatory response ranges from minimal to a marked neutrophilic infiltrate
- Granulomatous inflammation is occasionally seen
- Typical hyphae of *Aspergillus* are septate and branch at acute angles

Differential Diagnosis
- Other fungal infections (see Table 9-2)

MICROSCOPIC FINDINGS

The characteristic histologic lesion of aspergillosis is a nodular infarction consisting of a zone of ischemic necrosis centered on a blood vessel containing fungal organisms (Figs. 9-34 and 9-35). The fungal hyphae often extend outward from the infarct in parallel or radial arrays. Inflammatory response ranges from minimal to marked neutrophilic infiltrate; granulomatous inflammation is occasionally seen. The typical hyphae of *Aspergillus* are septate and branch at acute angles (Fig. 9-36).

DIFFERENTIAL DIAGNOSIS

The differential diagnosis consists primarily of other fungal infections (see Table 9-2).

PROGNOSIS AND THERAPY

Amphotericin B is the most commonly used antifungal agent for *Aspergillus* infection, particularly in neutropenic patients. Other useful antifungal agents include ketoconazole, fluconazole, and itraconazole.

MUCORMYCOSIS AND RELATED INFECTIONS

Mucor and related Zygomycetes (formerly phycomycetes) are ubiquitous soil fungi. They are uncommon pathogens in the GI tract and are seen predominantly in immunocompromised patients. These fungi usually

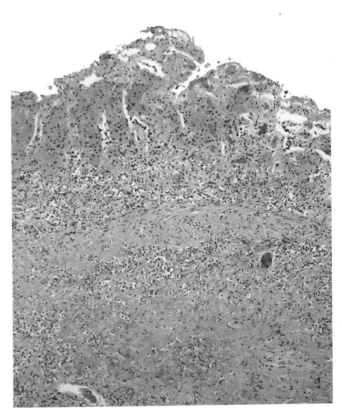

FIGURE 9-34
Aspergillosis. Note nodular focus of ischemic necrosis (H&E).

superinfect tissues that have been previously ulcerated; invasive disease is often fatal. Although many cases of GI phycomycosis are part of a disseminated fungal infection, infection limited to the GI tract has been described.

CLINICAL FEATURES

Immunocompromised patients, particularly those with diabetes or other causes of systemic acidosis, appear to be at increased risk for developing zygomycosis.

PATHOLOGIC FEATURES

GROSS FINDINGS

Any area in the colon may be involved, and the cecum is a common location in the large bowel. The gross features are similar to those produced by *Aspergillus* species. Ulcerative lesions are the most common gross manifestation, and ulcers containing these

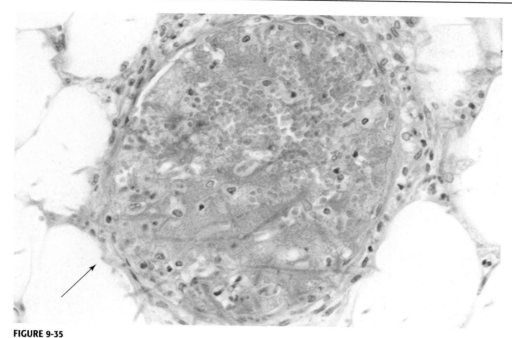

FIGURE 9-35

Aspergillus organisms penetrate a submucosal vessel (H&E).

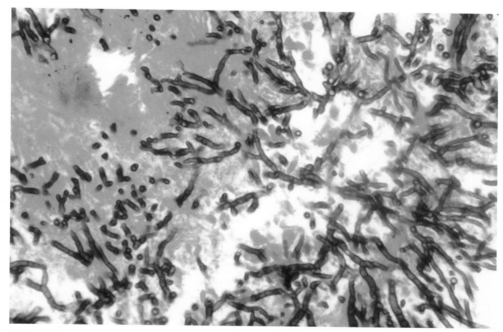

FIGURE 9-36

Aspergillus organisms have septate hyphae that branch at acute angles (GMS).

organisms tend to be large with rolled, irregular edges that may mimic malignancy. The fungal process often invades through the wall to involve and destroy other structures, and may produce large, obstructive masses. Similar to aspergillosis and candidiasis, if large vessels are penetrated and occluded by fungi, infarction may develop, and the gross picture is that of ischemia.

MICROSCOPIC FINDINGS

The inflammatory reaction and presence of intravascular thrombotic lesions are markedly similar to that seen in aspergillosis. Typical organisms have broad, ribbon-like, pauciseptate hyphae that branch randomly at various angles. Transected hyphae have optically clear centers in tissue sections (Fig. 9-37).

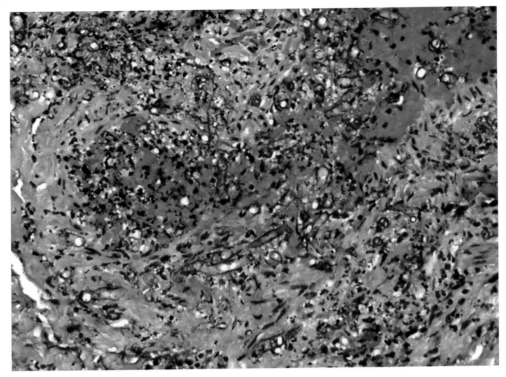

FIGURE 9-37
Mucor organisms, present within a vessel, have broad, ribbon-like pauciseptate hyphae with optically clear centers on cut section (H&E). *(Courtesy Dr. Neriman Gokden).*

MUCORMYCOSIS—PATHOLOGIC FEATURES

Gross Findings

- Similar to *Aspergillus* species, often mimicking infarction
- Ulcerative lesions are the most common gross manifestation, often large with rolled, irregular edges
- Process often invades through wall to involve and destroy other structures
- May produce large, obstructive masses
- If vessels are penetrated, produces ischemic picture

Microscopic Findings

- Inflammatory reaction and presence of intravascular thrombotic lesions are markedly similar to aspergillosis
- Typical organisms have broad, ribbon-like, pauciseptate hyphae that branch randomly at various angles
- Transected hyphae have optically clear centers in tissue sections

Differential Diagnosis

- Other fungi (see Table 9-2)

DIFFERENTIAL DIAGNOSIS

The differential diagnosis is that of other fungal infections (see Table 9-2).

PROGNOSIS AND THERAPY

Amphotericin B is the most commonly used antifungal agent in invasive mucormycosis.

HISTOPLASMOSIS

Histoplasma capsulatum is endemic to the central United States, but has been described in many nonendemic areas as well. It is most abundant in soil enriched with bat or avian droppings. Although disseminated histoplasmosis occurs in the majority of immunocompromised patients who contract the disease, immunocompetent patients may be affected as well, especially young children and elderly persons. GI involvement occurs in approximately 80% or more of patients with disseminated infection. Patients may initially present with signs and symptoms of GI illness and do not always have concomitant pulmonary involvement.

PATHOLOGIC FEATURES

GROSS FINDINGS

Any level of the colon may be involved. Gross lesions include ulcers, nodules, obstructive mass lesions, and normal mucosa (often in immunocompromised patients). A combination of these lesions is commonly seen in a single patient.

MICROSCOPIC FINDINGS

Histologic findings include diffuse lymphohistiocytic infiltrates (Fig. 9-38) and nodules, usually involving the mucosa and submucosa, with associated ulceration. Often these lesions are present overlying Peyer's patches. Discrete granulomas and giant cells are seen in only a minority of cases. In immunocompromised patients, large numbers of organisms may be seen with virtually no tissue reaction. Histoplasma organisms typically are small, ovoid, usually intracellular yeast forms with small buds at the more pointed pole (Fig. 9-39).

DIFFERENTIAL DIAGNOSIS

The differential diagnosis is primarily that of other fungal infections (see Table 9-2).

PROGNOSIS AND THERAPY

Amphotericin is the most commonly used antifungal agent in histoplasmosis.

CRYPTOCOCCUS

Cryptococcus neoformans is an unusual but important cause of GI infection, particularly in immunocompromised patients. Cryptococci have a global distribution and are abundant in avian (especially pigeon) habitats. Virtually all patients with GI cryptococcosis have hematogenously disseminated disease with multisystem organ involvement, and most have pulmonary and meningeal disease.

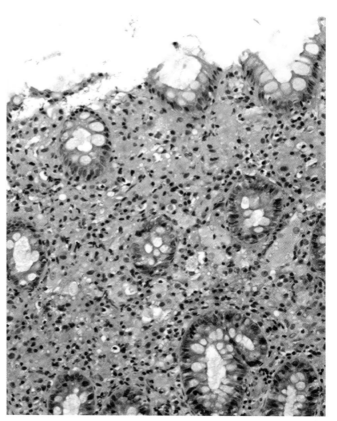

FIGURE 9-38

Histiocytic infiltrate in a colon biopsy from a patient with AIDS with disseminated histoplasmosis. Note "halo" around organism (H&E).

PATHOLOGIC FEATURES

GROSS FINDINGS

Grossly, cryptococcal infection may be present at any location in the colon. Endoscopic lesions include nodules and ulcers, sometimes associated with a thick white exudate; however, no mucosal abnormalities are present in many cases of GI cryptococcosis.

MICROSCOPIC FINDINGS

Histologic features include typical round-to-oval yeast forms with narrow-based budding; cryptococci may show considerable variation in size. Occasionally, cryptococci produce hyphae and pseudohyphae. Often a "halo" effect can be seen on H&E staining, representing the capsule of the organism. Both superficial and deep involvement may occur, and lymphatic involvement is frequent. The inflammatory reaction is variable and depends on the immune status of the host, ranging from a suppurative, necrotizing inflammatory reaction often with granulomatous features, to virtually no reaction at all in anergic hosts. The mucopolysaccharide capsular material stains with

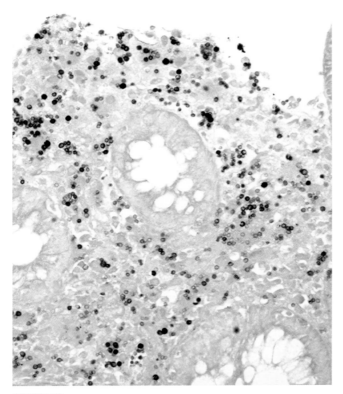

FIGURE 9-39
Fungal stain shows uniformly small yeast forms with buds at the more pointed pole, consistent with histoplasmosis (GMS).

CRYPTOCOCCUS—PATHOLOGIC FEATURES

Gross Findings
- Present at any location in the colon
- Endoscopic lesions include nodules and ulcers, sometimes associated with a thick white exudate
- No mucosal abnormalities are present in many cases

Microscopic Findings
- Round-to-oval yeast forms with narrow-based budding and considerable variation in size
- Often a "halo" effect can be seen on H&E staining, representing the capsule
- Both superficial and deep involvement may occur, and lymphatic involvement is frequent
- The inflammatory reaction ranges from a suppurative, necrotizing inflammatory reaction, often with a granulomatous feature, to virtually no reaction at all in anergic hosts
- Organisms are GMS positive; mucopolysaccharide capsular material stains with Alcian blue, mucicarmine, and colloidal iron

Differential Diagnosis
- Other fungal infections (see Table 9-2)

Alcian blue, Fontana-Masson, mucicarmine (Fig. 9-40), and colloidal iron; GMS stains are of course positive as well. Capsule-deficient cryptococcal infection may present a diagnostic challenge, but most have sufficient capsular material left to be seen on mucin stains.

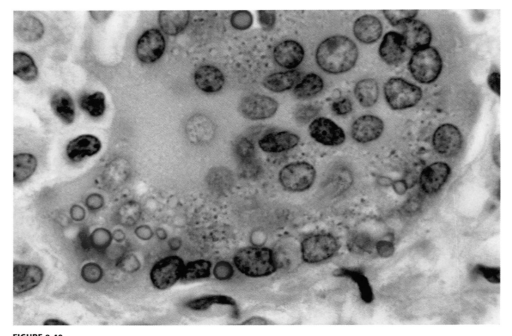

FIGURE 9-40
Cryptococcus within a giant cell (mucicarmine). *(Courtesy of Dr. George F. Gray Jr.)*

DIFFERENTIAL DIAGNOSIS

The differential diagnosis consists of other fungal infections (see Table 9-2).

PROGNOSIS AND THERAPY

Amphotericin B is the most commonly employed antifungal agent. Other fungal infections that are occasionally seen in the GI tract include *Blastomyces dermatididis, Paracoccidioides brasiliensis* (South American blastomycosis), *Pneumocystis carinii,* and *Fusarium.*

The differential diagnosis of fungal infections most often includes other infectious processes; occasionally Crohn's disease, ulcerative colitis, sarcoidosis, and ischemic colitis enter the differential as well. The bigger challenge, once a fungus has been identified, is to properly classify it. Although definite speciation must rely on culture techniques, some attempt can and should be made to classify the organisms on morphologic grounds (see Table 9-2). It is important to remember that fungi exposed to antifungal therapy or ambient air may produce bizarre and unusual forms. Helpful diagnostic aids, in addition to culture, include serologic assays, antigen tests, and immunohistochemistry.

■ PARASITIC INFECTIONS OF THE GASTROINTESTINAL TRACT PROTOZOA

ENTAMOEBA HISTOLYTICA

Approximately 10% of the world's population is infected with this parasite, and the prevalence is much higher in tropical and subtropical locations. Homosexual men are also at increased risk for harboring this pathogen.

CLINICAL FEATURES

Many infected patients are asymptomatic or have only vague, nonspecific GI complaints that may mimic irritable bowel syndrome. Symptomatic patients most commonly have diarrhea, abdominal cramps, and variable right lower quadrant tenderness; this may be referred to as "nondysenteric" amebiasis. Invasive disease, most often manifested as amoebic dysentery or liver abscess, reportedly occurs in less than 10% of infected persons. Amebic dysentery presents suddenly, approximately 1 to 3 weeks after exposure, with severe abdominal

---

AMEBIASIS—FACT SHEET

Definition
- Common protozoal infection, affecting approximately 10% of the population worldwide

Incidence and Location
- Any level of the colon or appendix; cecum most frequent

Clinical Features
- Many patients asymptomatic or with vague, nonspecific GI symptoms
- Some patients suffer fulminant colitis
- May form large inflammatory masses
- Homosexual men at increased risk for infection

Prognosis and Therapy
- Antiparasitic drugs such as metronidazole

---

cramps, tenesmus, fever, and diarrhea (which may be mucoid and/or bloody).

Complications of intestinal amebiasis include bleeding; perforation; dissemination to other sites, particularly the liver; fistula formation between the intestine and the skin, peritoneum, and urogenital tract; and toxic megacolon. The latter complication is often associated with corticosteroid use. Rarely, large inflammatory masses (amebomas) may be formed.

PATHOLOGIC FEATURES

GROSS FINDINGS

Small ulcers are the early lesion, which may coalesce to form large, irregular ulcers that are often "geographic" or serpiginous. Intervening mucosa is often normal. The ulcers have associated inflammatory exudate or adjacent inflammatory polyps. Ulcers may undermine adjacent mucosa to produce the classic "flask-shaped" lesion. The cecum is the most common site of involvement, but any level of the colon or appendix may be involved. Fulminant colitis resembling ulcerative colitis, PMC resembling that caused by *C. difficile,* and toxic megacolon have been described. Colonoscopy may be normal in asymptomatic patients or those with mild disease. Invasive disease generally produces more severe symptoms.

MICROSCOPIC FINDINGS

The earliest lesion is a mild neutrophilic infiltrate. In more advanced disease, ulcers are often deep, extending at least into the submucosa (Fig. 9-41), with undermining of adjacent normal mucosa. There is associated necroinflammatory debris; the organisms are generally

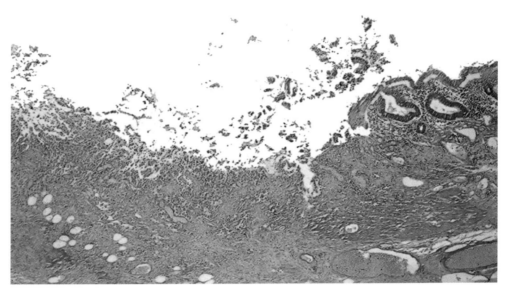

FIGURE 9-41

Colonic amebiasis. Deep ulcer with overlying exudate (H&E).

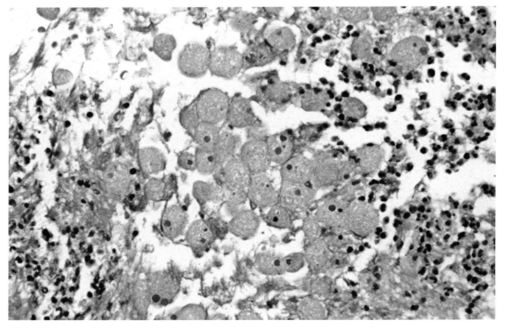

FIGURE 9-42

Entamoeba histolytica organisms have foamy cytoplasm and a round, eccentric nucleus. The presence of ingested red blood cells is pathognomonic of *E. histolytica* (H&E). *(Case courtesy of Dr. Rickey Ryals.)*

found within this purulent material (Fig. 9-42). Invasive amebas are occasionally seen within the bowel wall. The adjacent mucosa is usually normal, but may show gland distortion and inflammation. The organisms, which may be very few in number, resemble macrophages with foamy cytoplasm and a round, eccentric nucleus; the presence of ingested red blood cells is pathognomonic of *E. histolytica*. In patients who are asymptomatic or have mild symptoms, histologic changes may range from normal to a heavy mixed inflammatory infiltrate. Organisms may be particularly difficult (if not impossible) to find in these patients.

ANCILLARY STUDIES

Examination of stool for parasites is a helpful diagnostic test, and serologies are also available.

DIFFERENTIAL DIAGNOSIS

The differential diagnosis most often is that of amebas versus macrophages within an inflammatory exudate. Amebas are trichrome positive; in addition, macrophages stain with immunostains for α_1-antitrypsin and chymotrypsin, whereas amebas do not. Amebiasis can also be confused with Crohn's disease or ulcerative colitis, as well as other types of infectious colitis. The ciliate *Balantidum coli* produces a spectrum of clinical and pathologic changes similar to that of *E. histolytica*. However, *B. coli* organisms are distinguished from amebas by their larger size, kidney bean–shaped nucleus, and cilia (Fig. 9-43).

Two other species of amoeba, *E. dispar* and *E. moshkovskii*, which are histologically indistinguishable from *E. histolytica*, have recently received attention because they have been recovered from the stool of patients with GI symptoms. To date, there is no convincing evidence that *E. dispar* causes symptomatic GI disease, and many studies are confounded by coinfection with *E. histolytica* and other GI pathogens. Some authorities, however, do currently refer to the organism as "*E. histolytica-E. dispar*" complex, resulting from the high rate of coinfection. There are rare reports of symptomatic

infection with *E. moshkovskii*, although many of these are also confounded by coinfection with *E. histolytica* and other pathogens, and thus the true pathogenicity of this species remains controversial. In the context of a patient with symptomatic amebiasis and the microscopic identification of organisms with an accompanying tissue reaction, however, distinction between these species is rarely important for clinical management purposes.

PROGNOSIS AND THERAPY

Antiparasitic drugs such as metronidazole are effective against even invasive amebiasis.

FLAGELLATES

VISCERAL LEISHMANIASIS (KALA-AZAR) CAUSED BY *LEISHMANIA DONOVANI* AND RELATED SPECIES

The prevalence of leishmaniasis is increasing worldwide as a result of immigration, urbanization, and increased numbers of immunocompromised patients. It is endemic in more than 80 countries in Africa, Asia, South and Central America, and Europe. The causative parasite, *Leishmania*, is transmitted via sandfly bites.

CLINICAL FEATURES

GI involvement is generally part of widely disseminated disease. GI signs and symptoms include fever, abdominal pain, diarrhea, dysphagia, malabsorption, and weight loss.

PATHOLOGIC FEATURES

GROSS FINDINGS

Leishmania may be found anywhere in the colon. Endoscopic findings include normal examination, focal ulceration, and changes grossly consistent with enteritis.

MICROSCOPIC FINDINGS

Histologic changes in immunocompetent and immunocompromised persons are similar. Histologic features typically consist of macrophages within the lamina propria containing amastigotes. Often, an associated inflammatory infiltrate is absent. The amastigotes are round to oval, tiny organisms with a nucleus and kinetoplast in a "double-knot" configuration.

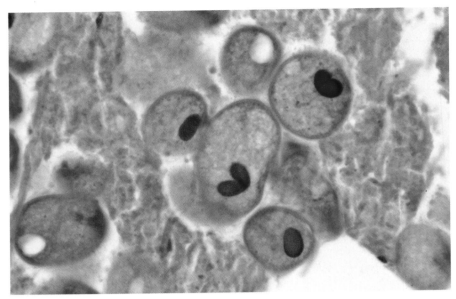

FIGURE 9-43
The ciliate *Balantidum coli* is distinguished from *Entamoeba histolytica* by its larger size, kidney bean–shaped nucleus, and cilia (H&E). *(Case courtesy of Dr. David Owen.)*

LEISHMANIASIS—FACT SHEET

Definition
- Parasitic infection transmitted by sandfly bites, endemic in more than 80 countries in Africa, Asia, South and Central America, and Europe

Incidence and Location
- Anywhere in bowel

Clinical Features
- Part of widely disseminated disease
- Fever, abdominal pain, diarrhea, dysphagia, malabsorption, and weight loss

Prognosis and Therapy
- Pentavalent antimony, amphotericin, pentamidine

LEISHMANIASIS—PATHOLOGIC FEATURES

Gross Findings
- Range from normal to focal ulceration, changes of enteritis

Microscopic Findings
- Macrophages within the lamina propria containing amastigotes
- Amastigotes are round to oval, tiny organisms with a nucleus and kinetoplast in a "double-knot" configuration
- Histologic changes in immunocompetent and immunocompromised persons are similar
- Inflammatory infiltrate is often absent

Differential Diagnosis
- *Histoplasma*
- *T. cruzi* (Chagas' disease)

ANCILLARY STUDIES

Serologic studies and immunohistochemistry may aid in diagnosis.

DIFFERENTIAL DIAGNOSIS

The differential diagnosis is primarily that of other parasitic and fungal infections, and *Leishmania* may be confused with similar organisms such as *Histoplasma* and *Trypanosoma cruzi*. All but *T. cruzi* lack a kinetoplast, and *Leishmania* is GMS, mucicarmine, and PAS negative. *T. cruzi* is seldom visualized in the GI tract, and the resultant inflammatory lesion affects the myenteric plexus rather than the lamina propria.

PROGNOSIS AND THERAPY

Pentavalent antimonial compounds are the first line of therapy in most cases. Other drugs such as amphotericin B and pentamidine are also used.

COCCIDIANS

Although coccidial infection is particularly important when considering diarrhea in a patient with AIDS, coccidians also are important pathogens in healthy persons. They are worldwide pathogens that are more common in, but not limited to, developing countries. Transmission is via the fecal-oral route, either directly or via contaminated food and water.

CLINICAL FEATURES

Coccidians often produce asymptomatic infections in both immunocompromised and healthy patients. All coccidians except microsporidia (which is thought to be limited to the immunocompromised) can cause diarrhea (often prolonged) in healthy patients, especially infants and children, travelers, and the institutionalized. Diarrhea may be accompanied by fever, weight loss, abdominal pain, and malaise. The stool does not usually contain red blood cells or leukocytes. In immunocompetent persons, infection is usually self-limited. Immunocompromised patients are at risk for chronic, severe diarrhea with malabsorption, dehydration, and death.

PATHOLOGIC FEATURES

GROSS FINDINGS

Endoscopic findings are usually absent or mild. When present, they may include mild erythema, mucosal granularity, mucosal atrophy, and mild erosions.

MICROSCOPIC FINDINGS

1. *Cryptosporidium parvum.* Although most commonly seen in the small bowel, *Cryptosporidium* may be seen in the colon as well. The characteristic appearance of the organism is a 2- to 5-mm basophilic spherical body protruding from the apex of the enterocyte (Fig. 9-44). It can be found in the crypts or at the surface. Associated mucosal changes include a mixed inflammatory infiltrate, and crypt abscesses. Organisms stain with the Giemsa stain. *Cryptosporidium* may be distinguished from most other coccidians by their unique apical location; although *Cyclospora* organisms are similar in appearance, they are much larger (8 to 10 mm).

2. *Toxoplasma gondii.* GI toxoplasmosis is primarily a disease of the immunocompromised. Intestinal involvement is a rare feature. Ulcers have been described in the bowel, with *Toxoplasma* organisms in the ulcer base. Both crescent-shaped tachyzoites and cysts containing bradyzoites may be seen within tissue sections.

3. *Microsporidia.* Enterocytozoon bieneusi and Encephalitozoon intestinalis are the most commonly seen in human infection. They are usually seen in the small bowel, but the colon and biliary tree may be affected. These stain with modified trichrome (Fig. 9-45), tissue Gram stain, and silver impregnation stains. *Microsporidia* can be very difficult to detect in H&E sections. The histologic features include a subtle vacuolization of the surface epithelium and a patchy lymphoplasmacytic infiltrate in the lamina propria. Sometimes *Microsporidia* will polarize within tissue biopsies, because the chitin-rich internal polar filament of the organism is birefringent under polarized light. However, this method is unreliable resulting from the unpredictability of spore birefringence, as well as variability depending on the microscope and light source used.

4. *Cyclospora cayetanensis* and *Isospora belli* are only rarely seen in the colon; they are usually found in the small bowel.

COCCIDIANS—FACT SHEET

Definition

- Parasitic infection causing chronic diarrhea, most often in immunocompromised patients; transmitted through fecal-oral route and contaminated food and water

Incidence and Location

- Most commonly small bowel; rarely colon

Clinical Features

- Chronic diarrhea, with or without fever, weight loss, abdominal pain, and malaise
- Stool lacks red blood cells and leukocytes
- Infection is self-limited in immunocompetent persons
- Immunocompromised patients are at risk for chronic, severe diarrhea with malabsorption, dehydration, death

Prognosis and Therapy

- *Cryptosporidium:* no effective treatment
- *Microsporidium:* some efficacy with drugs such as albendazole
- *Toxoplasmosis:* numerous effective antibiotics, especially sulfa drugs

---

COCCIDIANS—PATHOLOGIC FEATURES

Gross Findings

- Usually absent or mild
- Can have mild erythema, mucosal granularity, mucosal atrophy, and mild erosions

Microscopic Findings

- *Cryptosporidium parvum*
  - 2- to 5-mm basophilic spherical body protruding from the apex of the enterocyte
  - In the crypts or at the surface
  - Tissue reaction includes mixed inflammatory infiltrate, crypt abscesses
- *Toxoplasma gondii*
  - Almost always immunocompromised
  - Intestinal involvement is a rare feature
  - Both crescent-shaped tachyzoites and cysts containing bradyzoites can be seen
- *Microsporidia*
  - Tiny organisms in apex of enterocytes
  - Stain with modified trichrome, tissue Gram stain, and silver impregnation stains

Differential Diagnosis

- Primarily other coccidians

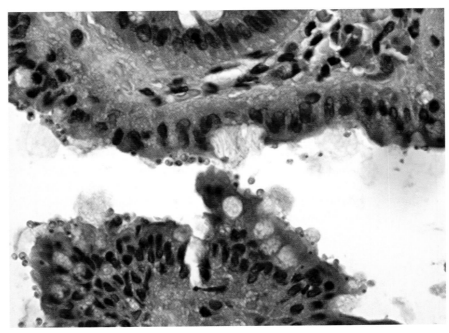

FIGURE 9-44

Colon biopsy from an AIDS patient. Numerous *Cryptosporidia* are seen bulging beneath the surface of enterocytes (H&E).

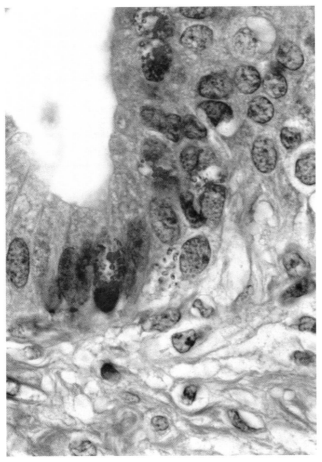

FIGURE 9-45

Tiny *Microsporidia* organisms are present within enterocytes, with minimal inflammatory response (modified trichrome).

ANCILLARY STUDIES

Although electron microscopy was once considered the gold standard for diagnosis of these organisms, it is expensive, subject to sampling bias, and not widely used. Examination of stool specimens may be helpful in many cases. Enzyme-linked immunosorbent assay techniques, immunohistochemistry, and PCR studies are available for many coccidians, although these tests are not widely available to the practicing pathologist.

DIFFERENTIAL DIAGNOSIS

The differential diagnosis is primarily between species of coccidians.

PROGNOSIS AND THERAPY

Most antimicrobial agents are ineffective against cryptosporidial infection, although antimotility agents may provide symptomatic relief. Agents, such as albendazole, are at least anecdotally effective against microsporidial infection in some studies. Antibiotics may be effective against *Cyclospora* and toxoplasmosis.

HELMINTHS (NEMATODES, TREMATODES, AND CESTODES)

Although the most common method of diagnosing GI helminth infections is examination of stool for ova and parasites, these organisms are occasionally seen in biopsy or resection specimens. GI helminths have a worldwide distribution, but their clinical importance varies with geographic region. They are more often a cause of serious disease in underdeveloped nations, because deficient sanitation systems, poor socioeconomic status, and hot, humid climates are predisposing factors. Helminthic infections are becoming an increasingly important problem in immunocompromised patients. The nutritional problems caused by helminths can be severe and even life-threatening, particularly in children. The anatomic site of infection is most often the small bowel, although the large bowel may certainly be involved.

The differential diagnosis of helminthic infections often involves differentiating between types of worm. Other entities to be considered include other causes of ulcerative inflammation, eosinophilic infiltration, and granulomatous inflammation, such as tuberculosis, amebiasis, allergic enteritides, and Crohn's disease.

NEMATODES

ENTEROBIUS VERMICULARIS (PINWORMS)

Pinworms are one of the most common parasites affecting humans. They have a worldwide distribution, but are more common in cold or temperate climates and developed countries. They are extremely common in the United States and Northwestern Europe. The infective larva-containing egg resides in dust and soil, and transmission is believed to be fecal-oral. School children and adolescents, especially those who live in institutions, have the highest prevalence of infection. The worms live and reproduce in the ileum, cecum, proximal colon, and appendix, and the female migrates to the anus to lay her eggs and die. The ability of *Enterobius* to cause colitis and actual mucosal damage is controversial. However, they have been noted to rarely invade the GI mucosa.

CLINICAL FEATURES

The eggs and worms produce the classic symptom of nocturnal pruritus ani. Many infections are asymptomatic, but heavy infections may cause abdominal pain, nausea, and vomiting. Appendicitis, vulvovaginitis, colitis, and peritoneal involvement have been described secondary to pinworm infection.

ENTEROBIASIS—FACT SHEET

Definition
- Common helminthic infection; rarely causes colitis

Incidence and Location
- Anus, appendix, large bowel

Clinical Features
- Perianal itching, primarily nocturnal
- Rarely, colitis and appendicitis

Prognosis and Therapy
- Antiparasitic drugs such as mebendazole

PATHOLOGIC FEATURES

GROSS FINDINGS

Grossly, the worms are 2 to 5 mm in length and may be seen with the naked eye (Fig. 9-46). Although the mucosa of the GI tract often appears normal upon examination, hemorrhage and ulceration are occasionally seen in invasive infection.

MICROSCOPIC FINDINGS

Although even invasive pinworms usually incite little or no inflammatory reaction, as discussed previously, an inflammatory infiltrate composed of neutrophils and eosinophils may occasionally be seen. Granulomas, sometimes with necrosis, may be seen as well, often associated with degenerating worms or eggs. These lesions have been described within the omentum and peritoneum, as well as in the appendix, anus, and colon in rare cases.

ENTEROBIASIS—PATHOLOGIC FEATURES

Gross Findings
- Worms are 2 to 5 mm in length
- Mucosa often appears normal on examination
- Hemorrhage and ulceration are occasionally seen in invasive infection

Microscopic Findings
- Usually little or no inflammatory reaction
- Rarely, an inflammatory infiltrate composed of neutrophils is present
- Granulomas, sometimes with necrosis, can be associated with degenerating worms or eggs
- Worm morphology: lateral ala with easily visible intestine and uterus (in the female); eggs are ovoid with one flat side, and have a bilayered refractile shell

Differential Diagnosis
- Other helminths

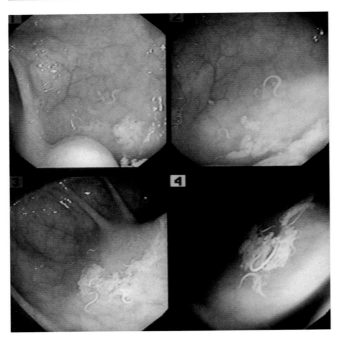

FIGURE 9-46

Pinworms are 2 to 5 mm in length and are easily visible on colonoscopy. *(Courtesy of Dr. William A. Webb.)*

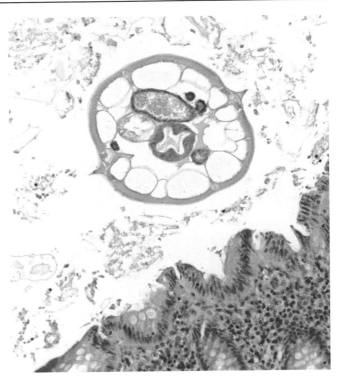

FIGURE 9-47

Pinworms have prominent lateral ala and an easily visible intestine (H&E).

ANCILLARY STUDIES

Stool examination for ova and parasites has a relatively low yield. Inspection of the perianal area for worms, and the anal "scotch tape test" are the most helpful diagnostic aids.

DIFFERENTIAL DIAGNOSIS

The differential diagnosis is primarily other types of worms. Pinworms have lateral ala (Fig. 9-47) with an easily visible intestine and uterus (in the female). The eggs are ovoid with one flat side, and have a bilayered retractile shell. It may be difficult to distinguish between primary *Enterobius* infection and infection complicating a preexisting inflammatory lesion such as an inflamed anal fissure.

PROGNOSIS AND THERAPY

Most infections clear spontaneously, although this may require several weeks. However, treatment with antiparasitic drugs such as mebendazole is recommended to prevent transmission to others, and for symptomatic cases.

ASCARIS LUMBRICOIDES (ROUNDWORM), *ANCYLOSTOMIASIS* (HOOKWORM), AND *TRICHURIS TRICHIURA* (WHIPWORM)

These worms are rarely a problem in diagnostic biopsies but may cause significant GI complications, including bleeding, malabsorption, anemia, obstruction, and diarrhea. *Ascaris* is one of the most frequent parasites in humans. It has a worldwide distribution but is most common in the tropics. These worms are ingested from soil contaminated from feces. Hookworms (*Necator americanus* and *Ancylostoma duodenale*) are a common parasite in virtually all tropical and subtropical countries. Whipworms are also a soil-borne helminth with a worldwide distribution.

CLINICAL FEATURES

Clinical findings in *Ascaris* infection are variable and include appendicitis, massive infection with obstruction and perforation, childhood growth retardation, and pancreaticobiliary obstruction. Hookworms attach to the intestinal wall and suck blood from villous capillaries, resulting in anemia. Other clinical symptoms include abdominal pain, diarrhea, hypoproteinemia, and an associated cough with eosinophilia as the worms migrate. Mesenteric adenitis secondary to hookworm infection has also been described. The anemia may lead to significant growth retardation in children. Whipworm infection is often asymptomatic, but infection may cause diarrhea, GI bleeding, malabsorption, anemia, and appendicitis.

PATHOLOGIC FEATURES

Ascaris organisms are very large worms (up to 20 cm) that may be identified endoscopically or at resection if obstruction occurs (Fig. 9-48). Tissue damage occurs primarily at attachment sites. Hookworms affect all levels of the GI tract. Endoscopically, the worms (about 1 cm in length) are visible to the naked eye. Pieces of worm may be visible on biopsy; although other histologic changes are usually minimal, an eosinophilic infiltrate is sometimes seen. Whipworms are found predominantly in the right colon and ileum. They may cause gross mucosal hemorrhage and ulceration; the worms are 3 to 5 mm long with a characteristic whiplike tail, and can be seen endoscopically. Histologically, the worms thread their anterior ends under mucosal epithelium, which may produce enterocyte atrophy and an associated mixed inflammatory infiltrate; crypt abscesses may be present as well. Whipworm infection also may rarely mimic Crohn's disease.

ANCILLARY STUDIES

Stool examination for ova and parasites is a helpful diagnostic test.

DIFFERENTIAL DIAGNOSIS

The differential diagnosis is primarily that of other helminthic infections. An ulcerative inflammatory process similar to Crohn's disease has been described associated with both whipworm and hookworm infection.

PROGNOSIS AND THERAPY

Antihelminthic treatment is recommended, and similar drugs may be used against all three worms. Intestinal obstruction (particularly in *Ascaris* infection) may require surgery. Iron supplementation may be required for infections causing anemia.

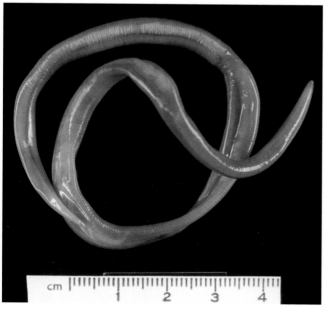

FIGURE 9-48

Ascaris organisms measure up to 20 cm in length and are easily seen with the naked eye.

STRONGYLOIDES STERCORALIS

This nematode has a worldwide distribution. In the United States, it is endemic in the Southeast, urban areas with large immigrant populations, and mental institutions. This infection occurs primarily in adults, many of whom are hospitalized, suffer from chronic illnesses, or are immunocompromised. *S. stercoralis* penetrates the skin, enters the venous system, travels to the lungs, and then migrates up the respiratory tree and down the esophagus to eventually reach the small intestine. The female lives in the small intestine and lays eggs there, thus perpetuating the cycle. This capability of autoinfection allows it to reside in the host and produce illness for upwards of 30 years.

CLINICAL FEATURES

Symptoms and signs include diarrhea, abdominal pain and tenderness, nausea, vomiting, weight loss, malabsorption, and GI bleeding. GI symptoms may be accompanied by rash, eosinophilia, urticaria, pruritus, and pulmonary symptoms. However, many patients are asymptomatic. *S. stercoralis* can disseminate in immunocompromised patients, causing severe and even fatal illness.

PATHOLOGIC FEATURES

GROSS FINDINGS

Lesions may be seen in the stomach, as well as the small and large intestines. Endoscopically, colonic findings include ulcers, which may be aphthoid, and pancolitis; features of PMC have also been reported.

MICROSCOPIC FINDINGS

Histologically, both adult worms and larvae may be found in the crypts (Figs. 9-49 and 9-50), but they may be difficult to detect. Adult worms typically have sharply pointed tails that may be curved. Other histologic features include ulcers (which may be fissuring), edema, and a dense eosinophilic and neutrophilic infiltrate. Granulomas may also be seen, often mixed with eosinophilic and neutrophilic infiltrates.

ANCILLARY STUDIES

Stool examination is the primary ancillary technique for diagnosis.

STRONGYLOIDIASIS—FACT SHEET

Definition
- Helminthic infection infecting the bowel; may cause fatal disseminated disease in immunocompromised patients

Incidence and Location
- Large bowel, small bowel, stomach

Clinical Features
- Diarrhea, abdominal pain and tenderness, nausea, vomiting, weight loss, malabsorption, and GI bleeding
- Often accompanied by rash, eosinophilia, urticaria, pruritus, and pulmonary symptoms
- Many patients are asymptomatic
- May disseminate in immunocompromised patients, causing fatal illness

---

STRONGYLOIDIASIS—PATHOLOGIC FEATURES

Gross Findings
- Ulcers, which may be aphthoid
- Pancolitis
- PMC rarely reported

Microscopic Findings
- Both adult worms and larvae may be found in the crypts
- Adult worms typically have sharply pointed tails that may be curved
- Histologic features include ulcers (which may be fissuring), edema, and a dense eosinophilic and neutrophilic infiltrate
- Granulomas may also be seen

Differential Diagnosis
- Other infectious processes, especially other helminthic infections
- Crohn's disease
- Ulcerative colitis
- PMC

DIFFERENTIAL DIAGNOSIS

The differential diagnosis is primarily that of other helminthic infections and infectious processes, although the histologic inflammatory pattern may mimic PMC, Crohn's disease, and ulcerative colitis.

PROGNOSIS AND THERAPY

Antihelminthic treatment with agents such as thiabendazole is required.

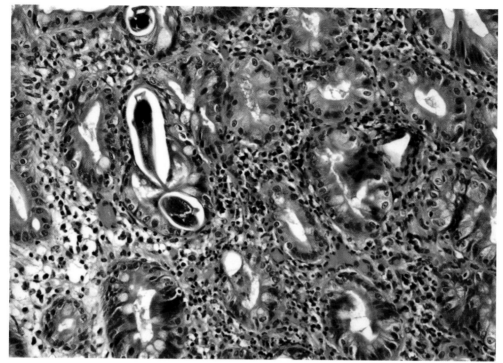

FIGURE 9-49

Strongyloides organisms within colonic crypts (H&E).

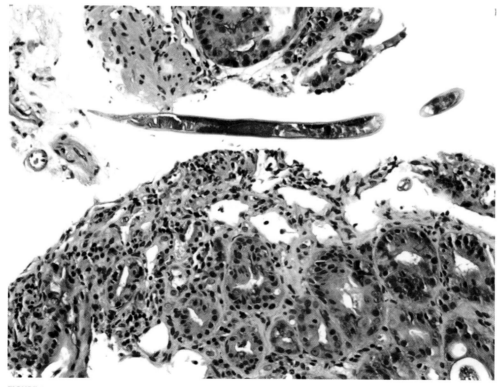

FIGURE 9-50

Strongyloides larva at the surface of the bowel (H&E).

ANISAKIS SIMPLEX (ANISAKIASIS) AND RELATED SPECIES

These nematodes parasitize fish and sea mammals, and humans generally ingest them when eating raw and pickled fish.

CLINICAL FEATURES

The most common clinical manifestations are those of acute gastric anisakiasis; however, colonic manifestations have been well described, presenting with abdominal pain and distention, often accompanied by peripheral eosinophilia. The allergenic potential of *Anisakis* species has also been recognized, and some patients with gastroallergic anisakiasis manifest both GI and hypersensitivity symptoms such as urticaria, angioedema, eosinophilia, and anaphylaxis.

PATHOLOGIC FEATURES

GROSS FINDINGS

The stomach is the most frequent site of involvement, although small bowel, colon, and appendix may also be involved. Endoscopic findings include mucosal edema, friability, hemorrhage, erosions, and ulcers. Sometimes larvae may be seen endoscopically.

MICROSCOPIC FINDINGS

Histologic findings include an inflammatory infiltrate rich in eosinophils, which often extends transmurally into serosal and mesenteric tissues. Eosinophilic microabscesses, granulomas, and giant cells may also be seen. The inflammatory changes may be centered around a worm. Larvae (ranging from 0.5 to 3.0 cm in length) are occasionally seen in tissue sections.

ANCILLARY STUDIES

No ancillary studies are helpful in anisakiasis, because worms and larvae are rarely seen in stool samples.

DIFFERENTIAL DIAGNOSIS

The differential diagnosis primarily includes other worms. The size and morphology of the worm usually confirm the diagnosis.

PROGNOSIS AND THERAPY

Endoscopic removal of the worm is the therapy of choice.

ANISAKIASIS—FACT SHEET

Definition
- Parasitic infection most often associated with consumption of raw fish

Incidence and Location
- Rare in colon and small bowel; common in stomach

Clinical Features
- Abdominal pain and distention
- Peripheral eosinophilia
- May cause gastroallergic anisakiasis, featuring both GI and hypersensitivity symptoms such as urticaria, angioedema, eosinophilia, and anaphylaxis

Prognosis and Therapy
- Endoscopic removal of worm

ANISAKIASIS—PATHOLOGIC FEATURES

Gross Findings
- Mucosal edema, friability, hemorrhage, erosions, and ulcers
- Larvae may be seen endoscopically

Microscopic Findings
- Inflammatory infiltrate rich in eosinophils, often extends transmurally into serosal and mesenteric tissues
- Eosinophilic microabscesses, granulomas, and giant cells may also be seen
- Inflammatory changes may be centered around a worm
- Larvae occasionally seen in tissue sections

Differential Diagnosis
- Primarily other helminths

TREMATODES

SCHISTOSOMIASIS

All species of *Schistosoma* are capable of causing significant GI disease. In addition, patients with *Schistosoma*-related liver disease may also have associated portal colopathy and GI bleeding.

CLINICAL FEATURES

Patients generally present with diarrhea (often bloody), accompanied by anemia, weight loss, and protein-losing enteropathy. More dramatic GI presentations have also been described, including profound dysentery-like illness, obstruction, perforation, intussusception, rectal prolapse, fistulas, and perianal abscesses.

PATHOLOGIC FEATURES

GROSS FINDINGS

Any level of the alimentary tract may be affected. Endoscopically, *Schistosoma* can cause a striking inflammatory polyposis (particularly in the distal colon) with associated mucosal granularity, friability, and punctate ulcers and hemorrhages.

MICROSCOPIC FINDINGS

Histologically, inflammatory polyps and mucosal ulcers with associated granulomatous inflammation and an eosinophilic infiltrate are typical. Eggs are occasionally seen in histologic specimens, and sometimes they are calcified. Remote disease may show only calcified eggs with no inflammatory infiltrate (Fig. 9-51).

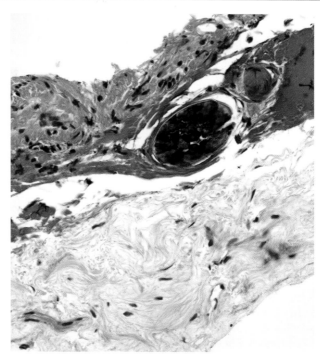

FIGURE 9-51
Remote colonic infection with schistosomes may show calcified eggs with no inflammatory reaction (H&E).

ANCILLARY STUDIES

Stool for ova and parasites is a helpful ancillary test. Serologic testing may also be helpful, especially outside of endemic areas. History of travel to an endemic area may be invaluable.

DIFFERENTIAL DIAGNOSIS

The differential diagnosis is primarily that of other helminthic infections, or other granulomatous infections if eggs or worms are not visible.

PROGNOSIS AND THERAPY

Antiparasitic agents, such as praziquantel, are the treatment for schistosomiasis.

OTHER MISCELLANEOUS HELMINTHIC INFECTIONS

The nematode *Angiostrongylus costaricensis*, endemic to Central America, may cause a dramatic, even fatal, ileocecal infection featuring large obstructive inflammatory masses with perforation and mesenteric vessel thrombosis. *Trichinella spiralis* is a rare cause of diarrhea. Esophagostomiasis, a parasitic disease generally seen in nonhuman primates, may form deep inflammatory masses predominantly in the right colon and appendix.

10

Idiopathic Inflammatory Bowel Disease

■ Theresa S. Emory, MD ■ Leslie H. Sobin, MD

Idiopathic inflammatory bowel diseases include the chronic crypt destructive colitides, chronic ulcerative colitis, and Crohn's disease. Ulcerative colitis and Crohn's disease differ in natural history, clinical and pathologic associations, effective therapies, and response to treatment. These differences, particularly with regard to recommended surveillance strategies and treatment options, underscore the importance of distinguishing between them. While classic cases can be separated, there may be gross, clinical, and histologic overlap of features not only between ulcerative colitis and Crohn's disease but also with other inflammatory conditions of the colon, resulting in an initial diagnosis of indeterminate colitis initially in up to 20% of cases of idiopathic inflammatory bowel disease.

■ ULCERATIVE COLITIS

Ulcerative colitis is a chronic crypt destructive inflammatory process of unknown cause characterized by a predominantly mucosal-based disease and clinically associated with exacerbations and remissions of bloody diarrhea.

CLINICAL FEATURES

Ulcerative colitis has a slightly higher incidence in males, and occurs at all ages, with the major peak incidence in the age range of 15 to 25 years and a minor peak in the seventh decade of life. There is a familial association, with up to 25% of the patients having another affected family member.

Clinically, ulcerative colitis is characterized by recurrent episodes of bloody diarrhea that can undergo spontaneous or therapy-induced remission. The initial presentation may be indolent in onset or may be severe and acute, presenting with toxic hemorrhagic colitis. The clinical diagnosis is rendered following the exclusion of infectious colitis.

ULCERATIVE COLITIS—FACT SHEET

Definition

- Chronic idiopathic inflammatory bowel disease with episodes of bloody diarrhea
- Histologically characterized by mucosal-based chronic crypt destructive colitis with continuous involvement from the rectum extending proximally

Incidence and Location

- Uncommon (4 to 20 per 100,000 population annually)
- Higher incidence in North America, Western Europe, South Africa

Gender, Race, and Age Distribution

- Incidence slightly higher in males than females
- Whites higher incidence than other ethnic groups
- Jews higher incidence than other religious groups
- Rare in first decade of life
- Major peak at 15 to 25 years of age
- Minor peak at 60 to 70 years of age
- Familial association: up to 25% have affected relative

Clinical Features

- Recurrent episodes of bloody diarrhea

Endoscopic Features

- Active phase: mucosa erythematous, bloody, friable, and granular
- Quiescent phase: mucosa granular with punctuate erythema; loss of haustral folds (tubelike appearance)
- Polyps: pseudopolyps (mucosal remnants) and inflammatory polyps in active disease and postinflammatory polyps in active or quiescent disease
- All phases: normal submucosal vascular network is lost

Prognosis and Therapy

- Cure: none
- Low mortality, high morbidity
- Treatment: anti-inflammatory and immunosuppressive drugs; surgery if not responsive
- Increased risk for dysplasia and adenocarcinoma
- Surveillance for dysplasia annually after 8 years
- Colectomy for fulminant disease (toxic colitis), high-grade dysplasia, DALM, and adenocarcinoma
- Ileal pouch anal anastomosis recommended

RADIOLOGIC FEATURES

Endoscopy has virtually replaced radiology in the diagnosis of inflammatory bowel disease. Features that may be seen radiographically in ulcerative colitis include continuous involvement of the colon with ulcers or polyps, no strictures, and the occasional finding of megacolon. Fistulas, "thumbprinting," and skip areas are not seen.

ENDOSCOPIC FEATURES

The gross endoscopic appearance of ulcerative colitis varies with the degree of activity, duration of disease, and response to therapy. It is characterized by diffuse disease, with rectal involvement extending proximally. In the more active phases the mucosa is typically erythematous, bloody, and friable, with a granular appearance (Fig. 10-1). Quiescent disease may appear granular with areas of punctuate erythema (Fig. 10-2). Pseudopolyps (mucosal remnants) and inflammatory polyps may be seen in active disease and postinflammatory polyps in active or quiescent disease (Fig. 10-3). In all cases, the normal submucosal vascular network is lost and is an important clue to the endoscopist that there is chronic colitis. In patients who have had repeated bouts of colitis, the normal haustral folds may be lost, giving the lumen a

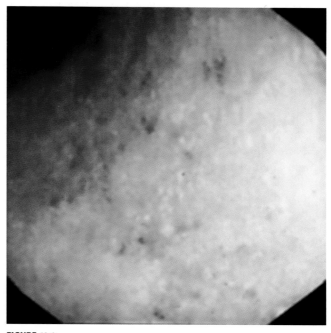

FIGURE 10-2
Relatively quiescent chronic ulcerative colitis. Mucosa is granular with minimal erythema and friability. Mucosal folds are flattened and the submucosal vascular pattern is lost.

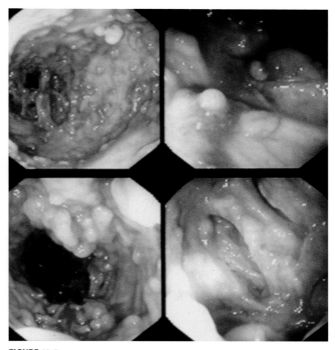

FIGURE 10-3
Chronic ulcerative colitis. Mucosa diffusely involved by polyps and areas of bridging.

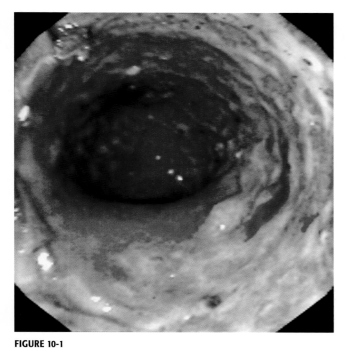

FIGURE 10-1
Endoscopic imagery of chronic ulcerative colitis. Diffuse erythema and granular appearance of active ulcerative colitis.

tubelike appearance. The transition between normal and abnormal mucosa is generally gradual but may be abrupt. Except for the occasional presence of focal cecal and appendiceal involvement, there is no loss of disease continuity and no skip lesions in ulcerative colitis.

PATHOLOGIC FEATURES

GROSS FINDINGS

The serosa is typically unremarkable. Longitudinal opening usually reveals a bowel wall that is of normal thickness, which opens with ease in the fresh state. Strictures are unusual. The mucosa may be flattened, bloody, and friable (Fig. 10-4) or may be granular with numerous polyps. The process grossly extends in a continuous manner from the rectum proximally and may involve the entire colon and appendix and even the terminal ileum (backwash ileitis). If the mucosal involvement extends proximally beyond the splenic flexure, it is designated as pancolitis; if it is confined to the colon distal to the splenic flexure, it is termed left-sided disease. Discontinuity is not a feature of ulcerative colitis except for focal cecal or appendiceal involvement.

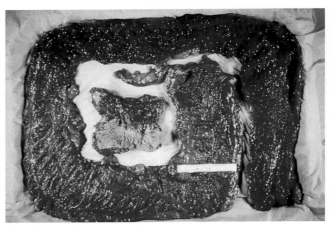

FIGURE 10-4
Resection ulcerative colitis. Diffusely hemorrhagic mucosa extends from the anorectal junction to the cecum. Bowel wall thickness is grossly normal.

ULCERATIVE COLITIS—PATHOLOGIC FEATURES

Gross Findings
- Unremarkable serosa
- Bowel wall of normal thickness
- Mucosa flattened, bloody, friable, and granular with variable numbers of polyps
- Continuous involvement from rectum proximally
- May progressively extend to involve entire colon and terminal ileum
- Focal cecal involvement may be present with distal disease

Microscopic Findings
- Biopsy
- Crypt architectural distortion
- Increased mucosal chronic inflammation
- Neutrophils, the hallmark of active disease, are located within crypt epithelium (cryptitis) and crypt lumens (crypt abscesses)
- Eosinophils may predominate
- Lymphoid aggregates commonly seen at mucosal–submucosal interface
- Regenerating epithelium is immature and does not contain mucin (mucin depletion)
- Biopsy fragments from the same topographic area typically show similar findings
- Inflammation usually more severe distally
- Resection
- Inflammatory process is confined predominantly to mucosal surface with abrupt interface with submucosa; no fissures
- Mucosa often congested
- Decreased numbers of crypts
- Crypts malformed: loss of the normal perpendicular, or "test tube" arrangement of crypts
- Pseudopolyps and postinflammatory polyps, sometimes bizarre in shape
- Submucosa without significant inflammation and lacks fibrosis
- Transmural chronic inflammation and lymphoid aggregates not present except in areas of deep ulceration (in toxic colitis)

Differential Diagnosis
- Infectious colitis
- Medication-induced colitis
- Ischemic colitis
- Crohn's disease

MICROSCOPIC FINDINGS

BIOPSY FINDINGS

Crypt architectural distortion and increased mucosal chronic inflammation are the two characteristic histologic findings (Fig. 10-5). The architectural distortion is the result of prior mucosal destruction and imperfect repair resulting in decreased numbers of crypts and branched malformed regenerated crypts. ("Crypt destructive colitis" refers to the distortion of regenerated crypts rather than active destruction of crypts resulting from cryptitis.) The chronic inflammatory cells consist of variable numbers of plasma cells, eosinophils, and lymphocytes, which expand the lamina propria and extend into the muscularis mucosae (basal plasmacytosis). Eosinophils may predominate. Lymphoid aggregates are commonly seen at the mucosal-submucosal interface. Neutrophils, the hallmark of active disease, are located within crypt epithelium (cryptitis) and crypt lumens (crypt abscesses), and fewer are seen within the lamina propria around the crypts (Fig. 10-6). The regenerating epithelium is immature and as such does not contain mucin, typical of a mature goblet cell (mucin depletion). Biopsy fragments from the same topographic area typically show similar findings. Inflammation is usually more severe distally.

Quiescent, or inactive, ulcerative colitis is characterized by the absence of neutrophils, slight architectural distortion, and mildly increased lymphoplasmacytic infiltrate (Fig. 10-7), sometimes associated with the presence of Paneth cells. Paneth cells are normal in the ascending colon but are considered an indicator of prior mucosal injury and repair in the distal colon.

Ileal involvement by ulcerative colitis ("backwash ileitis") occurs in patients who have severe pancolitis. Inflammation in the ileum is often mild, characterized by mild acute inflammation in the lamina propria and the crypt and villous epithelium. Chronic changes such as villus destruction and repair and pyloric metaplasia,

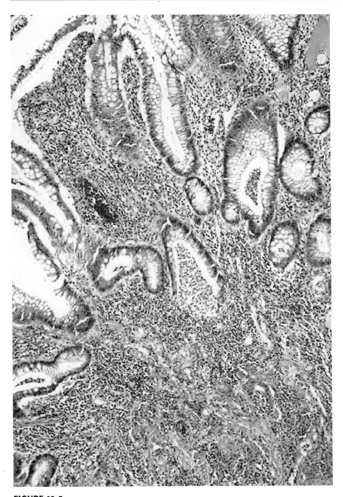

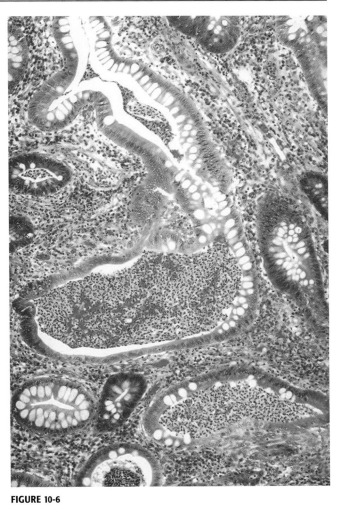

FIGURE 10-5

Endoscopic biopsy: ulcerative colitis. Crypt architectural distortion and branching. Crypt abscess extends into lamina propria; basal plasmacytosis.

FIGURE 10-6

Endoscopic biopsy: ulcerative colitis. Marked inflammation, crypt distortion, and crypt abscesses.

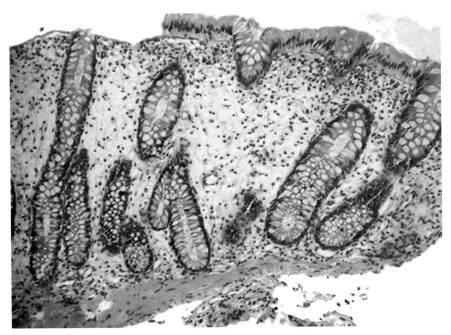

FIGURE 10-7

Ulcerative colitis. Quiescent colitis. Crypt distortion, minimal inflammation.

reminiscent of Crohn's disease, may be seen but are uncommon.

RESECTION FINDINGS

The inflammatory process is confined predominantly to the mucosal surface and has an abrupt interface with the submucosa (Fig. 10-8). The mucosa is, on low power, cellular, often congested, and has decreased numbers of crypts and loss of the normal perpendicular, or "test tube," arrangement of crypts. There may be lymphoid aggregates at the mucosal interface, which can be numerous. In areas of significant activity, ulcers can be adjacent to preserved mucosa. These mounds of residual mucosa surrounded by ulcer are termed pseudopolyps. With time, as the adjacent mucosa regenerates, the mound may protrude, forming a postinflammatory polyp, sometimes bizarre in shape (Fig. 10-9). The submucosa, while often edematous and congested, is typically without significant inflammation and lacks fibrosis. Transmural chronic inflammation and lymphoid aggregates are not present except in areas of deep ulceration, as seen when toxic colitis (toxic megacolon) occurs.

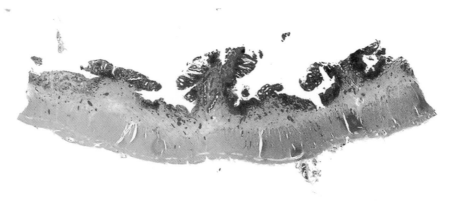

FIGURE 10-8
Low-power resection specimen shows diffuse mucosal inflammation that abruptly stops at the mucosa-submucosa interface. Mucosal remnants appear polypoid (pseudopolyps).

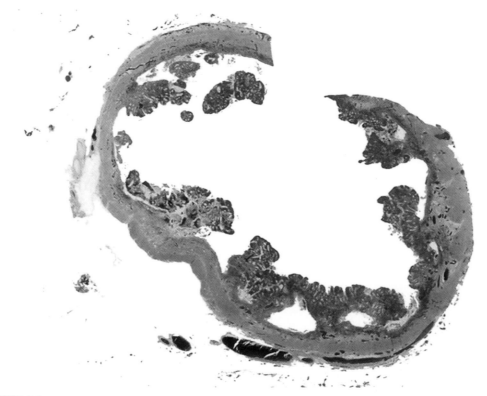

FIGURE 10-9
Ulcerative colitis low-power resection specimen shows diffuse involvement by inflammatory polyps and pseudopolyps with mucosal bridging. Inflammation is confined to the mucosa.

ANCILLARY STUDIES

No specific tests for ulcerative colitis are available. Initially, patients should be tested for infectious causes that are associated with long-standing and toxic colitis, particularly to exclude *Shigella, Salmonella,* and *Campylobacter jejuni.* Patients who have a flare-up of ulcerative colitis while being treated with immunosuppressives may also benefit from testing for cytomegalovirus infection, which can present with deep ulcers in the background of ulcerative colitis. Results of serologic tests for perinuclear antineutrophil cytoplasmic antibody (P-ANCA) are often positive in ulcerative colitis.

DYSPLASIA IN ULCERATIVE COLITIS/DALM (DYSPLASIA-ASSOCIATED LESION OR MASS)

Long-standing ulcerative colitis is associated with an increased risk for dysplasia and adenocarcinoma, even in patients with well-controlled, quiescent disease. Periodic colonoscopic examinations are used to survey for dysplasia and adenocarcinoma. Routine surveillance with biopsies is recommended annually for patients with extensive disease of more than 8 years' duration because there is an increasing annual incidence of adenocarcinoma. Biopsies are generally taken from the cecum, ascending colon, hepatic flexure, transverse colon, splenic flexure, descending colon, sigmoid colon, and rectum. The pathologist records evidence of colitis, activity, and the presence or absence of dysplasia.

GROSS FINDINGS

Dysplasia can be found in both flat, grossly undetectable, and raised mucosa, termed *DALM* (dysplasia-associated lesion or mass). There are no specific features grossly to distinguish between an inflammatory polyp and DALM.

MICROSCOPIC FINDINGS

Dysplasia in ulcerative colitis is characterized by both cytologic and architectural changes of dysplasia including nuclear hyperchromatism, enlargement, and irregularity. The cytoplasm of dysplastic epithelium is often eosinophilic while regenerative epithelium often has a basophilic "blush." Architecturally, there is crypt budding and crowding. Interestingly, dysplasia in ulcerative colitis may appear at the crypt base, in contrast to dysplasia in colonic adenomas, which begins at the surface. Cytologically, low-grade dysplasia is characterized by mild nuclear enlargement and hyperchromasia and small nucleoli. The cells maintain polarity and show mild nuclear overlap and irregularities (Fig. 10-10). High-grade dysplasia is characterized by more pronounced nuclear changes including nuclear pleomorphism, hyperchromasia, and overlap. Architecturally, there is loss of polarity, more crypt crowding complex glands, and glandular distortion (Fig. 10-11).

The presence of a raised dysplastic lesion in the background of ulcerative colitis is termed a *DALM*. Dysplasia can occur in inflammatory polyps (Fig. 10-12). Recent evidence supports differentiating between nonadenoma-like

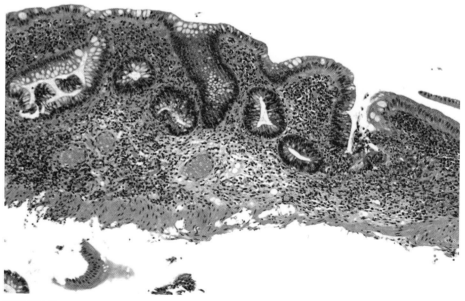

FIGURE 10-10

Dysplasia in ulcerative colitis. Crypt loss and distortion with dysplasia, predominantly at the crypt base, focally extending to the surface.

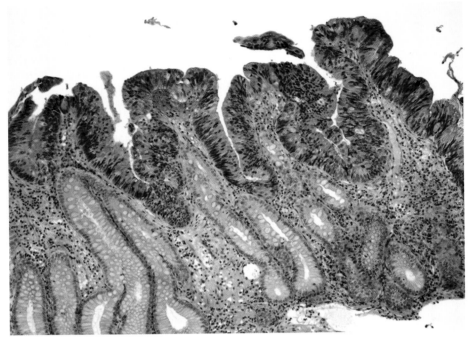

FIGURE 10-11
Dysplasia in ulcerative colitis, focally high grade. Hyperbasophilic enlarged nuclei, focal cribriform glands.

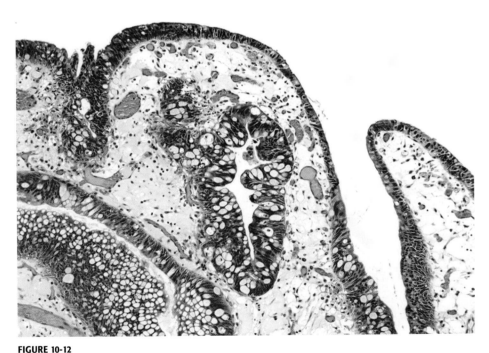

FIGURE 10-12
Dysplasia in ulcerative colitis. Inflammatory polyp with focal low-grade dysplasia. Stratification of nuclei and dystrophic goblet cells with low-grade dysplasia.

DALM and adenoma-like DALM. Nonadenoma-like DALMs are grossly large, irregular, or villiform without a stalk (Fig. 10-13). Colectomy is recommended regardless of the degree of dysplasia because there is often an underlying invasive adenocarcinoma that resulted in the mass. Dysplastic lesions that are endoscopically discrete, well circumscribed, pedunculated, and resemble an adenoma can be treated with polypectomy alone.

Some polypoid lesions in ulcerative colitis do not show the characteristic cytologic features of dysplasia but rather minimal atypia and a serrated appearance. Their relationship to inflammatory bowel disease is unclear.

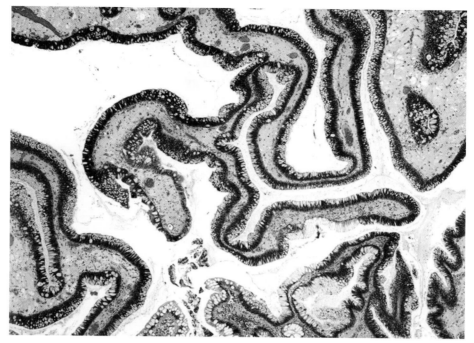

FIGURE 10-13

Dysplasia-associated lesion or mass (DALM). Villiform histology of nonadenoma-like DALM.

DIFFERENTIAL DIAGNOSIS

Ulcerative colitis must be distinguished from infectious colitis, medication-induced colitis, ischemic colitis, Crohn's disease, and pouchitis. Long-standing infectious colitis may have many of the features of ulcerative colitis, including increased chronic inflammation, neutrophils, loss of the inflammatory cell zone (plasma cells in the deep mucosa), and diffuse colonic involvement. A predominance of neutrophils within the lamina propria rather than within the crypt epithelium and overall architectural preservation support an infection over ulcerative colitis. The initial episode of ulcerative colitis may histologically appear similar to infectious colitis; therefore, infectious causes should be excluded prior to confirming a diagnosis of ulcerative colitis. Medications, particularly nonsteroidal anti-inflammatory drugs (NSAIDs) may present with focal acute colitis or one or many ulcers throughout the colon. Histologically, NSAID ulcers are typically abrupt, with no significant inflammation either in the area of ulceration or in the adjacent mucosa. Chronic ischemic colitis can be mistaken for ulcerative colitis, particularly because ischemia resulting from low vascular flow often affects the left colon. Because it may be intermittent, there may be abrupt episodes of ischemia that result in mucosal ulceration, which, following reperfusion, may become inflamed and show all of the architectural features of ulcerative colitis. Features that support ischemia include the age of the patient, location, ischemic involvement of the muscularis propria,

and, importantly, the lack of neutrophils destroying crypt epithelium. Crohn lesions that are characterized by crypt destruction are typically patchy, with areas that appear involved and uninvolved within single biopsy samples and among different fragments from one area. Typically there is not the diffuse crypt destruction seen in ulcerative colitis. Inflammation of the pouch, following proctocolectomy and ileoanal anastomosis, can mimic both ulcerative colitis and Crohn's disease with increased inflammation, architectural distortion, and Paneth cell metaplasia. Lack of crypt destruction and aphthous erosions as well as review of the previous material can help distinguish between pouchitis and inflammatory bowel disease.

PROGNOSIS AND THERAPY

There is no curative therapy for ulcerative colitis. The goals of treatment include inducing and maintaining remission, minimizing side effects, and improving the quality of life. Standard therapy includes anti-inflammatory drugs, specifically, the 5-aminosalicylic acid (5-ASA) compounds (sulfasalazine and other salicylates), which are effective in preventing exacerbations in patients in remission. Steroids, either topical (enemas) or systemic, are effective in treating acute exacerbations.

Most patients have mild to moderately active disease, which does not require colectomy. Mortality is uncommon, most commonly occurring in the first 2 years of disease as the result of severe fulminant disease (toxic colitis). Mortality may also be the result of disease-associated complications, including colorectal carcinoma, primary sclerosing cholangitis, therapeutic complications, and thromboembolic disease. Colectomy is required in up to 20% of patients, usually within the first 2 years resulting from fulminant disease. Colectomy is also performed following the detection of dysplasia or adenocarcinoma.

Patients who are detected to have adenocarcinoma as part of a surveillance program have a significantly better prognosis than those in whom carcinoma is detected following the development of clinical symptoms. Total colectomy is then indicated. Resection with subsequent ileoanal anastomosis allows the patient to have relatively normal bowel function by maintaining the anal sphincter following colectomy.

Additional long-term complications and associated conditions of ulcerative colitis include chronic anemia, hypoalbuminemia, sclerosing cholangitis, ankylosing spondylitis, arthritis, uveal disease, arthritis, vasculitis, and drug-associated complications.

■ CROHN'S DISEASE

Crohn's disease, also referred to as *regional enteritis, granulomatous enterocolitis,* and *terminal ileitis,* is a chronic relapsing and remitting inflammatory disease of unknown cause that is often multifocal and can affect any portion of the gastrointestinal tract. It is typically characterized by foci of glandular destruction, aphthous erosions, and serpiginous ulcers, as well as areas of transmural inflammation, fibrosis, and sometimes granulomas. Because of its transmural nature, fissures, sinuses, and fistulas may occur.

CLINICAL FEATURES

Crohn's disease has a slightly higher incidence in females, and occurs at all ages, with the major peak incidence between 20 and 30 years of age. The initial presentation may be indolent in onset or may be acute and severe. The symptoms are variable but often include cramping pain, typically localized to the right lower quadrant, nonbloody diarrhea, as well as fever, malaise, and anorexia. These findings may mimic acute appendicitis. Although the appendix may be involved with Crohn's disease, appendicitis, as a presenting feature, is considered extremely rare. Hemorrhage and hematochezia are uncommon, but chronic blood loss does occur as a result of erosions and ulcers. Patients with upper intestinal disease may present with dyspepsia, weight loss, hypoalbuminemia, and iron deficiency anemia, mimicking gluten-sensitive enteropathy (celiac sprue). Fistulas between organs (enterovaginal, enterovesical, and enterocutaneous) may result in the passage of blood, feces, pus, and air

---

CROHN'S COLITIS—FACT SHEET

Definition
- A chronic multifocal relapsing and remitting, progressive inflammatory disease of unknown cause that can affect any portion of the gastrointestinal tract
- Typically characterized by foci of glandular destruction, aphthous erosions, and serpiginous ulcers, as well as transmural inflammation, fibrosis, and granulomas in the small and large bowel

Incidence and Location
- Uncommon (5 to 20 per 100,000 population annually)
- Higher incidence in North Americans, Northern Europeans

Gender, Race, and Age Distribution
- Incidence slightly higher in females than males
- Whites higher incidence than other ethnic groups
- Higher incidence among Ashkenazi Jews than other groups
- Major peak at 20 to 30 years of age
- Minor peak at 60 to 70 years of age
- Familial association: approximately 10% have affected relative

Clinical Features
- Cramping pain, nonbloody diarrhea, fever, malaise, and anorexia
- Hemorrhage and hematochezia uncommon
- Upper intestinal disease: dyspepsia, weight loss, hypoalbuminemia, and iron deficiency anemia
- Fistulas, stenosis
- Anal and perianal fissures and fistulas
- Inflammatory changes can occur in joints, eyes, liver, and skin

Endoscopic Features
- Aphthous erosions
- Longitudinal ulcers (train track or rake ulcers) and adjacent unremarkable mucosa
- Cobblestoning
- Strictures
- Fissures and fistulas
- Terminal ileal involvement
- Submucosal vascular network lost
- Often rectal sparing

Prognosis and Therapy
- Cure: none
- Low mortality, high morbidity
- Treatment: anti-inflammatory and immunosuppressive drugs, monoclonal antibody to TN-Fα
- Surgery only for complications or if not responsive to medical therapy
- Increased risk for dysplasia and adenocarcinoma
- Surveillance for dysplasia not defined
- Ileal pouch anal anastomosis contraindicated

---

from the vagina, urethra, or skin. In some cases, fissuring necrosis with fistula formation is the main complication; in others, stenosis resulting from fibrosis predominates. Anal and perianal fissures and fistulas are features of many Crohn's disease cases, but rarely of ulcerative colitis. Inflammatory changes can occur in joints, eyes, liver, and skin. There is a familial association estimated to be approximately 10% of the patients having another affected family member.

RADIOLOGIC FEATURES

As with ulcerative colitis, endoscopy has replaced radiology in the diagnosis of Crohn's disease; however, visualization of small bowel lesions often requires radiologic imaging. Radiographic features typical of Crohn's disease include segmental constriction of the lumen, longitudinal ulcers, cobblestone appearance, and asymmetric ileal involvement. Fistulas and thumbprinting may also be demonstrated.

ENDOSCOPIC FEATURES

Because resection is limited to patients with disease complications, it is important for the pathologist to be familiar with the varied endoscopic findings of Crohn's disease because this can aid in arriving at the correct diagnosis. The gross endoscopic appearance of Crohn's disease is most consistently characterized as a multifocal process (Fig. 10-14). Aphthous erosions (Fig. 10-15), longitudinal ulcers (train track or rake ulcers) (Fig. 10-16), and adjacent areas of erythematous or grossly unremarkable mucosa are hallmarks. Additional endoscopic findings include cobblestoning (irregular mucosa resulting from alternating ulcers and edematous mucosa), strictures, and fissures. The ileum typically shows focal or asymmetric involvement by Crohn's disease. This may include erosions, ulcers, and/or stricture. The rectum is often not involved (unlike ulcerative colitis). Inflammatory polyps

may be present. Rarely, Crohn's disease may become confluent, involving the entire bowel, which can be diagnostically difficult for the endoscopist. In both Crohn's disease and ulcerative colitis, the normal submucosal vascular network is lost in the involved areas, assisting the endoscopist in the diagnosis of chronic colitis. There is little correlation between the endoscopic appearance and the clinical symptoms of the patient.

PATHOLOGIC FEATURES

GROSS FINDINGS

Resection is typically performed only in patients who have severe complications such as obstruction resulting from strictures, fistulas, perforation, severe chronic anemia, abscess, obstruction, or hemorrhage. Because the milder forms of the disease are not resected, the gross pathologic findings are prominent. The subserosal fat is often firm and contracted over areas of involvement, so-called "creeping fat." Longitudinal opening of the bowel may reveal areas with normal bowel wall thickness and other areas of the bowel that are firm, thickened, and pipelike (Fig. 10-17). Interloop adhesions occur. The mucosa may show a variety of changes, including aphthous erosions, longitudinal "rake" ulcers, cobblestoning, polyps, fissures, and fistulas (Fig. 10-18). The process is usually multifocal, often with rectal sparing, but may become confluent. When confluent, the firm pipelike nature of the bowel may help to distinguish Crohn's disease from ulcerative colitis, where fibrosis is unusual.

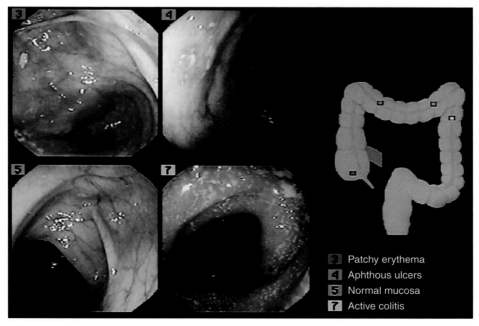

FIGURE 10-14

Crohn's enterocolitis. Multiple areas of involvement and skip areas. Cecal erythema, grossly normal proximal transverse colon, focal aphthous erosions distal transverse, erythema, and narrowing in the descending colon with loss of the submucosal vascular network.

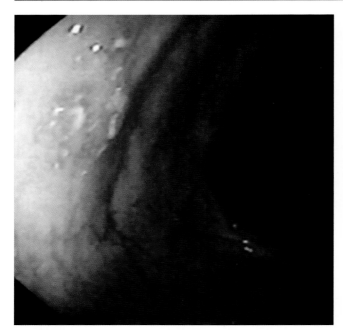

FIGURE 10-15

Crohn's enterocolitis. Aphthous erosions: small, irregular white mucosal erosions with erythematous borders.

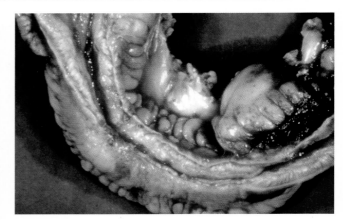

FIGURE 10-17

Crohn's enterocolitis. Narrow, constricted lumen with greatly thickened wall, "pipe stem" bowel.

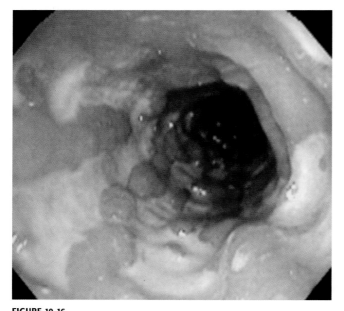

FIGURE 10-16

Crohn's enterocolitis. Longitudinal "rake" ulcers with intervening normal-appearing mucosa.

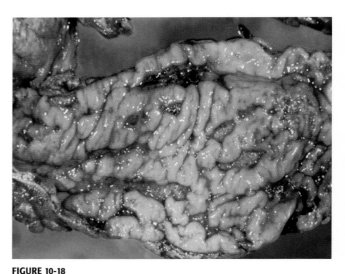

FIGURE 10-18

Crohn's enterocolitis. Resection specimen with longitudinal ulcers and intervening normal mucosa.

MICROSCOPIC FINDINGS

BIOPSY FINDINGS

Mucosal biopsies, although superficial, can show features that are suggestive of Crohn's disease. Discrete foci of inflammation often associated with neutrophils within crypts (cryptitis) and adjacent to histologically normal crypts are common. Aphthous erosions or ulcers, characterized by focal surface epithelial necrosis associated with a mixed chronic inflammatory infiltrate and sometimes associated with underlying lymphoid aggregates, are typical early lesions. Variability of inflammation within a single biopsy sample and among several biopsy fragments from the same anatomic location is also typical. The areas of inflammation show architectural changes of chronic crypt destructive colitis, while adjacent crypts may appear totally normal (Fig. 10-19). Granulomas are infrequently seen, but, when present, are poorly formed, non-necrotizing, and associated with chronic inflammation (Fig. 10-20).

When Crohn's disease involves the terminal ileum, findings include increased lamina propria inflammation, aphthous erosions, and flattened and broad villi. Pyloric metaplasia (mucinous glands, reminiscent of the antral or pyloric mucosa) indicates repeated bouts of inflammation and repair. One must remember that focal acute ileitis is most commonly caused by medications, particularly NSAIDs, rather than Crohn's disease. Medication-induced injury is usually not associated

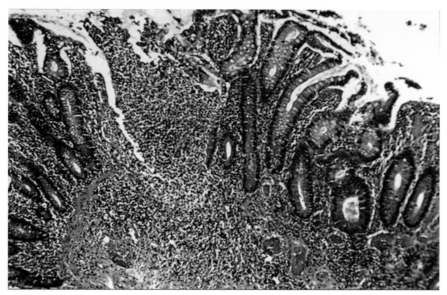

FIGURE 10-19
Endoscopic biopsy. Crohn's enterocolitis. Aphthous erosion: focal mucosal disruption with polymorphs over a lymphoid nodule. Adjacent crypts appear relatively normal.

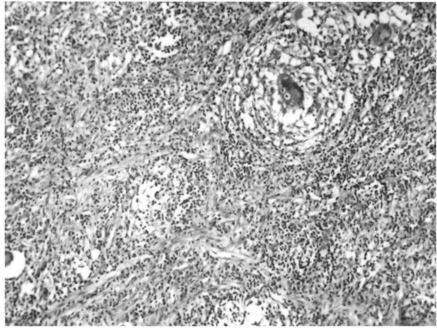

FIGURE 10-20
Crohn's enterocolitis. Poorly formed, non-necrotizing granuloma associated with marked chronic inflammation.

with increased lamina propria inflammation or pyloric metaplasia. Peyer's patches are a normal component of the terminal ileum, particularly in young individuals, and should not be mistaken for chronic inflammation. The mucosa over Peyer's patches may be distorted with flattened villi resulting from underlying expansion of lymphoid nodules in nonspecific reactive hyperplasia or from infections (e.g., yersiniosis).

If submucosa is present in the biopsy, there may be significant submucosal chronic inflammation, while the overlying mucosa may only be slightly expanded by

chronic inflammatory cells, a feature that is not seen in infectious colitis or ulcerative colitis. Submucosal fibrosis can also be a sequel to NSAID damage.

RESECTION FINDINGS

The inflammatory process is multifocal, with areas of submucosal fibrosis and transmural inflammation, including transmural lymphoid aggregates, which are a hallmark of Crohn's (Figs. 10-21 through 10-23). Lymphoid aggregates in the subserosa and submucosa are often oriented

CROHN'S COLITIS—PATHOLOGIC FEATURES

Gross Findings

- Subserosal fat firm and contracted over areas of involvement ("creeping fat")
- Areas of firm, thickened, and pipelike bowel
- Interloop adhesions
- Aphthous erosions
- Longitudinal "rake" ulcers
- Cobblestoning
- Inflammatory polyps
- Fissures
- Fistulas
- Multifocal
- Rectal sparing
- Occasional confluent involvement

Microscopic Findings

- Biopsy
- Discrete foci of inflammation and architectural changes adjacent to histologically normal crypts
- Aphthous erosions often associated with underlying lymphoid aggregates
- Variability of inflammation within a single biopsy and among several biopsy fragments from the same anatomic location
- Granulomas uncommon and, if present, are poorly formed, and associated with chronic inflammation
- Submucosal chronic inflammation disproportionate to that in the overlying mucosa
- Terminal ileal involvement: aphthous erosions, distorted, flattened villi, pyloric metaplasia
- Resection
- Ulcers separated by histologically normal edematous mucosa
- Fissures, sinuses, and fistulas
- Submucosal fibrosis
- Transmural inflammation
- Neural hyperplasia
- Lymphoid aggregates in subserosa and submucosa

Differential Diagnosis

- Infectious colitis
- Medication-associated colitis
- Ulcerative colitis
- Pouchitis

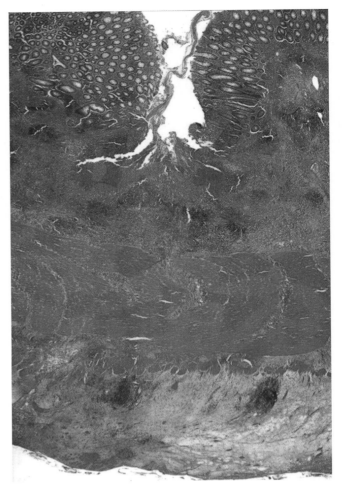

FIGURE 10-21

Resection specimen: Crohn's enterocolitis. Low power. Aphthous erosion associated with transmural inflammation and submucosal fibrosis.

to dilated lymphatics. Granulomas, when present, are typically poorly formed and may be located at any level of the bowel wall. Ulcers are typically longitudinally oriented, separated by histologically normal edematous mucosa. Fissures, sinuses, and fistulas with associated abundant inflammation may be seen. Transmural inflammation occurs away from deep ulcers, a feature helpful in distinguishing from ulcerative colitis. Neural hyperplasia is common in the submucosa and muscularis propria.

ANCILLARY STUDIES

No specific tests for Crohn's colitis are available. However, as with ulcerative colitis, exclusion of infectious etiologies is important, particularly *Yersinia* infection. A serologic test for anti–*Saccharomyces cerevisiae* antibody

(ASCA) appears to be promising; the results are positive in approximately 70% of patients with Crohn's disease and usually negative in ulcerative colitis patients. In cases in which there is difficulty distinguishing between ulcerative colitis and Crohn's colitis, performance of both ASCA and P-ANCA tests may help in the differential diagnosis because P-ANCA test results are positive in approximately 70% of patients with ulcerative colitis and in 10% to 30% of patients with Crohn's disease. There is overlap of results between Crohn's disease and ulcerative colitis, and although these tests may be helpful, further research is needed.

DIFFERENTIAL DIAGNOSIS

Crohn's colitis must be distinguished from infectious colitis, medication-associated colitis, and ulcerative colitis. The endoscopic finding of focal aphthous erosions of early Crohn's colitis may be similar to erosions caused by medications and infections. Histologically, the erosions of Crohn's colitis are associated with a chronic inflammatory infiltrate. Infectious colitis is characterized by a predominance of neutrophils rather than lymphocytes and plasma cells. Medication-induced (NSAIDs and others) erosions usually have negligible acute inflammation, and typically only a few neutrophils are seen in the area of erosion. The more advanced changes of Crohn's colitis, particularly discrete ulcers and masses seen endoscopically, must be distinguished from medications and infection. NSAID ulcers may be multiple and deep. They tend to be found on the top of mucosal folds and are circumferential rather than longitudinal. Biopsies often show fibrosis with only minimal inflammation. NSAID strictures may form; when these are circumferential, they appear like and are termed "diaphragms." Bowel wall thickening and heaped up masses may be seen in *Yersinia* infection, particularly in the terminal ileum and right colon. The presence of marked inflammation histologically with numerous granulomas and the clinical information of a mass or stricture may lead to a diagnosis of Crohn's disease in a patient with yersiniosis. Features that suggest *Yersinia* infection over Crohn's disease include numerous granulomas, granulomas centered in lymphoid follicles, and granulomas with central polymorph-rich suppuration. Any specimen with numerous granulomas should raise suspicion of infection over Crohn's disease.

Fulminant Crohn's colitis can be difficult or impossible to distinguish from ulcerative colitis in a mucosal biopsy specimen because many of the distinguishing features are deep to the mucosa. Furthermore, in fulminant (toxic) ulcerative colitis, inflammation may become transmural. In resection specimens, the most important features are the presence of transmural lymphoid aggregates and the presence of occasional poorly formed granulomas at all levels of the bowel wall. The effects of treatment can also cause diagnostic difficulty because treated ulcerative colitis may show areas of involved and uninvolved mucosa and variable degrees of activity. It is important to review original pretreatment material, if possible, to help distinguish between ulcerative colitis and Crohn's colitis because patients with ulcerative colitis are candidates for ileal pouch anal anastomosis and those with Crohn's disease are not, because of the high risk for pouch failure resulting from anastomotic breakdown. Patients who have undergone ileal pouch anal anastomosis following proctocolectomy for ulcerative colitis may develop inflammation in the ileal pouch, which can mimic Crohn's disease. The lack of crypt destruction and aphthous erosions and a review of the previous biopsies and the resection specimen can be helpful in avoiding a misdiagnosis of Crohn's disease. In some cases, serologic testing for P-ANCA and ASCA may be helpful.

PROGNOSIS AND THERAPY

There is no cure for Crohn's disease. The goals of treatment focus on inducing and maintaining remission, minimizing side effects, and improving the quality of life.

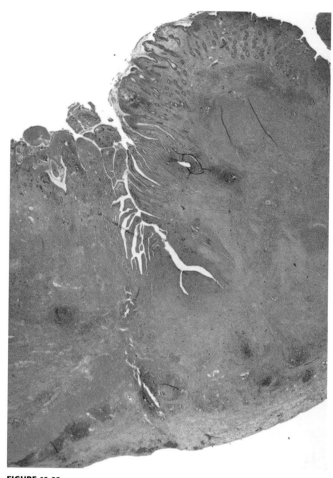

FIGURE 10-22

Resection specimen: Crohn's enterocolitis. Marked submucosal fibrosis associated with transmural and subserosal lymphoid aggregates. Fissuring ulceration.

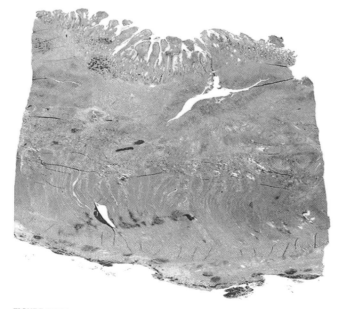

FIGURE 10-23

Resection specimen: Crohn's enterocolitis. Greatly thickened bowel wall with distorted mucosa, fissure, submucosal fibrosis, and transmural lymphoid aggregates.

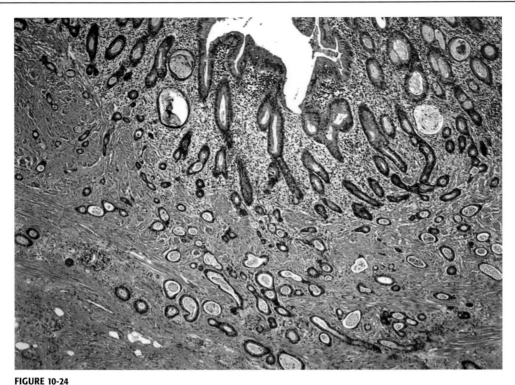

FIGURE 10-24
Adenocarcinoma arising in Crohn's disease. Well-differentiated adenocarcinoma arising in Crohn's disease extending into the bowel wall.

Standard therapy includes anti-inflammatory drugs, specifically the 5-ASA compounds (sulfasalazine and other salicylates) and steroids. Recently, infliximab, a monoclonal antibody against tumor necrosis factor-α, has been found to be helpful in treating acute episodes of Crohn's colitis, particularly fistulas and other complications. Budesimide, a topical steroid that is taken orally, has also been shown to be effective in treating ileal Crohn's disease. It is locally absorbed and metabolized in the liver, minimizing the systemic side effects seen with other steroids.

Surgery is reserved for those patients who have disease that is unresponsive to therapy, resulting in severe anemia, and to those cases in which there are complications such as obstruction, non–infliximab-responsive fistulas, sepsis, and carcinoma. Patients who have undergone surgical intervention are at increased risk for requiring additional surgery resulting from anastomotic complications such as strictures with resultant obstruction, anastomotic leaks, and fistulas.

Recent improvements in therapy have markedly decreased the mortality and morbidity associated with Crohn's disease. The most significant complications are seen in the first few years of disease, possibly because younger patients tend to have more active disease, perhaps resulting from an active immune system, which diminishes with age. The most common complications include perianal fistulas, toxic colitis, and anemia, as well as arthritis and drug-associated problems. It is interesting that patients who have strictures tend not to have fistulas and vice versa.

There is an increased risk for adenocarcinoma in patients with Crohn's disease, estimated to be 4 to 20 times more than those without Crohn's disease. Adenocarcinomas may arise in a morphologically normal bowel, in areas of stricture, and within fistula tracts, making diagnosis difficult. Multiple synchronous or metachronous adenocarcinomas may occur and involve the large and small intestines. Well-differentiated adenocarcinomas may arise in mucosa that has low-grade dysplasia or even questionable dysplasia and may take the form of deceptively bland glandular structures such as those reported by Levi and Harpaz (Fig. 10-24). Well-differentiated mucinous adenocarcinomas that arise in chronic anal fistulas can be difficult to distinguish from non-neoplastic fistula lining. Overall mortality for adenocarcinomas arising in Crohn's disease is high, approximately 80%. This may be caused by the similarities between symptoms of Crohn's disease relapse and symptoms of developing cancer, resulting in delayed diagnosis. Dysplasia does occur in patients with Crohn's disease, but no standard surveillance strategy has been advocated as a result of the technical difficulty in surveying the bowel. Unlike ulcerative colitis, resection is not always advocated for dysplasia because of the risk for postoperative complications.

11

Inflammatory/Descriptive/Iatrogenic Colitides

■ Joel K. Greenson, MD

■ COLLAGENOUS COLITIS

CLINICAL FEATURES

Patients with collagenous colitis (CC) present with a history of chronic watery diarrhea. Colonoscopy typically shows normal or near normal mucosa, although there are a few reports of linear mucosal tears that were thought to occur upon insufflation during endoscopy. This has been referred to as "cat scratch colon" because of the endoscopic appearance. In addition, there are rare reports of CC with pseudomembranes. Affected females largely outnumber males, and most patients are middle-aged or older.

It appears as though a luminal antigen or antigens are important in the pathogenesis of CC. Diversion of the fecal stream causes the histologic changes of CC to regress, while reestablishing the fecal stream induces a relapse. Studies have shown a strong association of CC with use of nonsteroidal anti-inflammatory drugs (NSAIDs) and with celiac disease. Other medications have also been associated with CC, including selective serotonin reuptake inhibitors (SSRIs), proton pump inhibitors, simvastatin, and lisinopril.

PATHOLOGIC FEATURES

At low power, biopsy specimens of CC often show a pink subepithelial "stripe" with an intact crypt architecture and an increase in superficial lamina propria mononuclear

---

COLLAGENOUS COLITIS—FACT SHEET

Definition
- Chronic nondistorting colitis with characteristic subepithelial collagen deposition and surface epithelial damage

Incidence and Location
- 1 to 2.3 per 100,000 population
- Generally involves the entire colon, but relative rectal or left-sided sparing can be seen
- Subepithelial collagen may be patchy

Gender, Race, and Age Distribution
- Female predominance (males to females, 1:8)
- Primarily affects middle-aged to older adults
- Mean age, 59 years

Clinical Features
- Chronic watery diarrhea with normal or near normal endoscopy

Prognosis and Therapy
- Most patients respond to symptomatic or anti-inflammatory therapy.

COLLAGENOUS COLITIS—PATHOLOGIC FEATURES

Gross Findings
- Usually normal gross appearance
- Rarely linear ulcers or pseudomembranes

Microscopic Findings
- Subepithelial collagen deposition (10 to 30 μm vs. normal 2 to 5 μm)
- May be patchy and spare the rectum/left colon
- Collagen encircles superficial capillaries and may have an irregular lower border; shown by trichrome stain
- Surface damage with increased intraepithelial lymphocytes
- Increased lamina propria plasma cells, often superficial
- Occasional foci of cryptitis or neutrophils in surface epithelium
- Little if any crypt distortion
- Paneth cell metaplasia may predict worse prognosis (refractory disease)

Differential Diagnosis
- Lymphocytic colitis
- Radiation colitis
- Ischemic colitis
- Mucosal prolapse/SRUS
- Ulcerative colitis
- Crohn's disease
- Normal mucosa with a thick basement membrane
- Enema effect

LYMPHOCYTIC COLITIS—FACT SHEET

Definition
- Chronic nondistorting colitis typified by increased intraepithelial lymphocytes and surface damage

Incidence and Location
- 3.1 per 100,000 population
- Generally involves the whole colon, but may have distal sparing

Gender, Race, and Age Distribution
- Males to females, 1:1
- Primarily affects middle-aged to older adults
- Mean age of onset 51 years

Clinical Features
- Chronic watery diarrhea with normal or near normal endoscopy

Prognosis and Therapy
- Most patients respond to symptomatic or anti-inflammatory therapy

LYMPHOCYTIC COLITIS—PATHOLOGIC FEATURES

Gross Findings
- Usually normal gross appearance

Microscopic Findings
- Surface damage with increased intraepithelial lymphocytes
- Increased lamina propria plasma cells, often superficial
- May have occasional foci of cryptitis or neutrophils in surface epithelium
- Little, if any, crypt distortion

Differential Diagnosis
- Collagenous colitis
- Resolving infectious colitis
- Colonic epithelial lymphocytosis associated with chronic food- or water-borne epidemics
- Crohn's disease
- Normal mucosa overlying a lymphoid aggregate
- Lymphocytic enterocolitis

intraepithelial lymphocytes there (Fig. 11-5). One should also recognize that normally there are more intraepithelial lymphocytes in the right colon compared with the left colon. A few foci of cryptitis or a rare crypt abscess may be seen in LC, but more neutrophilic inflammation than this suggests another diagnosis. Recently it was recognized that some cases of LC have less surface damage and more intraepithelial lymphocytes in the deeper crypt epithelium. Another variation of LC has been described with collections of histiocytes and poorly formed granulomas underneath the surface epithelium.

DIFFERENTIAL DIAGNOSIS

The differential diagnosis of LC is somewhat narrower than CC. The resolving phase of infectious colitis can mimic LC, because there can be surface damage and a modest increase in intraepithelial lymphocytes.

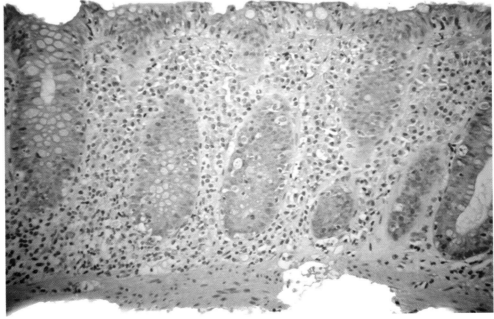

FIGURE 11-4

Lymphocytic colitis. This low-power view shows intact crypt architecture with a plasmacytosis of the lamina propria. Note the normal basement membrane and the increase in intraepithelial lymphocytes.

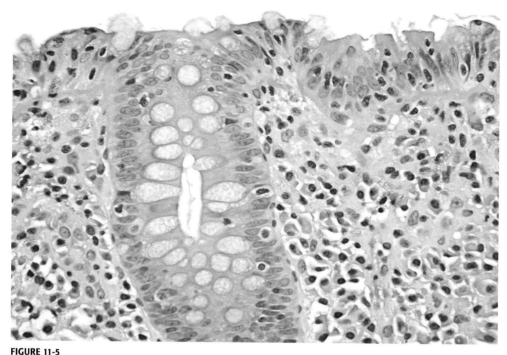

FIGURE 11-5

Lymphocytic colitis. This high-power view shows a marked increase in intraepithelial lymphocytes and a normal basement membrane (contrast with Figs. 11-1 through 11-3). Note the increase in lamina propria plasma cells and eosinophils.

Lymphocytic colitis-like changes have also been described in an outbreak of chronic diarrhea linked to the water supply on a cruise ship. This so-called colonic epithelial lymphocytosis seemed to have less surface damage than in LC. Reports have also been made of LC-like histology in patients with constipation as well as in patients with endoscopic abnormalities. Hence, it is important for the pathologist to make sure the clinical history is consistent with LC before making this diagnosis. There are also reported cases of Crohn's disease with patchy areas showing an LC-like pattern. Collagenous colitis may be confused with lymphocytic cases when only rectal biopsy samples are obtained or when the subepithelial collagen table in CC is patchy and fairly thin.

PROGNOSIS AND THERAPY

Therapy for LC is variable and is largely identical to that used for CC. Some patients' symptoms resolve spontaneously, while others may require over-the-counter diarrheals, bismuth subsalicylate, 5-aminosalicylic acid compounds, or immunosuppressants. Overall, the prognosis is good, because eventually most patients respond to some form of therapy. However, there is a small subset of patients who have LC and sprue-like changes in their small bowel biopsies that seem refractory to all therapy. These patients have been classified as having lymphocytic enterocolitis, although some investigators have raised the possibility that these patients have a lymphoproliferative disorder.

ISCHEMIC COLITIS

CLINICAL FEATURES

Ischemia can give rise to a wide range of clinical presentations depending on the duration and severity of the underlying pathology. While many cases of ischemia occur in older patients with known cardiovascular disease, ischemic colitis can also be seen in younger seemingly healthy people secondary to medications or previous abdominal surgery. Symptoms may range from transient bloody diarrhea or abdominal pain to a full-blown surgical emergency resulting from an infarcted bowel.

While lack of blood flow to the mucosa is the ultimate cause of ischemic colitis, there is a long list of conditions that can lead to this. Ischemic necrosis may be caused by atherosclerosis, low-flow states secondary to hypovolemia, vasculitis, adhesions, various drugs, and even long-distance running (Fig. 11-6). In some instances the drug may induce vasospasm (catecholamines, cocaine), while in other cases the medication may lead to thrombosis (estrogens). Enterohemorrhagic strains of *Escherichia coli* (such as *E. coli* O157:H7) can also cause an ischemic-type colitis, presumably resulting from fibrin thrombi that develop during this toxin-mediated infection.

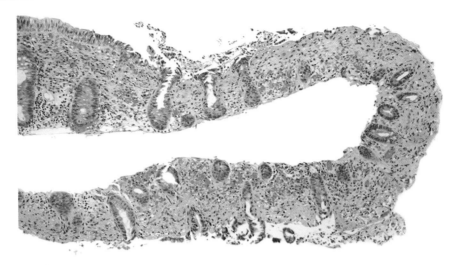

FIGURE 11-6
Ischemia. This low-power view shows superficial mucosal necrosis with loss of surface epithelium and preservation of deep portions of colonic crypts. There is hyalinization of the lamina propria with a paucity of inflammation.

ISCHEMIC COLITIS—FACT SHEET

Definition
- Damage to the colon secondary to decreased blood flow

Incidence and Location
- 3 per 10,000 population
- The splenic flexure and descending and sigmoid colon are the most common sites of ischemia, but any site in the colon can be involved
- The rectum is the least common site for ischemia

Gender, Race, and Age Distribution
- Males equal to females
- Most patients are older than 50 years, but younger patients and even children can have ischemia, depending on the underlying disease processes that may be involved

Clinical Features
- Presentation is variable depending on severity and underlying etiology
- Abdominal pain, bloody diarrhea, vomiting, and fever may be seen

Radiologic Features
- Barium enema shows "thumbprinting"
- CT can show "target lesions"
- Angiography can be used to identify vascular lesions

Prognosis and Therapy
- A majority of ischemic colitis cases resolve with supportive care, but 15% to 20% require surgical intervention
- Complications include perforation, peritonitis, and stricture formation

ISCHEMIC COLITIS—PATHOLOGIC FEATURES

Gross Findings
- Geographic ulcers or infarcts, pseudomembranes, submucosal edema, strictures

Microscopic Findings
- Superficial mucosal necrosis, hyalinized lamina propria, withered or atrophic crypts, pseudomembranes, chronic ulcers/strictures

Differential Diagnosis
- *Clostridium difficile* colitis
- Enterohemorrhagic *E. coli*
- NSAID damage
- Crohn's disease
- Radiation colitis
- Collagenous colitis
- Dysplasia

RADIOLOGIC FEATURES

The classic radiologic finding of ischemia on a barium enema study is that of "thumbprinting." This finding is produced by marked submucosal edema. Computed tomographic (CT) findings of circumferential bowel wall thickening may also be a marker for ischemia.

PATHOLOGIC FEATURES

GROSS FINDINGS

Ischemia typically shows geographic areas of ulceration that may have pseudomembranes. This is often accompanied by marked submucosal edema. Endoscopically this submucosal edema can be prominent enough to mimic a tumor or mass lesion. The watershed areas around the splenic flexure are the most common sites for ischemia, but nearly any site can be involved, including the proximal rectum. Chronic or healed ischemic lesions may form isolated strictures that resemble Crohn's disease.

MICROSCOPIC FINDINGS

Acute ischemic lesions of the colon show superficial mucosal necrosis that may spare the deeper portions of the colonic crypts (Fig. 11-7). The remaining crypts typically have a withered or an atrophic appearance. There may be striking cytologic atypia, to the point where care should be taken to avoid overcalling these reactive changes dysplastic. Ischemic colitis may often have pseudomembranes, as well as hemorrhage into the lamina propria and hyalinization of the lamina propria. A trichrome stain can be used to highlight the hyalinization of the lamina propria (Fig. 11-8). While cryptitis and crypt abscesses may be seen, these are usually not prominent. Depending on the severity of the decreased blood flow, these ischemic lesions may regress on their own or lead to perforation and/or stricture formation. The chronic phase of ischemia is often more difficult to diagnose, because the only histologic findings may be strictures and areas of submucosal fibrosis.

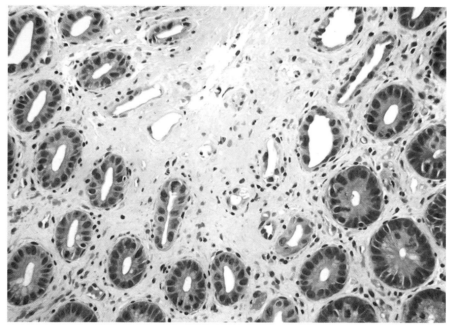

FIGURE 11-7

Ischemia. This high-power view shows atrophic-appearing "micro crypts," which are typical of ischemia. There is also a prominently hyalinized lamina propria. Note the marked regenerative atypia, which can be mistaken for dysplasia.

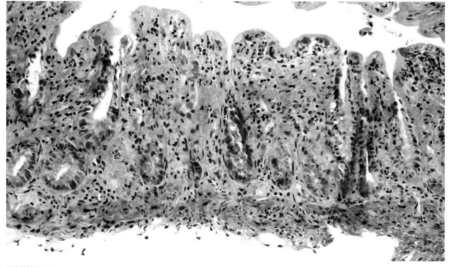

FIGURE 11-8

Ischemia, trichrome stain. This trichrome-stained section shows blue staining of the lamina propria in areas of hyalinization. This feature can help differentiate ischemia from *C. difficile* colitis.

PATHOLOGIC FEATURES

GROSS FINDINGS

The gross and endoscopic features of diversion colitis include erythema, friability, edema, and nodularity with aphthous ulcers.

MICROSCOPIC FINDINGS

Histologically, the nodularity seen grossly corresponds to large lymphoid aggregates with prominent germinal centers (Fig. 11-10). The remaining features of diversion colitis are variable. In some instances, the inflammation may mimic severe ulcerative colitis with crypt distortion and marked chronic inflammation of the lamina propria. In other cases, patchy cryptitis and aphthous lesions may mimic Crohn's disease (Fig. 11-11). As a result of the nonspecific nature of these histologic changes, it is imperative that the pathologist knows that he or she is looking at material from a diverted segment of colon (usually a Hartmann's pouch).

DIFFERENTIAL DIAGNOSIS

Because many people with diverted segments of colon have inflammatory bowel disease, the main differential diagnosis is generally that of recurrent Crohn's disease or ulcerative colitis. The aphthous lesions may also mimic infectious colitis. Definitive diagnosis requires the knowledge that the pathologic changes are occurring in a diverted segment.

PROGNOSIS AND THERAPY

Prognosis is excellent because diversion colitis completely regresses once the fecal stream is reestablished. If this is not possible, then the inflammation can be reversed by giving short chain fatty acids via enemas. Because diversion colitis is frequently asymptomatic, therapy is often not necessary.

colitis is often an incidental finding in asymptomatic patients, some patients may present with mucoid or bloody discharge or abdominal pain. The colitis occurs 3 to 36 months following bypass and completely regresses within 3 months of reestablishment of the fecal stream.

A deficiency of short chain fatty acids is thought to be the cause of diversion colitis. Short chain fatty acids are the main source of energy for colonocytes, and they are usually derived from fermentation of dietary starches by normal colonic bacterial flora. Once the fecal stream is diverted, dietary starches are no longer present. This lack of colonocyte nutrition leads to an inflammatory reaction. The inflammation can be reversed by giving short chain fatty acids via enemas several times a week, or by reestablishing the fecal stream.

RADIOLOGIC FEATURES

Double-contrast barium enemas detect the lymphoid follicular hyperplasia that is characteristic of diversion colitis.

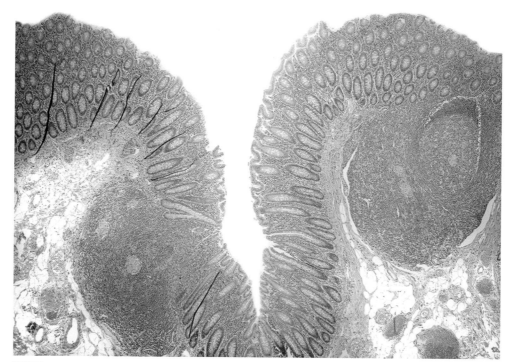

FIGURE 11-10

Diversion colitis. This low-power photomicrograph shows two expanded lymphoid aggregates (one with a large germinal center), which are typical of diversion colitis. The lamina propria also appears slightly hypercellular for the sigmoid colon.

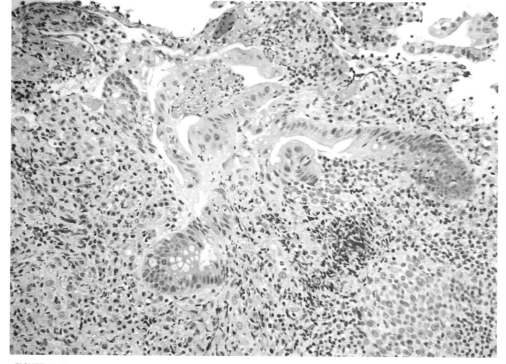

FIGURE 11-11

Diversion colitis. This high-power photomicrograph shows an aphthous lesion (erosion overlying a lymphoid aggregate). Note neutrophils in surface epithelium and luminal exudates.

■ DIVERTICULAR DISEASE–ASSOCIATED COLITIS

CLINICAL FEATURES

Diverticular disease is common among patients older than age 60 years, particularly in the sigmoid colon. Diverticular disease–associated colitis has been described as a chronic segmental colitis present in the distribution of the diverticula that mimics ulcerative colitis. This colitis is restricted to the mucosa and is not a manifestation of diverticulitis. Patients often present with hematochezia.

There is also a form of diverticulitis that mimics Crohn's disease. This form of colitis occurs in patients with diverticulitis who do not have evidence of Crohn's disease elsewhere in the gastrointestinal (GI) tract. The resection specimens demonstrate a Crohn's-like reaction to the diverticulitis.

PATHOLOGIC FEATURES

GROSS FINDINGS

Colonoscopic evaluation generally reveals patchy or confluent hyperemia, often accentuated on the crests of mucosal folds. The mucosa may appear granular, and an exudate is variably present. The distribution is predominantly descending colon and sigmoid, in the region of diverticular disease; the rectum is often spared.

MICROSCOPIC FINDINGS

Histologically one can find a range of changes in the mucosa, from a mild plasmacytosis and mild crypt distortion to a full-blown ulcerative colitis–like appearance. Cryptitis and crypt abscesses are typically seen (Figs. 11-12 and 11-13).

DIVERTICULAR DISEASE–ASSOCIATED COLITIS—FACT SHEET

Definition
- Segmental colitis resembling ulcerative colitis present in the distribution of diverticula

Incidence and Location
- Sigmoid colon with rectal sparing

Gender, Race, and Age Distribution
- Males equal to females
- Patients are generally 60 years of age or older

Clinical Features
- Patients typically present with hematochezia

Prognosis and Therapy
- Varies from fiber and antibiotics to anti-inflammatory therapies used for ulcerative colitis

---

DIVERTICULAR DISEASE–ASSOCIATED COLITIS— PATHOLOGIC FEATURES

Gross Findings
- Granular mucosa with exudates and crescentic hyperemia in distribution of diverticula

Microscopic Findings
- Cryptitis and crypt abscesses with increased lamina propria chronic inflammation and crypt distortion in distribution of diverticula

Differential Diagnosis
- Ulcerative colitis, Crohn's disease

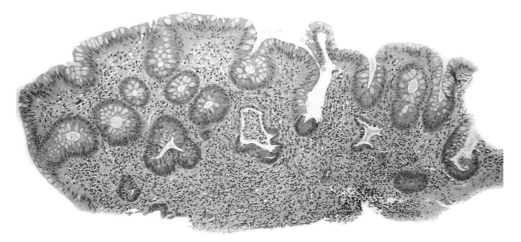

FIGURE 11-12

Diverticular disease–associated colitis. This low-power photomicrograph from the sigmoid colon shows crypt distortion and a chronically inflamed lamina propria. There is a crypt abscess in the center of the image. These changes resemble ulcerative colitis.

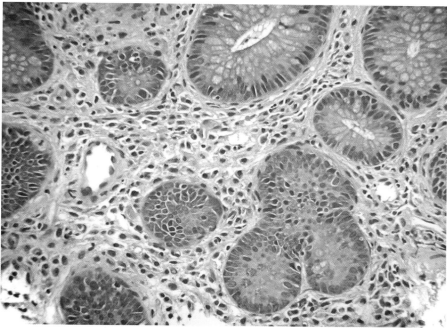

FIGURE 11-13

Diverticular disease–associated colitis. This high-power photomicrograph of the sigmoid colon shows a forked crypt with Paneth cell metaplasia and basal plasma cells, all features indicative of chronic colitis.

DIFFERENTIAL DIAGNOSIS

The main differential diagnosis is between diverticular disease–associated colitis and ulcerative colitis. The key to the correct diagnosis is to recognize that the distribution of disease is identical to the distribution of the diverticula. Crohn's disease is also in the differential diagnosis resulting from the presence of rectal sparing.

PROGNOSIS AND THERAPY

The treatment of diverticular disease–associated colitis varies from therapies aimed at diverticulitis (fiber and antibiotics) to anti-inflammatory therapies similar to those used for ulcerative colitis. Some cases are refractory to medical management and require surgical resection.

■ MUCOSAL PROLAPSE/SOLITARY RECTAL ULCER SYNDROME

CLINICAL FEATURES

Mucosal prolapse presents in a variety of clinical scenarios including those of solitary rectal ulcer syndrome (SRUS), diverticular disease (polypoid prolapsing mucosal folds), and at ostomy sites. SRUS most often occurs in young women with alternating diarrhea and constipation, pain or difficulty defecating, and rectal bleeding. The etiology is thought to be malfunction of the puborectalis muscle such that excessive straining on defecation results. This leads to mucosal prolapse that ultimately may ulcerate and form polypoid masses.

Prolapse polyps also occur in association with diverticular disease, at ostomy sites, and adjacent to other mass lesions, the common denominator being an abnormality that causes mucosal prolapse and resultant injury. When this process occurs at the anal verge and forms a polyp, it is also known as an *inflammatory cloacogenic polyp*. These other forms of mucosal prolapse are typically asymptomatic but are important to recognize so as not to be confused with adenomas or chronic inflammatory bowel disease.

RADIOLOGIC FEATURES

Anal endosonography and defecography can be used to make the diagnosis, with the latter being the gold standard. Prolapse polyps throughout the GI tract may be picked up on barium enemas.

PATHOLOGIC FEATURES

GROSS FINDINGS

Grossly, prolapse polyps are friable, ulcerated polyps with an irregular shape and a beefy, red appearance. The surface may be granular and ulcerated, and occasionally the polyps have an unusual brown color if they contain abundant

MUCOSAL PROLAPSE/SOLITARY RECTAL ULCER SYNDROME—FACT SHEET

Definition
- Benign fibroinflammatory process secondary to mucosal prolapse

Incidence and Location
- 1:100,000
- SRUS in anterior rectum
- Prolapsing polypoid mucosal folds at mouths of diverticula (sigmoid colon) and near colostomy and ileostomy stomas
- Inflammatory cloacogenic polyps at anal verge

Gender, Race, and Age Distribution
- Females more than males (SRUS)
- SRUS in young adults
- Prolapsing polypoid mucosal folds in older patients with diverticular disease (older than 60 years)

Clinical Features
- Alternating diarrhea and constipation, pain or difficulty defecating, and rectal bleeding

Radiologic Features
- Anal endosonography, defecography

Prognosis and Therapy
- Responds well to bulk laxatives and stool softeners
- May require rectopexy or resection

MUCOSAL PROLAPSE/SOLITARY RECTAL ULCER SYNDROME—PATHOLOGIC FEATURES

Gross Findings
- Friable ulcerated polyps/masses on anterior rectal wall or at mouths of diverticula and stomas

Microscopic Findings
- Fibromuscular hyperplasia of the lamina propria
- Hyperplastic regenerative epithelium
- Crypt distortion
- Ulcers

Differential Diagnosis
- Adenoma or carcinoma
- Chronic inflammatory bowel disease
- Peutz-Jeghers polyp

hemosiderin. Endoscopically these lesions can look quite threatening, because the mass lesions mimic carcinoma and the ulcerative lesions mimic Crohn's disease. SRUS is typically located on the anterior rectal wall between 4 and 10 cm from the anal verge, while prolapse polyps associated with diverticular disease are typically found in the sigmoid colon at the mouths of diverticula.

MICROSCOPIC FINDINGS

The characteristic finding in mucosal prolapse at any site is the presence of fibromuscular hyperplasia of the lamina propria. The presence of strands of smooth muscle growing perpendicular to colonic crypts is diagnostic of prolapse. Occasionally, the amount of fibrosis can overshadow the smooth muscle proliferation. The epithelium is often inflamed and ulcerated, and in some cases an ischemic appearance may be present complete with small pseudomembranes. There may be significant crypt architectural distortion. The lamina propria is often vascular, with numerous congested capillaries and hemosiderin deposition. The surface mucosa may be serrated and tufted with goblet cell hypertrophy. In polypoid cases, the mucosa often takes on a villiform configuration that can mimic a villous adenoma (Figs. 11-14 and 11-15). In some cases glands may become trapped in the submucosa, forming what is known as *colitis cystica profunda*.

DIFFERENTIAL DIAGNOSIS

Perhaps the most crucial differential diagnosis is between mucosal prolapse and colorectal neoplasia. SRUS can easily be misinterpreted as a villous adenoma or even an invasive carcinoma, with disastrous consequences for the patient (particularly if an anterior perineal resection is performed). It is important to evaluate the epithelium critically and notice that the changes are reactive/hyperplastic rather than dysplastic. Cases of SRUS with colitis cystica profunda may be mistaken for a well-differentiated mucinous carcinoma. Recognition that the lining epithelium in the cysts is not dysplastic is the key to an accurate diagnosis. Similarly, if the ulcerative component of SRUS is recognized without the characteristic fibromuscular hyperplasia of the lamina propria, an errant diagnosis of chronic inflammatory bowel disease may be rendered. A trichrome stain can be used to confirm the presence of fibromuscular hyperplasia.

Prolapsing polypoid mucosal folds may be confused with Peutz-Jeghers polyps caused by the increase in smooth muscle associated with prolapse. One can usually differentiate the two based on the lack of an arborizing architecture in the smooth muscle of prolapse polyps.

PROGNOSIS AND THERAPY

Prolapse changes are completely benign, and the patient outcome is determined by the underlying disorder. If diverticular disease–associated polyps cause problematic bleeding, they may be excised. Patients with SRUS may respond to nonsurgical management such as bulk laxatives and stool softeners. Patients with severe rectal prolapse may require surgical intervention.

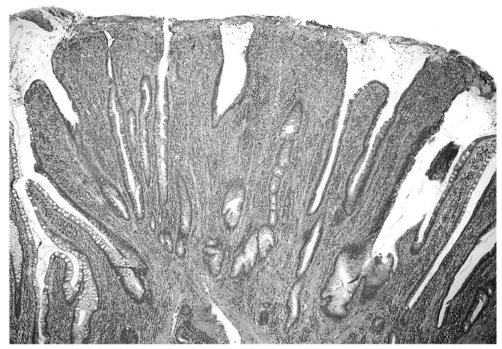

FIGURE 11-14
Mucosal prolapse/solitary rectal ulcer syndrome. This low-power photomicrograph of a solitary rectal ulcer shows villiform hyperplasia with surface ulceration. This villiform growth pattern can be mistaken for a villous adenoma. The base of the crypts is separated by proliferating smooth muscle.

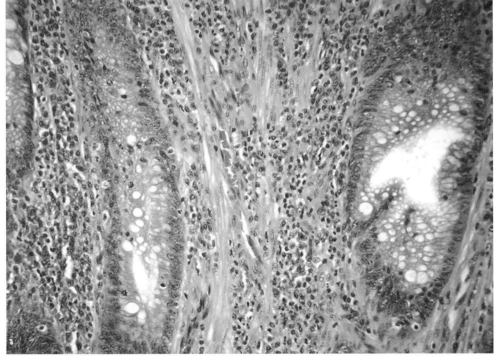

FIGURE 11-15
Mucosal prolapse/solitary rectal ulcer syndrome. This high-power view from the same lesion seen in Figure 11-14 shows smooth muscle twigs growing parallel to the colonic crypts. This smooth muscle proliferation is the hallmark of mucosal prolapse.

■ ALLERGIC PROCTOCOLITIS

CLINICAL FEATURES

Allergic proctocolitis is a disease of infants in the first year of life who develop an allergy to formula or breast milk. Occasionally the allergy is related to food ingested by the mother that is passed to the child via breast milk rather than the breast milk itself. These children present with blood-streaked stools, diarrhea, vomiting, or anemia.

PATHOLOGIC FEATURES

GROSS FINDINGS

Endoscopic features of allergic proctocolitis include focal erythema and friability, as well as rare ulcers or erosions.

MICROSCOPIC FINDINGS

The histologic features of allergic proctitis are often focal and may be subtle. The major finding is that of increased eosinophils, which can be in the lamina propria and within the epithelium and muscularis mucosae (Fig. 11-16). Studies from the northern United States (Boston) have found that the presence of greater than 60 eosinophils per 10 high-power fields

in the lamina propria correlates with allergic proctocolitis. Because the normal number of eosinophils in the lamina propria of the colon varies by geographic region, this number may be inappropriate in more southern climates, where eosinophil counts are higher. The distribution of eosinophils is also important because their presence in the epithelium and muscularis mucosae and at the periphery of lymphoid aggregates correlates with allergy. One may also find foci of cryptitis in allergic proctocolitis.

DIFFERENTIAL DIAGNOSIS

Allergic proctocolitis needs to be distinguished from infectious colitis, necrotizing enterocolitis, and colitis associated with Hirschsprung's disease. Because all of these conditions may show cryptitis, the diagnosis of allergy rests on finding abnormal numbers and distributions of eosinophils.

PROGNOSIS AND THERAPY

Treatment revolves around dietary manipulation to exclude whatever nutrient seems to be causing the symptoms. The prognosis is excellent, because most children outgrow this condition.

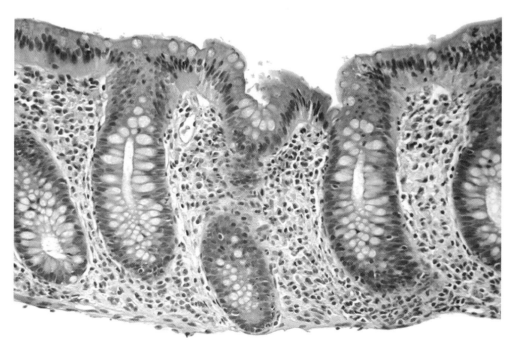

FIGURE 11-16

Allergic colitis. This medium-power photomicrograph of the left colon shows clusters of eosinophils in the lamina propria, as well as several intraepithelial eosinophils. While not overwhelming, this number of eosinophils may be all that is seen in infants with allergic colitis.

ALLERGIC PROCTOCOLITIS—FACT SHEET

Definition
- A disease of infants in the first year of life who develop an allergy to formula or breast milk

Incidence and Location
- 0.5% to 10% of pediatric population (lower in exclusively breastfed infants)
- Rectum most common site of involvement

Gender, Race, and Age Distribution
- Males equal to females
- Age: 1 month to 1 year

Clinical Features
- Blood-streaked stools, diarrhea, vomiting, and anemia

Prognosis and Therapy
- Change diet to eliminate allergen
- By age 3 years, most children outgrow the allergy

ALLERGIC PROCTOCOLITIS—PATHOLOGIC FEATURES

Gross Findings
- Focal erythema and friability, as well as rare ulcers or erosions

Microscopic Findings
- Greater than 60 eosinophils per 10 high-power fields in the lamina propria
- Eosinophils in the epithelium, muscularis mucosae, and at the periphery of lymphoid aggregates
- Cryptitis

Differential Diagnosis
- Infectious colitis, necrotizing enterocolitis, and colitis associated with Hirschsprung's disease

■ MYCOPHENOLATE MOFETIL COLITIS

CLINICAL FEATURES

Mycophenolate mofetil (MMF) is a drug used for immunosuppression, largely in patients who have undergone solid organ transplants. It is also used in bone marrow transplant patients to treat graft-versus-host disease (GVHD), and it may be used to help treat various autoimmune diseases. Patients taking MMF may present with a wide variety of GI complaints including diarrhea, abdominal pain, malabsorption, weight loss, and bleeding. Symptoms are more likely to occur if MMF therapy is started later after transplantation or if the patient has an elevated creatinine measurement.

PATHOLOGIC FEATURES

GROSS FINDINGS

Ulcers and erosions may be seen throughout the GI tract.

MICROSCOPIC FINDINGS

MMF damage in the colon is typified by apoptosis similar to GVHD (Fig. 11-17). In addition one may find dilated attenuated crypts containing a few eosinophils or neutrophils floating within the crypt lumen (Fig. 11-18). In severe cases, there may be crypt dropout with only small nests of residual endocrine cells in the lamina propria. Over time, a fair amount of crypt distortion may develop such that the changes mimic chronic inflammatory bowel disease (Fig. 11-19). Often the lamina propria appears hypocellular resulting from the immunosuppressive effects of MMF.

MYCOPHENOLATE MOFETIL COLITIS—FACT SHEET

Definition
- Damage to the colon secondary to the drug mycophenolate mofetil (CellCept)

Incidence and Location
- Incidence is unknown, but more likely if patient's creatinine level is elevated or if drug is started later in the transplant course
- Location can be anywhere in the GI tract

Gender, Race, and Age Distribution
- There are no predilections known for gender, race, or age

Clinical Features
- Diarrhea, abdominal pain, weight loss, bleeding

Prognosis and Therapy
- Rapid response once drug is discontinued or dose is lowered

MYCOPHENOLATE MOFETIL COLITIS—PATHOLOGIC FEATURES

Gross Findings
- Ulcers or erosions throughout GI tract

Microscopic Findings
- Apoptosis, dilated crypts with eosinophils/neutrophils, crypt distortion

Differential Diagnosis
- GVHD, chronic IBD, ischemia

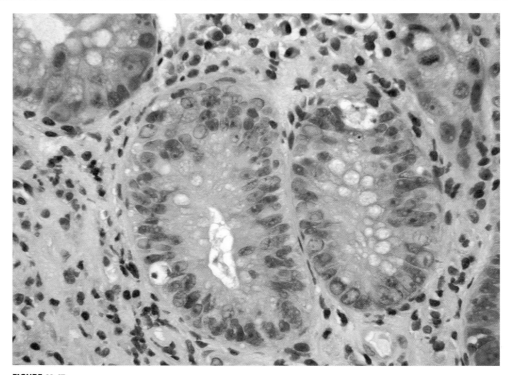

FIGURE 11-17
Mycophenolate mofetil colitis. This high-power photomicrograph shows a few apoptotic cells within the colonic crypts similar to the changes seen in mild graft-versus-host disease.

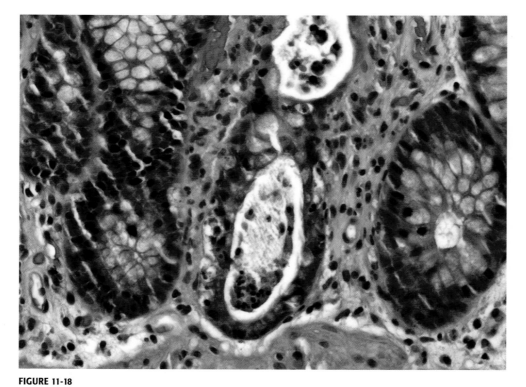

FIGURE 11-18
Mycophenolate mofetil colitis. This high-power photomicrograph shows a dilated crypt containing eosinophils and neutrophils. Such crypts are more typical of mycophenolate damage than graft-versus-host disease.

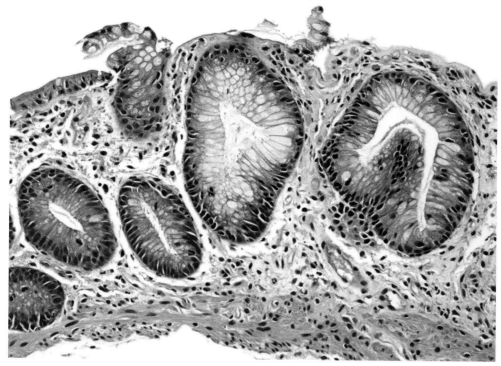

FIGURE 11-19

Mycophenolate mofetil colitis. This medium-power photomicrograph shows distorted crypts resembling quiescent inflammatory bowel disease.

DIFFERENTIAL DIAGNOSIS

GVHD can mimic MMF colitis to the point that they are indistinguishable. If the patient has had a bone marrow transplant, this can be problematic. In the author's experience, the presence of dilated crypts with eosinophils or neutrophils favors MMF over GVHD. In some cases the amount of crypt distortion can mimic quiescent ulcerative colitis. In addition, the amount of epithelial damage with minimal inflammation may also bring up the possibility of ischemia.

PROGNOSIS AND THERAPY

Discontinuing the drug or decreasing the dosage typically leads to rapid symptomatic improvement, often within 5 to 7 days.

■ NONSTEROIDAL ANTI-INFLAMMATORY DRUG (NSAID) COLITIS

CLINICAL FEATURES

NSAIDs have become ubiquitous in today's society, and doses as small as a baby aspirin a day can cause profound damage to the GI tract. Not only do these drugs have direct toxic effects on the mucosa, but they inhibit prostaglandin synthesis that helps protect the mucosa. Symptoms include abdominal pain, bloody diarrhea, iron deficiency anemia, and malabsorption. The risk of GI complications increases with dose, duration of therapy, age, and concurrent use of steroids or anticoagulants. It has been estimated that several thousand patients in the United States experience exsanguination from GI bleeding caused by NSAIDs each year. NSAIDs are also known to complicate or exacerbate ulcerative colitis and diverticular disease.

PATHOLOGIC FEATURES

GROSS FINDINGS

Ulcers and erosions may be seen throughout the GI tract. The terminal ileum and right colon, as well as the rectum (suppositories), are the most common sites of NSAID damage in the lower gut. Diaphragm disease is a rare complication most often seen in the small intestine, but this has also been reported in the colon.

MICROSCOPIC FINDINGS

A number of different patterns of mucosal damage in the colon have been reported with NSAIDs. Focal active colitis has been mentioned in several studies as being

NONSTEROIDAL ANTI-INFLAMMATORY DRUG COLITIS—FACT SHEET

Definition
- Damage to the colon secondary to NSAIDs

Incidence and Location
- Incidence is unknown, but 40% of those with NSAID damage have lower GI involvement
- Location can be anywhere in the GI tract, but terminal ileum, right colon, and rectum more common

Gender, Race, and Age Distribution
- Age older than 60 years increases risk of GI damage from NSAIDs

Clinical Features
- Abdominal pain, bloody diarrhea, iron deficiency anemia

Prognosis and Therapy
- May resolve with discontinuation of drug, but may require surgical or medical intervention
- Thousands die every year from massive GI bleeding secondary to NSAIDs

NONSTEROIDAL ANTI-INFLAMMATORY DRUG COLITIS—PATHOLOGIC FEATURES

Gross Findings
- Ulcers or erosions throughout GI tract
- Diaphragm disease

Microscopic Findings
- Focal active colitis, ischemic-like colitis, apoptosis, nonspecific ulcers/erosions

Differential Diagnosis
- Crohn's disease, resolving infection, ischemia

associated with NSAID use. Other articles have described a more mixed or lymphocytic infiltrate in the mucosa. Nonspecific ulcers/erosions are common, but crypt distortion like that seen in ulcerative colitis is generally not seen. There are also numerous reports of NSAIDs causing an injury identical to ischemic colitis as well. NSAIDs are also known to increase the amount of apoptosis seen in the gut/colon.

DIFFERENTIAL DIAGNOSIS

NSAID lesions in the terminal ileum and right colon can mimic Crohn's disease while the focal active colitis pattern mimics resolving infectious colitis. NSAIDs can also cause colonic lesions that are identical to ischemic colitis. History is of paramount importance in making the correct diagnosis.

PROGNOSIS AND THERAPY

Discontinuing the drug is the first line of defense, but patients may require surgical intervention for perforations, strictures, or bleeding ulcers. Metronidazole and sulfasalazine have been used as medical therapy. Misoprostol or proton pump inhibitors can be given with NSAIDs to protect the mucosal barrier (upper GI tract). Selective COX-2 inhibitors may cut down on NSAID damage in the gut.

■ CHEMOTHERAPY EFFECT/MUCOSITIS

CLINICAL FEATURES

Five percent to 15% of patients on chemotherapy develop mucositis; this number jumps to 30% to 40% when radiation is added to the regimen. It has been theorized that chemotherapy generates reactive oxygen species that damage epithelial cell DNA, leading to apoptosis and clonal cell death. However, recent evidence suggests that cytokine activation may also play a role in causing mucositis. Even though chemotherapy damage is much more common in the small bowel, stomach, and esophagus, the colon can still be affected. Diarrhea and bleeding (rather than nausea and vomiting) are related to colonic injury. Overall mucositis is a major cause of morbidity that often leads to infection and causes delay or decreased dosing of chemotherapy.

PATHOLOGIC FEATURES

GROSS FINDINGS

Ulcers and erosions are endoscopic findings typical of chemotherapy damage.

MICROSCOPIC FINDINGS

Chemotherapy leads to epithelial damage with little, if any, inflammation. There are usually attenuated crypts with apoptosis and the surviving cells have atypical hyperchromatic nuclei suggestive of cytomegalovirus (CMV) or herpes virus infection (Fig. 11-20). The atypia may also mimic dysplasia. In general, one can usually exclude viral infection, in that there are many cells with atypical nuclei, but none with classic viral inclusions.

CHEMOTHERAPY EFFECT/MUCOSITIS—FACT SHEET

Definition

- Damage to the colon secondary to chemotherapy

Incidence and Location

- 5 % to 15% of patients on chemotherapy
- More common in small bowel, stomach, and esophagus than colon

Gender, Race, and Age Distribution

- Female patients have more mucosal damage from 5-fluorouracil-based chemotherapy than males
- Mucositis is less common in African-Americans than in whites

Clinical Features

- Diarrhea, hematochezia

Prognosis and Therapy

- Major cause of morbidity
- No therapy except delay or decreased dosing of chemotherapy

CHEMOTHERAPY EFFECT/MUCOSITIS—PATHOLOGIC FEATURES

Gross Findings

- Ulcers or erosions throughout GI tract

Microscopic Findings

- Attenuated crypts with apoptosis and little inflammation
- Marked regenerative changes with nuclei resembling CMV inclusions

Differential Diagnosis

- CMV, GVHD, ischemia, dysplasia

DIFFERENTIAL DIAGNOSIS

As previously mentioned, the nuclear changes induced by chemotherapy often resemble CMV inclusions; however, exhaustive searching will not yield any classic inclusions despite finding many atypical cells. Immunostains can be helpful in excluding this possibility. In patients receiving bone marrow transplant, it generally takes 3 weeks for the apoptosis induced by conditioning chemotherapy to completely disappear. Therefore, extreme care should be taken in diagnosing GVHD before day 21 after transplantation. Chemotherapy effect can also mimic ischemia, in that both processes have epithelial damage with minimal inflammation. A hyalinized lamina propria favors the diagnosis of ischemia (as does a geographic distribution of disease).

PROGNOSIS AND THERAPY

Overall mucositis is a major cause of morbidity that often causes delay or decreased dosing of chemotherapy. It is also a frequent cause of secondary infection. While many treatment compounds are being studied, the only current therapy is supportive care and decreased or delayed dosing of chemotherapy.

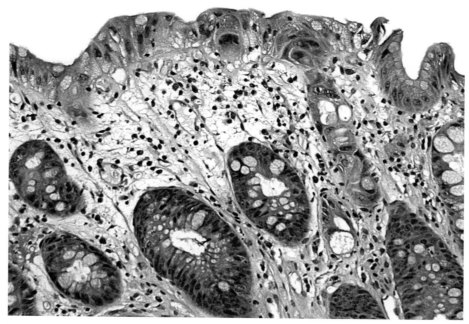

FIGURE 11-20

Chemotherapy effect. This medium-power photomicrograph shows reactive cytologic atypia, which raises the question of dysplasia, as well as viral infection.

■ GRAFT-VERSUS-HOST DISEASE

CLINICAL FEATURES

GVHD is an all too common complication of bone marrow transplantation that affects approximately 50% of patients. It can rarely be a complication of solid organ transplantation as well, especially with small bowel transplants. T-cells within the graft are responsible for GVHD, and attempts at decreasing the number of T-cells in transplants have reduced mortality associated with GVHD. In the gut, GVHD causes nausea, vomiting, and diarrhea, as well as abdominal pain and bleeding.

PATHOLOGIC FEATURES

GROSS FINDINGS

There are conflicting data on whether there is good correlation between endoscopic findings and histologic evidence of GVHD. One study reported 40% of normal-appearing mucosa showed GVHD histologically. In the author's experience, when abnormalities are seen endoscopically, there is a higher likelihood of finding severe GVHD.

MICROSCOPIC FINDINGS

Apoptosis is the hallmark of GVHD. Milder forms show only scattered apoptotic cells at the base of the crypts (Fig. 11-21), whereas severe GVHD may show a completely empty lamina propria with only small buds of endocrine cells present at the base of the mucosa. While a pathologic grading scale has been used to quantify the amount of damage, this has very limited clinical utility and hence a recent NIH consensus panel on GVHD recommended dropping the grading scale altogether. The real difficulty is determining what the minimal threshold for diagnosing GVHD should be. Because there are little data on this, some pathologists have arbitrarily decided that at least one apoptotic body per piece of tissue should be present before making the diagnosis. Cases with fewer apoptotic bodies may be considered indefinite for GVHD. Over time, the bowel may develop a scleroderma-like fibrosis that some have classified as chronic GVHD. This is very difficult to diagnose during life because it requires a resection. While the difference between acute and chronic GVHD used to be defined as occurring before or after 100 days, this does not correlate with pathologic changes, in that patients can have the same apoptotic damage several years after transplantation. Consequently, the term *acute GVHD* has largely been abandoned. The mucosa may show marked crypt distortion in the healing phase of severe GVHD. This can mimic quiescent inflammatory bowel disease.

GRAFT-VERSUS-HOST DISEASE—FACT SHEET

Definition
- Damage to the colon caused by donor lymphocytes after an allogeneic transplant

Incidence and Location
- 40% to 80% of bone marrow transplant patients get GVHD
- Much less common in solid organ (small bowel) transplant recipients
- Location can be anywhere in the GI tract
- Rectosigmoid may be best place for biopsy

Gender, Race, and Age Distribution
- There are no predilections known for gender, race, or age

Clinical Features
- Nausea, vomiting, diarrhea, abdominal pain, and bleeding

Prognosis and Therapy
- Chronic complications secondary to GVHD develop in 50% of patients
- Biggest cause of long-term morbidity and mortality
- Immunosuppressive therapy with steroids, MMF, cyclosporine, tacrolimus, and others

---

GRAFT-VERSUS-HOST DISEASE—PATHOLOGIC FEATURES

Gross Findings
- Unclear whether endoscopic abnormalities correlate with histologic GVHD

Microscopic Findings
- Apoptosis at base of crypts, loss of crypts with residual nests of endocrine cells
- May develop marked crypt distortion mimicking quiescent IBD

Differential Diagnosis
- Infections, chemotherapy effect, MMF, NSAIDs, sodium phosphate bowel preparations

---

DIFFERENTIAL DIAGNOSIS

Infections, NSAIDs, oral sodium phosphate bowel preparations, chemotherapy, and MMF can all cause apoptosis in the colon. CMV, adenovirus, HIV, and cryptosporidia are just a few of the infections that cause increased apoptosis. It is critical to exclude infections in cases of mild GVHD because the additional immunosuppressive therapy given to treat GVHD can have dire consequences. In some cases patients may have both infection and GVHD (particularly CMV). Although it is

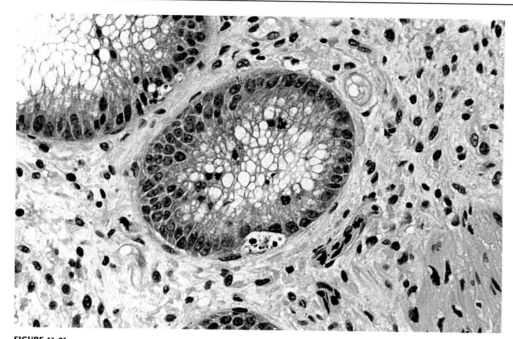

FIGURE 11-21

Graft versus host disease (GVHD). This medium-power photomicrograph shows a few apoptotic cells typical of mild GVHD.

hard to know how much apoptosis is too much to blame on an infection, loss of crypts may point to superimposed GVHD. As mentioned, biopsies taken from patients within 3 weeks of conditioning chemotherapy may show signs that mimic GVHD. Lastly, many bone marrow transplant patients now have their GVHD treated with MMF. The presence of dilated crypts with a few neutrophils or eosinophils helps point to MMF as the culprit.

PROGNOSIS AND THERAPY

GVHD is the largest cause of long-term morbidity and mortality in bone marrow transplant patients; about 50% of patients develop chronic problems related to GVHD. Treatment consists of a wide range of immunosuppressive drugs including steroids, MMF, cyclosporine, and tacrolimus.

12

Gastrointestinal Polyposis Syndromes

■ **Christine A. Iacobuzio-Donahue, MD, PhD**

The intestinal polyposis syndromes are responsible for less than 1% of all lower gastrointestinal (GI) tract malignancies but have provided vast insight into the genetic alterations that underlie GI neoplasia. Polyposis syndromes may be categorized into those that cause intestinal adenomatous polyps and those that cause nonadenomatous, or hamartomatous, polyps (Table 12-1). Syndromes that cause adenomatous polyps most commonly include familial adenomatous polyposis and its phenotypic variants, whereas syndromes that cause hamartomatous polyps include Peutz-Jeghers syndrome (PJS), juvenile polyposis syndrome, or Cowden's disease. Polyposis syndromes may also be classified as those that are hereditary and those that occur in a sporadic manner. Important information necessary to make a diagnosis of an intestinal polyposis syndrome includes the number and location of intestinal polyps, the patient's age, the patient's family history, and other clinical features of the patient that may identify him or her as having a polyposis syndrome.

TABLE 12-1
Classification of Gastrointestinal Polyposis Syndromes

Hereditary Polyposis Syndromes

Adenomas
Familial adenomatous polyposis coli
Attenuated familial adenomatous polyposis coli
Gardner's syndrome
Turcot's syndrome
MYH adenomatous polyposis coli
Hamartomatous
Peutz-Jeghers syndrome
Juvenile polyposis syndrome
Cowden's disease
Bannayan-Riley-Ruvalcaba syndrome
Devon family syndrome

Other

Hereditary mixed polyposis syndrome
Neurofibromatosis type 1
Multiple endocrine neoplasia type 2
Nonhereditary polyposis syndromes
Hyperplastic polyposis syndrome
Cronkhite-Canada syndrome
Lymphomatosis polyposis
Nodular lymphoid hyperplasia
Pneumatosis cystoides intestinalis
Colitis cystica profunda

■ FAMILIAL ADENOMATOUS POLYPOSIS

CLINICAL FEATURES

Familial adenomatous polyposis (FAP) is the most common intestinal polyposis syndrome, affecting approximately 1 in 10,000 individuals. It is characterized by the development of adenomatous polyps at an early age in association with numerous extracolonic manifestations. FAP is the prototype of any hereditary cancer syndrome because the risk for affected patients developing colon cancer approaches 100%.

In the fully developed form, hundreds to thousands of adenomatous polyps are present throughout the colorectum. Adenomas emerge at an average age of 16 years, and colon cancers occur at an average age of 39 years. Colonic adenomas develop in more than 95% of patients with FAP by the age of 35 years and, without treatment, 93% of all patients with FAP will develop colon cancer before age 50 years.

Upper GI polyps are also found in up to 100% of patients with FAP. Most are fundic gland polyps, although adenomatous polyps of the gastric mucosa may also occur. Duodenal adenomatous polyps also develop in more than 90% of patients with FAP, with up to a 10% lifetime risk for duodenal or periampullary cancer. Adenomas occurring within the small bowel have been reported, but symptoms or malignancy from adenomas in this region is unusual.

Extraintestinal manifestations in FAP are common and include osteomas, epidermoid cysts, fibromas, supernumerary teeth, odontomas, and congenital hypertrophy of the retinal pigmented epithelium. These lesions are usually asymptomatic and are not associated with malignant potential. One exception, however, is desmoid tumor, occurring in 10% of patients with FAP. Desmoid tumors are considered benign lesions but result in significant morbidity (and sometimes mortality) in half of patients who have them.

FAMILIAL ADENOMATOUS POLYPOSIS—FACT SHEET

Definition

- An autosomal dominantly inherited syndrome characterized by hundreds to thousands of adenomatous polyps throughout the colorectum and a variety of extracolonic manifestations

Incidence and Location

- Most common polyposis syndrome (1 in 10,000)
- 80% to 100% gene penetrance in affected families
- 30% of patients with FAP have spontaneous new mutations of the APC gene

Morbidity and Mortality

- Average age of colorectal cancer diagnosis is 39 years
- More than 90% of patients develop colorectal cancer by age 50 years
- 100% of patients have upper GI polyps, typically fundic gland polyps
- Age of adenoma and cancer onset is 10 years later for AFAP than for classic FAP

Gender, Race, and Age Distribution

- Males and females equally affected
- No racial or ethnic predominance
- Average age of onset in teens

Clinical Features

- Most patients asymptomatic until puberty
- Adenomas often present years before symptoms occur
- Most common symptoms are rectal bleeding (75% of patients) or diarrhea (63% of patients)
- Carcinomas develop on average 6 years after symptom onset
- Synchronous cancers (40% of patients) and metachronous cancers (70% of patients) common

Prognosis and Therapy

- 100% risk of colon cancer without intervention
- Only treatment is prophylactic total colectomy
- Following colectomy, most common cause of mortality is periampullary cancer (22% of patients)

FAMILIAL ADENOMATOUS POLYPOSIS—PATHOLOGIC FEATURES

Gross Findings

- Hundreds to thousands of adenomas evenly distributed throughout colorectum and appendix
- Adenomas tend to be larger in the rectosigmoid
- Adenomas range in size from microscopic (crypt adenomas) to pedunculated lesions greater than 1 cm in diameter
- The rectum is occasionally spared, particularly in AFAP
- Colorectal carcinomas may be multifocal
- No differences in the distribution or pathology of colorectal adenomas or carcinomas among sporadic or inherited forms

Microscopic Findings

- Grossly and histologically identical to sporadic adenomas
- Early adenomas consist of small tubules lined by adenomatous epithelium that may be unicryptal, bicryptal, or tricryptal lesions in grossly normal appearing mucosa
- When multiple crypts become involved by adenomatous epithelium, more typical polypoid configuration is seen grossly
- Continued proliferation results in pedunculated tubulovillous gross appearance
- AFAP more commonly associated with flat, depressed, or polypoid adenomas

Genetics

- As a result of homozygous inactivation of the APC gene on chromosome 5q
- Mutations within the mutation cluster region in exon 15 associated with classic FAP
- Mutations in the 5' region of the APC gene associated with AFAP

Differential Diagnosis

- Chronic IBD with pseudopolyposis
- Peutz-Jeghers syndrome
- Juvenile polyposis coli syndrome (JPS)

When the extraintestinal manifestations of FAP are particularly prominent, the condition may be referred to as *Gardner's syndrome.* An attenuated form of FAP (AFAP) is also well accepted, in which the average number of adenomatous polyps is approximately 30. Adenomas are typically present in a right colonic distribution, and adenomas and colon cancers arise an average of 10 years later than in the classic form of FAP. Turcot's syndrome refers to those patients with brain cancer (particularly medulloblastomas) and intestinal polyposis.

PATHOLOGIC FEATURES

GROSS FINDINGS

Adenomas develop throughout the entire colorectum and appendix. While they tend to be evenly dispersed, adenomas are relatively larger in the rectosigmoid, giving the appearance of a greater density of polyps in this region. In the classic and most dramatic form, the entire mucosa becomes carpeted with adenomatous polyps so that no intervening normal mucosa is recognizable (Fig. 12-1A and B). In these cases, the total number of adenomas present is greater than 100, often exceeding 1000. Colorectal carcinomas may be multifocal and show a relative predilection for the left colon. The adenomatous polyps in FAP typically demonstrate a range of sizes and shapes. Adenomas may vary from large, pedunculated tubulovillous adenomas greater than 1 cm in diameter, to flat, broad-based nodular adenomatous polyps, to microscopic foci less than 1 mm in diameter.

In patients with AFAP, the number of polyps present is typically less than 100 and preferentially involves the right colon (see Fig. 12-1C). Sparing of the rectum by adenomatous polyps may also indicate AFAP, as well as the presence of numerous flat adenomas in that patient.

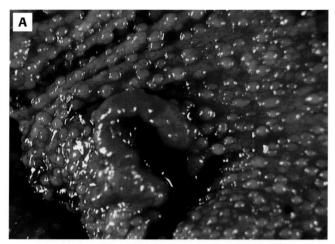

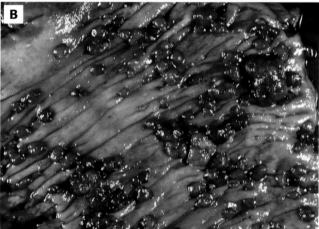

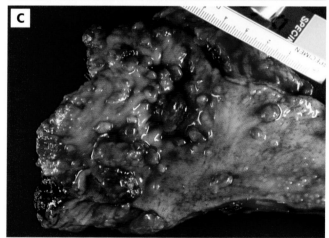

FIGURE 12-1

Familial adenomatous polyposis (FAP). **A,** In this specimen, the colonic mucosa is carpeted with thousands of dome-shaped adenomas of uniform size and distribution. An infiltrating carcinoma is present at the bottom right. **B,** In a different patient with FAP, adenomas show a wide variation in size and are clustered. Areas of intervening colonic mucosa without gross involvement are seen. **C,** In contrast to classic FAP, in which the entire colon is involved by adenomatous polyps, this colectomy specimen from a patient with known attenuated FAP shows approximately 30 adenomas all located within the cecum and proximal right colon.

MICROSCOPIC FINDINGS

The adenomas and carcinomas that arise in FAP are indistinguishable from their sporadic counterparts (Fig. 12-2A). Similar to sporadic adenomas and colorectal carcinomas, the incidence of malignancy is related to adenoma size and frequency. Single, double, or tricryptal adenomas are common in grossly normal mucosa (see Fig. 12-2B). The adenomas of AFAP show similar cytologic changes characteristic of adenomatous epithelium. However, in contrast to the adenomas of classic FAP, the adenomas of AFAP are more commonly flat, depressed, or polypoid adenomas. Specifically, in flat adenomas, the adenoma lacks a concave surface and may be seen as a plaque on the mucosal surface, whereas in depressed adenomas, the adenoma surface lies below the level of the adjacent normal mucosa.

Upper GI polyps are found in virtually 100% of patients with FAP, most commonly fundic gland polyps and adenomatous polyps of the small bowel (Fig. 12-3). The histologic features of fundic gland polyps in this condition are similar to their sporadic counterparts. Epithelial dysplasia is not an uncommon finding, characterized by nuclear enlargement, hyperchromasia, and loss of polarity within dilated oxyntic glands that extend to the polyp surface. However, high-grade dysplasia or frank carcinoma arising in a fundic gland polyp in FAP is rare. Adenomatous polyps within the small bowel are grossly and histologically similar to those that are sporadic in nature.

ANCILLARY STUDIES

Genetic testing for germline mutations in the adenomatous polyposis coli (*APC*) gene identifies 95% of patients with FAP. Germline mutations in the *MYH* gene have been reported in a subset of patients with polyposis coli, no germline *APC* mutation, and a family history compatible with recessive inheritance.

DIFFERENTIAL DIAGNOSIS

Few entities enter into the differential diagnosis of the classic form of FAP because polyposis syndromes are generally rare and the histopathologic features of this disease are diagnostic. Differentiation from other polyposis syndromes may become problematic in the absence of an appropriate clinical history.

PROGNOSIS AND THERAPY

The key to the management of FAP is to identify presymptomatic individuals, predominantly through screening of relatives of affected patients. The diagnosis

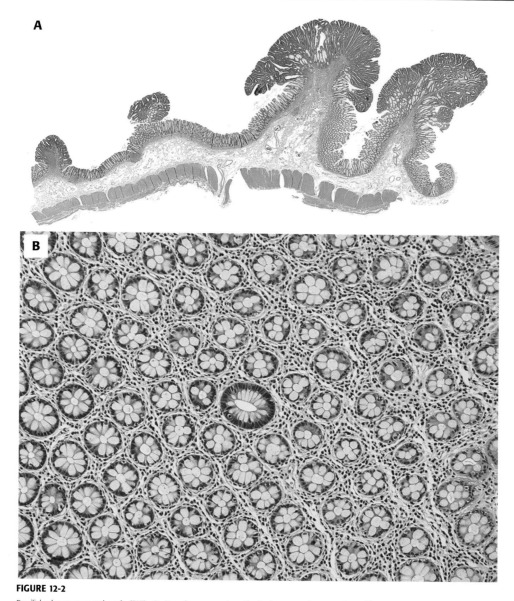

FIGURE 12-2

Familial adenomatous polyposis (FAP). **A,** Scanning power view of colonic mucosa from a patient with FAP reveals four different polypoid tubular adenomas in this area alone. **B,** Single crypt adenoma seen on cross section within an area of normal mucosa from a patient with FAP.

can easily be made or excluded by sigmoidoscopy or barium enema examinations performed annually beginning at 10 to 12 years of age with histologic confirmation of adenoma. Further workup of the colon is not required other than to rule out the presence of an infiltrating carcinoma. The development of an infiltrating carcinoma is inevitable by the age of 50 years in the absence of a total or subtotal proctocolectomy. Thus surgical management is recommended even in asymptomatic individuals who have not completed puberty.

Preservation of the rectum may be considered for those patients with few rectal polyps. However, this segment must be continuously monitored for the development of adenomas and carcinomas, in that some reports suggest more than 50% of patients will develop carcinomas in this region despite semiannual surveillance. A recent approach to the surveillance of the rectal stump is to treat these patients with nonsteroidal anti-inflammatory drugs such as sulindac. Patients who undergo prophylactic colectomy may still die of carcinomas arising in other sites, most commonly periampullary carcinomas. Thus evaluation of the upper GI tract is also necessary at the time of diagnosis of colonic disease and afterward every 1 to 3 years at least.

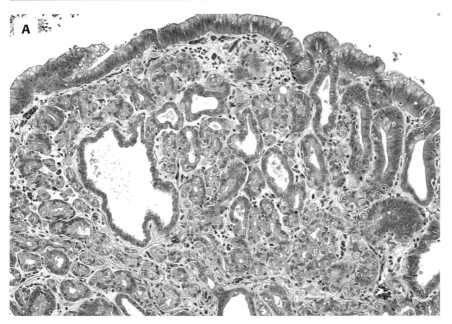

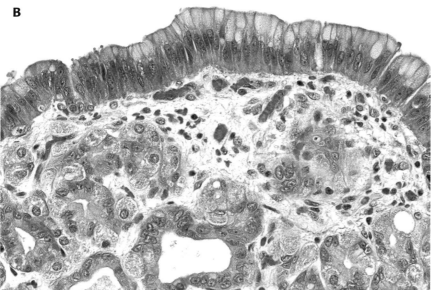

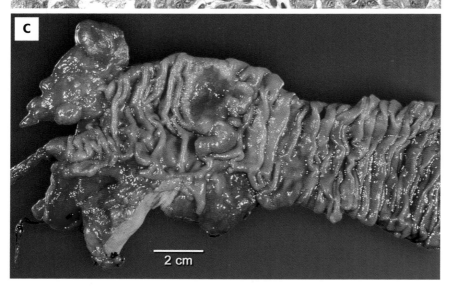

FIGURE 12-3

Familial adenomatous polyposis (FAP). **A,** Low-power view of a fundic gland polyp from a patient with FAP showing characteristic dilated oxyntic glands lined by parietal and chief cells. **B,** High-power view of surface epithelium reveals nuclear enlargement, hyperchromasia, and loss of polarity consistent with low-grade dysplasia. **C,** Large tubular adenoma identified by endoscopic surveillance of the duodenum in a patient who underwent prophylactic total colectomy 7 years earlier.

2 cm

PEUTZ-JEGHERS SYNDROME

CLINICAL FEATURES

PJS is the second most common form of intestinal polyposis, with an incidence approximately one tenth that of FAP. Similar to FAP, PJS is inherited in an autosomal dominant pattern. However, unlike FAP, the inherited dominant allele shows a variable and incomplete penetrance. PJS consists of two major and characteristic components: hamartomatous polyps involving the entire GI tract and pigmented macules involving the mucous membranes and skin.

The diagnosis of PJS can be made in infancy because most patients develop mucocutaneous pigmentation within 2 years, and small bowel hamartomatous polyps are frequently symptomatic. More than 95% of patients with PJS demonstrate pigmentation of the mucocutaneous membranes at birth, specifically around the nose, lips, buccal mucosa, hands and feet, genitalia, and perianal region (Fig. 12-4). The pigmentation of PJS can easily be distinguished from freckles because freckles are not present at birth, are sparse near the lips, and never involve the mucous membranes. While the pigmentation of the skin may fade, the melanin deposits of the buccal mucosa persist throughout life.

Benign complications of PJS predominate in the pediatric population. Jejunal and ileal hamartomatous polyps often produce intussusception, leading to a partial or total bowel obstruction. When located within the rectum, hamartomatous polyps may prolapse, resulting in torsion, infarction, and GI bleeding. In adults with PJS, morbidity and mortality are related to the development of cancer. Tumors can develop in multiple organ sites in addition to the GI tract, including the breast, lung, pancreas, uterus, ovary, cervix, and Sertoli cells of the testis. Unique ovarian neoplasms may affect up to 12% of female patients with this syndrome, whereas hormonally active Sertoli cell testicular tumors may occur in males. Breast cancers, often bilateral, may be found in young women, with the breast cancer risk not unlike that found for the *BRCA1* and *BRCA2* genes.

PATHOLOGIC FEATURES

GROSS FINDINGS

Hamartomatous polyps occur throughout the GI tract. In decreasing frequency, the most common sites of polyp formation are the jejunum, ileum, colon, stomach, duodenum, and appendix. Intestinal polyps are typically present in the dozens. They may be sessile or pedunculated, and often show a smooth, lobulated surface. The size of Peutz-Jeghers (PJ) polyps ranges from a few millimeters to several centimeters in diameter.

MICROSCOPIC FINDINGS

Although PJ polyps are not easily distinguished from adenomatous or inflammatory polyps based on their gross appearance, their histologic appearance is quite distinctive and characterized by a hyperplastic mature epithelium appropriate to the anatomic site and divided by broad bands of mature smooth muscle (Figs. 12-5 and 12-6). Small intestinal PJ polyps consist of crypts and villi of varying lengths divided by arborizing bands of smooth muscle. The muscle fibers commonly fan out from the center of the polyp to form a treelike appearance. The lamina propria is normal. Cells normally present within small bowel mucosa,

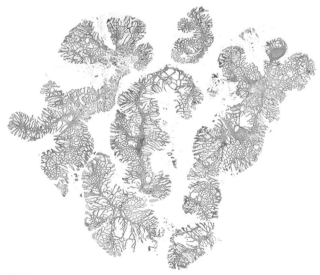

FIGURE 12-5

Whole-mount view of Peutz-Jeghers polyp. On low power, hamartomatous polyps have a characteristic leaf-like appearance and irregular surface.

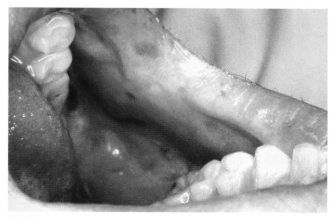

FIGURE 12-4

Mucosal pigmentation in Peutz-Jeghers syndrome.

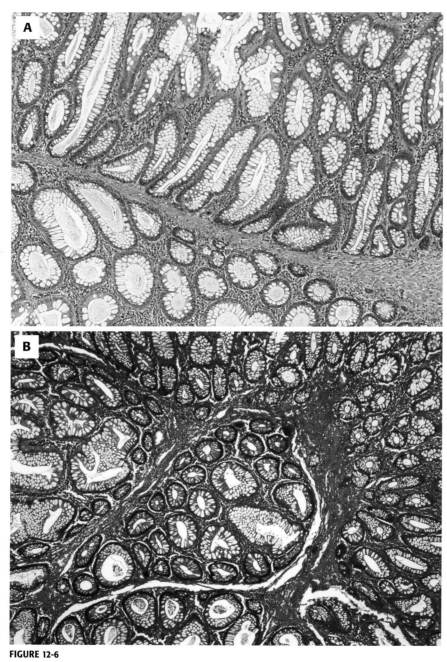

FIGURE 12-6

Peutz-Jeghers polyp. **A,** Histologic examination of the same polyp shown in Figure 12-5 reveals hyperplastic epithelium that is otherwise appropriate for the site of origin separated by broad bands of smooth muscle. **B,** A trichrome stain highlights the bands of smooth muscle that are characteristic of these polyps.

including absorptive enterocytes, Paneth cells, goblet cells, and argentaffin cells, are present within the hyperplastic epithelium of the PJ polyp (Fig. 12-7A and B). Erosion of the surface epithelium is common, particularly for larger polyps, and may be associated with reactive and regenerative epithelium containing prominent mitoses.

Colonic PJ polyps demonstrate similar histologic features, but less developed than those seen for their small bowel counterparts. Specifically, PJ polyps of the colon contain elongated, branched crypts that may simulate a villous architecture. Goblet cells are the predominant cell type lining the hyperplastic crypts, although absorptive cells may also be present (see Fig. 12-7C). The replication zone at the crypt base is relatively short, with mature cells predominantly lining the crypts. However, in the presence of surface erosion, this replication zone may become expanded as the epithelial cells become regenerative.

PEUTZ-JEGHERS POLYPOSIS—FACT SHEET

Definition

- An autosomal dominantly inherited syndrome characterized by GI hamartomatous polyps and pigmented macules of mucous membranes and skin

Incidence and Location

- 1 in 200,000 live births
- Second most common polyposis syndrome

Morbidity and Mortality

- Benign complications (intussusception and obstruction, torsion, infarction and bleeding) predominate in the pediatric population
- 73% incidence of malignancies involving the reproductive organs, breast, or GI tract in adult population

Gender, Race, and Age Distribution

- Males and females affected equally
- No racial or ethnic predilection
- Symptoms begin in infancy
- Average age of diagnosis of polyps is 25 years

Clinical Features

- Pigmented lesions of the mucous membranes develop by 2 years of age
- Hamartomatous polyps present throughout the intestinal tract, most commonly the small bowel (jejunum)
- Polyps typically number in the tens

Prognosis and Therapy

- 93% lifetime risk of cancer in both intestinal and extraintestinal organs
- Screening and regular surveillance of high-risk organs (GI tract, breast, pancreas, reproductive organs)

PEUTZ-JEGHERS POLYPOSIS—PATHOLOGIC FEATURES

Gross Findings

- Hamartomatous polyps present throughout the GI tract
- Small bowel the most common site of PJ polyps, followed by colon, stomach, duodenum, and appendix
- Sessile or pedunculated appearance
- Smooth, lobulated surface
- Wide size range (millimeters to several centimeters)

Microscopic Findings

- Hyperplastic epithelium appropriate to the site of origin divided by arborizing bands of mature smooth muscle
- Normal lamina propria
- Cellular constituents of normal GI mucosa (goblet cells, Paneth cells, absorptive cells, argentaffin cells) present within hyperplastic epithelium
- Surface commonly eroded with areas of regeneration

Genetics

- Inactivation of the STK11/LKB1 gene identified in up to 70% of affected families

Differential Diagnosis

- Sporadic hamartomatous polyp
- Other hamartomatous polyposis syndromes (juvenile polyposis or CD)
- Mucosal prolapse
- Filiform polyp of IBD

Arborizing bands of smooth muscle are less frequent in colonic PJ polyps than in the small bowel. Smooth muscle is not present in all polyps, particularly small lesions.

ANCILLARY STUDIES

Germline mutations in the *LKB1/STK11* tumor suppressor gene on chromosome 19p can be demonstrated in up to 70% of families with classic PJS.

DIFFERENTIAL DIAGNOSIS

A variety of neoplastic and inflammatory entities enter into the differential diagnosis of hamartomatous polyps of PJS, including juvenile polyps, mucosal prolapse, and filiform polyps of chronic inflammatory bowel disease (IBD). Small PJ polyps can be particularly difficult to differentiate from juvenile polyps. However, in contrast to juvenile polyps, PJ polyps are more common within the small bowel and do not have an inflamed lamina propria. Granulation tissue may be seen in association with both PJ and juvenile polyps, but in PJ polyps granulation tissue is typically present in association with surface erosion and histologic examination of deeper regions of the polyp reveals the lack of inflammation. The prominence of smooth muscle within PJ polyps may simulate that seen in mucosal prolapse disorders or filiform polyps. Differentiation from these entities relies on histologic examination of the overlying epithelium, which shows the presence of reactive epithelial changes of mucosal prolapse. In filiform polyps of IBD, the surface epithelium also shows features of chronic inflammation (crypt distortion, crypt atrophy) that may be seen in nonpolypoid mucosa as well.

PROGNOSIS AND THERAPY

The lifetime risk for developing cancer in individuals with PJS is estimated to be 93%, with a mean age of cancer diagnosis at 43 years. Although a variety of neoplasms have been reported, the greatest risk for cancer in patients with PJS is in the GI tract, particularly the colorectum, stomach, and pancreas. At this time, management of patients with PJS involves periodic surveillance of high-risk organs for which early detection and screening are reasonable.

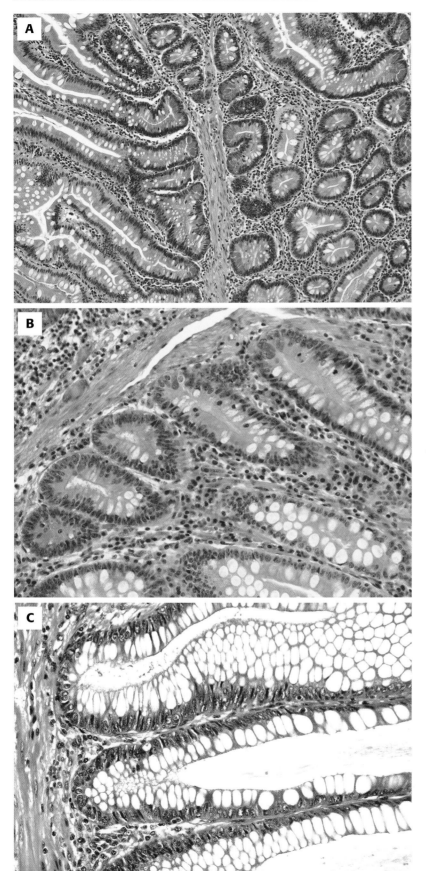

FIGURE 12-7

Peutz-Jeghers polyp. **A,** In small bowel Peutz-Jeghers polyps, the lining epithelium shows reactive and hyperplastic features. **B,** At higher power, the epithelium is seen to retain goblet cells, neuroendocrine cells, and Paneth cells within the bases of hyperplastic crypts. **C,** Peutz-Jeghers polyps that arise within the colon contain predominantly goblet cells. Scattered neuroendocrine cells are present at the crypt bases.

◼ JUVENILE POLYPOSIS SYNDROME

CLINICAL FEATURES

Juvenile polyposis coli syndrome (JPS) denotes multiple juvenile or inflammatory polyps distributed throughout the colon or GI tract. JPS is the third most common form of intestinal polyposis, accounting for 1 to 2 cases per 100,000 live births a year. JPS may occur sporadically or through autosomal dominant inheritance in affected kindreds. In the familial form, a family history can be elicited in up to 50% of affected patients.

Sporadic juvenile polyps are the most common type of polyp diagnosed in children and are estimated to be present in as many as 2% of asymptomatic children. Thus the criteria for a diagnosis of syndromic juvenile polyps are (1) greater than five juvenile polyps in the colon at one time, (2) the presence of extracolonic juvenile polyps, and (3) any number of juvenile polyps in a patient with a family history of juvenile polyposis. Sporadic juvenile polyps are often first diagnosed in

patients ranging from 1 to 10 years of age, with a peak incidence between 2 and 4 years of age. In contrast, patients with JPS tend to present at an older age, with a mean age of 9.5 years. Although sporadic juvenile polyps are found in both sexes, there is a slight male predominance in patients with JPS.

Two forms of JPS have been recognized: an autosomal dominantly inherited familial form with no associated congenital abnormalities and a nonfamilial form with associated congenital abnormalities. In the nonfamilial form, 20% of affected individuals show abnormalities such as congenital heart disease, hydrocephalus, or intestinal malrotation, among others. Digital clubbing and failure to thrive are also considered to be extraintestinal manifestations of JPS.

Children with JPS usually present with painless rectal bleeding. Less than 10% have symptoms such as abdominal pain, rectal prolapse or polyp extrusion, anal pruritus, constipation, or diarrhea. Extensive and extracolonic polyposis in the small bowel or stomach may cause GI and systemic dysfunction such as intussusception, protein-losing enteropathy, malabsorption, diarrhea, or significant hemorrhage.

PATHOLOGIC FEATURES

GROSS FINDINGS

Up to 90% of juvenile polyps are found in the rectum or rectosigmoid colon. The majority of juvenile polyps are solitary, although some series have reported that

---

JUVENILE POLYPOSIS SYNDROME—FACT SHEET

Definition
- Multiple juvenile or inflammatory polyps distributed throughout the colon or GI tract

Incidence and Location
- 1 in 100,000 live births

Morbidity and Mortality
- Most frequent presentation: painless rectal bleeding
- 10% of patients have abdominal pain, rectal prolapse, anal pruritus, constipation, or diarrhea
- Extensive extracolonic polyposis in the small bowel or stomach associated with GI intussusception or systemic dysfunction, such as protein-losing enteropathy and malabsorption
- Infants and young children may present with severe, even life-threatening protein-losing enteropathy

Gender, Race, and Age Distribution
- Males more than females
- No racial or ethnic predilection
- Mean age at diagnosis 9.5 years

Clinical Features
- GI polyposis is the predominant feature of the familial form of the disease
- Congenital abnormalities and extraintestinal manifestations frequent in the nonfamilial form of the disease

Prognosis and Treatment
- High risk for GI cancers
- Current management is screening and regular upper endoscopy and colonoscopic surveillance

---

JUVENILE POLYPOSIS SYNDROME—PATHOLOGIC FEATURES

Gross Findings
- More than 75% are pedunculated
- Average size 1 to 1.5 cm (range 0.2 to 4 cm)
- External surface is usually smooth or coarsely lobulated
- Cut surface shows grossly visible cystic spaces containing gray-to-yellow mucoid material

Microscopic Findings
- Prominent stroma with a mixed inflammatory infiltrate
- Cystically dilated glands lined by mature epithelium
- Eroded surface lined by inflamed granulation tissue
- Reactive and regenerative epithelium

Genetics
- Genetic inactivation of either *SMAD4* or *BMPR1A* gene in 50% of cases

Differential Diagnosis
- Sporadic juvenile/retention polyp
- Other hamartomatous polyposis syndromes (mainly PJS or CD)
- Inflammatory pseudopolyp arising in severe colitis
- Solitary rectal ulcer syndrome

one third to one half of cases may be multiple, perhaps reflecting variable extent of colonoscopic evaluation. Multiple juvenile polyps are usually separate or discrete, although occasionally multilobular or clustered polyps may be encountered (Fig. 12-8A). Their colonoscopic appearance ranges from relatively smooth homogeneous pale sessile polyps to large pedunculated polyps with a coarsely nodular surface. These pedunculated polyps may rotate on their stalks, causing ischemia and hemorrhage before autoamputation or avulsion. Surface granulation tissue is common, often with visible capillaries and venules and occasionally coated with exudates.

MICROSCOPIC FINDINGS

The histologic features of juvenile polyps are usually easily recognized. The classic juvenile polyp is a well-circumscribed mass that frequently displays an eroded surface (see Fig. 12-8B). In contrast to PJ hamartomatous polyps, juvenile polyps characteristically contain prominent stroma with a mixed inflammatory infiltrate (Fig. 12-9). Bands of smooth muscle, if present, are usually present in association with mucosal blood vessels. The smooth surface seen grossly corresponds to a cap of granulation tissue. Dilated cysts within the polyp are usually lined by mature epithelium appropriate for the

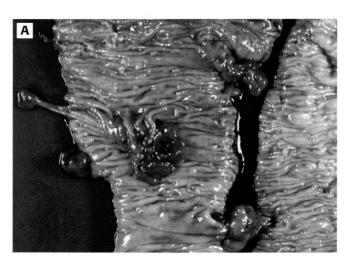

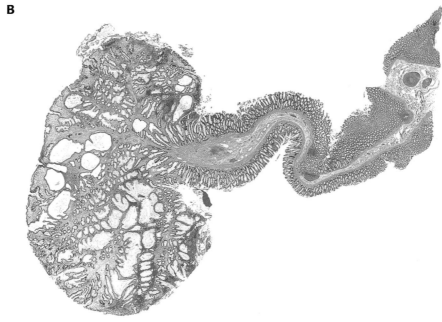

FIGURE 12-8

Juvenile polyposis syndrome. **A,** In this colectomy specimen from a young patient with juvenile polyposis syndrome, scattered polyps are present throughout the colorectum. Note the smooth glistening surface and prominent polyp stalk of the larger polyps. **B,** Whole-mount view of a polyp from the same patient. In contrast to the polyps of Peutz-Jeghers syndrome shown in Figure 12-5, juvenile polyps have a rounded contour. In addition, numerous cystically dilated glands can be appreciated below the polyp surface.

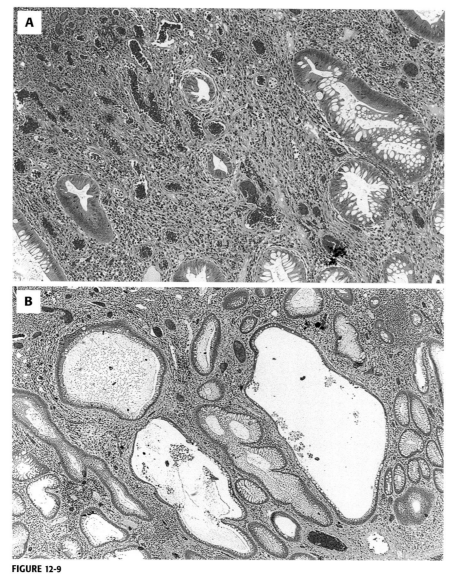

FIGURE 12-9

Juvenile polyp. **A,** The lamina propria, a prominent component of the polyp, contains numerous acute and chronic inflammatory cells, congested vessels, and granulation tissue. **B,** Cystically dilated glands that contain acellular debris are also typical findings of juvenile polyps.

site of origin. As a result of the inflammatory nature of juvenile polyps, the epithelium may show a range of cellular atypia varying from reactive changes to frank dysplasia and thus represents the most problematic histologic finding within a juvenile polyp (Fig. 12-10). The diagnosis of dysplasia in a juvenile polyp relies on the standard criteria for diagnosis of adenomatous change in the GI tract, including crowded, pseudostratified foci of columnar epithelium with granular cytoplasm, decreased cytoplasmic mucin, large hyperchromatic nuclei with prominent nucleoli, and increased mitoses. Patients with multiple polyps or a diagnosis of juvenile intestinal polyposis have an increased frequency of dysplastic change, and the change is more frequently graded as severe. Epithelial dysplasia, when it occurs in a juvenile polyp, is found more frequently in polyps exceeding 1 cm in diameter.

ANCILLARY STUDIES

Approximately 50% of families with JPS have a germline mutation in either the *SMAD4* gene or the bone morphogenic protein receptor 1A (*BMPR1A*) gene.

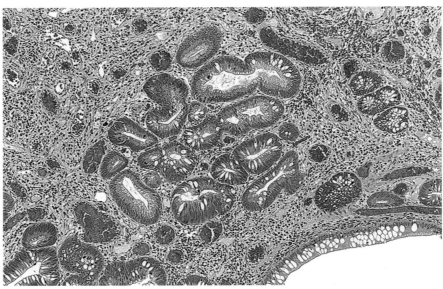

FIGURE 12-10

Juvenile polyp. Owing to the inflammatory nature of these polyps, reactive and regenerative epithelial changes are common and must be differentiated from adenomatous change.

DIFFERENTIAL DIAGNOSIS

The differential diagnosis of a juvenile polyp includes PJ hamartomatous polyps, inflammatory pseudopolyps, and solitary rectal ulcer syndrome. Differentiation from PJ polyps relies on recognition of the presence of an inflamed and prominent lamina propria and lack of broad bands of smooth muscle. Inflammatory pseudopolyps that arise in IBD or any other form of severe colitis are histologically similar to juvenile polyps. In these cases, examination of the surrounding nonpolypoid mucosa can identify the presence of colitis as the cause of the polyp formation. Solitary rectal ulcer syndrome can often be distinguished from juvenile polyps by fibrous replacement of the lamina propria (as opposed to the inflamed stroma characteristic of juvenile polyps) and smooth muscle ingrowth among colonic glands.

PROGNOSIS AND THERAPY

Patients with JPS have a significant risk for adenocarcinoma of the colon, as well as increased risk for gastric, duodenal, and pancreatic cancer. Upper endoscopy and pancolonoscopy screenings for affected patients should begin in adolescence. If multiple polyps are found, they should be removed with annual surveillance. All polyps should be submitted for histopathologic examination for the presence of dysplasia. If no polyps are identified, screening colonoscopy should be performed every 3 years. Colectomy may be necessary if polyps progress faster than colonoscopy surveillance or if premalignant dysplasia or malignant transformation is detected.

■ COWDEN'S DISEASE

CLINICAL FEATURES

Cowden's disease (CD), also known as *multiple hamartoma syndrome,* is an autosomal dominant syndrome characterized by extraintestinal hamartomas, frequently involving the face and oral cavity with associated GI hamartomatous polyposis anywhere from the esophagus to colon. Facial trichilemmomas, acral keratoses, papillomatous papules, and mucosal lesions are considered strict diagnostic criteria for CD. Macrocephaly; carcinomas of the breast, thyroid, or endometrium; and Lhermitte-Duclos disease are major criteria, and GI hamartomas are minor criteria.

CD is poorly described in young children. Progressive macrocephaly, scrotal-appearing tongue, and mild to moderate mental retardation suggest the diagnosis of CD in this age group. In contrast, commonly described features of CD in adult patients include facial anomalies, fibrocystic and neoplastic breast disease, cysts of the genitourinary system, facial papules and trichilemmomas, multiple skin tags, various neurologic abnormalities, endocrine abnormalities, and an increased risk for various types of neoplasia. The facial lesions are often trichilemmomas (lichenoid and verrucous papules), the oral mucosal lesions (gingiva and buccal mucosa) are often fibromas, and hyperkeratoses are seen on the hands and feet. Breast lesions occur in almost half of all adult patients, ranging from fibrocystic disease to cancer, commonly ductal carcinoma. Thyroid disease is the most common abnormality, occurring in up to 68% of patients.

The macrocephaly, multiple lipomas, and hemangiomata syndrome (MMLH) is currently considered a phenotypic variant of CD. MMLH is characterized by ileal and colonic juvenile polyps in association with macrocephaly, developmental delay, lipomatosis, hemangiomatosis, and pigmented macules on the glans penis. MMLH encompasses the previously described Bannayan-Riley-Ruvalcaba syndrome and the Myhre-Riley-Smith syndromes, an inherited autosomal dominant disorder that primarily affects men. As the clinical features of CD and MMLH overlap, both syndromes may occur within the same family.

PATHOLOGIC FEATURES

GROSS FINDINGS

Polyps associated with CD and MMLH tend to be small and not easily visualized. They may occur anywhere from the esophagus to the rectum, but the distal large intestine is most commonly affected.

MICROSCOPIC FINDINGS

Intestinal polyps in CD include juvenile polyps, PJ polyps, lipomas, lymphoid polyps, hyperplastic polyps, leiomyomas, and ganglioneuromas. Juvenile polyps are most common, with distinctive histologic features that include disorganization and proliferation of the muscularis mucosa, prominent lamina propria, and normal overlying colonic epithelium (Fig. 12-11).

ANCILLARY STUDIES

Approximately 80% of families with CD have a germline mutation in the *PTEN* gene. Kindreds with features of both CD and MMLH syndromes tend to be positive for *PTEN* germline mutations.

DIFFERENTIAL DIAGNOSIS

Due to the prominence of extraintestinal manifestations of CD, few entities enter into the differential diagnosis. Ganglioneuromatosis of the colon has been described in association with CD, a feature also known to occur in neurofibromatosis type 1. However, the distinctive extraintestinal manifestations of both CD and neurofibromatosis should allow a correct classification of the patients' disease.

PROGNOSIS AND THERAPY

Patients with CD have a significantly higher risk for breast tumors, including fibroadenomas and lipomatosis. Breast carcinoma, the most common malignancy

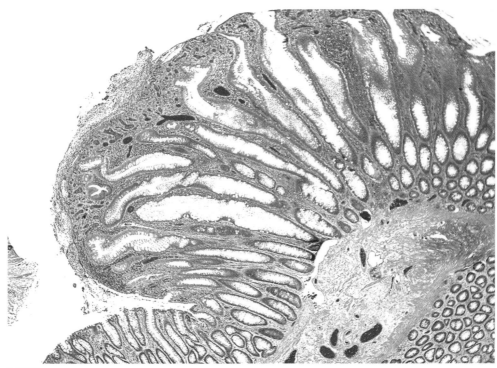

FIGURE 12-11
Cowden's syndrome. The polyp is similar in appearance to those that arise in juvenile polyposis syndrome. However, as shown in this example, the polyps of Cowden's syndrome tend to be small and contain splaying of the muscularis mucosa at the base of the lesion.

in CD, affects up to 50% of female patients. Thus once a diagnosis of CD is made, regular surveillance for breast cancer is indicated. There is no increased risk for GI cancer in CD.

■ CRONKHITE-CANADA SYNDROME

CLINICAL FEATURES

Cronkhite-Canada syndrome (CCS) is a nonhereditary form of diffuse GI polyposis affecting adults, presenting with rapidly progressive diarrhea and malabsorption. In addition to GI polyposis, affected patients show changes of the integumentary system, including skin hyperpigmentation, vitiligo, alopecia, and dystrophic changes of the nails.

The average age of onset is in the fifth to sixth decade of life. A slight male predominance is found. All racial and ethnic groups are affected. The most common presenting symptoms are diarrhea, protein-losing enteropathy, weight loss, abdominal pain, and anorexia. Laboratory findings are notable for hypoproteinemia, particularly hypoalbuminemia, hypocalcemia, hypomagnesemia, anemia, guaiac-positive stool, and severe electrolyte deficiency. The mortality rate is 60% and results from severe protein and electrolyte losses from the intestinal tract.

PATHOLOGIC FEATURES

GROSS FINDINGS

GI polyps are located anywhere from the esophagus to the rectum. In severe cases, the entire mucosal surface of affected sites is involved. Polyps are most frequent in the stomach and colon, followed by the duodenum, ileum, and jejunum. Grossly, the polyps of CCS vary from a subtle nodularity of the mucosal surface to large, edematous fronds of mucosa resulting from the presence of large cystically dilated glands within an edematous stroma (Fig. 12-12A).

MICROSCOPIC FINDINGS

The histologic appearance of CCS polyps is related to the site of origin. In all sites, polyps are typically broad-based sessile lesions with no recognizable stalk. In the colon, CCS polyps are histologically similar to juvenile polyps with cystically dilated glands lined by mature epithelium within an inflamed and edematous stroma. In the stomach, gastric CCS polyps resemble hyperplastic polyps and often show corkscrew-shaped glands, foveolar pits, and smooth muscle fibers extending into the lamina propria (see Fig. 12-12B and C). In the small intestine, the lesions are similar, although the degree of inflammation and

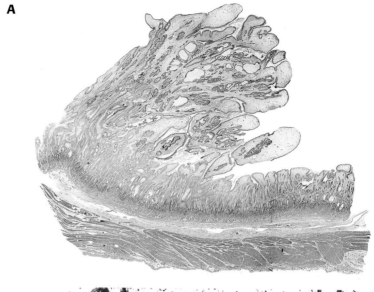

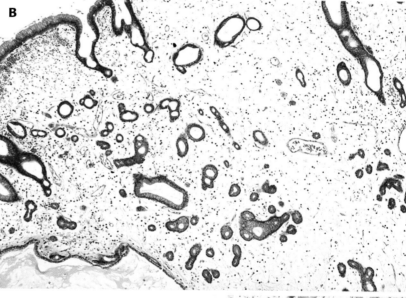

FIGURE 12-12

Gastric mucosal polyp in Cronkhite-Canada syndrome. **A,** Whole-mount view. The polyp is broad-based and characterized by large, edematous fronds of mucosa. **B,** Higher-power view of the polyp shows prominent edema of the lamina propria. The epithelial glands are hyperplastic and reactive in appearance. **C,** High-power view of intervening nonpolypoid mucosa shows similar findings (i.e., prominent lamina propria edema and reactive epithelium).

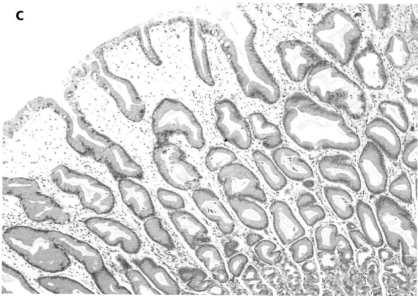

CRONKHITE-CANADA SYNDROME—FACT SHEET

Definition
- A rapidly progressive form of diffuse GI polyposis associated with protein-losing enteropathy and malabsorption

Incidence and Location
- Rare

Morbidity and Mortality
- 60% mortality rate if untreated

Gender, Race, and Age Distribution
- Male predominance
- Average age at diagnosis in sixth to seventh decades of life
- No racial predilection

Clinical Features
- Diarrhea, protein-losing enteropathy, weight loss, abdominal pain, and anorexia
- Laboratory findings notable for hypoalbuminemia, hypocalcemia, hypomagnesemia, and severe electrolyte deficiencies

Prognosis and Therapy
- Rapidly progressive and fatal (60% mortality) if untreated
- Management is largely supportive (aggressive nutritional support or antibiotics)

CRONKHITE-CANADA SYNDROME—PATHOLOGIC FEATURES

Gross Findings
- Diffuse polyposis affecting any portion of GI tract

Microscopic Findings
- Broad-based sessile polyp with prominent edema
- Normal epithelium

Differential Diagnosis
- Inflammatory/retention polyps
- JPS
- Ménétrier's disease

edema tends to be greater and the lesions may involve the full thickness of the bowel wall.

DIFFERENTIAL DIAGNOSIS

The distinction of the polyps of CCS from JPS can be difficult and often relies on the clinical history. Microscopic features to support a diagnosis of CCS are (1) the polyp lacks a stalk, (2) the intervening mucosa is also abnormal, and (3) the degree of edema is in excess of that typically seen in juvenile polyps. In some cases, the confluence of polyps may simulate the giant mucosal folds characteristic of Ménétrier's disease.

PROGNOSIS AND THERAPY

The malabsorption syndrome is progressive and may be fatal without specific therapy. A variety of medical and surgical measures have been used to treat patients with this syndrome, including corticosteroids, antibiotics, and surgical resection. However, aggressive nutritional support in the form of calories, nitrogen, lipids, fluids, electrolytes, vitamins, and minerals appears the most important factor associated with a favorable outcome. Antibiotics appear beneficial when bacterial overgrowth is a contributing factor to the malabsorption syndrome.

■ HYPERPLASTIC POLYPOSIS SYNDROME

CLINICAL FEATURES

Hyperplastic polyposis syndrome (HPS) is an entity characterized by the development of multiple hyperplastic polyps throughout the GI tract in association with an elevated risk for colorectal neoplasia. In contrast to sporadic hyperplastic polyps that tend to be solitary and located in the rectosigmoid, hyperplastic polyposis is defined as (1) greater than five hyperplastic polyps at one time proximal to the sigmoid colon, two of which are greater than 10 mm in diameter, (2) any number of hyperplastic polyps proximal to the sigmoid colon in a first-degree relative of a patient with HPS at least one of which has large size (>1 cm), or (3) 30 or more hyperplastic polyps of any size but evenly distributed throughout the colorectum. Serrated adenomatous polyposis (hyperplastic polyps with cytologic features of adenomatous transformation) is likely a phenotypic variant of this syndrome. Families with documented inheritance of HPS have been described but account for the minority of cases.

PATHOLOGIC FEATURES

GROSS FINDINGS

The number of polyps is often in the tens and usually does not exceed 100. They are virtually always sessile. Although often less than 1 cm in diameter, large polyps that are several centimeters in diameter have been reported (so-called giant hyperplastic polyps) (Fig. 12-13). The gross appearance can range from obvious polypoid lesions to very subtle protuberances that mimic a thickened mucosal fold. Unlike sporadic hyperplastic polyps that are confined to the rectosigmoid, polyps in hyperplastic polyposis are located proximal to the rectosigmoid colon or are evenly distributed throughout the colorectum.

HYPERPLASTIC POLYPOSIS—FACT SHEET

Definition

- Numerous hyperplastic polyps throughout the colorectum, including large hyperplastic polyps (>10 mm) and location proximal to sigmoid colon

Incidence and Location

- Rare

Morbidity and Mortality

- Related to increased risk for colorectal neoplasia

Gender, Race, and Age Distribution

- Males equal to females
- No known ethnic or racial predilection
- Average age at diagnosis in the fifth to seventh decades of life

Clinical Features

- Family history of colon cancer
- Proximal colon cancers more common

Prognosis and Therapy

- Frequent surveillance by colonoscopy as a result of elevated risk for colon cancer
- Colectomy may be indicated if number of polyps too numerous for adequate surveillance

HYPERPLASTIC POLYPOSIS—PATHOLOGIC FEATURES

Gross Findings

- Up to 100 polyps distributed throughout the colorectum, more commonly in the proximal colon
- Sessile growth pattern
- <1 cm in diameter

Microscopic Findings

- Hyperplastic polyps with mild cytologic atypia (nuclear enlargement, upper crypt mitoses)
- Architectural atypia (free-floating goblet cells, papillary infoldings extending to crypt bases, perpendicular crypts)
- Serrated adenomas (hyperplastic polyps with adenomatous epithelium)
- Mixed hyperplastic-tubular adenomas

Genetics

- Low levels of microsatellite instability frequently observed in hyperplastic polyps
- Frequent G:C→T:A transversions in *KRAS* or *BRAF* suggest HPS is related to MYH deficiency

Differential Diagnosis

- Sporadic hyperplastic polyps
- Familial adenomatous polyposis
- Hereditary mixed polyposis syndrome

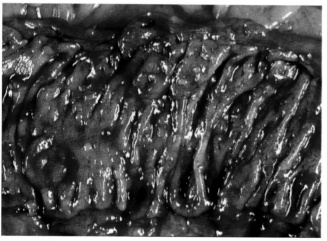

FIGURE 12-13

Colectomy specimen from a patient with hyperplastic polyposis syndrome. Numerous sessile polyps are seen that are irregularly distributed and show a wide variation in size. Note that the polyps are similar in color and texture to intervening normal mucosa.

MICROSCOPIC FINDINGS

The spectrum of polyps in HPS includes hyperplastic polyps, sessile serrated adenomas, mixed hyperplastic-tubular adenomas, and tubular adenomas. Hyperplastic polyps and sessile serrated adenomas are most common. At low power, the hyperplastic polyps of HPS are histologically similar to sporadic hyperplastic polyps, except for their larger size and proximal location (Fig. 12-14A). They contain elongated colonic crypts lined by epithelial cells with a papillary configuration and are composed of well-differentiated goblet and absorptive cells. Sessile serrated adenomas are similar in appearance to their sporadic counterparts, characterized by upper crypt mitoses, nuclear atypia, and architectural distortion with associated free-floating goblet cells, prominent papillary infoldings that extend to the base of the colonic crypts, and perpendicularly oriented crypts (see Fig. 12-14B through D). When the cytologic atypia in a serrated lesion is particularly prominent, the polyp is better classified as a mixed hyperplastic/adenomatous polyp.

ANCILLARY STUDIES

Low levels of microsatellite instability have been reported in association with HPS, and more recently MYH defects have also been implicated. However, genetic testing of HPS patients for microsatellite instability or MYH genetic status is currently not performed.

DIFFERENTIAL DIAGNOSIS

Endoscopically, this syndrome mimics familial adenomatous polyposis. Histologic examination reveals that the majority of polyps have features more typical of hyperplastic polyps or sessile serrated adenomas.

13

Epithelial Neoplasms of the Colorectum

■ Christine A. Iacobuzio-Donahue, MD, PhD

A large variety of neoplasms may occur in the colorectum, a reflection of the complexity of this organ and its cellular components. This chapter focuses primarily on those neoplasms arising from the epithelial and neuroendocrine cells of the colorectum (Table 13-1). Epithelial neoplasms that arise as a component of a polyposis syndrome are discussed in Chapter 12.

■ HYPERPLASTIC POLYPS

CLINICAL FEATURES

Hyperplastic polyps are the most commonly encountered polyp in the adult colorectum. They are found with increasing frequency in individuals older than 40 years of age, are more common in men than in women, and are more common in westernized populations. Because of their small size, hyperplastic polyps are asymptomatic and often detected incidentally at sigmoidoscopy or colonoscopy.

Most patients with adenomatous polyps have coexistent hyperplastic polyps. This observation has prompted the suggestion that hyperplastic polyps are a biomarker of an increased risk for neoplasia. However,

TABLE 13-1

Histopathologic Types of Colorectal Carcinoma Recognized by the World Health Organization

Adenocarcinoma
Mucinous adenocarcinoma
Signet ring carcinoma
Small cell carcinoma
Adenosquamous carcinoma
Squamous cell carcinoma
Undifferentiated carcinoma

the vast amount of evidence to date indicates that conventional hyperplastic polyps have no preneoplastic potential, and the finding of a hyperplastic polyp during sigmoidoscopy is not an indication for colonoscopic examination. Patients with adenomatous or carcinomatous transformation occurring in a hyperplastic polyp have been reported, usually in association with large polyp size (> 1 cm), or location within the proximal colon. However, recent data indicate that these lesions are most likely the result of sporadic microsatellite instability (MSI), and are better classified as sessile serrated adenomas (SSAs), a distinct form of colorectal neoplasm that does have neoplastic potential.

PATHOLOGIC FEATURES

GROSS FINDINGS

Grossly, hyperplastic polyps are dome-shaped nodules that rarely grow beyond 5 mm in diameter. They are often multiple and are most frequently found in the sigmoid colon and rectum. Hyperplastic polyps are most commonly found on the crest of mucosal folds and are similar in color to the surrounding normal mucosa.

MICROSCOPIC FINDINGS

Hyperplastic polyps contain elongated colonic crypts lined by epithelial cells with a pseudopapillary configuration and are composed of well-differentiated goblet and absorptive cells (Fig. 13-1). The papillary infoldings are most prominent in the upper half of the crypts, resulting in the characteristic "saw-toothed" or serrated appearance. The number of absorptive cells lining the crypts is greater than the number of goblet cells, and these crypts contain ample eosinophilic cytoplasm and a prominent brush border. Apical mucin vacuoles may be present within the absorptive cells. Mitoses are not

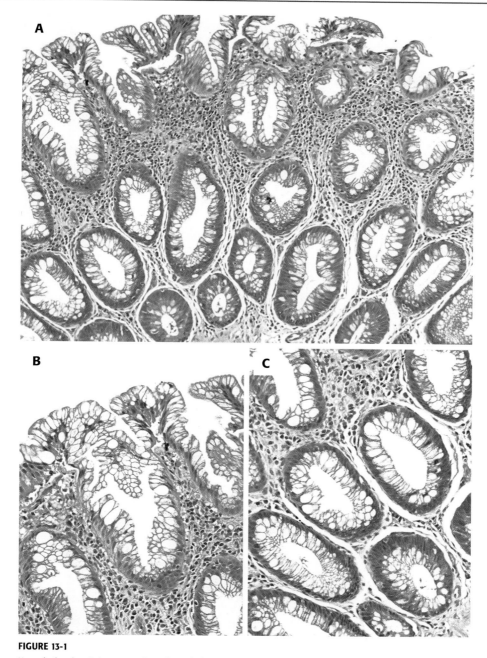

FIGURE 13-1

Hyperplastic polyp. **A,** Low-power view, microvesicular type. The serrated appearance of the upper crypts is evident at low power. The lamina propria is normal. **B,** High-power view of polyp surface. The nuclei are small and basally located, and the cytoplasm of the lining epithelium has a "frothy" appearance resulting from mucin-containing vesicles. Scattered goblet cells are also present, but account for the minority of epithelial cells within the polyp. **C,** High-power view of polyp base showing mild nuclear enlargement, prominent nucleoli, and scattered mitoses. Note that the crypt bases are smaller in diameter than the crypt surfaces.

uncommon but are confined to the bottom half of crypts. The subepithelial collagen layer is thickened, best appreciated at the polyp surface. At the crypt base, the muscularis mucosa often shows splaying of the muscle fibers, with fibers extending into the lamina propria and surrounding individual crypts. The nuclei of epithelial cells range from small and hyperchromatic to slightly enlarged with a prominent nucleolus. Scattered Paneth or endocrine cells may also be seen within the crypt bases (Fig. 13-2).

Three histologic subtypes of hyperplastic polyp have been described. They include the microvesicular cell type (see Fig. 13-1), the goblet cell type (Fig. 13-3), and the mucin-poor type (Fig. 13-4). Microvesicular type hyperplastic polyps are the most common, and likely equate to the classically recognized hyperplastic polyp. They are best distinguished by their microvesicular mucin with few goblet cells, some dystrophic goblet cells, and mild nuclear atypia. Goblet cell type polyps are noted by elongated crypts with prominent goblet cells and minimal

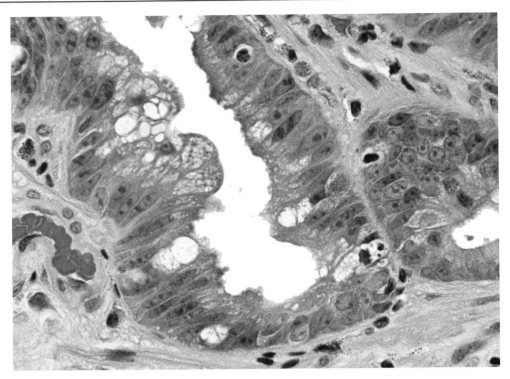

FIGURE 13-2

Hyperplastic polyp. Mild nuclear atypia may be present in a hyperplastic polyp, seen as enlarged nuclei with fine chromatin pattern and one or more prominent nucleoli. However, crowding of nuclei is minimal. At the base of crypts, scattered endocrine cells are also present.

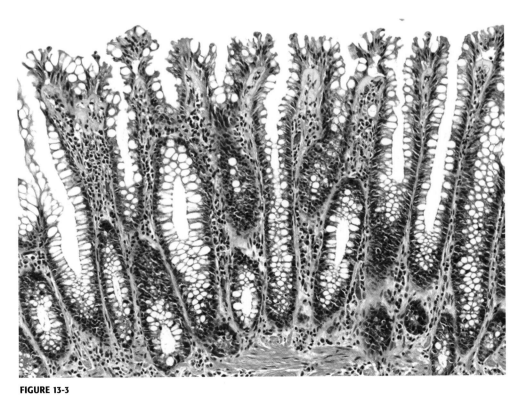

FIGURE 13-3

Goblet cell hyperplastic polyp. In this morphologic variant, the crypts are elongated and the epithelium is composed predominantly of goblet cells. Serrations of the epithelium are minimal, mostly present at the polyp surface.

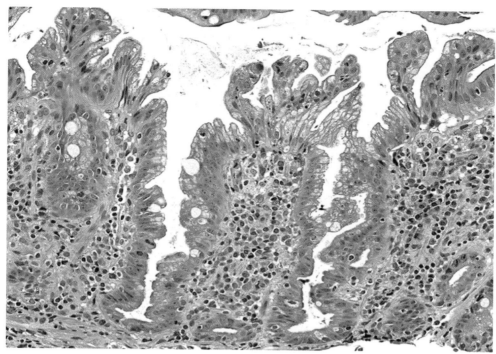

FIGURE 13-4

Mucin-poor hyperplastic polyp. In this morphologic variant, the crypts are uniformly dilated from surface to base, with the serrated epithelium lining the crypts composed of small cells with minimal intracytoplasmic mucin and rare goblet cells. Mild nuclear atypia is present. The epithelial changes are reminiscent of regenerative changes following mucosal injury.

serrations of the epithelium (see Fig. 13-3). Finally, mucin-poor polyps are the least common and have features suggestive that they are regenerative in nature (see Fig. 13-4). The epithelial cells are small with minimal cytoplasm, lack neuroendocrine cells, and show varying amounts of crypt dilatation. However, as a result of their crypt dilatation, some investigators have regarded mucin-poor hyperplastic polyps as morphologic variants of SSAs. At this time, however, there is no evidence that a distinction among these types of hyperplastic polyp has any clinical significance. The most important features to distinguish conventional hyperplastic polyps from an SSA are the lack of architectural distortion and the normal distribution of proliferating epithelial cells.

HYPERPLASTIC POLYPS—FACT SHEET

Definition
- Metaplastic proliferation of differentiated colonic epithelium with no malignant potential

Incidence and Location
- Most common non-neoplastic polyp
- 10% to 20% of asymptomatic patients

Morbidity and Mortality
- No elevated risk for neoplasia

Gender, Race, and Age Distribution
- Incidence increases with age
- Male more than female
- No racial or ethnic associations

Clinical Features
- Asymptomatic
- Incidental finding at endoscopy

Prognosis and Therapy
- Polypectomy only indicated to distinguish from adenomatous polyps by histologic examination

---

HYPERPLASTIC POLYPS—PATHOLOGIC FEATURES

Gross Findings
- Small sessile polyp (< 5 mm) grossly indistinguishable from a small tubular adenoma
- Rectosigmoid colon most common location

Microscopic Findings
- Crypt elongation with micropapillary appearance of epithelium
- Well-differentiated goblet and absorptive cells
- Mitoses restricted to crypt bases

Differential Diagnosis
- Mucosal prolapse
- Reactive epithelial changes
- Tubular adenoma

DIFFERENTIAL DIAGNOSIS

Other lesions with serrated epithelial features can mimic a hyperplastic polyp, including inflammatory cloacogenic polyps (ICPs), which often show prominent serrated epithelial changes of the surface epithelium. Features to distinguish ICPs from hyperplastic polyps include the polyp location at the anal verge, presence of smooth muscle ingrowth, reactive epithelial changes, and lamina propria hemorrhage and fibrosis. In some cases, a hyperplastic polyp may show areas of erosion with associated reactive epithelial changes, also raising the concern of a sessile serrated adenoma. The presence of surface maturation and lack of cytologic atypia should rule out this possibility.

PROGNOSIS AND THERAPY

Hyperplastic polyps do not have malignant potential. Because they may be endoscopically similar in appearance to small adenomatous polyps, hyperplastic polyps are often removed by polypectomy solely to distinguish them on histologic grounds from adenomatous polyps.

■ SESSILE SERRATED ADENOMAS

CLINICAL FEATURES

Sessile serrated adenomas are an entity that has been recognized only within the past decade as a pathologic lesion distinct from hyperplastic polyps. Recognition of these lesions has largely stemmed from the observations that (1) patients with hyperplastic polyposis, a disorder characterized by numerous hyperplastic polyps, have an increased risk for colorectal neoplasia and (2) sporadic right-sided hyperplastic polyps more commonly contain a variety of genetic alterations, including MSI and increased gene methylation, than their left-sided counterparts. Part of the reason for discrepancies in the literature are that these lesions have been called by a variety of names, including *serrated polyp with atypical proliferation, giant hyperplastic polyps, large hyperplastic polyps, mixed hyperplastic/adenomatous polyps, sessile serrated polyps, serrated adenomas,* and *inverted hyperplastic polyps.*

Formal evaluations of the clinical features of SSAs indicate that they represent approximately 10% of all lesions with serrated epithelial architecture encountered at endoscopy. The most common age at diagnosis is in the sixth to seventh decade of life, similar to that for classic adenomatous polyps.

PATHOLOGIC FEATURES

GROSS FINDINGS

As their name indicates, SSAs are always sessile. They can arise anywhere within the colorectum but are predominantly located in the proximal colon. They show a wide size range and may reach several centimeters in diameter, hence the former designation as "giant hyperplastic polyps." The gross appearance can range from obvious polypoid lesions to subtle protuberances that mimic a thickened mucosal fold. Small SSAs are indistinguishable from conventional hyperplastic polyps or classic adenomatous polyps.

MICROSCOPIC FINDINGS

Two major morphologic features distinguish SSAs from conventional hyperplastic polyps: architectural distortion and abnormal proliferation. Architectural features that are characteristic of SSAs include crypt dilatation, horizontal orientation of deep crypts, serrations of crypt epithelium extending to the crypt bases, and inverted crypts (Fig. 13-5). Abnormal proliferation in SSAs is characterized by nuclear atypia that extends to the mid and upper crypts (as opposed to conventional hyperplastic polyps where atypia, if present, is confined to the crypt base), asymmetric proliferation within crypts, prominent nucleoli, and mitoses in upper crypts

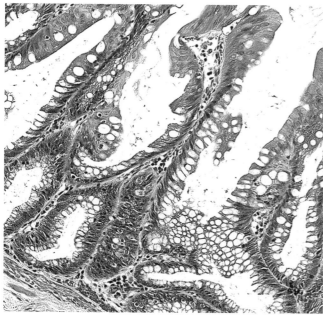

FIGURE 13-5

Sessile serrated adenoma. Unlike conventional hyperplastic polyps shown in Figure 13-1, sessile serrated adenomas show widening of the crypt bases relative to the surface, complexity of crypts including papillary structures, and serrated epithelial changes extending to the crypt bases.

(Fig. 13-6). The basement membrane is not thickened, and the muscularis mucosa does not extend into the lamina propria as described for conventional hyperplastic polyps. Both neuroendocrine cells and Kulchitsky cells are decreased to absent. Cytologic features are less of a distinguishing feature of SSAs than of conventional hyperplastic polyps and include dystrophic goblet cells, irregular distribution of goblet cells, increased apoptosis, and excessive luminal mucin.

Mixed hyperplastic/adenomatous polyps are thought to represent conventional epithelial dysplasia arising within an SSA and thus are part of a histomorphologic continuum of these lesions. In these cases, the serrated changes of an SSA are present but with clear cytologic evidence of conventional epithelial dysplasia, including nuclear enlargement, loss of polarity extending to the polyp surface, and nuclear pleomorphism (Fig. 13-7).

ANCILLARY STUDIES

Immunohistochemical labeling does not have a routine role in the diagnosis of SSAs at this time, in that as no markers have demonstrated the appropriate sensitivity to discriminate a small SSA from a hyperplastic polyp. MUC6 has been reported to be a marker of SSAs, although this finding has not been validated in independent studies. By contrast, abnormal nuclear labeling for beta-catenin has been shown to be specific marker of serrated polyps with neoplastic potential (Fig. 13-8A). However, because nuclear labeling is only found in 29% of SSAs compared with 100% of SSAs with foci of conventional epithelial dysplasia, its role is limited as a diagnostic tool in early polyps. Similarly, some SSAs have been shown to have loss of hMLH1 protein expression, consistent with the increased rate of MSI reported for these polyps, although the loss of hMLH1 expression also occurs in the setting of conventional epithelial dysplasia or carcinoma arising in an SSA, limiting its utility as a diagnostic marker (see Fig. 13-8B).

DIFFERENTIAL DIAGNOSIS

The main entity in the differential diagnosis of an SSA is a conventional hyperplastic polyp or a traditional serrated adenoma, particularly for left-sided lesions. Recognition of a lack of cytologic atypia, normal proliferation, thickened subepithelial basement membrane, and presence of neuroendocrine cells should aid in diagnosis as a hyperplastic polyp. Traditional serrated adenomas have a polypoid or villiform growth pattern, as well as ectopic crypt formations.

PROGNOSIS AND THERAPY

Recognition and differentiation of an SSA from a hyperplastic polyp are of clinical importance, because SSAs are associated with an increased risk for colorectal neoplasia,

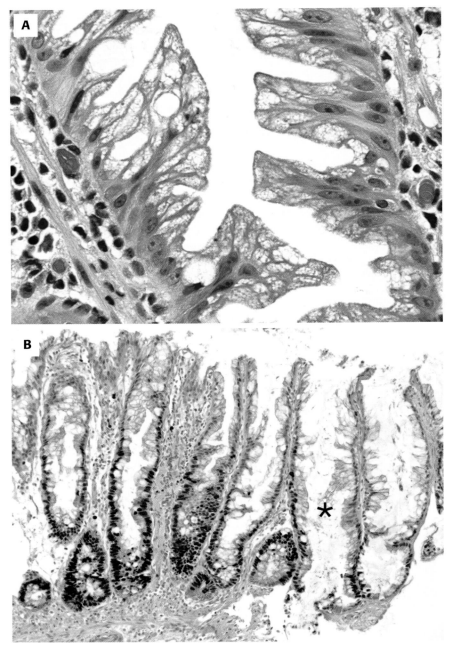

FIGURE 13-6

Sessile serrated adenoma. **A,** Nuclear atypia may be seen as enlarged nuclei with a fine chromatin pattern and one or more prominent nucleoli. In the absence of true adenomatous features, the atypia is not unlike that encountered in a conventional hyperplastic polyp. **B,** Asymmetric proliferation demonstrated by Ki-67 immunostain. In the crypt noted by an asterisk, nuclear staining extends more than halfway up the left side of the crypt in contrast to the right side, in which nuclear staining is confined to the base.

A

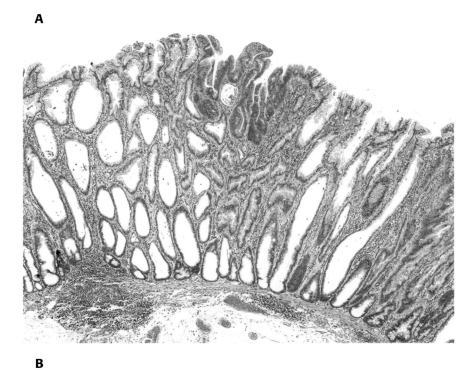

B

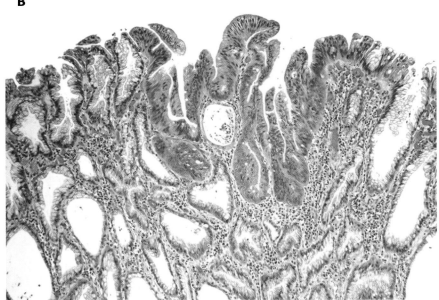

FIGURE 13-7

Conventional epithelial dysplasia arising in a sessile serrated adenoma. Low-power **(A)** and high-power **(B)** views of conventional epithelial dysplasia arising in a large sessile serrated adenoma, recognized by its nuclear crowding, nuclear enlargement, pencillate nuclei, loss of nuclear polarity, and loss of differentiation.

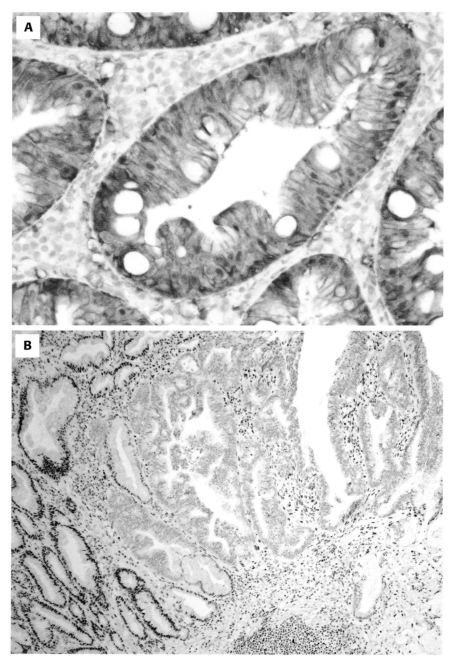

FIGURE 13-8

Immunohistochemical labeling for beta-catenin and hMLH1 in sessile serrated adenomas. **A,** Nuclear accumulation of beta-catenin protein within the epithelial cells of a sessile serrated adenoma. This polyp did not have associated conventional epithelial dysplasia. **B,** Loss of hMLH1 protein labeling within regions of conventional epithelial dysplasia and infiltrating carcinoma arising in a sessile serrated adenoma. Note the retention of hMLH1 labeling in the residual sessile serrated adenoma in the left side of the image.

while hyperplastic polyps are not. The absolute risk for neoplastic transformation in an SSA remains an area of uncertainty. However, an association is recognized between MSI colorectal cancers and serrated adenomas, with up to 6% of colorectal cancers found in association with these lesions. The need for SSAs to be diagnosed and reported is thus of critical importance to aid in the development of management guidelines. In the absence of these data, management as for classic adenomatous polyps is likely the most appropriate course of action.

■ TRADITIONAL SERRATED ADENOMAS

CLINICAL FEATURES

Traditional serrated adenomas (TSAs) are a subset of colorectal polyps with the architectural and cytologic features that overlap both tubular adenomas and hyperplastic polyps. Whereas the initial descriptions of these polyps likely also included SSAs, leading to diagnostic confusion, more recent evidence has definitely shown that they are a pathologically and genetically distinct entity from both tubular adenomas and sessile serrated adenomas. For this reason, the clinical features and incidence of TSAs at endoscopy are unknown but will likely be revealed in the coming years. It is estimated that TSAs are less prevalent than SSAs, with an average age at diagnosis in the seventh decade of life, similar to that for classic adenomatous polyps and SSAs. They are slightly more common in males, and there is no racial predominance.

TRADITIONAL SERRATED ADENOMAS—FACT SHEET

Definition
- Epithelial neoplasms with features of both a serrated polyp and tubular adenoma and associated risk for colorectal neoplasia

Incidence and Location
- Unknown

Morbidity and Mortality
- Actual risk for progression to carcinoma unknown

Gender, Race, and Age Distribution
- Slight male predominance
- No known racial predominance
- Average age at diagnosis in seventh decade of life

Clinical Features
- Usually asymptomatic
- Symptoms related to larger polyp size
- Associated with sporadic microsatellite instability

Prognosis and Therapy
- Routine surveillance indicated caused by increased risk for colorectal neoplasia

---

PATHOLOGIC FEATURES

GROSS FINDINGS

Traditional serrated adenomas most commonly arise in the left colon. Their gross appearance is typically of a polypoid growth that may or may not have villiform features, and they range in size from 0.5 to 2 cm in diameter. Small TSAs are indistinguishable from conventional hyperplastic polyps, and large TSAs may be difficult to distinguish from a classic adenomatous polyp.

MICROSCOPIC FINDINGS

TSAs have features of both a classical tubular adenoma and a serrated polyp. The architectural features that are similar to tubular adenomas include polypoid or villiform growth of tubular glands with an intervening normal lamina propria. Cytologic features that are similar to tubular adenomas include nuclear enlargement, nuclear crowding, pencillate nuclei, loss of nuclear polarity, and loss of goblet cells and apical mucin. In addition, TSAs have a pronounced serrated epithelial architecture, ectopic crypt formations, and eosinophilic cytoplasm. Ectopic crypt formations followed by cytoplasmic eosinophilia are the most specific features of a TSA (Fig. 13-9).

DIFFERENTIAL DIAGNOSIS

The main entities in the differential diagnosis of a TSA are sessile serrated adenomas and classical tubular adenomas. Sessile serrated adenomas can be recognized by their sessile growth pattern and the presence of crypt dilatation, horizontal orientation of deep crypts, serrations of crypt epithelium extending to the crypt bases, and

---

SESSILE SERRATED ADENOMAS—PATHOLOGIC FEATURES

Gross Findings
- Polypoid growth
- Size ranges up to 2 cm
- Left colon distribution

Microscopic Findings
- Villiform growth
- Serrated epithelium in association with nuclear and cytologic atypia
- Ectopic crypt formations
- Eosinophilic cytoplasm

Differential Diagnosis
- Sessile serrated adenoma
- Tubular adenoma

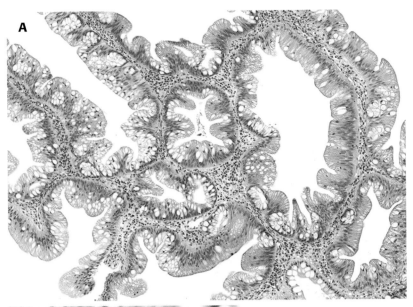

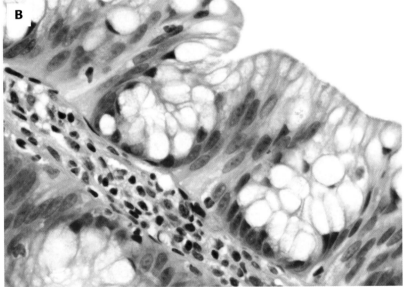

FIGURE 13-9

Traditional serrated adenoma. **A,** In addition to the serrated appearance of the epithelium, there is clear evidence of adenomatous change characterized by nuclear enlargement, crowding, pseudostratification, and atypia. Ectopic crypt formations are also a prominent feature. **B,** High-power view of ectopic crypt formations, seen as the abnormal development of crypts specifically within the epithelium, with the base of the crypt juxtaposed to the basement membrane. **C,** In this example of a traditional serrated adenoma, the adenomatous features are particularly prominent and are associated with eosinophilia of the neoplastic epithelium.

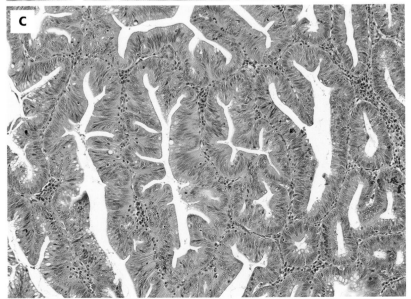

inverted crypts. Sessile serrated adenomas are also more commonly located in the right colon. Tubular adenomas can be recognized by their lack of serrated epithelium. Neither sessile serrated adenomas nor classical tubular adenomas have ectopic crypt formations that are a specific feature of TSAs.

PROGNOSIS AND THERAPY

The absolute risk for neoplastic transformation in a TSA is unknown. However, as high-grade dysplasia or carcinoma has been found in association with TSAs, they are best managed as for classic adenomatous polyps.

■ ADENOMATOUS POLYPS

CLINICAL FEATURES

The prevalence of large intestinal adenomas varies in different parts of the world. Adenomas are common in westernized countries, present in up to 60% of individuals in autopsy studies. In contrast, adenomas in underdeveloped countries are uncommon, found in only 5% of the population. Adenomas are of clinical importance because they can develop into an infiltrating carcinoma, a notion supported by extensive epidemiologic data. The incidence of adenomas parallels the incidence of colorectal cancer, and countries with high rates of colorectal cancer also have high rates of colorectal adenoma. Clinical data in support of the neoplastic potential of adenomas relate to adenoma size, adenoma type, and the presence of high-grade dysplasia. Infiltrating carcinoma is found in 5% of all adenomas and is more commonly found in adenomas greater than 1.0 cm in diameter, with villous morphology and with coexistent areas of high-grade dysplasia. Four factors have been described in association with the formation of colorectal adenomas: environment, genetics, diet, and host factors.

ENVIRONMENT

Colorectal adenomas show wide geographic variations in frequency among industrialized nations. They are most common in North America, Western Europe, New Zealand, and Australia. Variations in incidence are also found within industrialized nations. For example, in the US, colorectal cancer is most frequently diagnosed in the Northeast and least commonly in rural regions of the Southeast.

GENETICS

The genetic factors that contribute to colorectal carcinogenesis are perhaps the best understood for any tumor type (Table 13-2). Patients with a high risk for developing colorectal cancer are those with an inherited predisposition to colorectal adenoma formation (i.e., familial adenomatous polyposis), patients with chronic inflammatory bowel disease (IBD; particularly ulcerative colitis), or patients with a family history of colon cancer (as in hereditary nonpolyposis colon cancer [HNPCC]). Hereditary polyposis syndromes account for 1% of all colorectal cancers, whereas HNPCC accounts for up to 10% of all newly diagnosed cases of colorectal carcinoma.

TABLE 13-2

Molecular Genetic Pathways of Colorectal Carcinogenesis

	Sporadic Colorectal Carcinoma			Hereditary Colorectal Carcinoma		
Molecular Pathway	Clinical Phenotype	Histopathology	Genetics	Clinical Phenotype	Histopathology	Genetics
Chromosome instability (CIN)	Left-sided predominant cancers	Tubular, tubulovillous, and villous adenomas Moderately differentiated adenocarcinomas	Somatic inactivation of *APC*, p53	Familial adenomatous polyposis	Innumerable tubular, flat, and crypt adenomas	Germline *APC* inactivation
Microsatellite instability (MSI)	Right-sided predominant cancers	Sessile serrated adenomas Large (>1 cm) hyperplastic polyps Mixed hyperplastic/ adenomatous polyps Mucinous carcinomas	Hypermethylation, microsatellite instability by somatic inactivation of DNA repair enzymes	Hereditary nonpolyposis colorectal cancer	Mucinous and poorly differentiated cancers; lymphocytic infiltrates	Germline hMLH1 or hMSH2 inactivation

DIET

The relationship of diet to colorectal cancer risk is a topic of enormous interest and debate. Nonetheless, the role of dietary factors in the development of colorectal adenomas and carcinoma is generally accepted, and thought to relate to diets that are high in animal fat and protein and low in fiber or vegetables. High-fat diets may increase colorectal cancer risk resulting from increased calories, or as a surrogate marker for high animal protein contents such as red meat. Low-fiber diets also show a relationship to colorectal cancer, possibly resulting from decreased stool transit time and thus increased exposure of the intestinal epithelium to potential carcinogens. Green leafy vegetables and fruits are a rich source of antioxidants and vitamins; diets low in these foods are also associated with increased cancer risk. Additional dietary factors thought to increase colorectal cancer risk include increased alcohol consumption, particularly beer.

HOST FACTORS

A variety of host factors related to colorectal cancer risk include obesity, smoking history, and occupational exposures. Bile acid turnover in association with gut microflora metabolism is also related to tumor incidence. For example, fecapentaenes, a product of the gut microflora, are potent mutagenic compounds found in human feces that are correlated with colorectal carcinogenesis.

ADENOMATOUS POLYPS—FACT SHEET

Definition
- Dysplastic neoplasms of intestinal epithelium with the potential for transformation to invasive carcinoma

Incidence and Location
- Common finding in patients living in industrialized countries

Morbidity and Mortality
- Related to risk for malignant progression
- Infiltrating carcinoma more common in adenomas greater than 1 cm in diameter, with villous morphology, and located in left colon

Gender, Race, and Age Distribution
- Males more than females
- More common in African American population
- Average age at diagnosis in sixth decade of life

Clinical Features
- Associated with high-fat, low-fiber diet
- More common in patients with prior adenomas or positive family history

Prognosis and Therapy
- Left-sided adenomas are a biomarker for elevated colorectal cancer risk
- Routine surveillance indicated to remove metachronous adenomas

---

PATHOLOGIC FEATURES

GROSS FINDINGS

Adenomas smaller than 1 cm in diameter tend to be evenly distributed throughout the colorectum. In contrast, adenomas 1 cm or larger in diameter are more commonly found in the sigmoid colon and rectum. In general, the polyp size is correlated with the histologic type. Among adenomas smaller than 1 cm in diameter, more than 90% are tubular adenomas, 7% are tubulovillous, and 2% are villous. In contrast, only 50% of adenomas larger than 2 cm are tubular, whereas 38% are tubulovillous and 12% villous. Grossly, colorectal adenomas may appear pedunculated, sessile, or flat (Fig. 13-10). However, in addition to showing polyp size, polyp architecture also shows a relationship to the histologic pattern. For example, tubular adenomas are most often pedunculated, and villous adenomas are most often sessile, although exceptions do occur.

Tubular adenomas range in size from individual crypt adenomas to large exophytic lesions several centimeters in diameter. Small adenomas (1 to 3 mm) are round, dome-shaped lesions with a smooth surface; they are grossly indistinguishable from hyperplastic polyps. Larger tubular adenomas may become polypoid with a lobulated surface and a stalk at the base of the lesion. The stalk can range in length from millimeters to more than a centimeter. With growth of the adenoma, the color may become reddish or darker than the surrounding mucosa. In addition to the surface lobulations, areas of hemorrhage may be present resulting from erosion of the surface epithelium. In contrast, villous adenomas are commonly sessile lesions with a broad base and grossly evident papillary architecture.

ADENOMATOUS POLYPS—PATHOLOGIC FEATURES

Gross Findings
- Pedunculated or sessile growth pattern
- Pancolonic distribution
- Larger adenomas (>1 cm) more often left sided

Microscopic Findings
- Tubular adenomas contain complex networks of branching dysplastic glands
- Villous adenomas contain dysplastic glands growing in long, finger-like projections
- Crowded, enlarged nuclei with prominent nucleoli
- Decreased apical mucin
- Frequent mitoses
- High-grade dysplasia associated with crowding of glands, cribriform glands, and complete loss of nuclear polarity

Genetics
- Complex genetic alterations
- Frequent alterations of *APC*, *KRAS*, and *Tp53*

Differential Diagnosis
- Reactive epithelial changes

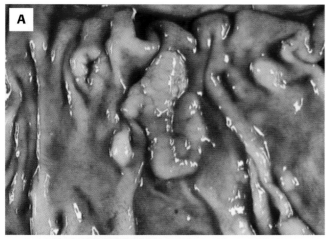

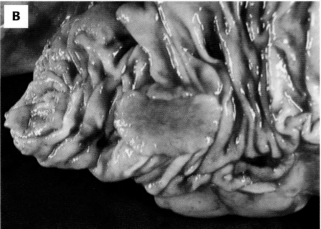

FIGURE 13-10

Adenoma: gross features. **A,** Tubular: The polyps have a dome-shaped surface. The largest polyp in the center also shows subtle lobulations. **B,** Villous: The polyp grows as a flat plaque with slightly raised edges.

Flat adenomas are a morphologic type of adenoma with a propensity for development of high-grade dysplasia while still small. They are thought to be precursors of deep, penetrating colorectal carcinomas. Grossly, they appear as flat or slightly raised plaques on the mucosal surface with a central depression and a size rarely greater than 1 cm.

MICROSCOPIC FINDINGS

Regardless of the gross features of adenomatous polyps, the cytologic features are the same (Fig. 13-11). Cytologic features of the adenomatous epithelium include nuclear enlargement (cigar-shaped nuclei), nuclear hyperchromasia, prominent nucleoli, loss of apical mucin, and pseudostratification of nuclei extending from the crypt bases to surface epithelium (loss of polarity). Apoptoses may be prominent, and mitoses are frequent. Neutrophilic infiltration of the epithelium may also be seen, not to be confused with active inflammation of an inflammatory polyp.

The earliest recognizable lesion is an aberrant crypt focus that can be seen with the aid of a dissecting microscope.

These foci represent adenomatous transformation within an individual colonic crypt, seen as an enlarged crypt or dilated crypt lumen whose opening protrudes above the mucosal surface. Continued proliferation by the adenomatous cells leads to branching, budding, and infolding of the epithelium, causing mucosal elevations so that grossly visible polyps may be seen by endoscopy (tubular adenomas; see Fig. 13-11BC). Neoplastic glands may cluster at the luminal half of the polyps, with normal-appearing colonic crypts present at the polyp base. With further increases in size, the adenomatous polyps may become pedunculated and show associated mucosal prolapse changes typical of a polyp stalk, including heme-laden macrophages, fibrosis, and herniation of adenomatous glands into the stalk. The lamina propria intervening among adenomatous glands is normal.

By definition, all adenomas are low-grade dysplastic lesions. Although the World Health Organization and the National Polyp Study both used a three-tiered classification of epithelial dysplasia (mild, moderate, and severe dysplasia), in practice most pathologists grade adenomas as low-grade or high-grade dysplasia. Low-grade dysplasia corresponds to the cytologic features described previously for adenomatous epithelium, whereas high-grade dysplasia encompasses additional architectural and cytologic changes (Fig. 13-12). Architecturally, the crypts within areas of high-grade dysplasia show increasing complexity, seen as irregular branching, gland budding, and cribriform formations. Cytologically, the nuclei show severe atypia (enlarged, hyperchromatic, and vesicular nuclei with prominent nucleoli) and complete loss of polarity reaching the luminal surface of the epithelium. Mitoses are prominent and cytoplasmic mucin is absent.

Flat adenomas are in essence tubular adenomas that lack a polypoid growth or exophytic growth pattern. These lesions, by definition, are never more than twice the thickness of the adjacent normal colonic epithelium (Fig. 13-13). Rather than the complex branching of adenomatous glands, villous adenomas show tall, finger-like projections of adenomatous epithelium with a central fibrovascular core that extends from the polyp base to the surface (Fig. 13-14). Villous lesions are defined as those that contain at least 80% or more of a villous component.

A variety of cell types may be encountered in adenomas, including Paneth cells, goblet cells, or endocrine cells (Fig. 13-15). The finding of these cell types in an adenomatous polyp reflect the ability of the neoplastic cells to partially differentiate into a variety of cell types. Goblet cells within adenomatous polyps are often dystrophic, seen as free-floating goblet cells or goblet cells with atypical nuclei. Endocrine cells are present in at least half of adenomas and can best be discerned with the use of special stains. Paneth cells are present in 10% of adenomas, recognized for their characteristic eosinophilic granules. Some adenomas may contain foci of squamous metaplasia, osseous metaplasia, melanocytes, or gastric type epithelium.

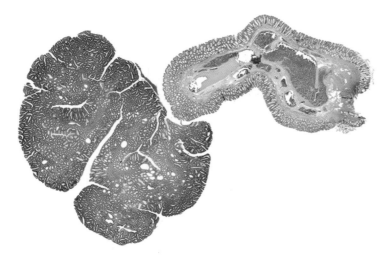

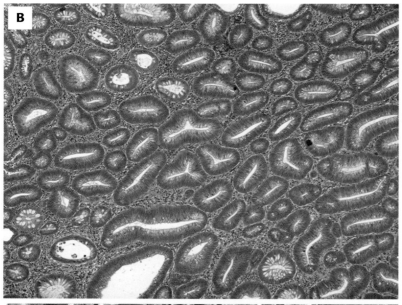

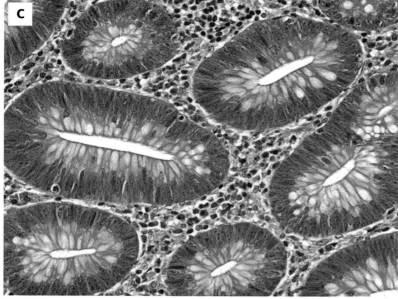

FIGURE 13-11

Tubular adenoma. **A,** Scanning power view of tubular adenoma. The polyp head is composed of crowded adenomatous glands. A large cleft is present, corresponding to the lobular gross appearance typical of tubular adenomas. In this example, the polyp also contains a prominent stalk. **B,** A higher-power view of the polyp head demonstrates the presence of crowded uniform tubular structures with normal intervening lamina propria. **C,** The cytologic features of adenomatous glands with low-grade dysplasia include nuclear enlargement and elongation ("cigar-shaped nuclei"), nuclear crowding, pseudostratification, multiple prominent nucleoli, frequent mitoses, and loss of apical mucin.

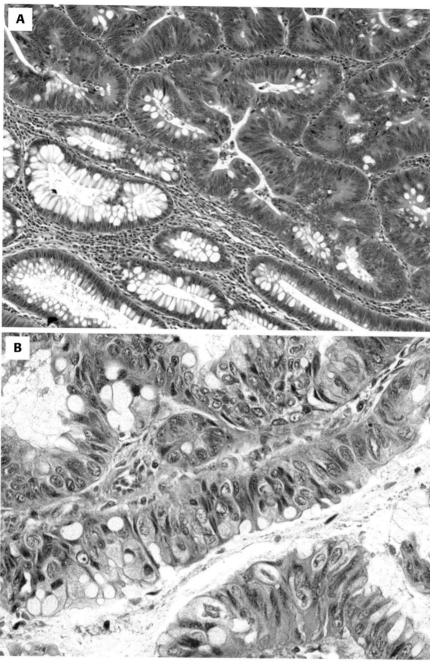

FIGURE 13-12

High-grade dysplasia. **A,** In contrast to low-grade dysplasia present in the bottom left, the adenomatous glands grow in a complex pattern that includes cribriforming of glands. Apical mucin is completely lost, and the nuclei show complete loss of polarity. **B,** High-power view of high-grade dysplasia in an adenomatous polyp. The nuclei show complete loss of polarity and marked pleomorphism. Numerous atypical goblet cells are also present in this example.

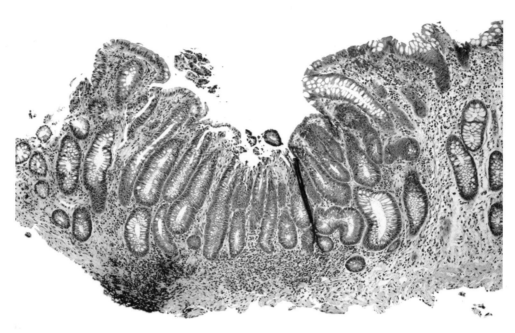

FIGURE 13-13

Flat adenoma. In contrast to the exophytic growth pattern typical of tubular adenomas, flat adenomas have a concave surface and do not exceed twice the thickness of the adjacent normal mucosa.

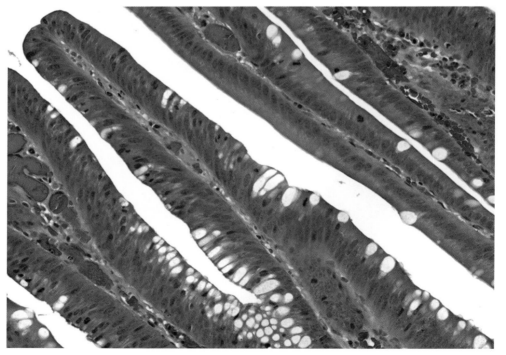

FIGURE 13-14

Villous adenoma. In contrast to the growth pattern of tubular adenomas, villous adenomas are characterized by slender papillae containing a fibrovascular core and lined by adenomatous epithelium.

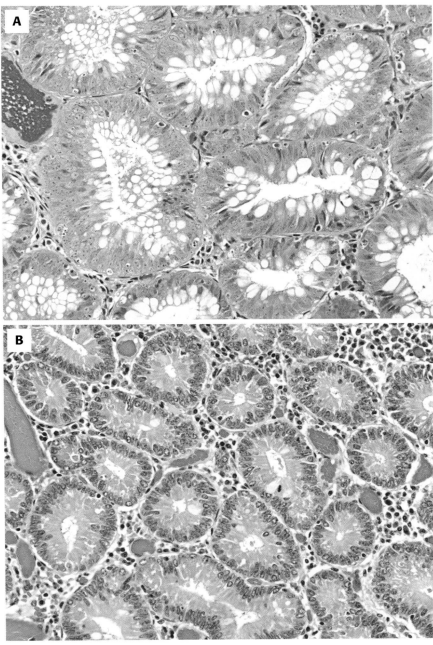

FIGURE 13-15

Adenomatous polyp variants. **A,** In a subset of adenomatous polyps, goblet cells may be numerous. At higher power, atypia of the goblet cells can be appreciated as atypical goblet cells, free-floating goblet cells, and goblet cell mitoses. **B,** Atypical Paneth cells are not uncommon in adenomatous polyps, recognized by their large eosinophilic granules.

DIFFERENTIAL DIAGNOSIS

Any pathologic entity in the colorectum in which the epithelium undergoes reactive changes can enter into the differential diagnosis with an adenomatous polyp, including hyperplastic polyps, mucosal prolapse disorders, and inflammatory polyps. In all cases, recognition of the lack of cytologic atypia and presence of surface maturation should lead to the correct diagnosis.

Pseudoinvasion is defined as the situation when the adenomatous epithelium of the polyp becomes misplaced into the submucosal tissue, mimicking invasive carcioma (Fig. 13-16). This phenomenon is most common in polyps arising in the rectosigmoid colon and that have a well-defined stalk. Pseudoinvasion is not uncommon and is important to distinguish from true invasion so that a mistaken diagnosis of cancer is avoided and unnecessary surgery not performed. Pseudoinvasion can be recognized by the fact that the displaced glands do not

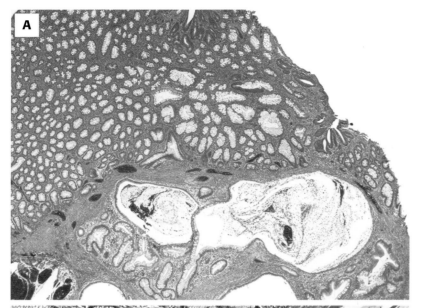

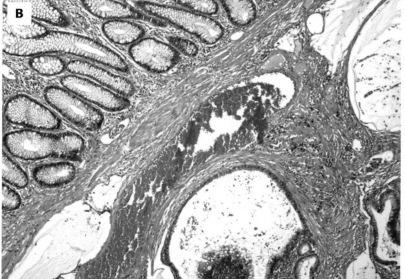

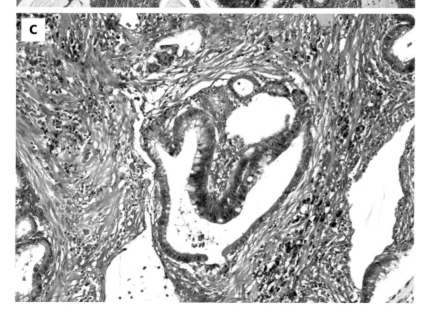

FIGURE 13-16

Pseudoinvasion of an adenomatous polyp stalk. **A,** Low-power view. Note the cystically dilated glands that are surrounded by normal lamina propria. **B,** High-power view of pseudoinvasion demonstrating dilated vasculature and heme-laden macrophages throughout the lamina propria surrounding herniated glands. **C,** High-power view of a herniated adenomatous gland in an area of pseudoinvasion. There is no desmoplastic response to the epithelium, and the surrounding stroma is fibrotic with evidence of both recent and remote hemorrhage (heme-laden macrophages) into the stalk.

elicit a desmoplastic reaction, are surrounded by normal lamina propria with fresh hemorrhage or heme-laden macrophages, and often show cystic dilatation, gland rupture, and mucin extravasation.

PROGNOSIS AND THERAPY

The prevention of colorectal cancer can largely be attained by effective screening for adenomatous polyps before they develop the ability to invade. Screening recommendations vary depending on each individual patient's risk, with high-risk patients defined as those with a known inherited predisposition to colorectal carcinoma, a personal history of colorectal adenomas or carcinoma, or a history of IBD. Patients without these risk factors should be screened beginning at age 50 and older with annual fecal occult blood testing (FOBT) or sigmoidoscopy. Individuals with negative screening results need not have another screening procedure for 5 years. Removal of adenomatous polyps has been shown to reduce mortality from colorectal cancer up to 85%. Moreover, when carcinomas have been found as part of a screening procedure, they are more often at a favorable clinical stage. Thus effective reductions in mortality result from early identification of cancers.

In contrast to the finding of intramucosal adenocarcinoma in an adenomatous polyp (infiltrating cancer limited to the lamina propria) that has no metastatic potential, a malignant polyp is one in which an infiltrating carcinoma is present and has invaded the submucosal tissue. It is important to differentiate among high-grade carcinoma or intramucosal carcinoma and infiltrating adenocarcinoma that has invaded beyond the muscularis mucosa into submucosal tissue, because the latter requires surgical intervention. Diagnosis of infiltrating carcinoma in an endoscopically removed polyp is dependent on a variety of factors, including fixation, plane of sectioning, and method of endoscopic removal (piecemeal or one piece). Piecemeal polypectomy results in multiple fragments of adenomatous tissue that precludes an evaluation of the margin of resection. In contrast, in polyps in which the margin can be evaluated, a negative margin is defined as one in which the infiltrating carcinoma is greater than or equal to 2 mm from the cauterized margin. When evaluating a malignant polyp, one should comment on the margin status (if possible), grade of cancer, and presence or absence of venous invasion. The common course of management for any infiltrating carcinoma in a polyp that reaches the margin, is grade III (poorly differentiated), or shows lymphatic/venous invasion is surgical management (Fig. 13-17). In the absence of these findings, polypectomy can be considered curative.

A significant area of interest in the past decade relates to the chemoprevention of colorectal adenoma formation. Chemopreventive agents of interest include antioxidants, nonsteroidal anti-inflammatory agents, and supplemental calcium. Aspirin and other anti-inflammatory agents have been shown to prevent the development and progression of colorectal adenomas, while calcium is thought to reduce intestinal proliferation and alters the metabolism of intestinal bile acids.

◼ COLORECTAL ADENOCARCINOMA

CLINICAL FEATURES

Colorectal carcinoma is among the most common neoplasms affecting industrialized nations. It is the third most frequently diagnosed cancer in the United States among both men and women, with an estimated 150,000 new cases each year. Colorectal carcinoma is also the third most common cause of cancer deaths in the United States among men and women, with an estimated 56,000 patients dying of colorectal carcinoma in the year 2004.

The lifetime risk for developing colorectal cancer is approximately 6% and is greater for men than women. The risk for development of colorectal cancer increases significantly after the age of 40 years in both men and women, with the average age of diagnosis in the seventh decade of life. Colorectal cancer risk also varies by location within the colorectum. In low-risk countries, right-sided cancers are more common, whereas in high-risk countries, left-sided cancers are more common. These statistics largely reflect the incidence of colon cancer, because the incidence of rectal cancer is fairly constant among high- and low-risk countries. Right-sided cancers are more common as patients age, particularly in women. The distribution of colorectal cancer also shows a relationship to race, in that 35% of African-Americans have right-sided cancers compared with only 24% of white patients. Sixty percent of whites develop sigmoid cancers as compared with 36% of African-Americans.

Family history is particularly important in assessing colorectal cancer risk, especially in patients younger than 50 years. Genetic factors play a role in at least 10% of patients, and epigenetic factors such as IGF2 loss of imprinting may account for an additional 10% of colorectal cancers in patients with a positive family history. HNPCC is the prototype of an autosomal dominant inherited colon cancer family syndrome, which is responsible for 10% of cases of colorectal carcinoma diagnosed each year. In contrast to gastrointestinal polyposis syndromes in which risk of carcinoma is related to the development of innumerable adenomas, HNPCC is not associated with increased colorectal adenoma formation. HNPCC is classified as either type I (Lynch syndrome I), in which affected patients inherit a predisposition for the development of early-onset right-sided colon cancers, or type II (Lynch syndrome II), in which in addition to colorectal cancers there is an increased predisposition for extracolonic cancers as well, including cancers of the

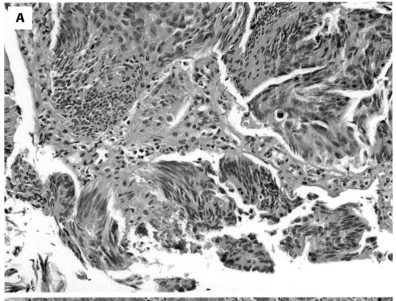

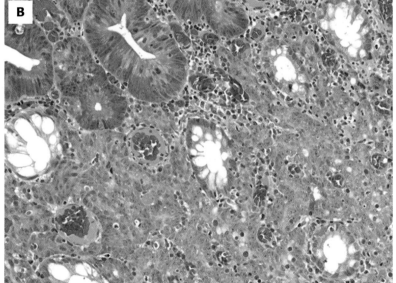

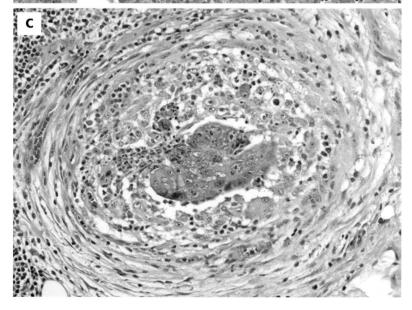

FIGURE 13-17

Malignant features in an adenomatous polyp. **A,** Infiltrating carcinoma extending to the cauterized margin of resection. **B,** Poorly differentiated carcinoma arising in an adenomatous polyp. Residual adenomatous glands are seen at the top of the image. **C,** Angiolymphatic invasion in a malignant adenomatous polyp.

COLORECTAL ADENOCARCINOMA—FACT SHEET

Definition
- Malignant neoplasm of colorectal epithelium

Incidence and Location
- Third most common cancer in industrialized nations

Morbidity and Mortality
- Responsible for 20% of cancer deaths
- 5-year survival rate 55% to 60%

Gender, Race, and Age Distribution
- Males more than females
- More common among African-American populations
- Average age at diagnosis in seventh decade of life (fifth decade for HNPCC)

Clinical Features
- High-risk populations include patients with positive family history or history of IBD
- 10% of colorectal cancers resulting from HNPCC
- Proximal and mucinous carcinomas associated with younger age, female gender, MSI

Prognosis and Therapy
- Prognosis related to clinical stage and tumor differentiation
- Surgical resection most effective treatment for early stage (T1 and T2)
- Adjuvant therapy recommended for advanced-stage carcinomas

COLORECTAL ADENOCARCINOMA—PATHOLOGIC FEATURES

Gross Findings
- Polypoid, fungating, or ulcerated appearance
- Larger tumors more common in proximal colon
- Circumferential growth (apple-core lesions) more common in left colon

Microscopic Findings
- Adenocarcinomas of well, moderate, or poor differentiation
- Prominent desmoplastic response
- Abundant eosinophilic necrotic debris within gland lumens
- Mucinous carcinomas associated with extracellular mucin production and mucin pools

Genetics
- Sporadic carcinomas associated with *APC, KRAS,* and *Tp53* alterations
- 10% of carcinomas caused by hereditary factors (HNPCC)

Immunohistochemistry
- Strong cytokeratin (AE1/AE3, CK20, and CAM5.2) positivity in sporadic carcinomas
- Variable CK20 positivity in MSI-high carcinomas
- CEA positive
- Abnormal p53 nuclear accumulation

Differential Diagnosis
- Metastatic carcinomas
- Endometriosis

---

genitourinary tract. Muir-Torre syndrome is considered by some experts to be a variant of Lynch syndrome II. The Amsterdam criteria for a diagnosis of HNPCC include (1) colorectal cancer in at least three family members, at least one of which is a first-degree relative of the other two; (2) colorectal cancer in at least two successive generations; and (3) the development of colorectal cancer before the age of 50 years in at least one of the affected family members. The mean age of cancer diagnosis among affected patients is in the fourth decade of life, and first-degree relatives of patients with HNPCC have up to a sevenfold increased risk for developing colorectal cancer in their lifetime.

The average age at diagnosis of cancer in patients with HNPCC is 45 years, at least 20 years younger than the general population. Eighty percent of colorectal carcinomas in patients with HNPCC are diagnosed before age 50 years. Synchronous and metachronous colon cancers are common among patients with HNPCC and affect up to 25% of patients with this syndrome. The number of adenomas in patients with HNPCC is not increased, although the time for progression from adenoma to carcinoma appears accelerated.

The estimated time for development of an infiltrating carcinoma from a small adenoma is 10 years. Thus most patients do not have specific clinical symptoms to alert the clinician to the presence of a lesion. Initial symptoms may

be vague and nonspecific, such as weight loss or malaise, whereas up to 12% of patients are entirely asymptomatic at the time of diagnosis. Of those patients who are symptomatic, clinical presentation may be related to location of the carcinoma within the colorectum. Cancers of the cecum and right colon are often polypoid; thus cancers in this location may remain clinically silent because they rarely cause obstruction or bleeding and the proximal bowel can accommodate large, bulky tumors. In contrast, left colon cancers may present with changes in bowel habits such as diarrhea, tenesmus, incontinence, or a decrease in stool caliber as the carcinoma grows and obstructs the lumen. Regardless of location, half of all patients present with rectal bleeding, which may be the result of frank hemorrhage or found by FOBT. Dark or maroon stools may indicate proximal location. Abdominal pain is also a presenting complaint in 50% of patients, more common in colon cancers than rectal cancers.

PATHOLOGIC FEATURES

GROSS FINDINGS

Grossly, colon cancers may be polypoid, exophytic, ulcerative, diffusely infiltrating, or obstructing, producing a circumferential narrowing of the bowel lumen

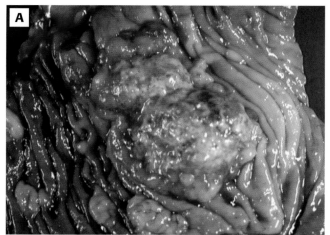

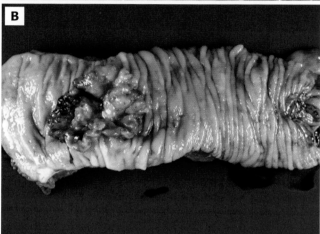

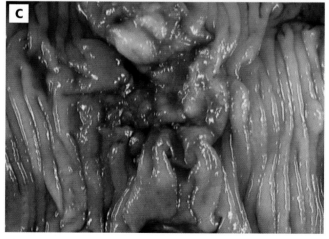

FIGURE 13-18

Colorectal carcinoma. **A,** Polypoid carcinoma. The carcinoma is bulky and occupies the intestinal lumen. **B,** Fungating carcinoma. The carcinoma shows a combination of exophytic growth and central ulceration. **C,** Ulcerating carcinoma. The carcinoma grows in an infiltrative and constricting manner. This form of carcinoma is more common in the left colon and responsible for the "apple-core" appearance of infiltrating carcinomas on barium enema.

(Fig. 13-18). Polypoid cancers are papillary, lobular masses that protrude into the lumen and are more common in the cecum and right colon. In contrast, ulcerative carcinomas deeply invade into the colon wall with an edge that is barely discernable from the adjacent mucosa. Ulcerative carcinomas are more common within the left colon or rectum. Fungating tumors show a mixture of these two patterns, characteristically seen as a central ulcerated crater with a raised, rolled edge. Fungating tumors rarely cause obstruction. Adenocarcinomas arising in the left and descending colon often produce growth that involves the circumference of the bowel, resulting in constriction. They may appear irregularly round, with raised edges and a central deep core. These lesions show the characteristic apple-core lesion on barium contrast radiographs. Except for their circumferential growth, they are similar to ulcerating carcinomas.

On cut surface, infiltrating carcinomas are white in color with indistinct edges, owing to the host desmoplastic response. Involvement of the muscularis propria by infiltrating carcinoma usually results in thickening of the bowel wall. Continued invasion through the bowel wall may involve contiguous structures, including loops of small bowel, bladder, or stomach. In some cases, central necrosis and ulceration may result in bowel perforation, resulting in peritonitis. Mucinous carcinomas are typically glistening as a result of the prominent extracellular mucin, and may show foci of gelatinous material.

MICROSCOPIC FINDINGS

The vast majority of colorectal cancers are adenocarcinomas. Adenocarcinomas are graded according to the degree of gland formation, with well-differentiated cancers showing predominantly ($> 75\%$) uniform tubule formation, similar to adenomatous epithelium (Fig. 13-19A). In well-differentiated carcinomas, the nuclei retain their polarity despite their obvious cytologic atypia. Moderately differentiated cancers retain the ability to make tubules, but architecturally they may be composed of a mixture of simple and complex glands (see Fig. 13-19B). Poorly differentiated cancers show minimal gland formation ($< 25\%$), often seen as sheets of cytologically malignant cells, with a complete loss of nuclear polarity (see Fig. 13-19C). More than 80% of colorectal adenocarcinomas are moderately differentiated and are associated with large regions of eosinophilic staining necrotic material within neoplastic glands, known as "dirty necrosis" (Fig. 13-20).

Mucinous (colloid) adenocarcinomas account for 10% of all colon cancers and 30% of rectal cancers. They are more common among patients with HNPCC or sporadic carcinomas arising in association with an SSA. The definition of a mucinous carcinoma is any carcinoma in which at least 50% of the lesion is mucinous. Mucinous carcinomas have a characteristic appearance, seen as cytologically malignant glands that are disrupted by abundant extruded intraluminal mucin, acellular mucin pools, and mucin pools containing free-floating malignant cells (Fig. 13-21A). Signet ring cancers are included in the designation of mucinous adenocarcinomas, with the

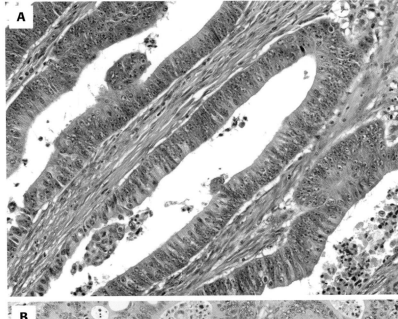

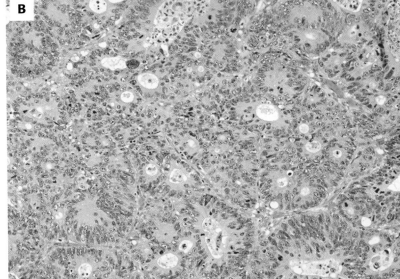

FIGURE 13-19

Colorectal carcinoma. **A,** Well-differentiated carcinoma. The neoplasm forms uniform gland structures, and the nuclei are localized to the basal half of the neoplastic cells. **B,** Moderately differentiated carcinoma. The neoplasm is composed of complex glandular structures, with loss of polarity of the nuclei. Most colorectal carcinomas are moderately differentiated. **C,** Poorly differentiated carcinoma. The carcinoma shows minimal to no gland formation.

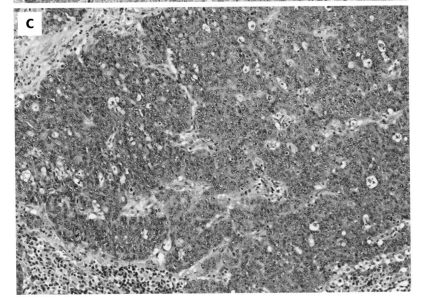

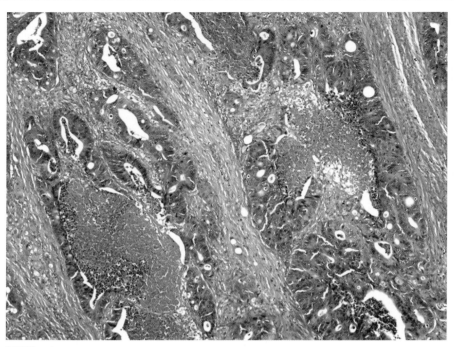

FIGURE 13-20

Dirty necrosis. Tumor necrosis is a common feature of infiltrating carcinomas arising in the colorectum, seen as abundant eosinophilic acellular debris within infiltrating glands.

exception that the mucin is intracellular (see Fig. 13-21B). The diagnosis of a mucinous carcinoma as signet ring type is dependent on findings of more than 50% of signet ring cells, seen as poorly differentiated tumor cells with copious intracytoplasmic mucin.

ANCILLARY STUDIES

Immunohistochemically, colorectal adenocarcinomas are virtually always positive for broad-spectrum and low-molecular-weight cytokeratins (AE1/AE3, CAM5.2), EMA, and carcinoembryonic antigen (CEA). They are consistently positive for cytokeratin (CK) 20, variably positive for CK7, and negative for vimentin.

DIFFERENTIAL DIAGNOSIS

A variety of metastatic neoplasms may involve the colorectum, including prostate, breast, stomach, and ovarian cancers and melanoma. The lack of associated adenomatous epithelium combined with the gross findings should be diagnostic. Immunohistochemical stains for appropriate markers (PSAP for prostate; CK7 for breast, ovary, or stomach; or S-100 for melanoma) may also indicate the primary tumor of origin, whereas colorectal carcinomas are almost universally CK20 and CEA positive.

Involvement of the colorectum by endometriosis is common among women of child-bearing age (up to 20%

of patients with endometriosis). Endometriomas involving the colon form ill-defined masses involving the subserosal tissue and muscularis propria, although lesions that protrude into the intestinal lumen have been reported. Histologic examination reveals the presence of normal mucosa overlying endometrial glands and stroma, which should be differentiated from adenocarcinoma glands with desmoplasia.

PROGNOSIS AND THERAPY

Colorectal cancer accounts for up to 20% of all cancer deaths. Death from colorectal carcinoma is uncommon among patients younger than 30 years but increases dramatically in patients older than age 50 years. The 5-year survival rate for colon cancer is 55% to 60%. The incidence is declining, partially resulting from improved measures of screening and removal of adenomatous polyps. Mortality rates are slightly different among different ethnic groups. Both Hispanic and African-American populations tend to present with a higher stage of disease for both colon and rectal cancer when compared with other ethnic populations.

Pathologists play a major role in the management of colorectal carcinoma by proper staging, which provides the clinician with critical information regarding prognosis and choice of adjuvant therapy. Features that should be addressed in pathology reports include no less than the presence or absence of carcinoma, the histologic type and grade, presence or absence of lymphatic invasion, and

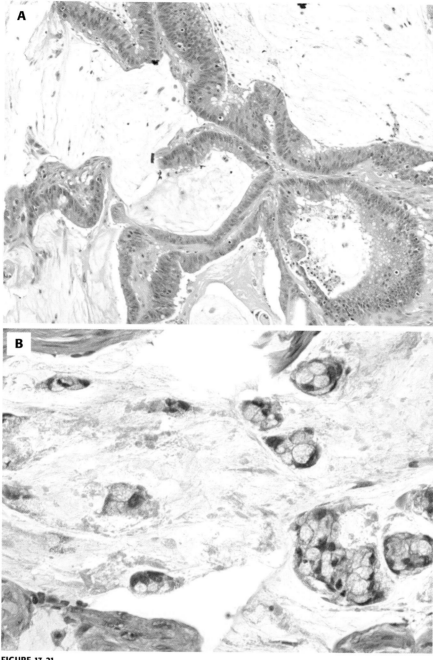

FIGURE 13-21

Mucinous features in colorectal carcinoma. **A,** Mucinous carcinoma. The neoplastic glands produce copious extracellular mucin that ruptures the glands and extrudes into the surrounding stromal tissue. **B,** Signet ring carcinoma. In this histologic variant of mucinous carcinoma, the mucin is intracellular within one or more cytoplasmic vacuoles that push the nucleus to the cell periphery.

resection margin. Histopathologic features associated by multivariate analyses to be independent predictors of prognosis include differentiation, presence of endocrine cells, Crohn's-like reaction, and tumor budding. Adjuvant therapy significantly improves the survival of patients with stage III colon cancer, particularly adjuvant 5-fluorouracil and levamisole. Radiotherapy may be used to treat rectal cancers preoperatively or postoperatively or to treat recurrent disease. Reductions in local recurrence and death have also been shown for stage II and III rectal cancers using a combination of 5-fluorouracil and radiation therapy.

Despite the higher incidence of poorly differentiated cancers in HNPCC, HNPCC patients have a better prognosis than patients without HNPCC, with a 5-year survival rate of 65% in patients with HNPCC. Mucinous carcinomas are of clinical significance because they are more common in young patients and are associated with preexisting villous adenomas, areas of villous dysplasia in ulcerative colitis, anorectal fistulas, or prior pelvic irradiation. Mucinous carcinomas are also more aggressive than their nonmucinous counterparts, because they show more extensive lymph node involvement, they are often diagnosed at an advanced stage, and they recur more frequently.

■ NEUROENDOCRINE NEOPLASMS

CLINICAL FEATURES

Neuroendocrine neoplasms can arise anywhere throughout the colorectum. They constitute a range of clinicopathologic entities ranging from well-differentiated neuroendocrine tumors (carcinoid tumors) to aggressive neuroendocrine carcinomas. Because neuroendocrine neoplasms arise from cells of the diffuse neuroendocrine system, they are related to medullary carcinoma of the thyroid, pheochromocytoma, and pancreatic neuroendocrine tumors. They occur in 9% of patients with multiple endocrine neoplasia syndrome type 1.

Well-differentiated carcinoid tumors of the gastrointestinal tract account for up to 95% of all carcinoid tumors. Within the gastrointestinal tract, carcinoid tumors comprise 20% of all gastrointestinal neoplasms and 6% of colorectal neoplasms. The incidence is estimated to be up to 8 per 100,000 individuals. The average age at diagnosis is in the sixth to seventh decade of life. They are more common in females than males, and are more common in African-Americans as compared with other races.

At least half of all carcinoid tumors are discovered as an incidental finding. The clinical presentation depends on the location of the tumor. Clinical symptoms associated with colonic neuroendocrine neoplasms are usually vague (weight loss, abdominal pain) or related to the mass effect from bulky aggressive lesions. Symptoms related to rectal neoplasms include pain, rectal bleeding, and diarrhea, usually resulting from mechanical trauma

associated with passage of feces over the polyp surface. Early lesions are polypoid and have an excellent prognosis, while more aggressive lesions appear ulcerated and present similar to conventional adenocarcinomas located within the same region. Carcinoid syndrome is uncommon even in the presence of liver metastases.

PATHOLOGIC FEATURES

GROSS FINDINGS

Of those neuroendocrine neoplasms that occur in the large intestine, the most commonly affected site is the rectum, followed by the cecum. This distribution parallels the presence of endocrine cells in the large intestine. They usually occur singly, although in a minority of patients multiple carcinoids may occur, appearing as areas of endocrine micronodules, particularly within the rectum. Grossly, they present as a submucosal mass with normal overlying mucosa. Their size can range from small nodules 2 to 3 mm in diameter to large lesions in excess of 5 cm. Larger tumors are more commonly encountered in the proximal colon. On cut surface, they are yellow to white in color and homogeneous. In some patients, the overlying mucosa may show areas of erosion and frank ulceration, usually vassociated with high-grade aggressive neuroendocrine

NEUROENDOCRINE NEOPLASMS—PATHOLOGIC FEATURES

Gross Findings

- Submucosal mass with yellow-tan appearance on cut surface
- Most commonly found in right colon or rectum

Microscopic Findings

- Uniform small round cells with rare mitotic figures
- Fine, speckled chromatin pattern
- Solid, ribbon-like, trabecular or nesting growth patterns

Immunohistochemistry

- Positive for synaptophysin and NSE
- Variably positive for chromogranin, serotonin, glucagons, gastrin, or somatostatin
- Variably positive for CEA
- Rectal lesions frequently positive for PSAP (> 80%)

Differential Diagnosis

- Poorly differentiated colorectal carcinoma
- Lymphoid neoplasms (particularly small biopsies)
- Metastatic carcinomas

carcinomas. Areas of hemorrhage or necrosis may also be seen, indicative of a higher-grade lesion.

MICROSCOPIC FINDINGS

The morphologic features of large intestinal neuroendocrine neoplasms are similar to those arising in other locations. Well-differentiated neuroendocrine neoplasms (classic carcinoid tumors) are composed of uniform round or polygonal cells with uniform, round nuclei; central prominent nucleoli; and a speckled chromatin pattern ("salt and pepper" nuclei; Fig. 13-22A). Necrosis is absent. The tumor may grow in any number of patterns, such as solid, nesting, trabecular, ribbon-like, or acinar (see Fig. 13-22B through D). High-grade neuroendocrine carcinomas show marked cytologic and nuclear atypia in association with other features related to malignant behavior, including size greater than 2 cm, two or more mitoses per 10 high-power fields, necrosis, and invasion of angiolymphatics or the overlying colorectal mucosa (Figs. 13-23 and 13-24).

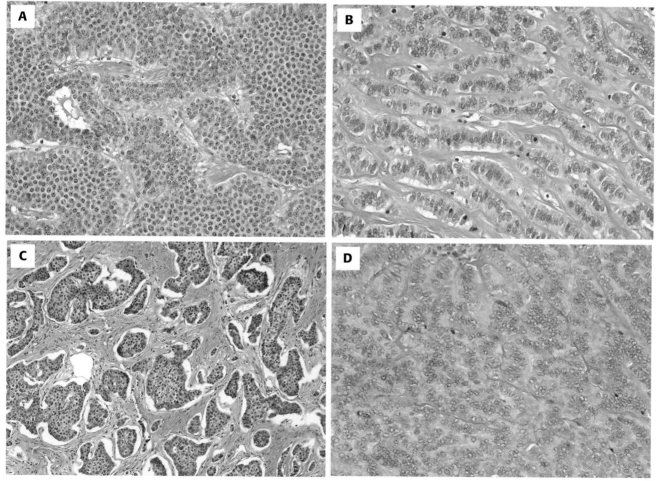

FIGURE 13-22

Carcinoid tumor. **A,** Well-differentiated neuroendocrine neoplasm with solid growth pattern. The tumor is composed of small uniform cells with eosinophilic cytoplasm, centrally located round nuclei with finely dispersed chromatin, and prominent nucleoli. Delicate vessels are present within the tumor stromal tissues. **B,** Carcinoid tumors may also grow in patterns described as ribbon-like, nesting **(C),** and trabecular **(D).**

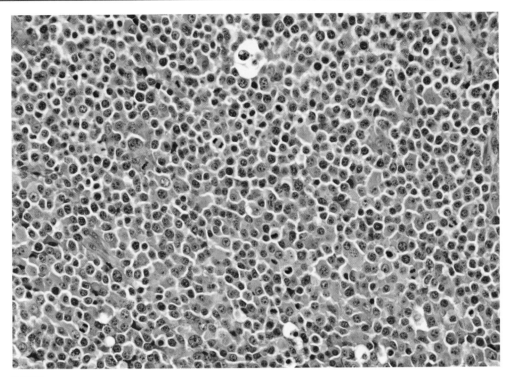

FIGURE 13-23
High-grade carcinoid tumor. In this example, in addition to the finely dispersed chromatin and prominent nucleoli, the nuclei show marked atypia and pleomorphism. Mitoses and apoptotic debris are abundant and the neoplasm grows in solid sheets.

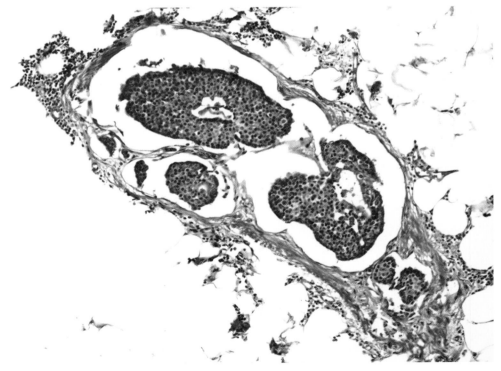

FIGURE 13-24
Carcinoid tumor. Despite the well-differentiated appearance and uniformity of cells, angiolymphatic invasion indicates a higher likelihood for malignant behavior.

ANCILLARY STUDIES

ELECTRON MICROSCOPY

Ultrastructural studies are able to demonstrate secretory granules of variable morphologic appearance with features of both goblet cells and endocrine cells.

IMMUNOHISTOCHEMISTRY

Immunohistochemical stains are frequently positive for synaptophysin (Fig. 13-25), neuron-specific enolase (NSE), and broad-spectrum cytokeratins (AE1/AE3) in colorectal neuroendocrine neoplasms, whereas chromogranin stains are variably positive in large intestinal tumors. Immunostains for vimentin are usually negative.

DIFFERENTIAL DIAGNOSIS

Because neuroendocrine neoplasms are typically submucosal in location, their identification within submucosal tissue in a rectal biopsy specimen may raise the concern of prostate cancer in male patients. Immunohistochemical staining for prostate-specific antigen (PSA) and PSAP can be helpful, although 80% of rectal carcinoids express PSAP. In addition, the uniform appearance of the neuroendocrine cells can be suggestive of a lymphoid neoplasm, whereas the solid growth pattern can be suggestive of a poorly differentiated

carcinoma. In all cases, immunohistochemical for classic carcinoid markers are most useful to differentiate these possibilities, such as synaptophysin and NSE.

PROGNOSIS AND THERAPY

The malignant behavior of a neuroendocrine neoplasm cannot be based solely on histology, and the presence of metastatic disease is the only proof of malignancy. However, neoplasms that behave in a malignant fashion have indicated so at the time of diagnosis. Features associated with a malignant phenotype include size greater than 2 cm, two or more mitoses per 10 high-power field, and invasion of angiolymphatics, or the overlying colorectal mucosa. The 5-year survival rate for colonic neuroendocrine tumors is 42%, whereas for rectal tumors it is 72%. Neoplasms without these features should be considered benign and are effectively treated by adequate surgical resection. No adjuvant treatments have yet proven beneficial.

■ UNCOMMON FORMS OF COLORECTAL CANCER

Small cell carcinoma is a rare variant of colorectal cancer, accounting for less than 1% of all cases. Histologically these carcinomas are identical to small cell carcinomas of the lung (oat cell carcinomas). They have an extremely poor prognosis, with almost all cases presenting with

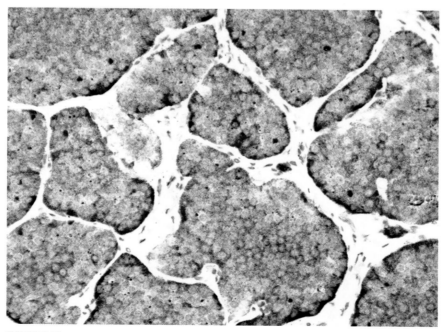

FIGURE 13-25

Synaptophysin labeling of carcinoid tumor. Synaptophysin is expressed by all neuroendocrine tumors of the gastrointestinal tract. Immunostaining reveals uniform cytoplasmic labeling.

lymph node or liver metastases. One third of small cell carcinomas arise in a preexisting adenoma.

Undifferentiated carcinoma, also known as *medullary carcinoma,* is another rare form of colorectal carcinoma, accounting for less than 1% of all colorectal neoplasms. They are characterized by the complete lack of glandular structures or other features to indicate cellular differentiation (Fig. 13-26). Undifferentiated carcinomas are composed of solid sheets of tumor cells with syncytial growth pattern and pushing borders. A marked lympho-plasmacytic infiltrate may be present in the peritumor region. These cells are fairly round, with regular nuclei and abundant eosinophilic cytoplasm, raising the question of a neuroendocrine carcinoma. However, IHC stains commonly positive in neuroendocrine carcinoma are negative. Undifferentiated carcinoma is significantly associated with HNPCC.

Squamous carcinomas of the colorectum are exceedingly rare. They occur most commonly in the setting of chronic schistosomiasis infection of the colon but have also been reported in association with ulcerative colitis and irradiation to the pelvis. Diagnosis of a primary colorectal squamous carcinoma may be made if there are no other sites of squamous cancer in the body and no involvement of cloacogenic or squamous mucosa. Prognosis is the same stage for stage with conventional adenocarcinomas.

Finally, rare cases of carcinosarcoma, adenocarcinoma with areas of choriocarcinoma, hepatoid adenocarcinoma, or clear cell carcinoma have been reported.

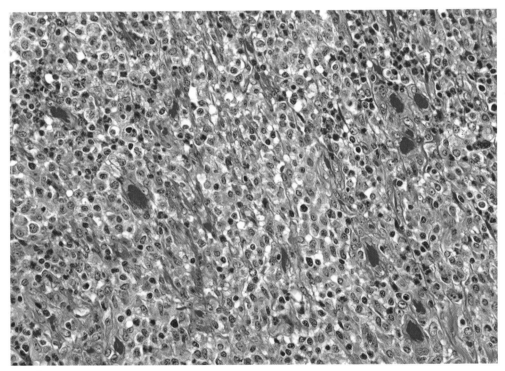

FIGURE 13-26
Undifferentiated (medullary) carcinoma. The carcinoma grows as sheets of undifferentiated cells. Lymphocytes are scattered among the neoplastic cells.

14

Molecular Diagnostics in Gastrointestinal Pathology

■ **Athanasios C. Tsiatis, MD** ■ **James R. Eshleman, MD, PhD**

Molecular diagnostics is a field of medicine that applies molecular biology techniques to the diagnosis of disease. Molecular diagnostics includes traditional methods such as cytogenetics, as well as encompassing the emerging fields of genomics and proteomics in personalized medicine. This chapter reviews the pertinent molecular methods that are commonly used in molecular diagnostics, and their most common applications in the field of gastrointestinal pathology.

■ POLYMERASE CHAIN REACTION

The polymerase chain reaction (PCR) is a method that takes one small region among a 3-billion base-pair genome and produces a billion copies of it. Two major advances that permitted the widespread application of PCR were the use of thermostable DNA polymerases such as *Taq* polymerase and the development of an instrument to cycle between temperatures, a so-called thermocycler. PCR is a fundamental method used in a variety of molecular diagnostic assays and is briefly reviewed here.

The requirements for a PCR reaction include genomic DNA (the template), two primers (short sequences of DNA approximately 18 to 20 nucleotides long) that are complementary to the genomic DNA and that flank the genetic region of interest, a DNA polymerase, and free nucleotides. A thermocycler carries out the three requisite reaction steps: denaturation, annealing, and extension (Fig. 14-1A). During the denaturation phase, the sample is elevated to a high temperature to denature the double-stranded genomic DNA. The thermocycler then lowers the temperature to allow primers to anneal to these single-stranded complementary DNA molecules. The temperature is then raised to a middle temperature for the polymerase to extend the primers by incorporating nucleotides as it replicates the template strands. These steps are sequentially repeated 25 to 40 times where each cycle produces two copies for every input

copy, thereby resulting in exponential amplification of the desired region (see Fig. 14-1B). PCR is a required step to identify disease-causing mutations in patients with hereditary gastrointestinal cancer syndromes, to identify carcinomas with microsatellite instability, and to identify gene mutations that influence response to therapies, among others.

■ *KRAS* AND *BRAF* GENOTYPING

KRAS and *BRAF* are signaling molecules that play critical downstream roles in the epidermal growth factor receptor (EGFR) signaling pathway by regulating cellular proliferation, motility, and survival. In normal cells, activation of the EGFR receptor leads to phosphorylation of tyrosine residues within its intracytoplasmic domain, and via intermediary proteins such as Grb and Sos leads to activation of KRAS and other downstream signaling components with resultant changes in cellular proliferation and migration. KRAS activation is then rapidly deactivated to its inactive form, thus terminating the signals initiated by ligand binding to the EGFR receptor. By contrast, mutations in *KRAS* or *BRAF* in cancer cells lead to the constitutive and uncontrolled activation of this signaling pathway independent of binding by growth factor ligands to EGFR, resulting in uncontrolled proliferation and growth (Fig. 14-2). Point mutations at codons 12, 13, and 61 in *KRAS* or at codon 600 in *BRAF* mimic the activated state of these signaling pathway intermediates, and for this reason these mutations are associated with resistance to and lack of clinical benefit from anti-EGFR immunotherapy. Thus determinations of the *KRAS* and *BRAF* mutation status in a colorectal carcinoma has become common practice to guide therapeutic options regarding anti-EGFR immunotherapy in patients with metastatic colon cancer.

Commonly used laboratory methods to detect these and other disease-associated mutations include conventional Sanger sequencing, pyrosequencing, and real-time

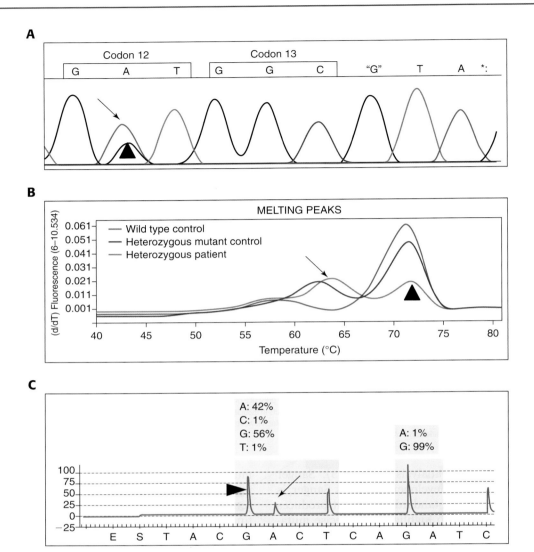

FIGURE 14-3

KRAS mutation is commonly detected by conventional Sanger sequencing **(A)**, real-time PCR with melting curve analysis **(B)**, or pyrose-quencing **(C)**. *Arrows* designate the mutant allele, and *arrowheads* the wild type allele. The most common *KRAS* mutation seen in primary and metastatic colon cancer is the G12D mutation.

were identified using the protein truncation test. More recently, however, full gene sequencing has become the standard diagnostic test. The location of the mutation in the *APC* gene may play a role in which clinical phenotype manifests. For example, mutations within the mutation cluster region in exon 15 are associated with classic polyposis, whereas mutations at the extreme ends of the *APC* gene are associated with attenuated FAP, a condition with equally high penetrance, but patients usually have fewer than 100 adenomatous polyps. Another *APC* mutation, I1307K, is a missense mutation typically found in Ashkenazi Jewish patients and confers a two- to five-fold increase in risk for the development of colon cancer. In addition to FAP, at least five other predisposition syndromes also increase the risk of colorectal cancer.

Additional syndromes for which molecular diagnostics play a crucial role are Peutz-Jeghers syndrome, an autosomal dominant inherited syndrome characterized by mucocutaneous pigmentation ("spots and polyps"), small bowel hamartomas and a greatly elevated risk of colon and pancreatic cancer, juvenile polyposis syndrome, an autosomal dominant inherited syndrome associated with the presence of juvenile polyps throughout the gastrointestinal tract that also predisposes to the development of colorectal cancer, and hereditary pancreatic cancer that is associated with germline mutations in the *BRCA2* or *PALB2* genes. Identification of individuals with an inherited susceptibility to gastrointestinal cancer is therefore important because it provides the patient with opportunities for medical and surgical interventions before the

TABLE 14-1
Hereditary Gastrointestinal Cancer Syndromes

Syndrome	Gene (Chromosome)	Clinical Phenotype	Testing Methodology	Mode of Inheritance
Familial adenomatous polyposis	*APC* (5q21)	>100 tubular adenomas	Sequencing	Dominant
I1307K mutation (Ashkenazi Jewish)	*APC* (5q21)	2- to 5-fold elevated risk of colon cancer	Sequencing	Dominant
Attenuated familial adenomatous polyposis	*APC* (5q21)	<100 tubular adenomas	Sequencing	Dominant
Hereditary nonpolyposis colon cancer	*hMLH1* (3p21) *hMSH2* (2p22) *hPMS2* (7p22) *hMSH6* (2p16)	Right-sided colorectal carcinomas, MSI-H	Microsatellite analysis, IHC, sequencing	Dominant
MutY-associated polyposis	*hMYH* (1p34)	<100 tubular adenomas	Sequencing	Recessive
Juvenile polyposis syndrome	*SMAD4/DPC4* (18q21) *BMPR1A* (10q22)	1 or more juvenile polyps	Sequencing	Dominant
Peutz-Jeghers syndrome	*LKB1/STK11* (19p13)	Mucocutaneous pigmentation, small bowel hamartomas, pancreatic cancers (IPMN)	Sequencing	Dominant
Familial atypical mole malignant melanoma syndrome	*CDKN2A* (9p21)	Melanoma and pancreatic cancer	Sequencing	Dominant
Familial pancreatic cancer	*BRCA2* (13q12)	Pancreatic, breast, and ovarian cancer	Sequencing	Dominant
Hereditary diffuse gastric cancer	*CDH1* (16q22)	Diffuse-type gastric cancers	Sequencing	Dominant

development of disease. In some instances, inherited mutations lead to an increased risk of cancer due to increased inflammation. For example, patients with hereditary pancreatitis syndrome have a 50- to 80-fold increased risk of pancreatic cancer due to chronic pancreatitis caused by inherited mutations in the *PRSS1* or *SPINK1* genes, and patients with hereditary hemochromatosis due to mutations in *HFE, HJV,* or *HAMP* have an increased risk of hepatocellular carcinoma due to chronic hepatitis in the setting of iron overload.

■ MICROSATELLITE INSTABILITY

Microsatellites, also known as short tandem repeats (STRs), are repetitive DNA elements in which the repeating unit is only one to six bases long, and the units are repeated 10 to 60 times. The repetitive nature of microsatellites renders them inherently unstable during normal cellular replication, leading to insertion or deletion of bases within these regions. However, normal cells possess a system of DNA mismatch repair (MMR) enzymes that rapidly corrects these errors to maintain microsatellite length. These MMR repair enzymes are encoded by the *mutL homolog 1* (*hMLH1*), *postmeiotic*

segregation increased 2 (*hPMS2*), *mutS homolog 2* (*hMSH2*), and *mutS homolog 6* (*hMSH6*) genes.

Individuals with hereditary nonpolyposis colon cancer syndrome (HNPCC, or Lynch syndrome) have an increased predisposition to colorectal and other extraintestinal cancers due to the inheritance of a mutated MMR gene. HNPCC represents approximately 2% to 5% of all colorectal cancers and has an autosomal dominant mode of transmission with approximately 80% to 90% penetrance. Of known MMR genes, *hMLH1* and *hMSH2* most commonly harbor the germline mutations that cause HNPCC, followed by a much smaller mutation incidence in *hMSH6* and *hPMS2*. Loss of the second copy of this MMR gene in the carcinoma of an HNPCC patient leads to the loss of DNA repair capacity during replication, resulting in the rapid development of mutations throughout the cancer genome in both noncoding microsatellite sequences and coding regions of genes. This phenomenon is known as *microsatellite instability*, or MSI. Histopathologic features suggesting MSI in colorectal tumors include mucinous or signet ring cell features, intense lymphocytic infiltrate, a medullary growth pattern, right-sided tumor location, and age younger than 50 years (see also Chapter 13). Even though these features are incorporated into the revised Bethesda criteria (Table 14-2), there is no single histologic feature

TABLE 14-2

Revised Bethesda Guidelines for Testing Colorectal Tumors for Microsatellite Instability

1. Colorectal cancer diagnosed in a patient who is younger than 50 years of age.

2. Presence of synchronous, metachronous colorectal, or other HNPCC-associated tumors,* regardless of age.

3. Colorectal cancer with MSI-H[†] histology[‡] diagnosed in a patient who is younger than 60 years of age.[§]

4. Colorectal cancer diagnosed in one or more first-degree relatives with an HNPCC-related tumor, with one of the cancers being diagnosed in a patient who is younger than 50 years of age.

5. Colorectal cancer diagnosed in two or more first- or second-degree relatives with HNPCC-related tumors, regardless of age.

---

*Hereditary nonpolyposis colorectal cancer (HNPCC)-related tumors include colorectal, endometrial, stomach, ovarian, pancreas, ureter and renal pelvis, biliary tract, and brain (usually glioblastoma as seen in Turcot syndrome) tumors, sebaceous gland adenomas and keratoacanthomas in Muir-Torre syndrome, and carcinoma of the small bowel.

[†]MSI-H, microsatellite instability-high in tumors refers to changes in two or more of the five National Cancer Institute–recommended panels of microsatellite markers.

[‡]Presence of tumor infiltrating lymphocytes, Crohn's-like lymphocytic reaction, mucinous/signet-ring differentiation, or medullary growth pattern.

[§]There was no consensus among the Workshop participants on whether to include the age criteria in guideline 3; participants voted to keep younger than 60 years of age in the guidelines.

From Umar A, Boland CR, Terdiman JP, et al: Revised Bethesda Guidelines for Hereditary Nonpolyposis Colorectal Cancer [Lynch Syndrome] and Microsatellite Instability. J Nat Cancer Inst 2004; 96:261–268.

that accurately predicts MSI. Adenomatous colorectal polyps are less frequently affected by MSI than colorectal carcinomas, even in patients with bona fide HNPCC, although they may be useful in the context of a significant family history.

MSI evaluation typically involves manual microdissection of tumor and normal tissue from submitted formalin-fixed paraffin embedded tissue sections followed by DNA isolation, a PCR using primers directed at amplifying a number of microsatellite markers and analysis of the PCR products by capillary electrophoresis for patterns of MSI. Electropherograms from both tumor and normal tissue are usually compared when conducting this analysis. The two most commonly used panels are a Promega Microsatellite Analysis System and a reference panel recommended by a National Cancer Institute (NCI)-sponsored consensus committee. The Promega system consists of five mononucleotide markers, whereas the NCI-sponsored reference panel consists of three dinucleotides and two mononucleotides. However, mononucleotide markers show the greatest sensitivity for MSI. MSI is diagnosed when microsatellite lengths are shifted from the germline pattern (Fig. 14-4A), indicating a change in size (addition or deletion of bases). Three possible data interpretations exist: MSI-high (MSI-H), MSI-low (MSI-L), and microsatellite stable (MSS). When five markers are used, a tumor that shows MSI in greater than or equal to two loci is considered MSI-H, one that shows MSI in a single locus is termed MSI-L, and one that shows no MSI at any locus is diagnosed MSS (see Fig. 14-4B).

Immunohistochemical labeling for MMR proteins represents an alternative and rapid approach to MSI screening (Fig. 14-5). Negative labeling for an MMR protein in a carcinoma compared to the normal cells within the same paraffin section indicates a loss of function and generally correlates well with the presence of MSI. Thus it can be used as a surrogate for evaluating for MMR enzyme mutations. MMR IHC is also of value in that it allows the clinician to order DNA sequencing on the gene most likely to be defective based on its immunolabeling patterns. However, positive immunolabeling for an MMR protein does not indicate the protein's functional status and thus does not preclude the possibility of a pathogenic missense mutation causing loss of function (detected as MSI by microsatellite analysis) while retaining antigenicity.

A
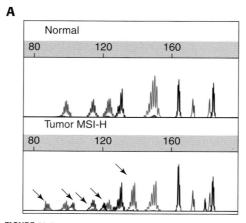

B
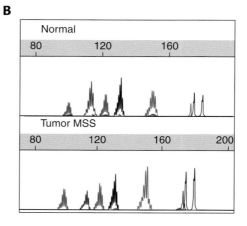

FIGURE 14-4

Microsatellite analysis of PCR products amplified from unstable and stable colon cancers. **A,** When analyzed, shifts in PCR product microsatellite length can be seen in the tumor (*arrows*) showing microsatellite instability-high (MSI-H). **B,** Paired normal and tumor samples showing no shift in microsatellite length of PCR products and therefore diagnosed as microsatellite stable (MSS).

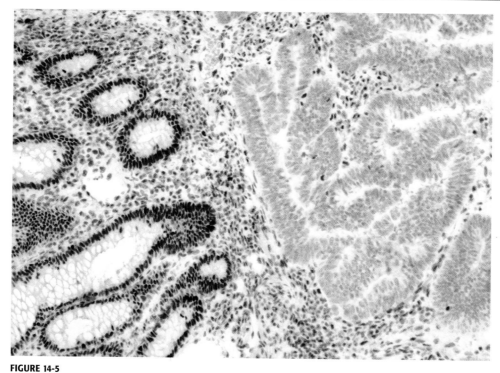

FIGURE 14-5

Immunohistochemical labeling for MLH1 protein expression in a patient with a germline MLH1 mutation.

In the diagnostic setting, reflex testing of colorectal tumors for MSI evaluation is becoming increasingly common to address a variety of patient management issues. In guidelines set forth by the NCI Workshop on Microsatellite Instability for Cancer Detection and Familial Predisposition, MSI is defined as "a change of any length due to either insertion or deletion of repeating units, in a microsatellite within a tumor when compared to normal tissue" (see Table 14-2). The identification of carcinomas with MSI in association with specific MMR gene mutations can thus have significant implications on entire families, prompting genetic screening, and leading to increased disease surveillance in individuals carrying the mutated allele. NCI recommendations for families with an individual (the proband) who has an MSI-positive tumor, yet who has a negative genetic mutation screen, include counseling the proband and at-risk members as if HNPCC had been confirmed and beginning a high-risk surveillance program.

MSI testing may also be useful for prognosis and response to chemotherapy. Patients with an MSI-H tumor have been shown not to clearly benefit from 5-fluorouracil (5-FU) chemotherapy and, in several studies, may actually have shorter disease-free survival when treated with 5-FU alone. Recent studies raise the possibility that MSI-H status predicts a better response to adjuvant therapy when irinotecan is administered. Patients with MSI-H stage II colorectal cancer have an improved survival relative to that of other patients.

15

Pathology of the Anus

■ **David Baewer, MD, PhD** ■ **Carol Adair, MD**

■ INFLAMMATORY PROCESSES AND NON-NEOPLASTIC LESIONS

A number of inflammatory and infectious processes may affect the anal canal; the histologic findings of anal fissures and ulcers, abscesses, and fistulas are not particularly distinctive and are discussed only briefly. Infectious agents that can affect the anorectum include human papillomavirus (HPV; discussed later in the condyloma and squamous dysplasia sections), herpes simplex virus (HSV), *Treponema pallidum* (syphilis), chlamydia, *Neisseria,* and *Enterobius vermicularis.* These infectious lesions are described in depth in Chapter 9. Lesions such as inflammatory cloacogenic polyps and anal Crohn's disease, as well as degenerative and reactive lesions such as hemorrhoids and anal tags, are considered in depth.

Anal fissures are thought to result from tearing of the anal mucosa during the passage of large or hard stools; individuals with low dietary fiber intake appear to be at increased risk for developing fissures. Even though anal fissures may be seen in any age group, they are especially common in young, otherwise healthy, adults, with no gender preference. The typical symptoms are pain during or after defecation and the passage of bright red blood per anus, separate from the stool. The bleeding is usually minor. Fissures are typically located in the posterior midline of the anal canal from the dentate line to the anal verge and are pear shaped on direct examination. Most represent superficial injuries and heal spontaneously within 6 weeks with dietary modification to increase fiber and with stool softeners; however, some fissures persist and progress to a larger, deeper chronic anal ulcers. Chronic fissures and ulcers may develop subsequent to childbirth, usually in the anterior midline of the anal canal. The treatment of chronic lesions is aimed at reducing spasm of the internal anal sphincter and pressure in the anal canal. This may be accomplished by surgical dilation or sphincterotomy or, more recently, by the use of organic nitrates, calcium channel blockers, α-adrenergic antagonists, β-adrenergic agonists, or botulinum toxin. Histologic examination is rarely used in the assessment of acute anal fissures; chronic lesions may be examined via biopsy to exclude inflammatory bowel disease or an underlying malignancy. The microscopic appearance is not distinctive, demonstrating the usual features of a mucosal ulcer. Chronic fissures may be associated with other anal abnormalities, including hemorrhoids, and the so-called sentinel tag, a fibroepithelial polyp resulting from hypertrophy of the anal papilla at the proximal end of the lesion.

Suppurative disease of the anal canal is thought to derive from infection of an anal duct, beginning as an abscess, with the duct providing the framework for the formation of a fistula from the perianal soft tissues to the anal canal. The purulent process can also tract along various planes in the anorectal area to give rise to ischiorectal abscesses when it tracts along the internal and external sphincter muscles, as well as intramuscular or "submucosal" abscesses when the infection tracks superiorly between the muscle layers of the anorectal wall. Histologic features of abscesses and fistulas include acute and chronic inflammation, granulation tissue, and fibrosis; a foreign body giant cell reaction to fecal material may be present. Although most abscesses and fistulas are infectious or idiopathic, they may develop in patients with Crohn's disease, hidradenitis suppurativa, or carcinoma.

CROHN'S DISEASE

Inflammatory bowel disease is discussed in depth in Chapter 10. Ulcerative colitis of the anus is histologically nonspecific and is usually characterized by superficial acute inflammation. On occasion, patients exhibit anal fissures, abscesses, or fistulas, but these are uncommon findings. Crohn's disease, on the other hand, commonly affects the anal canal, exhibits a distinctive microscopic appearance, and is often complicated by the inflammatory lesions discussed previously.

CLINICAL FEATURES

The incidence of anal involvement in Crohn's disease is approximately 25% of patients with small bowel disease and 50% to 80% of patients with colonic disease. Even though anal involvement usually is concurrent with or

CROHN'S DISEASE—FACT SHEET

Definition

- A chronic idiopathic ulceroinflammatory process that may involve any portion of the gastrointestinal tract, as well as extraintestinal sites

Incidence and Location

- Anal involvement in 25% of patients with small bowel disease; in 50% to 80% of patients with colonic disease
- Precedes intestinal disease in 20% to 36% of patients
- Anal canal, perianal skin

Morbidity and Mortality

- High morbidity with high relapse rate after therapy

Gender, Race, and Age Distribution

- No gender predominance
- Whites of Anglo-Saxon descent most often affected
- Any age affected; most common in third and fourth decades of life
- Possible familial predisposition in some cases

Clinical Features

- Symptoms vary with type of lesion: perianal pain, bleeding, bloody diarrhea, sepsis, incontinence
- Manifestations: fissures; anal tags and hemorrhoids; deep anal ulcers; abscesses; fistulas; anorectal strictures; rarely carcinomas

Prognosis and Therapy

- Anal lesions poorly responsive to usual medical therapy for intestinal Crohn's disease, such as steroids and aminosalicylates
- Antibiotics, immunomodulators (e.g., cyclosporin A, azathioprine) useful in managing fistulas
- Surgical: drainage of abscesses, fistulotomy, flap or graft repair of fistulas, resection of intestinal disease, proctectomy
- Prognosis guarded; high relapse rate makes "cure" unlikely, regardless of therapeutic modality

CROHN'S DISEASE—PATHOLOGIC FEATURES

Gross Findings

- Spectrum of lesions from reddened, eroded mucosa to abscesses and fistulas in anal canal
- Thickened perianal skin, may have fistulous openings
- "Sentinel tag," a fibroepithelial polyp

Microscopic Findings

- Abscesses and fistulas nonspecific, with acute and chronic inflammation and granulation tissue
- Key feature suggesting Crohn's disease is sarcoid-like granulomata in the mucosa, especially immediately adjacent to the epithelium

Differential Diagnosis

- Mycobacterial infection
- Sarcoidosis
- Adenocarcinoma arising in fistula

PATHOLOGIC FEATURES

GROSS FINDINGS

Crohn's disease of the anal canal and perianal region has a spectrum of gross appearances, from reddened, eroded mucosa to abscesses and fistulas, all of which may be seen in settings not associated with inflammatory bowel disease. External clues include thickened and discolored perianal skin, fissures, fistulous openings in or around the anal canal, and prominent anal tags. Multiplicity of lesions is a common finding.

MICROSCOPIC FINDINGS

Although the gross findings are nonspecific in perianal Crohn's disease, the presence of sarcoid-like granulomata closely associated with the anal mucosa is highly suggestive of the diagnosis (Fig. 15-1). Many anal biopsies of patients with Crohn's disease, however, demonstrate only acute or chronic inflammation and reactive changes in the mucosa.

DIFFERENTIAL DIAGNOSIS

Idiopathic anal abscesses, fissures, and fistulas may be difficult to distinguish from anal Crohn's disease in a patient without an established diagnosis of inflammatory bowel disease, especially when sarcoid-like granulomata are missing. Foreign body giant cells, common in idiopathic fistulas, abscesses, and other anal inflammatory lesions, should not be overinterpreted as evidence of Crohn's disease. If granulomatous inflammation is present, tuberculosis should be considered in the

follows the diagnosis of intestinal Crohn's disease, in 20% to 36% of patients, perianal lesions precede intestinal disease. Perianal manifestations of Crohn's disease include fissures (21% to 35% of patients), anal tags and hemorrhoids, deep anal ulcers (2% to 5%), abscesses (23% to 62%), fistulas (6% to 34%, most often anovaginal), anorectal strictures, and carcinomas (0.7%). The clinical presentation reflects the particular type of perianal lesion and may include perianal pain, bloody diarrhea, incontinence, and sepsis.

Crohn's disease may manifest at any age, but most patients are diagnosed in the third and fourth decades of life. White individuals of Anglo-Saxon descent are the most frequently affected, and some familial cases suggest a genetic predisposition. It is postulated that Crohn's disease represents an abnormal immune response to gastrointestinal flora, although proof of this theory is lacking; there has been some evidence for the role of probiotic therapy.

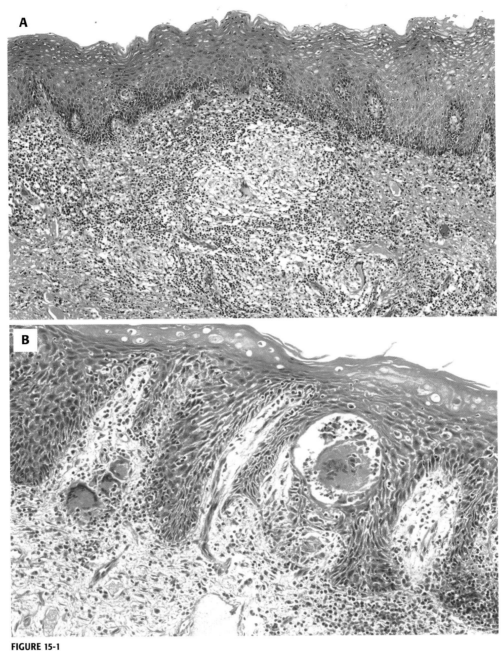

FIGURE 15-1

Crohn's disease. **A,** At low power, small granulomata are seen in a background of chronic inflammation beneath the surface squamous epithelium. **B,** At high power, the close proximity of the multinucleated giant cells to the epithelium is typical of perianal Crohn's disease.

differential diagnosis but is usually characterized by caseating granulomata and positive acid-fast stains or mycobacterial cultures.

The incidence of anal carcinoma arising in Crohn's disease is small. In particular, adenocarcinoma developing in a chronic fistula is described in the background of anal Crohn's disease; those patients who have severe inflammatory disease in this region are most at risk. There is virtually no increase in the incidence of squamous cell carcinoma between patients with Crohn's disease and the general population.

PROGNOSIS AND THERAPY

A variety of medical and surgical treatments are available for the perianal lesions of Crohn's disease, especially abscesses and fistulas. These lesions are typically nonresponsive to steroids and oral aminosalicylates, which are mainstays of therapy for intestinal Crohn's disease. Antibiotics are frequently successful in controlling abscesses and fistulas, although relapse is common after cessation of therapy. Immunomodulators, such as mercaptopurine, azathioprine, methotrexate, and cyclosporin A, have also demonstrated favorable results in managing fistulas, but again relapse is common. Surgical drainage of an abscess is the most common operative procedure in the management of perianal Crohn's disease and is usually semiemergent for elimination of the septic focus. Abscesses are often followed by fistulas, which may require placement of drains or diversion of the fecal stream to allow clearing of the underlying infection. Definitive surgical therapy for a Crohn's disease fistula is controversial due to the risk for poor wound healing and incontinence. Operative procedures include fistulotomy, placement of flaps or grafts to repair the defect, resection of proximal intestinal disease, a permanent diverting colostomy, and, as a last effort, proctectomy.

The prognosis for patients with perianal Crohn's disease is, as with intestinal disease, guarded. There is a high incidence of recurrence of lesions, and "cure" is not a realistic goal in most cases; quality-of-life issues must be considered a high priority in the management of these patients.

INFLAMMATORY CLOACOGENIC POLYP; MUCOSAL PROLAPSE SYNDROME

Inflammatory cloacogenic polyps are considered to be part of the spectrum of manifestations of mucosal prolapse, which includes solitary rectal ulcer syndrome, rectal prolapse, intussusception, and rectocele. The clinical features and, to some degree, the pathologic changes of these disorders are similar, suggesting a common etiology. The inflammatory cloacogenic polyp is thought to result from mucosal prolapse, which produces local trauma and ischemic injury followed by inflammation, repair, and regenerative changes. The polyps usually develop along the anterior aspect of the anorectal junction, where the loosely attached rectal mucosa meets the more firmly seated anal mucosa.

CLINICAL FEATURES

Inflammatory cloacogenic polyps occur at the anterior anorectal junction. They may be seen in any age group but are most common in middle age, with no gender predominance. While they commonly present with bright red rectal bleeding, other symptoms associated with mucosal prolapse syndrome may be noted. These include rectal pain, passage of mucus, excessive straining, tenesmus, and constipation or diarrhea.

PATHOLOGIC FEATURES

GROSS FINDINGS

Inflammatory cloacogenic polyps are frequently diagnosed by biopsy; intact lesions may be either sessile or pedunculated, ranging in size from 1 to 2 cm. They are indistinguishable from tubular adenomas. The surface may be eroded or may demonstrate a patchy exudate.

INFLAMMATORY CLOACOGENIC POLYP—FACT SHEET

Definition

- A manifestation of mucosal prolapse syndrome (solitary rectal ulcer syndrome) characterized by a hyperplastic and ulcerative lesion in the anal canal

Incidence and Location

- Estimated annual incidence 1 to 3.6 per 100,000, for solitary rectal ulcer syndrome, of which this is a subset
- Anterior wall of anorectal junction

Morbidity and Mortality

- Chronic disorder, requiring conservative approach to manage patient discomfort
- Rare instances of massive hemorrhage

Gender, Race, and Age Distribution

- Males equal to females, or slight female predominance
- Occurs at any age, but 80% younger than 50 years; average age 49 years
- Less common in cultures with high dietary fiber content

Clinical Features

- History of straining with defecation, constipation (55%) or diarrhea, rectal bleeding, rectal pain, tenesmus
- Some patients with underlying psychological disorder, such as obsessive-compulsive disorder

Prognosis and Therapy

- Chronic disorder, frequently recurs after therapy
- Medical therapy includes increase in dietary fiber, topical treatment with human fibrin sealant, biofeedback, psychological counseling, pelvic floor exercises
- Surgical treatment last resort due to high recurrence rate

INFLAMMATORY CLOACOGENIC POLYP—PATHOLOGIC FEATURES

Gross Findings

- Sessile or pedunculated polyp
- Surface erosion, ulceration, or adherent exudative fibrin cap

Microscopic Findings

- Surface erosion with adherent cap of fibrin and neutrophils
- Granulation tissue with reactive atypia and reparative changes (may be marked)
- Villiform architectural changes in the glandular mucosa
- Ingrowth of fibromuscular tissue into lamina propria
- Hyperplastic epithelial alterations with irregular branching of glands
- Underlying colitis cystica profunda with mucus-filled epithelial-lined cysts may be present

Differential Diagnosis

- Colonic adenoma
- Adenocarcinoma
- Dysplasia

MICROSCOPIC FINDINGS

The key features of inflammatory cloacogenic polyps are surface erosion or ulceration with underlying granulation tissue, reactive and reparative alterations, and hyperplastic glandular epithelium. The reparative surface epithelium is often thinned and flattened, with nuclear enlargement and prominent nucleoli. The lack of dysplastic nuclear changes readily distinguishes these inflammatory polyps from tubular and villous adenomas.

A fibrinous inflammatory exudate forms a cap on the surface of the polyp, overlying a bed of granulation tissue (Fig. 15-2). The lamina propria of the underlying mucosa is altered by the proliferation of fibromuscular tissue; the smooth muscle cells are particularly conspicuous by their presence above the muscularis mucosa. The glandular structures appear disorderly and may be dilated and branched or cystic. In some instances the surface of the polyp assumes a villous configuration. Glandular epithelial hyperplasia is present, with glands lined by columnar epithelium with an abundance of mucinous cytoplasm, folding and protruding into the crypt lumen. Colitis cystica profunda may be present, with distorted cystic glands filled with mucin embedded in the fibromuscular stroma deep to the mucosa.

DIFFERENTIAL DIAGNOSIS

Inflammatory cloacogenic polyps with florid proliferative changes may be mistaken for villous adenomas, especially in small biopsy specimens. The progression from very proliferative and perhaps somewhat atypical epithelium deep in the crypts to mature and orderly surface epithelium in the inflammatory cloacogenic polyp contrasts with the deep and surface dysplasia of the adenoma. The presence of a surface cap of fibrin and granulation tissue may also suggest the inflammatory nature of this lesion.

Cases with underlying colitis cystic profunda can be especially treacherous; the underlying fibromuscular stroma that replaces the normal elements of the lamina

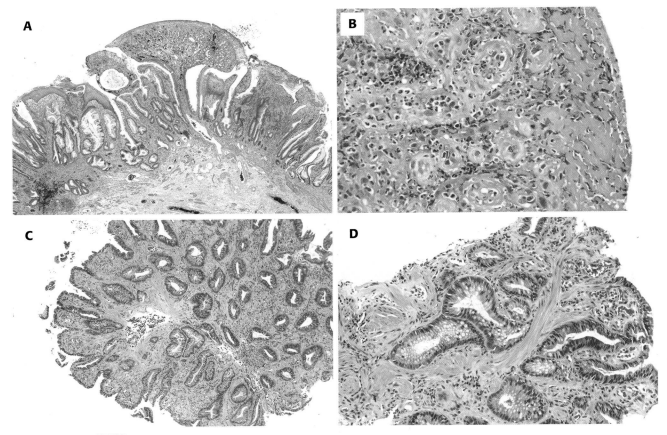

FIGURE 15-2

A, A low-power overview demonstrates the ulcer with a cap of fibrin and granulation tissue at the squamocolumnar junction. Note the irregular epithelial infoldings in the glands, indicative of hyperplastic change, and cystically dilated glands. **B,** At high power, the granulation tissue underlying the fibrin cap has florid vascular proliferation with enlarged reactive endothelial cells. **C,** The surface of the polyp exhibits a somewhat villous pattern, and the usual loose connective tissue and lymphoplasmacytic infiltrate of the lamina propria has been largely replaced by fibromuscular tissue. **D,** At high power, smooth muscle cells extend into the lamina propria immediately adjacent to the glandular epithelium.

propria can be suggestive of a desmoplastic reaction. This combination of findings may mimic an invasive adenocarcinoma.

A few cases with histologic changes identical to mucosal prolapse syndrome have been described in association with an invasive carcinoma. In most of the cases these changes were detected in superficial biopsy specimens and the carcinoma was infiltrating the underlying submucosa. The mechanism for the mucosal prolapse-like changes is postulated to be localized ischemia related to the malignancy.

PROGNOSIS AND THERAPY

Simple removal is generally adequate treatment of an inflammatory cloacogenic polyp. The underlying abnormality of rectal prolapse syndrome, however, must be addressed separately. Such treatment might include dietary modification with increased fiber and fluid intake, pelvic floor exercises, use of laxatives, and psychological counseling, reserving surgery as a last option. Surgical approaches aim at fixation of the rectal mucosa but may aggravate the underlying cause of the syndrome in some cases.

HEMORRHOIDS AND ANAL TAGS

The impact of hemorrhoids on the well-being of humans is evident through historical references from every age, from ancient Egypt to the Age of Enlightenment. The gravity of the problem is reflected by the designation of St. Fiacre as the patron saint of hemorrhoid sufferers. Many theories regarding the cause of hemorrhoids have been espoused over the centuries, including, in the last century, that they represent hyperplasia or varicosities of the mucosal venous plexus. Current evidence, however, suggests that hemorrhoids represent a "sagging" or "slippage" of the normal cushions of hemorrhoidal fibrovascular tissue found in the anal canal. The large venous channels seen in hemorrhoids are no different from those seen in the normal submucosal connective tissue; rather, changes seem to occur in the fibromuscular supportive tissue of these cushions. Once the slippage begins, it is apparently exacerbated by the stress of defecation and increased pelvic pressure.

"Internal" hemorrhoids arise in the anal canal and are subclassified on the basis of whether they prolapse out of the canal and on the persistence of the prolapse. Hemorrhoids that are permanently prolapsed are prone to thrombosis and infarction. External hemorrhoids are contiguous with the normal venous plexus located below the dentate line. Thrombosis is also common in external hemorrhoids.

Anal tags are polypoid masses of anal mucosa, usually squamous type, with underlying submucosal

tissue; these correspond to cutaneous fibroepithelial polyps or "skin tags." They lack the vascular component of hemorrhoids but are often clinically mistaken for such.

CLINICAL FEATURES

Hemorrhoids are a common problem, although the true incidence is difficult to determine because patients often refrain from seeking medical attention. They appear to be evenly distributed between the sexes, with most people seeking medical assistance during middle age. The incidence of hemorrhoids is not increased in individuals with portal hypertension. Symptomatic hemorrhoids are a common complaint during pregnancy, although the actual incidence is not known. Factors that may account for the apparent increase in symptoms during pregnancy include hormonal influences, constipation, pelvic pressure and congestion, and increased blood volume.

The most common complaint associated with hemorrhoids is painless bleeding, which is usually minor. Anal discomfort or pain on defecation may be noted. Infarction or thrombosis results in acute exacerbations of pain and usually requires more urgent medical attention.

PATHOLOGIC FEATURES

GROSS FINDINGS

Hemorrhoids are edematous masses of pale connective tissue covered by gray to tan mucosa. Infarcted or thrombosed hemorrhoids are dark purple and firm. Sectioning reveals dilated vascular spaces, frequently with evidence of thrombosis. Typical excised hemorrhoidal tissue measures a few centimeters in aggregate.

Anal tags are covered by thin tan mucosa; the cut surface may be edematous and soft or dense and fibrotic. The prominent dilated vessels of hemorrhoidal tissue are absent.

MICROSCOPIC FINDINGS

The epithelial lining of hemorrhoids may be columnar, transitional, or nonkeratinizing squamous type. The submucosa contains dilated thick-walled vessels and thin sinusoidal spaces in a loose and often edematous fibrous tissue, sometimes with chronic inflammation (Fig. 15-3). Thrombosis is common, and hemosiderin deposits in the connective tissue indicate previous trauma and hemorrhage. Organization of intravascular thrombi may produce cellular masses of granulation tissue, which nearly obliterate vascular lumina. When the intravascular proliferation is florid, it may suggest a neoplastic lesion, such as angiosarcoma or Kaposi's sarcoma;

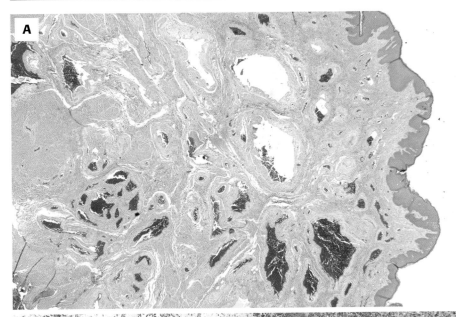

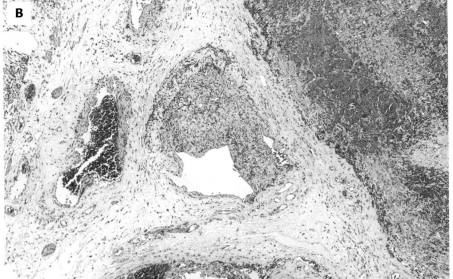

FIGURE 15-3

A, Low-power view demonstrating a typical hemorrhoid, in this case covered by squamous epithelium. The submucosa contains thick-walled dilated blood vessels in a loose fibroconnective tissue, actually normal morphology for the anal region. **B,** A thrombosed hemorrhoid has areas with intravascular granulation tissue that is quite cellular. This low-power pattern confirms that the cellular proliferation is within multiple larger vessels and represents a reactive process. **C,** At high power, the intravascular granulation tissue may appear alarming due to the intense cellularity and nuclear enlargement of the reactive endothelial cells. This should not be interpreted as a vascular neoplasm. It is important to consider the low-power pattern.

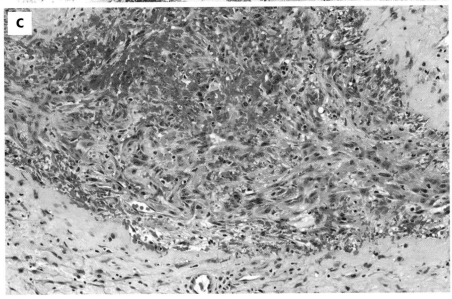

HEMORRHOIDS AND ANAL TAGS—FACT SHEET

Definition

- Enlarged and edematous masses of hemorrhoidal (perianal) soft tissue associated with the anal mucosa, thought to result from slippage or sagging of the normal tissue in this region

Incidence and Location

- Variable data, incidence reported from 4.4% to 36%
- More than 1000 physician visits per 100,000 population per year in the United States and United Kingdom

Morbidity and Mortality

- Not a significant cause of mortality, but a common cause of discomfort and expense

Gender, Race, and Age Distribution

- Males equal to females, although males more likely to seek medical attention
- Historical evidence in virtually all cultures
- Wide age range, peaking in middle age and declining thereafter

Clinical Features

- Painless bleeding most common symptom; also anal discomfort on defecation
- Acute pain exacerbations with thrombosis and infarction
- Commonly symptomatic during pregnancy
- Anal tags are merely fibroepithelial polyps; may be associated with hemorrhoids or other anal disease as a reactive process

Prognosis and Therapy

- Medical therapy is primary approach: increases in dietary fiber, injection sclerotherapy, banding, ablative photocoagulation, electrocoagulation, laser ablation, and cryotherapy
- Surgical therapy is reserved for the 5% to 10% who fail conservative measures
- Surgical excision should include only symptomatic hemorrhoidal tissue to protect continence
- Recurrence rate fairly high

HEMORRHOIDS AND ANAL TAGS—PATHOLOGIC FEATURES

Gross Findings

- Usually 1 to 3 cm in diameter
- Edematous masses of pale connective tissue covered by thin gray-to-tan mucosa
- Infarcted or thrombosed hemorrhoids are dark purple and firm
- Cut surface with dilated vascular spaces, some with thrombi
- Anal tags are edematous or firm masses of pale connective tissue covered by thin tan mucosa

Microscopic Findings

- Epithelium columnar, transitional, or squamous
- Submucosa with edematous stroma and dilated thick-walled vessels and thin sinusoidal spaces
- Vessels may contain thrombi, with intravascular and perivascular hemosiderin deposits and intravascular granulation tissue, often with marked reactive changes
- Anal tags have thin squamous epithelium over edematous stroma, without dilated vasculature

Differential Diagnosis

- Gross differential diagnosis includes neoplasms such as melanoma and squamous cell carcinoma among others
- Histologic differential diagnosis of thrombosed hemorrhoids with organization includes angiosarcoma and Kaposi's sarcoma

DIFFERENTIAL DIAGNOSIS

Although the clinical differential diagnosis of hemorrhoids includes neoplastic lesions such as condyloma, squamous cell carcinoma, and melanoma, the histologic differential diagnosis is limited. As noted previously, hemorrhoids with organizing thrombi may be associated with florid intravascular granulation tissue, suggesting a vascular neoplasm.

PROGNOSIS AND THERAPY

Although hemorrhoids may be a great nuisance to humanity, the extent of their morbidity is rather circumscribed. Thrombosis or infarction may lead to acute pain requiring surgical excision, but there are many treatment options available to most patients. These include simple increases in dietary fiber content, injection sclerotherapy and banding to induce fibrosis and fixation of the sagging tissue, and ablative techniques such as photocoagulation, electrocoagulation, laser ablation, and cryotherapy. Surgical excision is reserved for the 5% to 10% of patients who fail more conservative measures. Excision of only symptomatic hemorrhoidal tissue is favored to maintain continence; enlarged asymptomatic hemorrhoidal tissue should be left alone. There is no advantage to the traditional three-position hemorrhoidectomy procedure, which removes the right lateral, left lateral, and anterior hemorrhoidal tissue.

the low-power pattern highlights the intravascular distribution within large vessels and the underlying thrombosis with recanalization indicative of a reactive process. Excised hemorrhoidal tissue should always be examined microscopically to exclude an inflammatory, infectious, or neoplastic process with a clinical appearance mimicking hemorrhoids, or an associated epithelial dysplasia, although such findings are rare (<2%).

Anal tags resemble cutaneous fibroepithelial polyps, with a squamous epithelial lining over loose fibrovascular submucosal tissue. They lack dilated veins and sinusoids, containing instead smaller branching thin-walled vessels (Fig. 15-4). The stroma contains fibroblastic cells, which may be small, inconspicuous spindle cells or, especially if the lesion has been traumatized or irritated, enlarged stellate cells with bizarre or multiple nuclei. Such stellate cells are evenly distributed within the collagenous stroma and reflect a reactive or reparative atypia of no clinical significance.

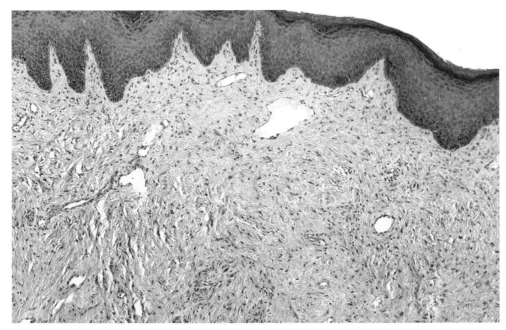

FIGURE 15-4

The anal tag is a type of fibroepithelial polyp: loose fibrovascular tissue covered by squamous epithelium. The plump fibroblastic cells in the submucosa may be enlarged due to irritation, but the even distribution of the cells suggests that they are not neoplastic. The vasculature is delicate, unlike the thick dilated vessels of a hemorrhoid.

Anal tags are easily removed by a snare or snip excision. They are significant only for cosmetic concerns and for potential clinical resemblance to a hemorrhoid or neoplasm.

■ NEOPLASTIC LESIONS

HIDRADENOMA PAPILLIFERUM

Hidradenoma papilliferum is an uncommon benign cutaneous neoplasm that is almost exclusively seen in the vulvar and perianal region. Although traditionally considered a cutaneous (sweat gland) adnexal tumor, there is convincing morphologic and immunohistochemical evidence to support development from ectopic mammary tissue.

CLINICAL FEATURES

Most examples have occurred in white women in the fourth to sixth decades of life. The most common site involved is the labium majus; other sites include the labium minus, interlabial sulcus, clitoris, posterior fourchette, mons pubis, and perineum; perianal examples are rare. The typical lesion is a few millimeters in diameter, although rare cases up to 2 cm have been described. They are located in the dermis, with no surface epithelial connection in most cases. Rarely surface erosion or ulceration may be present.

PATHOLOGIC FEATURES

GROSS FINDINGS

A small excisional biopsy specimen is usually received, demonstrating a dermal nodule covered by unremarkable skin. As noted previously, rare cases are associated with epidermal erosion or ulceration. The cut surface of the lesion is usually tan to brown and, in larger examples, may have a papillated appearance. The lesion is unencapsulated but circumscribed.

MICROSCOPIC FINDINGS

Microscopically the lesion has a complex papillary pattern of fibrovascular cores, sometimes within a cystic structure (Fig. 15-5). The papillae are lined by a double layer: a luminal layer of cuboidal to low columnar epithelial cells with faintly eosinophilic cytoplasm demonstrating occasional apical snouts (decapitation secretion), overlying a flattened myoepithelial layer. The luminal cells may be slightly pleomorphic and stratified. The lesion is within the dermis but may be accompanied by erosion or ulceration of the epidermis. A lymphoplasmacytic inflammatory infiltrate is common.

DIFFERENTIAL DIAGNOSIS

Although hidradenoma papilliferum is characterized by a distinctive histologic pattern, an erroneous diagnosis of adenocarcinoma may be made on a small biopsy. The

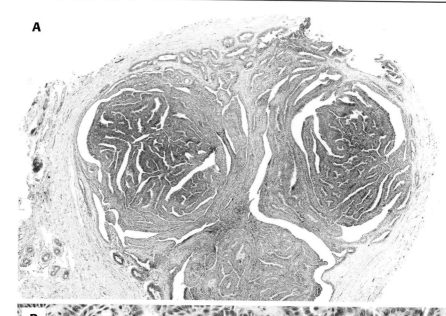

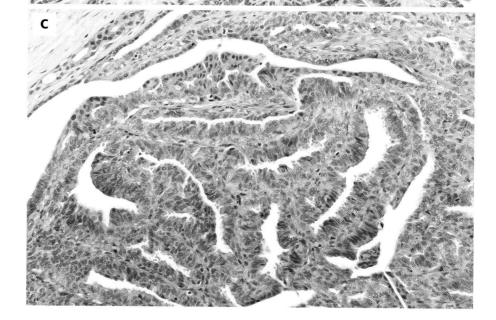

FIGURE 15-5

Hidradenoma papilliferum. **A,** A low-power view demonstrates an intracystic complex papillary proliferation with a lobulated appearance. **B,** At medium power, the lesion is characterized by fibrovascular cores and by a two-cell lining: the luminal secretory cells are columnar, with eosinophilic cytoplasm, with evidence of apical snouting; the flattened myoepithelial cells are visible between the secretory cells and the fibrovascular cores. **C,** A high-power view illustrates the crowding and stratification that may be present in the columnar cell component; this is not considered a worrisome feature in hidradenoma papilliferum.

HIDRADENOMA PAPILLIFERUM—FACT SHEET

Definition
- Benign cutaneous neoplasm thought to originate from either sweat glands or ectopic breast tissue

Incidence and Location
- Incidence uncertain—uncommon at any site
- Most occur in labium majus; other sites include labium minus, interlabial sulcus, clitoris, posterior fourchette, mons pubis, perineum, and perianal region

Morbidity and Mortality
- Benign lesion with limited morbidity, readily treated

Gender, Race, and Age Distribution
- Exclusively in females
- Fourth to sixth decades of life most frequent
- Most occur in whites

Clinical Features
- Dermal nodule covered by intact skin in most cases
- Occasionally skin eroded or ulcerated
- May be discovered incidentally on gynecologic examination

Prognosis and Therapy
- Benign lesion; conservative excision usually curative
- Extremely rare reports of possible malignant change

HIDRADENOMA PAPILLIFERUM—PATHOLOGIC FEATURES

Gross Findings
- Firm, ill-defined mass within dermis, with normal or ulcerated overlying skin
- Cut surface yellow-tan to brown
- Size ranges from few millimeters (typical) to 2 cm (rare)

Microscopic Findings
- Complex papillary pattern with arborizing fibrovascular cores
- Double cell lining: outer low columnar cells with apocrine snouting; inner flattened myoepithelial cells
- Chronic inflammation common
- No connection with epidermis

Differential Diagnosis
- Gross differential diagnosis: cutaneous cyst, hemorrhoids, polyps, carcinoma (if ulcerated)
- Histologic differential diagnosis includes adenocarcinoma

findings, but anal lesions may present with perianal discomfort and bleeding. The lesions vary in size; they are located in the dermis or subcutis and are covered by normal skin.

PATHOLOGIC FEATURES

GROSS FINDINGS

Although most granular cell tumors are small, but they may reach 5 cm in diameter. They are firm and poorly circumscribed, usually submucosal; occasional examples present as polypoid masses. The perianal skin or mucosa of the anal canal may be involved; one case within the internal anal sphincter has been reported.

MICROSCOPIC FINDINGS

Granular cell tumors often are observed growing in and around peripheral nerves. They are composed of large round to ovoid cells with abundant brightly eosinophilic, and slightly refractile, granular cytoplasm (Fig. 15-6). The cell borders are distinct; the nucleus is round, with a dense chromatin pattern, and is usually centrally placed within the cell. The cytoplasmic granules are small and uniform in size, admixed with occasional large eosinophilic droplets. The cytoplasm is positive for periodic acid-Schiff reagent and is diastase resistant. If the tumor is close beneath an epithelial surface, such as skin or squamous mucosa, the overlying epithelium may proliferate, with pseudoepitheliomatous hyperplasia sometimes mimicking squamous cell carcinoma. Mitotic figures are rare.

presence of the double epithelial-myoepithelial layer should prevent this mistake. The clinical differential diagnosis is more extensive, including cutaneous cysts, hemorrhoids, and polyps; ulcerated examples may suggest malignancy.

PROGNOSIS AND THERAPY

Hidradenoma papilliferum is a benign lesion that is adequately treated by conservative excision. There are reports of malignant transformation to adenocarcinoma or adenosquamous carcinoma, but this must be exceedingly rare.

GRANULAR CELL TUMOR

A granular cell tumor is a benign tumor of nerve sheath, or Schwann cell, origin, common in the skin, upper respiratory tract, and gastrointestinal tract, but rather rare in the anal region.

CLINICAL FEATURES

Granular cell tumors lack specific clinical features; rather, the presentation is generally due to the effects of a mass relative to its location. They may be incidental

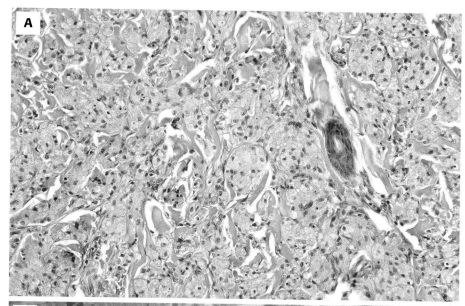

FIGURE 15-6

Granular cell tumors. **A,** A medium-power view demonstrates closely packed round to polygonal cells with distinct cell borders. The cytoplasm is eosinophilic and granular; the nuclei are round, with homogeneous dense chromatin. **B,** At high power, the eosinophilia and granularity of the cytoplasm are more obvious. **C,** Pseudoepitheliomatous hyperplasia of the overlying squamous epithelium may be so florid as to suggest a well-differentiated squamous cell carcinoma, especially on a small biopsy. It is important always to look for the cells of granular cell tumor in the submucosal tissue when considering a diagnosis of squamous cell carcinoma in a small biopsy specimen from this location.

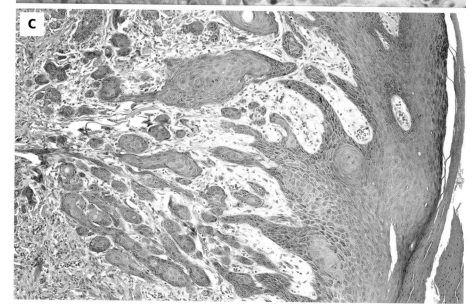

GRANULAR CELL TUMOR—FACT SHEET

Definition
- A benign neoplasm of Schwann cell origin, characterized by granular eosinophilic cytoplasm due to abundant cytoplasmic lysosomes

Incidence and Location
- Common in skin, upper respiratory tract, and gastrointestinal tract but rare in the anal region
- May be in submucosa or in perianal skin

Morbidity and Mortality
- Almost always benign, with excellent cure rate following conservative excision
- Malignant examples are rare but may metastasize

Gender, Race, and Age Distribution
- Females more than males
- No clear racial difference; multiple lesions more common in blacks
- Can occur at any age but most in adults

Clinical Features
- Anal lesions present as polyps or subcutaneous or submucosal nodules
- Symptoms related to effect of mass; some ulcerate and cause rectal bleeding or perianal discomfort
- May be mistaken for hemorrhoids

Prognosis and Therapy
- Complete conservative excision
- Low recurrence rate with adequate excision

GRANULAR CELL TUMOR—PATHOLOGIC FEATURES

Gross Findings
- Firm yellow-to-white, submucosal, subcutaneous, or polypoid mass, poorly circumscribed
- Size usually 1 to 2 cm but may be up to 5 cm

Microscopic Findings
- Large round cells with abundant eosinophilic granular cytoplasm and occasional large eosinophilic cytoplasmic droplets
- Dark, homogeneous, centrally placed nuclei; inconspicuous nucleoli
- Distinct cell borders
- Cytoplasmic granules PAS positive and diastase resistant
- Overlying skin or squamous mucosa may demonstrate pseudoepitheliomatous hyperplasia.

Ultrastructural Findings
- Electron microscopy rarely used for diagnosis
- Large number of lysosomes correlates with cytoplasmic granules

Immunohistochemistry
- S-100 protein positive

Differential Diagnosis
- Squamous cell carcinoma (if pseudoepitheliomatous hyperplasia present)
- Alveolar soft part sarcoma
- Adult rhabdomyoma

ANCILLARY STUDIES

IMMUNOHISTOCHEMISTRY

The tumor cells are usually positive with S-100 protein immunohistochemistry, which, combined with periodic acid-Schiff with diastase (PASD), is the most frequently used study for confirmation of the diagnosis. Other immunohistochemical study results reported as positive in granular cell tumor include laminin, inhibin, calretinin, and myelin basic protein.

ELECTRON MICROSCOPY

The cytoplasm of tumor cells is filled with an abundance of lysosomes, which impart the granular appearance on light microscopy.

DIFFERENTIAL DIAGNOSIS

Considerations in the differential diagnosis of granular cell tumor include rhabdomyoma, a benign tumor with skeletal muscle differentiation, and alveolar soft part sarcoma, a malignant neoplasm of uncertain histogenesis.

Rhabdomyoma is composed of round cells with eosinophilic cytoplasm and superficially bears a striking resemblance to granular cell tumor. However, the presence of multiple nuclei, peripherally placed, and readily identified cross-striations usually makes the distinction clear on closer examination. Rhabdomyomas are positive for immunohistochemical markers of muscle differentiation, including desmin, muscle-specific actin, Myo D1, and myoglobin.

Alveolar soft part sarcoma is also characterized by round large cells with abundant granular eosinophilic cytoplasm. The classic alveolar pattern and the degree of nuclear atypia, with vesicular nuclei and prominent nucleoli, should exclude granular cell tumor from the differential diagnosis. Like granular cell tumor, alveolar soft part sarcoma has cytoplasmic positivity for PASD, but the pattern is more coarsely granular to crystalline; the tumor cells are sometimes, but not reliably, positive for smooth muscle and sarcomeric actin, desmin, and other markers of muscle differentiation.

PROGNOSIS AND THERAPY

Granular cell tumors require conservative local excision for cure in most instances. Rare cases of malignant behavior are reported, with metastatic disease; these lesions are characterized by mitotic activity and nuclear pleomorphism.

CONDYLOMA

Condyloma is a common lesion of the anogenital region, caused by HPV (usually low-risk genotypes 6 and 11), with a low propensity for progression to malignancy, but with an etiologic kinship to premalignant and malignant squamous epithelial lesions. Even though the classification of condyloma as an infectious process versus a neoplastic process might be controversial, it is discussed here to emphasize the spectrum of HPV-induced lesions of the anus and the differential diagnostic distinction among them.

CLINICAL FEATURES

Condyloma is the most common manifestation of sexually transmitted HPV. The incidence and demographics of anal condylomata parallel the recent increase in anal cancers, particularly among young males.

Anal condylomata, like genital lesions, are found in sexually active adults of both genders, but with a high incidence in males who practice receptive anal intercourse, whether bisexual or homosexual. Other associations that increase the incidence of anal condylomata include human immunodeficiency virus (HIV) seropositivity, immunosuppression in the organ transplant population, cigarette smoking, alcohol use, other sexually transmitted diseases (including cervical intraepithelial neoplasia in females), and low socioeconomic status. Most patients present with visible or palpable polypoid perianal lesions.

PATHOLOGIC FEATURES

GROSS FINDINGS

Condylomata are white to skin-colored rubbery lobulated polypoid masses ranging in size from a few millimeters to 2 cm or more; they are often reminiscent of cauliflower florets (Fig. 15-7). Large lesions should prompt a thorough histologic assessment to exclude verrucous carcinoma.

MICROSCOPIC FINDINGS

Condylomata are characterized by a papillary proliferation of acanthotic squamous epithelium overlying elongated rete ridges, which may develop arborizing fibrovascular cores, with variable surface keratinization (Fig. 15-8). Koilocytotic features are usually most evident in the superficial layers of the epithelium, where enlarged cells with one or two, and occasionally more, nuclei are observed. The koilocytes are defined by a large central cytoplasmic vacuole that contains the central nucleus or nuclei; the rim of the vacuole is outlined by a ribbon-like

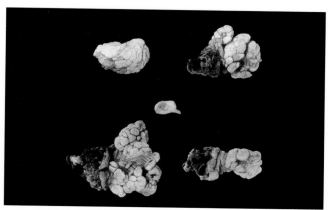

FIGURE 15-7

Condyloma acuminatum is characterized by exophytic rubbery to firm lobulated or warty cutaneous nodules. They usually appear paler than the normal skin, often light gray to white, bearing a striking resemblance to cauliflower florets. *(From Turk JL, ed. Royal College of Surgeons slide atlas of pathology, alimentary system. London, Gower Medical, 1986, with permission.)*

condensation of cytoplasm. The nuclei are often either slightly hyperchromatic or pyknotic and may have an irregular raisin-like contour. There is slightly disordered nuclear polarity in the areas of koilocytotic change. The lower layers of epithelial cells exhibit basal cells one to three cells deep, with orderly maturation above them. Mitotic figures, if present, are restricted to the basal zone in ordinary condylomata.

In lesions treated with podophyllin, there may be more atypia, along with individual cell keratinization, and mitotic figures above the basal zone. These features do not imply a more aggressive lesion given the history of topical treatment.

Dysplasia arising within condylomata should be reported as described in the following discussion of squamous dysplasia/anal intraepithelial neoplasia (AIN). Mild dysplasia and condyloma are essentially synonymous, much as the term *low-grade squamous intraepithelial lesion of the cervix* encompasses HPV-cytopathic effect/condyloma.

ANCILLARY STUDIES

MOLECULAR PATHOLOGY

The detection of HPV DNA has been well documented in anal condylomata, most frequently using chromogenic in situ hybridization techniques; polymerase chain reaction (PCR)-based techniques are also available and are extremely sensitive. HPV types 6 and 11 are found in typical condylomata (Fig. 15-9), while types 16 and 18 have been identified in both typical condylomata and in lesions with high-grade dysplasia, underscoring the link between HPV types 16 and 18 and the progression of disease.

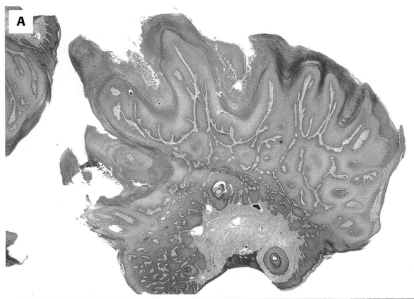

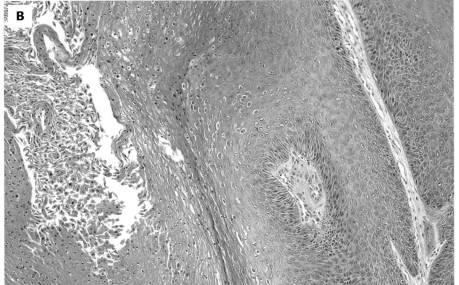

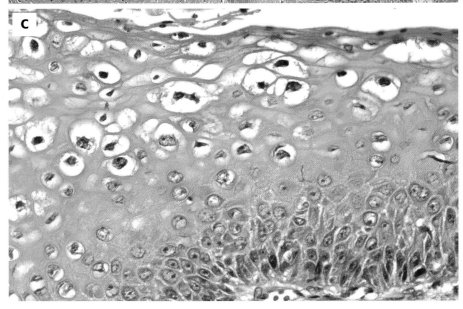

FIGURE 15-8

A, At low power, the warty papillomatous pattern of condyloma is readily apparent. Note the overlying hyperkeratosis. In this case tangential sectioning should be distinguished from the downward pushing invasion of a verrucous carcinoma. This lesion is quite small, unlike the usual verrucous carcinoma. **B,** A medium-power view reveals the orderly maturation of the squamous epithelium and the koilocytotic changes at the surface. **C,** At high power, the cytoplasmic vacuoles or cavities of koilocytes are seen. Note the presence of binucleated cells and the irregular nuclear contours in the koilocytes.

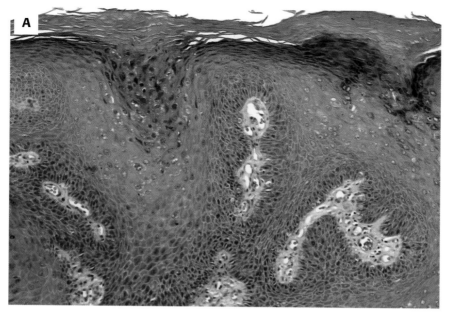

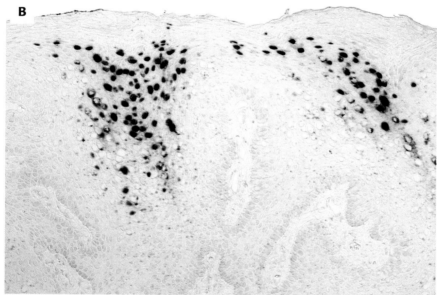

FIGURE 15-9
A, An example of a typical condyloma, AIN I. **B,** Positive for in situ hybridization for HPV 6/11.

DIFFERENTIAL DIAGNOSIS

Condyloma acuminatum should be distinguished from the so-called giant condyloma of Buschke-Lowenstein, which is believed to be a verrucous carcinoma, with a propensity for recurrence and locally destructive growth. Any very large condylomatous lesion should be scrutinized for subtle evidence of invasion, with a "pushing" border extending into the underlying stroma. The histologic similarity between mundane condyloma and verrucous carcinoma may make distinction virtually impossible on a biopsy. Clinical behavior may be the best indicator of the true nature of these lesions.

Clinically banal condylomata may harbor areas of high-grade dysplasia/AIN, particularly in high-risk populations. These findings should be reported and should prompt processing of all tissue.

CONDYLOMA—FACT SHEET

Definition

- Exophytic papillomatous lesion of squamous epithelium caused by HPV, with low propensity for progression to malignancy

Incidence and Location

- Most common manifestation of infection with HPV. High incidence in general population, with marked increase in young males in past two decades
- Anal condylomata are particularly common in males who practice anal-receptive intercourse.

Morbidity and Mortality

- Most condylomata are completely benign, although they may occasionally become very large, especially in the immunosuppressed population.
- Recurrence is frequent, but malignant transformation is uncommon in clinically typical condylomata, most of which are associated with the low-risk HPV genotypes (6 and 11).

Gender, Race, and Age Distribution

- Formerly higher in females; the incidence in young males is increasing, particularly in the homosexual population
- No clear racial predilection is identified, but low socioeconomic status is clearly linked to a higher incidence.
- The age range is broad, encompassing sexually active males and females
- Other associations with the incidence of anal condylomata include HIV seropositivity, immunosuppression in the transplant population, cigarette smoking, alcohol use, and other sexually transmitted diseases

Clinical Features

- Most patients present with visible or palpable polypoid lesions
- Very large lesions may become ulcerated
- Coexisting lesions of the vulva are common in women, as is the presence of cervical intraepithelial neoplasia; penile lesions are frequently encountered in males

Prognosis and Therapy

- Most condylomata are associated with nononcogenic HPV genotypes and pursue a benign course
- Immunosuppressed individuals, including organ transplant patients, HIV-positive patients, and particularly those with a low CD4 count, have a high risk for recurrence and development of high-grade intraepithelial neoplasia in association with anal condylomata.
- Primary treatment is with topical agents such as podophyllin for usual condylomata; extensive lesions may require intralesional interferon.
- Surgical excision reserved for persistent or recurrent lesions

CONDYLOMA—PATHOLOGIC FEATURES

Gross Findings

- Exophytic polypoid cauliflower-like tan to white lesions of the perianal skin
- Lesions frequently multiple
- Size ranges from a few millimeters to 2 cm or larger

Microscopic Findings

- Papillary proliferation of acanthotic squamous epithelium overlying elongated rete ridges that may develop into fibrovascular cores
- Koilocytes with large perinuclear "cavities"; pyknotic and round or irregularly shaped "raisin-like" nuclei are present in upper layers of epithelium
- Binucleated or multinucleated cells common
- All levels of epithelium demonstrate orderly maturation, with some possible atypia in the basilar two to three layers
- Mitoses limited to basal zone
- If podophyllin has been used, more atypia, individual cell keratinization, and mitotic figures above the basal zone may be noted.
- If moderate or severe dysplasia is present, it should be reported

Genetics

- HPV DNA detected by in-situ hybridization or PCR (most sensitive)
- HPV 6 and 11 found in typical condylomata
- HPV 16 and 18 found in typical condylomata and in those with high-grade AIN

Immunohistochemistry

- p16 used as surrogate for high-risk HPV infection

Differential Diagnosis

- High-grade AIN
- Verrucous carcinoma

PROGNOSIS AND THERAPY

Initial treatment of anal condyloma is generally a medical approach and includes topical agents such as podophyllin for small lesions and intralesional interferon in cases of extensive disease. Surgical removal is reserved for persistent or extensive lesions and is often necessary in immunosuppressed patients. The recurrence rate following surgical removal of anal condyloma is markedly increased in patients who are immunosuppressed due to HIV seropositivity, leukemia, and organ transplantation. In HIV-positive patients, low CD4 counts impart an especially high risk for recurrence. Intralesional interferon has been used in conjunction with surgical treatment to reduce postsurgical recurrence.

The incidence of HPV-associated high-grade AIN is increasing in homosexual males with HIV disease. HPV DNA is detectable in the vast majority of HIV-positive men, with genotypes similar between HIV-positive and HIV-negative men. The increased incidence of AIN in HIV-infected individuals despite a lack of increase of high-risk genotypes may reflect immune hyporesponsiveness against the virus and the inability to clear the infection, as is the usual clinical course in immunocompetent patients.

SQUAMOUS DYSPLASIA: BOWEN'S DISEASE AND ANAL INTRAEPITHELIAL NEOPLASIA

Squamous cell dysplasia of the anal canal and perianal skin has been variously termed *anal intraepithelial neoplasia (AIN), anal canal intraepithelial neoplasia, anal squamous intraepithelial neoplasia, squamous dysplasia,* and *Bowen's disease.* It is considered a precursor of invasive squamous cell carcinoma and has many epidemiologic, clinical, and pathologic similarities to cervical and vulvar intraepithelial neoplasia, which frequently accompany it. The term *Bowen's disease* has typically been applied to squamous intraepithelial neoplasia occurring in the marginal or perianal skin, similar to Bowen's disease in other cutaneous sites. Epidemiologic and demographic differences between squamous dysplasia arising from the anal canal's transitional-type epithelium and the distinctly squamous epithelium of the anal margin and perianal skin make location an important consideration; for clarity, therefore, Bowen's disease will refer to squamous dysplasia of the perianal skin or anal margin, whereas AIN describes dysplasia of the anal canal.

CLINICAL FEATURES

Bowen's disease of the anal margin and perianal skin occurs in middle-aged and older individuals, with a 2:1 female predominance. It is roughly four times more common in whites than in African-Americans. The dominant complaint is perianal itching; other symptoms include slight bleeding or induration. Although previous studies suggested a high incidence of internal malignancies associated with Bowen's disease, more recent investigations indicate no significant link between the two. Associated perianal disease has included hemorrhoids, fistulas, and condyloma; other HPV-linked lesions such as vulvar and cervical intraepithelial neoplasia are also commonly seen.

AIN of the anal canal usually occurs in the transitional epithelium above the dentate line. There is a strong association with HPV infection, particularly HPV types 16 and 18. High-grade AIN is most common in HIV-positive homosexual men, but 5% to 30% of cases occur in HIV-negative homosexual men. High-grade AIN is rare in heterosexual men. High-grade AIN is increased in women who are HIV positive and is also linked to anal intercourse and concomitant abnormal cervical cytology. In patients with acquired immunodeficiency syndrome (AIDS), the risk for high-grade AIN increases as the CD4 count decreases and as the plasma HIV RNA viral load increases. Immunosuppression in solid organ transplant patients also increases the risk for high-grade AIN.

PATHOLOGIC FEATURES

GROSS FINDINGS

Most specimens received for evaluation of squamous dysplasia are small biopsy specimens; therefore, gross features are rarely observed by the pathologist. Clinically, high-grade dysplasias involving the perianal skin are similar to areas of Bowen's disease in other cutaneous sites—a reddish scaly patch or plaque at the anal

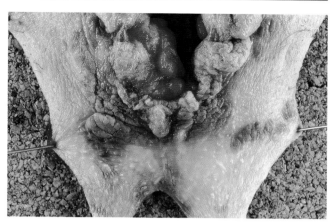

FIGURE 15-10

Squamous dysplasia/Bowen's disease. This large excisional specimen is from a female patient with extensive anogenital Bowen's disease. The lesions were most extensive in the vulva, with purplish placquelike lesions. Thinner reddish patches are present in the perianal skin; these represented areas of high-grade dysplasia microscopically. *(Courtesy of Dr. P. Vasallo.)*

margin (Fig. 15-10). Lesions involving the transitional mucosa within the anal canal are colposcopically similar to squamous intraepithelial lesions of the cervix. Excisional biopsies of either region should be evaluated for clear margins, by inking and specifying margin locations. AIN is also seen in polypoid condylomata, as well as in the flat lesions described previously.

MICROSCOPIC FINDINGS

The histologic appearance of squamous dysplasia of the anal canal and perianal skin are similar to their correlates in the cervix and vulva. The lesions may be divided into three grades: mild dysplasia (AIN I), moderate dysplasia (AIN II), and severe dysplasia (AIN III) (Fig. 15-11). As with squamous intraepithelial lesions of the cervix, grade I is classified as low grade, while grade II and grade III lesions are designated as high grade. Mild dysplasia (AIN I) is characterized by nuclear atypia and lack of orderly maturation of the cells in the lower third of the epithelium; the abnormality involves the lower two thirds of the epithelium in moderate dysplasia (AIN II); and in severe dysplasia (AIN III) the dysmaturation and nuclear changes involve the full epithelial thickness. In high-grade dysplasia, mitotic figures, sometimes atypical, are often seen well above the basal layer. Koilocytotic changes typical of HPV-related effect may be seen in the upper epithelial layers, especially in lesions of the perianal skin and in the polypoid lesions of condyloma acuminatum.

ANCILLARY STUDIES

IMMUNOHISTOCHEMISTRY

Immunohistochemical stains to demonstrate the presence of HPV antigens are not routinely used because immunohistochemistry is much less sensitive than in situ hybridization. However, detection of p16 as a

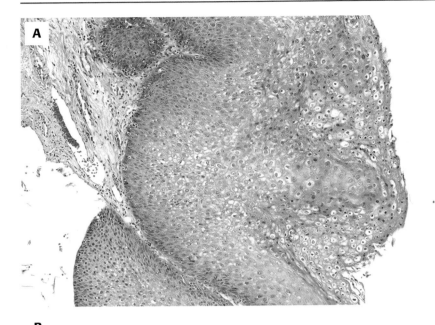

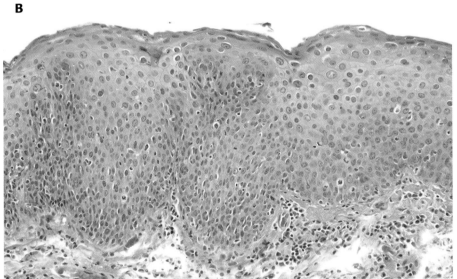

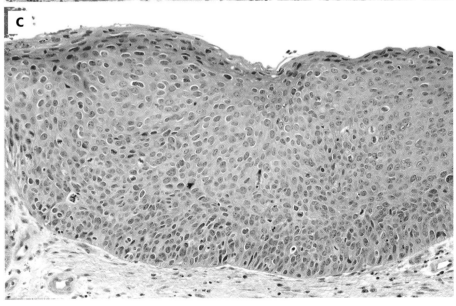

FIGURE 15-11

A, Anal intraepithelial neoplasia, grade I, has expansion of the basal layer with disorderly maturation in the lower third of the epithelial thickness. Koilocytotic change with cytoplasmic vacuolation and some loss of cellular polarity are evident in the superficial layers of the epithelium. **B,** Anal intraepithelial neoplasia, grade II, is characterized by nuclear crowding and lack of maturation in the lower one to two thirds of the epithelial thickness. **C,** Anal intraepithelial neoplasia, grade III, is defined by nuclear crowding and atypia, with loss of maturation, involving greater than two thirds of the epithelial thickness. Very atypical nuclei and mitotic figures may extend far above the basal zone. In this example there is virtually no maturation—the nuclei appear to float within a syncytial sea of cytoplasm, lacking distinct cell borders, even in the uppermost layers of the epithelium.

SQUAMOUS DYSPLASIA—FACT SHEET

Definition

- A precursor of invasive squamous cell carcinoma, also known as anal intraepithelial neoplasia (AIN) and Bowen's disease

Incidence and Location

- True incidence of AIN in the general public is unknown because only high risk populations are screened for dysplasia and the lesions of the anal canal are usually asymptomatic
- The incidence of AIN in HIV-negative men who have sex with men (MSM) is 17%, whereas HIV-infected MSM have a rate of 52%
- The prevalence of anal squamous dysplasia in HIV-negative women is approximately 8% and in HIV-positive women 26% (based on one population study)
- Bowen's disease refers to squamous dysplasia of the perianal skin
- AIN encompasses cutaneous and anal canal lesions

Morbidity and Mortality

- Little or no morbidity associated with anal dysplasia
- 2% to 5% of dysplasias of perianal skin (Bowen's disease) progress to invasive carcinoma
- Progression rate of low-grade to high-grade dysplasia of anal canal is about two thirds for HIV-infected MSM and one third in HIV-negative MSM over 2 years

Gender, Race, and Age Distribution

- Males more than females, 2:1 for perianal skin lesions
- Homosexual men have a higher incidence of dysplasia of the anal canal
- More common in whites (four times higher than in blacks for perianal cutaneous lesions)
- Perianal cutaneous lesions (Bowen's disease) in middle-aged and older adults
- Anal canal lesions in young sexually active males, especially if HIV positive

Clinical Features

- Perianal cutaneous dysplasia presents with perianal itching, slight bleeding, or induration.
- Anal canal squamous dysplasia asymptomatic
- High risk for anal canal lesions in HIV-positive homosexual patients who practice anal-receptive intercourse
- Perianal cutaneous lesions visible: reddish, scaly patches
- Anal canal lesions detectable by anoscopy and anal cytology

Prognosis and Therapy

- Progression to invasive squamous cell carcinoma low (2% to 5% for cutaneous lesions, probably similar for anal canal lesions)
- Both perianal cutaneous and anal canal squamous dysplasia require conservative excision and close follow-up.
- Anal canal cytology with reflex high-resolution anoscopy may be helpful in monitoring high-risk populations.

SQUAMOUS DYSPLASIA—PATHOLOGIC FEATURES

Gross Findings

- Cutaneous lesions on excisional specimen are reddish, tan, scaly patches; frequently multiple
- Anal canal lesions usually seen only as biopsy specimens
- Commonly associated with typical polypoid condylomata

Microscopic Findings

- Dysplasia characterized by nuclear enlargement, increased nuclear-to-cytoplasmic ratio, loss of polarity, and lack of orderly maturation
- Grading
- Mild dysplasia—dysmaturation involves lower third of the epithelial thickness
- Moderate dysplasia—dysmaturation in lower two thirds of epithelium
- Severe dysplasia—dysmaturation and nuclear abnormalities through entire epithelial thickness
- Koilocytotic change common in upper epithelial layers, especially in mild dysplasia
- Moderate and severe dysplasia unified as high-grade squamous intraepithelial neoplasia in some classifications
- Mitotic figures limited to basal zone in mild dysplasia; above basal zone in high-grade lesions

Molecular Studies

- PCR and fluorescent in situ hybridization frequently positive for HPV types 6 and 11 in low-grade lesions; types 16 and 18 in high-grade lesions
- Risk for developing invasive carcinoma higher with HPV 16 and 18
- Overexpression of c-myc linked to increased risk for invasive carcinoma

Immunohistochemistry

- HPV antigens for genotypes 16 and 18 common in high-grade lesions; types 6 and 11 in low-grade lesions
- Less sensitive than molecular studies

Differential Diagnosis

- Bowenoid papulosis
- Paget's disease
- Melanoma in situ

surrogate marker for high-risk HPV infection is often performed (Fig. 15-12).

MOLECULAR PATHOLOGY

Although not necessary for histologic diagnosis of AIN, in situ hybridization and PCR techniques have been used in the epidemiologic study of these lesions and invasive squamous cell carcinomas. The finding of HPV DNA in the majority of invasive anal cancers (HPV types 16, 18, 6, and 33) and in patients with AIN (HPV types 11, 6, 16, 70, and 31) is strong evidence of a causal relationship, supported by the demographics and clinical findings of patients with AIN and squamous cell carcinoma. Overexpression of the c-myc oncogene has also potentially been linked to the likelihood for developing invasive carcinoma.

DIFFERENTIAL DIAGNOSIS

Bowenoid papulosis may be histologically confused with AIN of the perianal skin and anal margin, although the clinical features are usually quite distinctive.

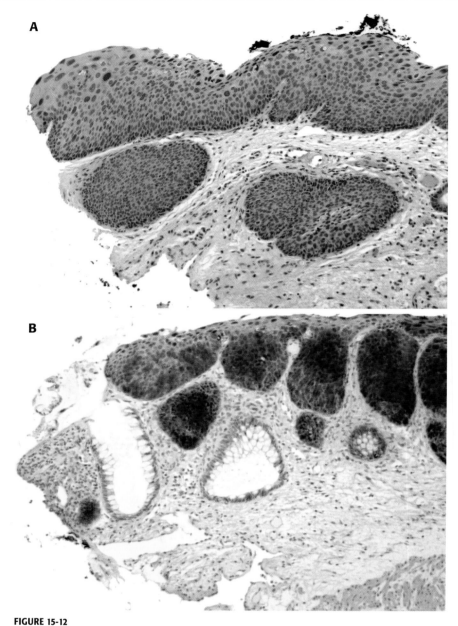

FIGURE 15-12

An example of anal intraepithelial neoplasia (AIN), grade III **(A),** with positive immunostaining for p16, a surrogate marker for high risk HPV infection **(B).**

Bowenoid papulosis is seen primarily in young adults and is characterized by reddish to violaceous papules. Although they are more commonly encountered in the penis or scrotum, they may occur in the perianal region. Typically associated with HPV, bowenoid papulosis is often seen in the company of classic condyloma acuminatum. It is often found in sexual partners of women with cervical intraepithelial neoplasia, and cases associated with squamous cell carcinoma have been reported. These findings suggest that bowenoid papulosis is part of a clinicopathologic spectrum of HPV-related lesions that include AIN and squamous cell carcinoma of the anal region. In spite of these similarities, the clinical behavior of bowenoid papulosis is usually innocuous, with resolution either spontaneously or following local excision or biopsy or topical therapy.

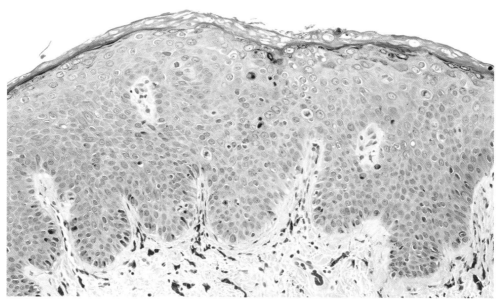

FIGURE 15-13

This is an example of bowenoid papulosis, presenting with clusters of small papules involving the penis and perianal skin. Although the lesion has dyskeratotic cells, atypical nuclei and mitotic figures well above the basal zone, simulating high-grade AIN, note the orderly maturation and lack of nuclear crowding. These features, as well as the clinical appearance, aid in distinguishing bowenoid papulosis from high-grade AIN.

The histologic features of bowenoid papulosis superficially resemble those of AIN and Bowen's disease, with highly atypical nuclei scattered throughout the epithelial thickness (Fig. 15-13). Closer examination of bowenoid papulosis, however, reveals an orderly background of maturation in contrast to the haphazard distribution of nuclei within the epithelium of AIN/Bowen's disease. Fewer dysplastic cells and mitotic figures are noted in bowenoid papulosis as well. Sparing of the pilosebaceous units and involvement of the upper zone of the eccrine glands by dysplastic cells is typical of bowenoid papulosis, whereas the opposite pattern is generally seen in AIN/Bowen's disease.

Paget's disease and melanoma may both resemble squamous dysplasia, especially perianal Bowen's disease. The two entities are readily distinguished from AIN by mucicarmine or PAS positivity in Paget's disease and by staining for S-100, HMB-45, MITF, and melan-A in malignant melanoma.

PROGNOSIS AND THERAPY

As presumptive precursor lesions of invasive squamous cell carcinoma with variable potential for progression, Bowen's disease and intraepithelial neoplasia of the anal canal require conservative excision and close follow-up. That said, however, the rate of progression of Bowen's disease of the perianal skin is only approximately 2% to 5%. Therapeutic modalities used in the management of perianal Bowen's disease include cryotherapy, CO_2 laser ablation, topical 5-fluorouracil (5-FU), argon laser therapy, and photodynamic therapy; however, the treatment of choice is wide local excision.

The progression rate of anal canal dysplasia is also apparently quite low. Assessment of other risk factors for invasive squamous cell carcinoma, such as receptive anal intercourse, high-risk HPV infection, HIV/AIDS, other immunosuppressive states, other sexually transmitted diseases, and presence of cervical squamous intraepithelial neoplasia in females, should be taken into consideration. Patients at risk may benefit from anal swab cytology as a part of their clinical monitoring.

SQUAMOUS CELL CARCINOMA

Squamous cell carcinoma of the anal margin or perianal skin is similar to that occurring in other cutaneous sites. These lesions represent only 15% of anal cancers. Squamous cell carcinoma of the anal canal is more common, comprising 75% to 80% of malignant anal tumors. Until the most recent World Health Organization (WHO) classification, the anal canal tumors were subclassified as large-cell keratinizing, large-cell nonkeratinizing, and basaloid types. In the intervening decade, therapy has shifted from radical surgery to combined modality therapy using chemotherapy and radiation, with diagnosis usually based on a small biopsy specimen. It is likely, therefore, that the biopsy may not be representative of the entire histologic picture; in addition, many tumors demonstrate a mixture of patterns. For these reasons, and for the lack of a clear association of pattern with differences in clinical behavior, the current WHO classification suggests that the broader term *squamous cell carcinoma* be used for these tumors. Three subtypes with distinctive histologic features are recognized: verrucous carcinoma, which is discussed later, and squamous cell carcinoma with mucinous microcysts and small cell (anaplastic) carcinoma, both of which are associated with a less favorable prognosis.

CLINICAL FEATURES

Although squamous cell carcinoma of the anal margin and anal canal usually occurs in the sixth and seventh decades of life, there has been a demographic shift in the past two decades, with an increase in the young adult population, particularly among patients with immune deficiencies. The average age of diagnosis in HIV-infected individuals is in the fourth decade of life. Females are affected approximately twice as often as males. The overall incidence of the disease, although it is still rare, has increased dramatically in recent decades. The risk is higher among urban populations, and it is higher in the black population than among whites. The risk for disease is particularly low among Asians and Pacific Islanders.

The global incidence of invasive anal cancer is up to 2.8/100,000 in men and 2.2/100,000 in women. The incidence in men who have sex with men is 35/100,000, which doubles in those infected with HIV to approximately 70/100,000. Other associated risk factors include multiple sexual partners, receptive anal intercourse, and presence of other sexually transmitted diseases. As the preceding risk factors might suggest, HPVs are detected in the majority of squamous cell carcinomas of the anus, especially those occurring in the anal canal.

A strong link to tobacco smoking has been noted in women but is less definitive in men. Immunosuppression due to causes other than HIV infection, such as renal transplantation, also increases risk. Hemorrhoids, fissures, fistulas, abscesses, and inflammatory bowel disease are not associated with an increase in incidence of squamous cell carcinoma.

Squamous cell carcinomas of the perianal skin are usually ulcerated lesions with rolled borders, which may present with pain, itching, or slight bleeding. Any nonhealing ulcer of the perianal skin should be examined via biopsy to exclude malignancy.

The initial presentation of an anal canal lesion may be nonspecific, resulting in delayed diagnosis. Minor anal bleeding, pain, discharge, altered bowel habits, pelvic pain, discomfort in sitting, anal fissure or fistula, and incontinence (from involvement of the anal sphincter) may be noted. A mass lesion is often evident on digital examination. Clinical evaluation typically includes rigid proctoscopy for biopsy, assessment for inguinal lymphadenopathy,

computed tomography or magnetic resonance imaging to evaluate other lymph node groups (inferior mesenteric, inferior rectal, and internal iliac), colonoscopy to exclude extension from a primary rectal tumor, and endoanal ultrasonography to assess depth of invasion.

PATHOLOGIC FEATURES

GROSS FINDINGS

Anal margin carcinomas, typically treated by excision, are usually ulcerated, with rolled borders. It is uncommon to see an intact lesion from the anal canal because chemotherapy and radiation are the preferred therapeutic modalities; they are typically ulcerated, with raised borders as well (Fig. 15-14). Radical surgical intervention is reserved for persistent or recurrent tumors following combined modality therapy; in such specimens the tumor may not be grossly evident. Careful and extensive sampling may be necessary to demonstrate the lesion; areas of induration or mucosal thickening are of particular concern and should be selected for histologic examination.

MICROSCOPIC FINDINGS

The typical histology of anal margin lesions is a well-differentiated keratinizing squamous cell carcinoma, as is seen in other cutaneous sites (Fig. 15-15). Squamous cell carcinomas of the anal canal may demonstrate one predominant pattern but are more often characterized by a varied histologic appearance (Fig. 15-16).

Two cell types are commonly encountered: the large-cell type and the basaloid cell type. The large-cell type is characterized by large polygonal cells with pale eosinophilic cytoplasm; centers of lamellar keratinization within islands of tumor may be present, as well as individual cell keratinization. Large areas without keratinization represent the pattern previously described

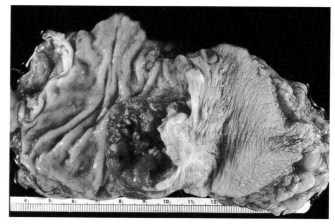

FIGURE 15-14

Squamous cell carcinoma arising at the area of the dentate line, with the typical ulcerated sessile mass with rolled borders. *(Courtesy of Dr. P. Vasallo.)*

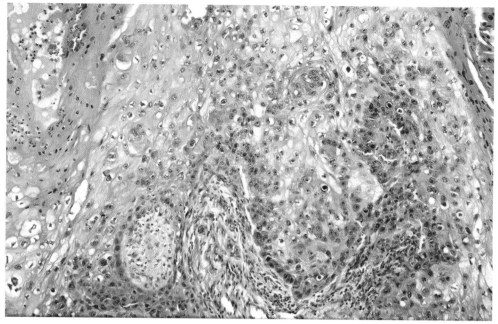

FIGURE 15-15

A squamous cell carcinoma of the anal margin/perianal skin. Tumors in this location are usually of the keratinizing type, identical to cutaneous squamous cell carcinoma. Note the moderate nuclear atypia and the readily apparent squamous differentiation with a mosaic-like arrangement of large cells with eosinophilic cytoplasm and adjacent areas of acellular keratinous material.

as large-cell nonkeratinizing squamous cell carcinoma. The cells of the basaloid pattern are small, with a high nuclear-to-cytoplasmic ratio and nuclear palisading at the periphery of tumor islands, resembling basal cell carcinoma of the skin. There is frequently a transition from one pattern to another, with a spectrum of variations in between, reemphasizing the logic of the unifying term *squamous cell carcinoma.* The infiltrative pattern of these tumors may be irregular and associated with marked desmoplasia or rounded, with pushing borders. A lymphoplasmacytic inflammatory infiltrate is variably present. Worthy of distinction are two subtypes of squamous cell carcinoma that are associated with a less favorable prognosis. The first is squamous cell carcinoma with mucinous microcysts or mucoepidermoid carcinoma, which is characterized by the presence of glandular or cystic spaces containing mucin, demonstrated by Alcian blue or PASD stains. The other form of squamous cell carcinoma with a poor prognosis is small cell (anaplastic) carcinoma. In this subtype, the small cells have a high nuclear-to-cytoplasmic ratio, nuclear molding, a high mitotic rate, and prominent apoptosis. Small cell (anaplastic) carcinoma, a poorly differentiated form of basaloid squamous cell carcinoma of the anal canal, is distinctive from the neuroendocrine tumor small cell undifferentiated carcinoma, which may arise in the rectum and extend into the anal canal. Immunohistochemical stains are helpful in making this distinction. Rare examples of spindle cell carcinoma, or sarcomatoid squamous cell carcinoma, have been reported in this area.

ANCILLARY STUDIES

IMMUNOHISTOCHEMISTRY

Immunohistochemical stains are not often needed in making a diagnosis of squamous cell carcinoma of the anal region, except at the poorly differentiated end of the spectrum, when the differential diagnosis may include small cell neuroendocrine carcinoma of the anus, melanoma, or, rarely, lymphoma. In such cases, neuroendocrine markers (e.g., chromogranin and synaptophysin), markers of melanocytic differentiation (e.g., S-100 protein, melan-A, HMB-45, and tyrosinase), or markers for phenotyping lymphoid lesions and cytokeratin would be helpful. The surrogate marker p16 for high risk HPV infection could also be used.

MOLECULAR PATHOLOGY

HPV DNA is of great interest in cases of anal squamous cell carcinoma because of its presumptive etiologic association; HPV DNA is identified in the vast majority of anal squamous cell carcinomas. PCR studies for high- and low-risk HPV genotypes have demonstrated that types 16 and 18 are prime culprits.

HPVs increase the risk for anal carcinoma by inactivating the tumor suppressor protein p53 at the gene level and at the protein level. Genetic alterations include point mutations or deletions in chromosome 17p.

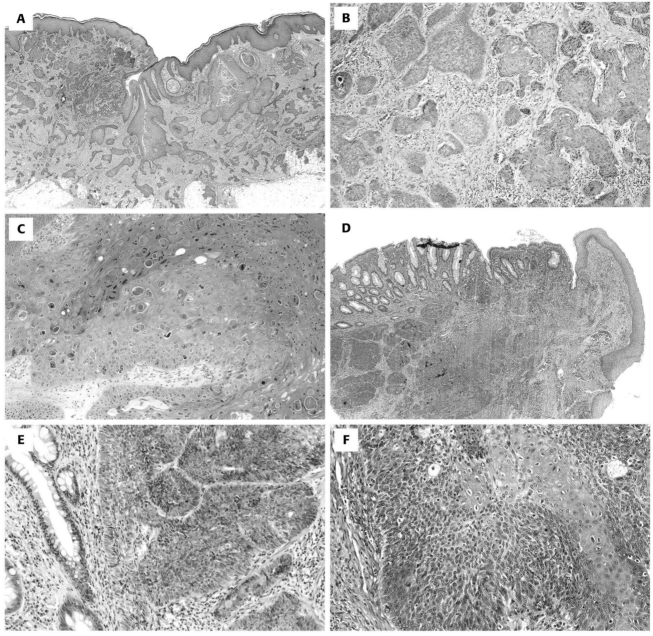

FIGURE 15-16

A, A low power view of squamous cell carcinoma with mixed large-cell and basaloid cell types. The basaloid areas are on the left; on the right the pattern is a keratinizing squamous cell type with keratinous cysts within some of the tumor islands. **B,** At higher power, the distinction between the basaloid pattern and the keratinizing large-cell pattern is more obvious. **C,** The large-cell pattern demonstrates squamous differentiation in this case, with a mosaic-like arrangement of large polygonal cells with eosinophilic cytoplasm, markedly atypical nuclei, scattered dyskeratotic cells, and acellular keratinous material. **D,** A case with a purely basaloid pattern, arising at the squamocolumnar junction, has large lobulated nests of cells. **E,** The same case as seen in **(D),** at a higher power, with small cells with a high nuclear-to-cytoplasmic ratio and scant basophilic cytoplasm. Note the nuclear palisading at the periphery of the cellular islands. **F,** Another case of squamous cell carcinoma demonstrates a transition from a large cell to a basaloid pattern.

Another pathway of p53 inactivation involves viral protein E6, produced by the high-risk HPV. E6, when bound to a specific cellular protein, causes proteolytic degradation of p53. In addition to the alterations in p53 activity, the E7 protein of high-risk HPV binds to the retinoblastoma gene (pRb), which normally restricts the proliferative activity of the basal epithelium, leading to an increase in epithelial proliferation. This double assault, with increased epithelial cell proliferation and decreased apoptosis following DNA injury, leads to an increased risk for developing squamous cell carcinoma in the anal region.

Another genetic abnormality that may be involved in anal carcinogenesis includes c-myc amplification,

SQUAMOUS CELL CARCINOMA—FACT SHEET

Definition

- Invasive malignant neoplasm demonstrating one or several patterns of squamous differentiation

Incidence and Location

- Squamous carcinoma of anal margin/perianal skin: 15% of anal cancers
- Squamous carcinoma of anal canal: 75% to 80% of anal cancers
- Worldwide incidence increasing, especially among HIV-positive individuals
- Uncommon, with 3400 new cases annually

Morbidity and Mortality

- Anal margin (cutaneous) lesions: 5-year survival rate of 70% to 89%
- Anal canal lesions: 5-year survival rate of 60% to 86%
- Morbidity reduced with advent of combined modality therapy for anal canal lesions, often eliminating need for abdominoperitoneal resection

Gender, Race, and Age Distribution

- Females more than males, 2:1
- Increase in young males over past two decades, especially HIV-positive individuals
- Higher incidence among urban populations
- More common in blacks than in whites; very low incidence in Asians and Pacific Islanders
- Demographic shift in progress from elderly females to young adult males

Clinical Features

- Symptoms include pain, itching, slight bleeding, nonhealing ulcer, anal discharge, altered bowel habits, discomfort in sitting, anal fissure, fistula, and incontinence
- Risk factors: multiple sexual partners, anal-receptive intercourse, presence of other sexually transmitted diseases, tobacco smoking in women, immunosuppression, HIV seropositivity

Prognosis and Therapy

- Anal margin cancers may metastasize to inguinal lymph nodes
- Anal canal cancers may metastasize to perirectal, iliac, or inguinal lymph nodes
- Wide local excision may be adequate for anal margin carcinomas smaller than 3 cm, followed by inguinal radiation therapy; yields 5-year survival rates of 70% to 89%
- Combined modality therapy (chemotherapy with radiation therapy) usually eliminates the need for radical resection in anal canal cancers; yields 5-year survival rates of 60% to 86%
- Abdominoperitoneal resection used as salvage procedure for recurrence or persistence following combined modality therapy; yields 3- to 5-year survival rates of 44% to 100%

SQUAMOUS CELL CARCINOMA—PATHOLOGIC FEATURES

Gross Findings

- Anal margin carcinomas ulcerated with rolled borders
- Anal canal carcinomas rarely observed; diagnosis by biopsy only
- In salvage surgery for anal canal carcinoma, tumor may not be grossly evident; sample area of induration or mucosal thickening

Microscopic Findings

- Anal margin carcinomas: well-differentiated squamous cell carcinoma with irregular infiltrative pattern most common
- Anal canal carcinomas have varied histologic patterns and two predominant cell types: (1) large cells with or without evidence of keratinization and (2) basaloid cells
- One cell type may predominate, or an admixture of patterns may be seen
- Anal canal carcinomas may demonstrate irregular infiltration with desmoplasia or rounded pushing margins
- Two more aggressive patterns: small cell (anaplastic) carcinoma and squamous cell carcinoma with mucinous microcysts

Molecular Studies

- HPV DNA identified in most anal squamous cell carcinomas
- PCR most sensitive—HPV types 16 and 18 most often identified
- Genomic hybridization demonstrates gains in chromosomes 3q, 17, and 19, with losses in 4p, 11q, and 18q
- Expression of p53, retinoblastoma gene protein, and c-erb B2 has no prognostic significance

Differential Diagnosis

- Generally not problematic
- In small biopsy samples, a basaloid-predominant pattern may require immunohistochemistry to exclude melanoma, small cell undifferentiated carcinoma extending from the rectum, and lymphoma

DIFFERENTIAL DIAGNOSIS

The differential diagnosis of squamous cell carcinoma of the anal region is generally not problematic; however, a small biopsy specimen with tumor exhibiting a predominantly basaloid pattern may require further investigation to exclude melanoma, small cell undifferentiated carcinoma extending from the rectum, and lymphoma (particularly when crush artifact is present). As discussed previously, immunohistochemical studies are quite effective in sorting out this differential diagnostic group.

PROGNOSIS AND THERAPY

Surgery is the preferred approach for tumors of the external anal margin. Small lesions (smaller than 3 cm) are generally managed effectively by wide local excision with a 1-cm margin. Larger and more invasive lesions may require abdominoperineal resection and radiation with or without chemotherapy. The squamous cell

which occurs in one third of anal squamous cell carcinomas. Genomic hybridization studies have demonstrated gains in chromosomes 3q, 17, and 19, with losses in chromosomes 4p, 11q, and 18q. Expression of p53, retinoblastoma gene protein, and c-erb B2 do not appear to have prognostic significance.

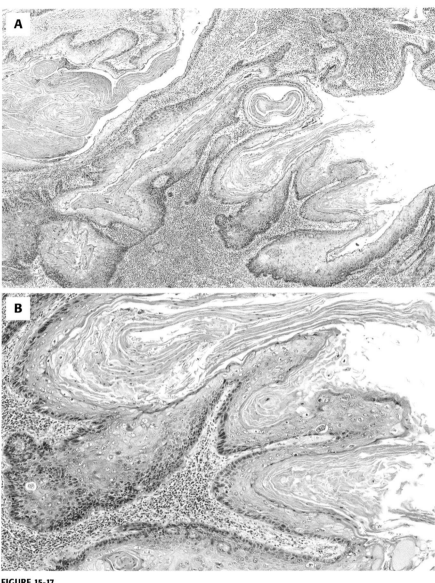

FIGURE 15-17

Verrucous carcinoma. **A,** At low power the papillomatous pattern with abundant surface keratinization and innocuous-appearing cytology are evident. Note the downward projections of the neoplasm into the submucosal connective tissue, with associated chronic inflammation. This is the typical "pushing" invasion of verrucous carcinoma. There is no desmoplastic reaction. **B,** A high-power view highlights the lack of significant nuclear atypia in this lesion, as well as the orderly pattern of maturation. There is no loss of polarity or nuclear crowding except in the lower two to three layers of the basal zone. Mitotic activity is not present above this basal zone.

atypia, it should be classified as squamous cell carcinoma (Fig. 15-18).

PROGNOSIS AND THERAPY

As might be anticipated, the overlap among verrucous carcinomas, large condylomata, and squamous cell carcinomas in the literature over the past several decades makes definitive statements regarding behavior of verrucous carcinoma difficult. Perianal verrucous carcinomas, like their counterparts in other parts of the body, seem to be locally destructive without metastasis. Lesions that metastasize should be classified as squamous cell carcinoma. Among the reported cases of "giant condyloma," as many as 50% were noted to contain areas of "malignant transformation" or "squamous cell carcinoma"; further investigation of such lesions is needed to clarify their place in the prognostic spectrum. Using the current WHO recommendations, these would be classified as squamous cell carcinoma.

The treatment of choice for verrucous carcinoma is wide local excision. For particularly large or locally destructive lesions, more aggressive surgery may be required. Radiation and chemotherapy have been used in cases of local recurrence when resection is not feasible. Although wide local excision may be curative, morbidity and mortality related to verrucous carcinoma are the result of locally aggressive behavior.

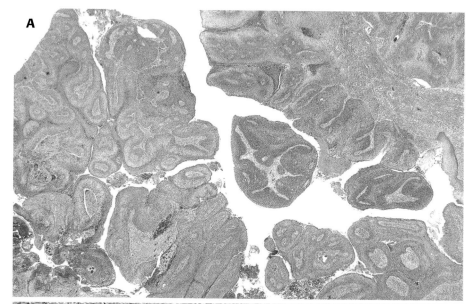

FIGURE 15-18

Verrucous carcinoma. **A,** This example of usual squamous cell carcinoma has a papillomatous exophytic pattern that grossly resembled condyloma or verrucous carcinoma. **B,** At high power the surface epithelium demonstrates marked cytologic atypia, with loss of polarity, nuclear crowding, lack of maturation, and absence of clearcut cell borders. This degree of atypia excludes a diagnosis of verrucous carcinoma. Note also the small invasive islands of tumor in the submucosa. **C,** Areas of this squamous cell carcinoma had the typical irregular infiltrating islands of tumor in a desmoplastic stroma, in contrast to the "pushing" invasive pattern of verrucous carcinoma.

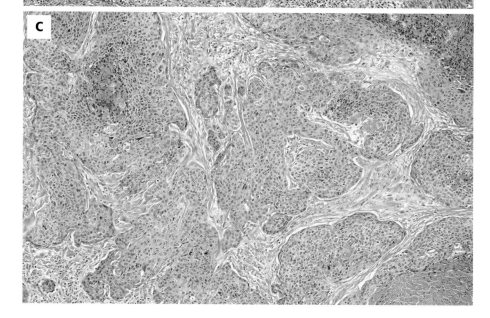

regional visceral organs. Although each hypothesis can be supported by some of the clinical scenarios and histopathologic findings in perianal Paget's disease, it is likely that this disease represents a histologic pattern expressed by a spectrum of related entities, with prognosis defined by the presence or absence of an accompanying invasive component or associated carcinoma in an adjacent organ.

PAGET'S DISEASE

Extramammary Paget's disease of the perianal region is an intraepithelial form of adenocarcinoma with many clinical and pathologic similarities to mammary Paget's disease; however, recent investigations have highlighted differences between the mammary and extramammary forms of the disease, as well as heterogeneity among cases of perianal Paget's disease. Whereas pure intraepithelial Paget's disease is encountered in the perianal region, many cases are associated with an invasive component or with an underlying visceral adenocarcinoma. The origin of Paget's disease has not been determined; proposed sources of the intraepidermal malignant glandular cells have included (1) in situ transformation of an intraepidermal pluripotential stem cell, (2) ectopic sweat gland cells within the epidermis, (3) intraepidermal spread of tumor cells from eccrine or apocrine gland carcinomas, and (4) epidermotropic spread of tumor cells from cancers in

CLINICAL FEATURES

Most cases of perianal Paget's disease represent extension from lesions of the vulva, the most common site of extramammary Paget's disease, and occur in postmenopausal white women. Paget's disease limited to the perianal region is rare, with relatively small numbers available for study even from large cancer centers. If cases associated with vulvar disease are excluded, there is no clear gender predilection; most cases occur from the sixth through the ninth decades of life.

Although Paget's disease has a typical clinical appearance, the rarity of the disease and its resemblance to a variety of benign dermatologic disorders may result in delayed diagnosis and treatment. Early lesions appear as erythematous, scaly patches and are typically pruritic; erosions or ulcers may develop. The size of the clinical lesion may be deceptive, with microscopic extension of neoplastic cells beyond the visible abnormality.

PAGET'S DISEASE—FACT SHEET

Definition

- Intraepithelial form of adenocarcinoma that may or may not have an underlying component of invasive adenocarcinoma

Incidence and Location

- Most cases of perianal Paget's disease represent extension from lesions of the vulva
- Isolated perianal Paget's disease is rare, with few cases available for study

Morbidity and Mortality

- In the 50% to 80% associated with a rectal adenocarcinoma, the prognosis reflects that of the rectal tumor
- In limited Paget's disease with no underlying rectal carcinoma, outcome is dependent on presence of an invasive component
- Morbidity related to extent of wide local excision required for limited Paget's disease or by the complications of radical surgery for an underlying rectal adenocarcinoma

Gender, Race, and Age Distribution

- Majority of cases in females because most extend from vulvar lesions
- Predominantly whites affected
- Women: postmenopausal age group; men: middle aged to older adult

Clinical Features

- Erythematous, scaly patches; lesion may extend beyond visible abnormality
- Vulvar lesions often present
- Most common complaint is pruritus
- Symptoms may be secondary to underlying rectal adenocarcinoma

Prognosis and Therapy

- For limited Paget's disease, wide local excision is indicated, with a favorable prognosis
- Recurrences usually addressed by reexcision
- Limited Paget's disease with dermal invasion has a less favorable prognosis and may metastasize
- If Paget's disease is associated with rectal adenocarcinoma, the stage of the primary carcinoma determines the prognosis
- The adenocarcinoma is usually in the distal rectum and often is associated with soft tissue extension, which is associated with a poor outcome

PAGET'S DISEASE—PATHOLOGIC FEATURES

Gross Findings

- Erythematous patches, irregular in shape and variable in extent
- If an underlying invasive component is present, whether from a rectal carcinoma, an eccrine or apocrine adenocarcinoma, or an invasive form of Paget's disease, the dermis may be indurated or may contain pools of mucin

Microscopic Findings

- The squamous epithelium is infiltrated by large cells with pale cytoplasm in a haphazard "pagetoid" arrangement
- Paget cells may have a central vesicular nucleus with prominent nucleolus or signet ring morphology
- Cytoplasm amphophilic or slightly basophilic
- Paget cells may be single or in clusters, or may form intraepithelial glands
- Paget cells may infiltrate the dermis and may extend into the cutaneous adnexal structures
- An obvious invasive adenocarcinoma may be present beneath the area of Paget's disease
- Mucin stains such as mucicarmine, Alcian blue, and PAS-diastase are helpful in demonstrating the glandular nature of the Paget cells

Immunohistochemistry

- CK7+/CK20+/GCDFP−: Most often signet ring morphology Paget's disease, with associated rectal adenocarcinoma
- CK7+/CK20−/GCDFP+: Usually classic Paget's disease without underlying rectal adenocarcinoma

Differential Diagnosis

- Melanoma
- Squamous cell carcinoma in situ (pagetoid Bowen's disease)
- Artifactually vacuolated epidermal squamous cells

PATHOLOGIC FEATURES

GROSS FINDINGS

Initial diagnosis is usually made on a small specimen such as a punch biopsy; however, wide excisional specimens may demonstrate scaly, erythematous patches or plaques or, less commonly, erosions or ulcers. If an invasive component is present, the dermal or submucosal tissue may appear indurated or nodular or may contain mucinous material.

MICROSCOPIC FINDINGS

The squamous epithelium in Paget's disease is infiltrated by large cells with abundant cytoplasm that stand out by virtue of their dissimilarity with the squamous epithelial cells and by their rather haphazard arrangement within the epithelium. There is often an intact layer of basal cells at the dermal-epidermal junction. Two cytologic types of Paget cells have been described: the classic Paget cell (Fig. 15-19) has abundant pale or amphophilic cytoplasm, a centrally placed nucleus, vesicular chromatin, and a conspicuous nucleolus, whereas the signet ring type Paget

Many cases of perianal Paget's disease are associated with synchronous or metachronous rectal adenocarcinoma. The frequency of this association is difficult to determine accurately because studies often fail to distinguish limited perianal Paget's disease from perianal disease associated with vulvar Paget's disease. A landmark review of cases by Helwig and Graham found an underlying rectal adenocarcinoma in 80% of patients with perianal Paget's disease, while a more recent study by Goldblum and Hart identified this association in 5 of 11 patients. A diagnosis of Paget's disease in the perianal region should prompt a thorough search for a rectal carcinoma.

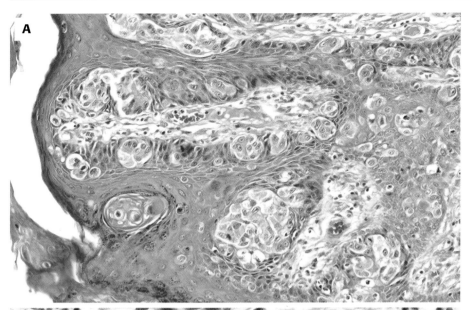

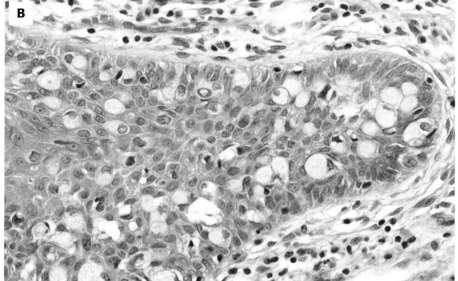

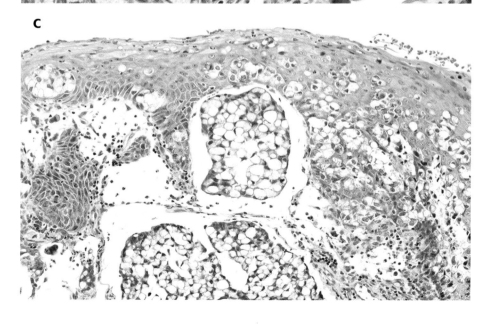

FIGURE 15-19

A, Classic Paget's cells have abundant pale to amphophilic cytoplasm and a centrally placed vesicular nucleus with conspicuous nucleolus. They are scattered singly and in small clusters throughout the squamous epithelium. **B,** The signet cell type of Paget cell has abundant intracytoplasmic mucin that pushes the nucleus to the periphery of the cell. **C,** An example of Paget's disease associated with a mucin-producing adenocarcinoma with prominent signet ring cells was located at the anorectal junction. The Paget cells in this case are also of the signet ring type, which is more often associated with an underlying invasive adenocarcinoma of visceral origin.

cell has a nucleus displaced and compressed by a large cytoplasmic mucin droplet. The Paget cells may infiltrate the epithelium as single cells or in clusters, or they may form intraepithelial glandular structures. Intraepithelial glands are more often associated with the signet ring type of Paget cell and may contain necrotic material as is commonly seen in colonic adenocarcinoma. The Paget cells may also involve cutaneous adnexal structures such as pilosebaceous units and eccrine and apocrine ducts.

An underlying eccrine or apocrine adenocarcinoma may be identified in some cases. Many cases of perianal Paget's disease are associated with anorectal adenocarcinoma. There appears to be some association of signet ring–type Paget cells and intraepithelial lumina with necrosis with increased likelihood of synchronous or metachronous anorectal adenocarcinoma. Rarely, Paget cells appear to directly infiltrate the perianal stroma, so-called invasive Paget's disease.

The squamous epithelium in incisional or excisional biopsy samples of Paget's disease may demonstrate a spectrum of proliferative changes that may initially suggest another diagnosis. The epidermis is typically acanthotic, hyperplastic, or papillomatous. Parakeratosis, hyperkeratosis, erosion, or ulceration may alter the epidermal surface.

ANCILLARY STUDIES

HISTOCHEMISTRY

Traditional histochemical stains are helpful in the differential diagnosis of Paget's disease. The Paget cells contain acid mucopolysaccharides and stain with mucicarmine, Alcian blue (pH 2.5), and PASD (Fig. 15-20).

IMMUNOHISTOCHEMISTRY

Two patterns of staining have been described in perianal Paget's disease (Fig. 15-21). In some cases the Paget cells are positive for cytokeratin (CK) 7 and CK20 but negative for gross cystic disease fluid protein (GCDFP). This staining pattern is also typical of mucinous colorectal adenocarcinoma and the CK7+/CK20+/GCDFP− cases of Paget's disease are more often associated with the signet ring–type Paget cell morphology and with an associated rectal carcinoma.

Other cases demonstrate immunohistochemical findings consistent with sweat gland differentiation: CK7+/CK20−/GCDFP+. This immunophenotype is commonly seen with the classic type Paget cell morphology and absence of rectal adenocarcinoma.

DIFFERENTIAL DIAGNOSIS

Chief considerations in the differential diagnosis of Paget's disease are the other intraepithelial neoplasms with pagetoid features. Paget's disease may be mistaken for Bowen's disease, or AIN, by hematoxylin and eosin stain alone. Mucin stains are helpful in confirming the diagnosis of Paget's disease in such cases (Fig. 15-22). The presence of melanin in neoplastic cells is not proof of melanoma because both Paget cells and the dysplastic cells of Bowen's disease may contain melanin pigment. S-100, HMB-45, MITF, and MART-1 immunostaining is useful in distinguishing melanoma from Paget's disease.

Occasional artifactually vacuolated cells in the epidermis may mimic Paget cells. However, their orderly

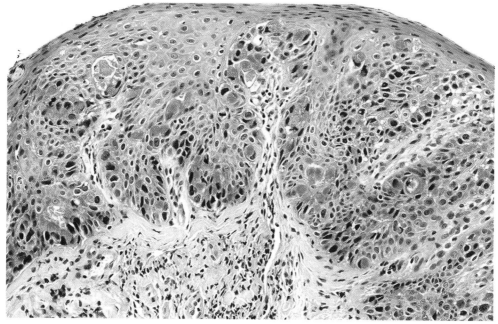

FIGURE 15-20

Paget cells contain acid mucopolysaccharides and stain with mucin stains such as periodic acid-Schiff/diastase (illustrated here) and mucicarmine.

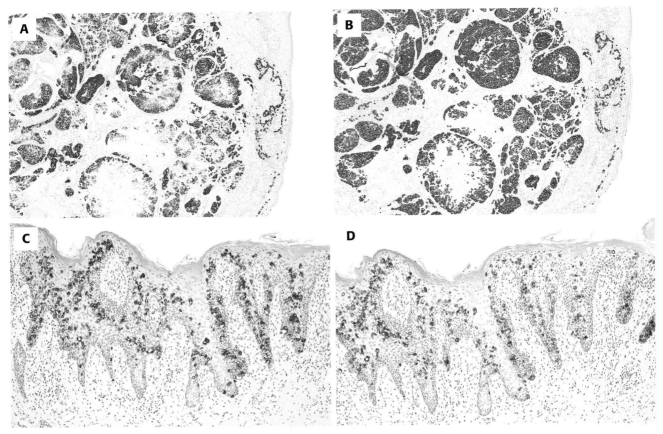

FIGURE 15-21

A, Paget's disease with underlying mucinous adenocarcinoma is positive for cytokeratin 7 (CK7) and for CK20 **(B).** Gross cystic disease fluid protein (GCDFP) did not stain the Paget cells or the underlying invasive tumor. **C,** Paget's disease without an underlying invasive adenocarcinoma was positive for CK7 and for GCDFP **(D).** CK20 did not stain the Paget cells in this case.

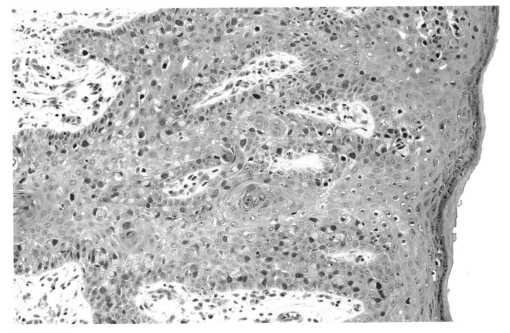

FIGURE 15-22

Biopsy from a case of Paget's disease with underlying adenocarcinoma was performed after combined modality therapy (radiation and chemotherapy). There was squamous atypia associated with the radiation therapy; however, a mucicarmine clearly demonstrates residual Paget cells within the epithelium.

distribution within the epidermis, as well as their innocuous cytologic features, generally confirm their innocence.

PROGNOSIS AND THERAPY

Clinical, histologic, and immunohistochemical findings, as noted previously, suggest that there are two forms of perianal Paget's disease: one with predominance of signet ring type Paget cells, CK7+/CK20+/GCDFP− phenotype, and frequent association with rectal adenocarcinoma, and the other with classic Paget cells, CK7+/CK20±/GCDFP− phenotype, and absence of colorectal cancer.

Paget's disease with rectal adenocarcinoma has a poor prognosis, and therapy is driven by the rectal cancer, which requires radical surgical intervention and, frequently, adjuvant therapy. The rectal lesions are frequently located in the distal rectum, and often are associated with extension into the perianal soft tissues. Local recurrence, regional lymph node metastasis, and distant metastasis account for the poor outcomes in this form of Paget's disease.

Patients with limited perianal Paget's disease, with no associated colorectal carcinoma, have a favorable prognosis following wide local excision, which is the treatment of choice. Local recurrences of Paget's disease are generally treated with reexcision. If dermal invasion by the Paget cells of the epidermis or adnexal structures occurs, the lesion, of course, has metastatic potential and the prognosis is adversely affected.

ADENOCARCINOMA

Adenocarcinomas of the anal canal are uncommon, accounting for approximately 0.1% of all gastrointestinal cancers; the paucity of cases makes generalizations with regard to prognosis and optimal therapy difficult. WHO recognizes two major groups of adenocarcinomas: those arising in the anal colorectal type mucosa (often extensions of rectal adenocarcinomas), with features essentially identical to colorectal adenocarcinoma, and extramucosal perianal adenocarcinomas of the anal glands with overlying non-neoplastic mucosa. The extramucosal perianal adenocarcinomas include anal gland adenocarcinomas and adenocarcinomas within anorectal fistulas; these two lesions may be histologically indistinguishable.

CLINICAL FEATURES

The clinical features of anal adenocarcinomas do not differ significantly from those of anal squamous cell carcinoma. Bleeding, pain, a palpable mass,

incontinence, and other changes in bowel habits are common presenting complaints.

The majority of adenocarcinomas involving the anal canal represent extension of a low rectal carcinoma downward into the anal canal. These lesions can be distinguished from true mucosal adenocarcinoma of the anus by demonstrating neoplastic changes in the surface epithelium of the distal rectum. A minority of such adenocarcinomas arise in the colonic-type mucosa of the anal canal above the dentate line. Colonoscopy may distinguish the point of origin for smaller tumors; however, it may be impossible to determine whether a large adenocarcinoma is of rectal or anal origin.

Perianal adenocarcinomas comprise between 3% and 11% of all anal carcinomas. The patient may present with anal pain, bleeding (due to ulceration of the overlying mucosa), or a mass. These tumors may grow slowly and occasionally present as a buttock mass. Diagnosis is often delayed. Patients may also have a history of chronic abscesses or fistulas, some associated with Crohn's disease.

The average age at diagnosis in one of the few series of anal adenocarcinomas was 59 years, with a range of 38 to 84 years. A male predilection was noted.

PATHOLOGIC FEATURES

GROSS FINDINGS

Adenocarcinoma arising in the anal mucosa is characterized by the exophytic, often ulcerated, red, fleshy mass lesion typical of colonic adenocarcinomas (Fig. 15-23). Location in the anal canal is mostly posterior with half of the tumors associated with fistulas. If possible, the site of origin in the anal canal should be confirmed by gross examination and by discussion with the surgeon.

Extramucosal (perianal) adenocarcinoma lacks surface epithelial involvement, presenting as a submucosal mass with overlying non-neoplastic mucosa. The cut surface of the tumor often demonstrates abundant mucinous material. There may be evidence of an anal fistula or sinus in some cases; gross findings of inflammatory bowel disease may be seen in those cases associated with Crohn's disease.

MICROSCOPIC FINDINGS

Adenocarcinoma arising in anal colorectal mucosa is histologically identical to adenocarcinomas elsewhere in the colon. They often have a tubulovillous surface pattern, with a deep infiltrative component, but may demonstrate any of the patterns seen in colorectal adenocarcinoma.

Extramucosal, or perianal adenocarcinoma is distinguished by the non-neoplastic surface epithelium lining the anal canal and overlying the lesions. The surface mucosa may be ulcerated and may exhibit

ADENOCARCINOMA—FACT SHEET

Definition

- Malignant neoplasm with glandular differentiation, either arising in the anal mucosa with features identical to colorectal adenocarcinoma, or extramucosal perianal adenocarcinomas with non-neoplastic overlying mucosa. Extramucosal adenocarcinomas include anal gland adenocarcinomas and adenocarcinomas arising within fistulous tracts.

Incidence and Location

- 3% to 11% of all anal carcinomas
- Majority of adenocarcinomas involving the anus represent extension from a rectal primary
- Distinguished by associated surface epithelial dysplasia; occasional true anal canal tumors exhibit this morphology, arising in the colonic-type epithelium of the anal canal above the dentate line

Morbidity and Mortality

- High level of morbidity due to locally destructive disease
- Stage is primary prognostic indicator; less favorable prognosis than squamous cell carcinoma of the region

Gender, Race, and Age Distribution

- Males equal to females
- No clear racial or geographic predominance
- Average age 59 years (range 38 to 84 years)

Clinical Features

- Symptoms include bleeding, pain, a palpable mass, incontinence, and other changes in bowel habits
- Perianal adenocarcinomas may grow slowly and present with a soft tissue mass of the buttock
- Diagnosis is often delayed

Prognosis and Therapy

- Rarity of cases makes prognostication and confirmation of optimal therapy difficult
- Treatment includes abdominoperitoneal resection with preoperative or postoperative combined modality therapy (chemotherapy plus radiation)
- Prognosis highly stage dependent

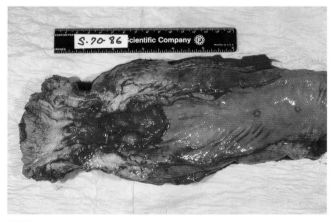

FIGURE 15-23

An adenocarcinoma arising in the distal rectum and involving the anal canal. The histology was that of the usual tubulovillous pattern of colonic adenocarcinoma. The ulcerated fleshy red mass is typical of carcinomas of mucosal origin.

ADENOCARCINOMA—PATHOLOGIC FEATURES

Gross Findings

- Adenocarcinoma arising in anal mucosa: exophytic, ulcerated, fleshy mass similar to usual colorectal adenocarcinoma
- Extramucosal perianal adenocarcinoma: no surface epithelial involvement; submucosal mass, the cut surface often with mucinous appearance

Microscopic Findings

- Adenocarcinoma arising in anal mucosa: surface epithelial dysplasia adjacent to invasive component
- Tubulovillous pattern common, with necrosis, similar to usual colorectal adenocarcinoma
- Extramucosal perianal adenocarcinoma associated with non-neoplastic surface mucosa; mucinous type adenocarcinoma with islands of cytologically bland tumor cells in pools of extracellular mucin is the most common pattern seen in association with fistulas
- Haphazardly arranged small glands with scant mucin production, in the perianal stroma, with no surface mucosal component are most diagnostic of anal gland carcinoma

Immunohistochemistry

- Mucinous-type adenocarcinomas usually seen in extramucosal perianal adenocarcinomas are most often CK7+/CK20−
- Adenocarcinomas with surface epithelial involvement and colorectal pattern are usually CK7−/CK20+

Differential Diagnosis

- Colorectal carcinoma extending from lower rectum

histologic features of inflammatory bowel disease. Although these tumors are thought to include two groups—those associated with a fistula and those arising in anal glands—they are not histologically or immunohistochemically distinctive. Adenocarcinomas associated with fistulas are most often of the mucinous type, with abundant extracellular mucin containing islands of atypical glandular epithelium; these may be referred to as perianal mucinous (colloid) adenocarcinoma. Origin of adenocarcinoma from anal glands is extremely difficult to document, and use of a histologically distinct definition of anal gland adenocarcinoma has not been widely adopted. Hobbs and colleagues from the Armed Forces Institute of Pathology have suggested that tumors with haphazardly arranged small glands in the perianal stroma with scant mucin and no surface mucosal component are most likely of anal gland origin (Fig. 15-24).

ANCILLARY STUDIES

IMMUNOHISTOCHEMISTRY

Immunostaining for CK7 and CK20 has been studied in the various patterns of adenocarcinoma of the anal region. Although not particularly necessary for

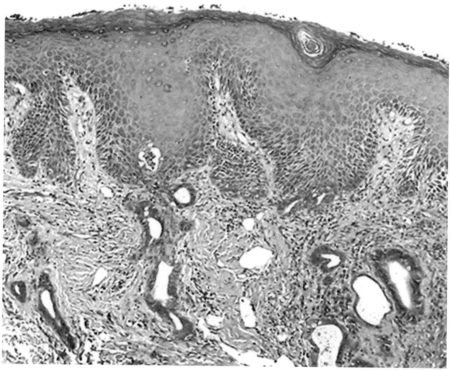

FIGURE 15-24

This perianal adenocarcinoma (anal gland or anal duct carcinoma) lacks surface mucosal abnormalities grossly and histologically. The tumor is characterized by haphazardly arranged small glands with scant mucin production, in the perianal stroma, with no surface mucosal component.

prognostic purposes, they may provide some evidence to suggest different sites of origin for these neoplasms. The mucinous type of adenocarcinoma, most often seen in association with fistulas in ano, are generally CK7+/CK20+. Typical tubulovillous colorectal-type carcinomas are CK7−/CK20+. Most adenocarcinomas of the small glandular type with scant mucin (of possible anal gland origin) are CK7+/CK20−.

DIFFERENTIAL DIAGNOSIS

The differential diagnosis of adenocarcinomas of the anal canal is relatively limited, except in very poorly differentiated examples; in such cases, melanoma, lymphoma, and poorly differentiated squamous cell carcinoma would be considered. Immunohistochemical stains may be used to exclude lymphoma and melanoma. Because squamous cell carcinomas of the anal canal may have areas of mucin production or may contain glandular structures, it may be impossible to classify poorly differentiated carcinomas with certainty. The distinction in these cases is not absolutely critical because both squamous cell carcinoma and adenocarcinoma are staged using the same American Joint Committee on Cancer system (see Table 15-1).

Distinction among the preceding three groups of anal canal adenocarcinomas does not appear to have prognostic significance. Colorectal adenocarcinomas extending into the anal canal from the distal rectum are considered rectal neoplasms and are usually recognized by clinical assessment rather than by pathologic examination.

PROGNOSIS AND THERAPY

The rarity of anal adenocarcinomas makes prognostication and recommendations for optimal therapy difficult. Stage is the primary prognostic indicator; stage for stage, adenocarcinoma has a less favorable prognosis than squamous cell carcinoma with a 5-year survival of less than 20%.

Treatment has included abdominoperineal resection with preoperative or postoperative combined modality therapy (radiation and chemotherapy). It is not known whether a more limited surgical approach with combined modality therapy, such as has been very effectively used in the treatment of anal canal squamous cell carcinoma, would provide acceptable results.

MELANOMA

Although the anorectum is the most common alimentary tract site for primary malignant melanoma, it is, nevertheless a rare tumor in this location, representing less than 1% of colorectal malignancies.

CLINICAL FEATURES

The mean age of diagnosis of anal melanoma is 63 years, with a range of 23 to 83 years. It is twice as common in women as in men and is usually seen in whites. Only a few cases have been reported in African Americans and Asians. The most common presenting symptom is rectal bleeding, which is seen in 55%. Other complaints include pain, changes in bowel habits, pruritus, tenesmus, and an inguinal mass associated with lymph node metastasis. Up to 26% of patients have metastatic disease at the time of diagnosis.

PATHOLOGIC FEATURES

GROSS FINDINGS

Anal melanomas are frequently polypoid (Fig. 15-25) and may be easily mistaken for benign lesions such as anal tags or hemorrhoids, sometimes resulting in a delay in diagnosis. Brown or black pigmentation, if present, suggests the diagnosis, but approximately one third are amelanotic. Size varies considerably, ranging from 3 mm to 3.5 cm. Although depth or thickness of the tumor is usually documented in the pathology report, it has no prognostic significance. Small lesions may be covered by intact mucosa; larger lesions are often ulcerated. The lesions often occur at the transitional zone of the anal canal where melanocytes are most likely to be encountered.

MICROSCOPIC FINDINGS

The microscopic appearance of anal melanoma does not differ significantly from its cutaneous counterpart. An in situ component with junctional nests and pagetoid

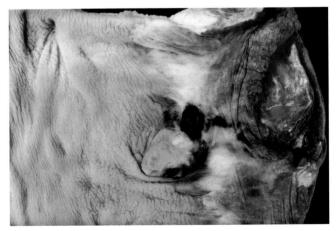

FIGURE 15-25

The polypoid morphology of this tumor is common in malignant melanoma of the anorectum. Note the variegated tan-to-black mottled appearance due to the presence of melanin in portions of the lesion. *(From Turk JL, ed. Royal College of Surgeons slide atlas of pathology, alimentary system. London, 1986, Gower Medical, with permission.)*

intraepithelial spread is common (Fig. 15-26), especially in nonulcerated lesions, a feature that suggests primary mucosal origin. The invasive component of the neoplasm may contain epithelioid, polygonal cells, spindle cells, or an admixture of both. The epithelioid cells often have eosinophilic granular cytoplasm, variably pleomorphic nuclei, frequent mitotic figures, and prominent nucleoli. Pigmented tumors may demonstrate brown-to-black melanin in tumor cells as fine, dusty-appearing pigment or as more coarse and refractile clumps in melanophages (non-neoplastic histiocytic cells scattered in and around the neoplasm). Tumor depth or thickness (Breslow's level) is measured using an ocular micrometer.

ANCILLARY STUDIES

IMMUNOHISTOCHEMISTRY

As with melanomas in any site, immunohistochemistry may be vital in making the diagnosis, especially in tumors lacking an adjacent junctional melanocytic proliferation (Fig. 15-27). S-100, HMB-45, melan-A, and tyrosinase are useful markers of melanocytic differentiation. Even though S-100 is the least specific, it is the most sensitive, making it a mainstay in the differential diagnostic workup of potential anal melanomas. HMB-45 is specific, but the staining may be focal; melan-A generally provides more diffuse staining of tumor cells and has been useful as a confirmatory stain in conjunction with a positive S-100 result. MITF is specific for melanocytes; it is a nuclear stain that is useful when there is extensive cytoplasmic melanin pigmentation. Immunoreactivity for CD117 (c-Kit) has been shown in up to 86% of anal/rectal mucosal melanomas.

MOLECULAR PATHOLOGY

PCR studies for *C-KIT* mutations may be useful because *C-KIT* is mutated in 15% to 22% of mucosal melanomas, but mutation does not correlate perfectly with immunohistochemical CD117 reactivity. Many of the identified mutations have been associated with dramatic responses to tyrosine kinase inhibitor therapy (such as with imatinib).

ELECTRON MICROSCOPY

The widespread availability and cost effectiveness of immunohistochemical staining in the differential diagnosis of poorly differentiated, pleomorphic, or spindle cell neoplasms have made electron microscopy almost obsolete in this regard. If the occasion to perform electron microscopy arises, it can provide helpful evidence to support a diagnosis of melanoma. The distinctive ultrastructural feature is the premelanosome, an elongated membrane-bound structure with an internal lamellar pattern. As the premelanosomes mature, they accumulate melanin pigment, which

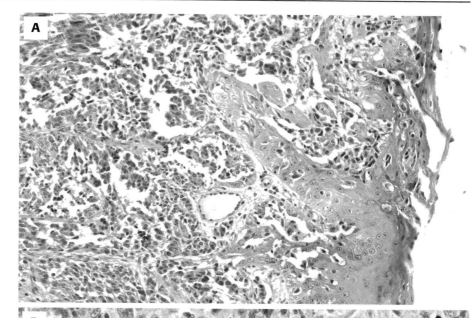

FIGURE 15-26

A, Low-power view demonstrates an in situ component of melanoma overlying the invasive tumor. Note the pagetoid spread of individual atypical melanocytes in a haphazard fashion through the squamous epithelium. **B,** At higher power two cellular patterns are evident. Here the epithelioid-type cells are large and polygonal, with abundant pale eosinophilic cytoplasms and large nuclei. Mitotic figures are common; faint deposits of fine brown melanin pigment are seen. **C,** In other areas of the same tumor the cells assume an elongated spindled pattern. Again, note the frequent mitoses and a hint of melanin pigment.

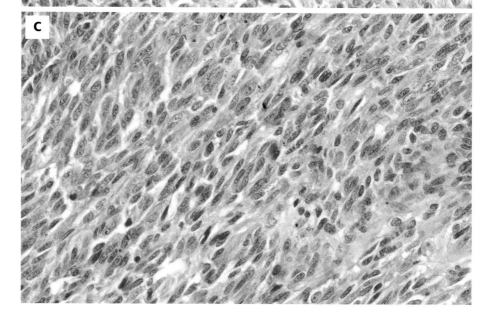

MELANOMA—FACT SHEET

Definition

- Malignant tumor of melanocytic origin usually primary to the anal mucosa
- Metastatic melanoma should also be considered if an in situ component is not identified

Incidence and Location

- Less than 1% of colorectal malignancies
- Anorectum most common alimentary tract site for primary melanoma

Morbidity and Mortality

- Virtually uniformly fatal, with few long-term survivors
- Death usually due to disseminated disease rather than local recurrence

Gender, Race, and Age Distribution

- Females more than males, 2:1
- Mean age at diagnosis 63 years (range 23 to 83 years)
- Most occur in whites; only rare cases in Asians and African Americans

Clinical Features

- Most common symptom is rectal bleeding
- Other symptoms include pain, changes in bowel habits, pruritus, tenesmus, and an inguinal mass associated with lymph node metastasis
- Metastatic disease common at time of diagnosis

Prognosis and Therapy

- Prognosis very poor; 5-year survival rates of 6% to 22%
- 26% of patients have metastatic disease at time of presentation
- Mean survival after appearance of metastatic disease is 6 months
- No survival benefit from abdominoperitoneal resection over wide local excision
- Wide local excision currently favored to decrease morbidity from radical surgery
- Tyrosine kinase inhibitors have been successful in patients with *C-KIT* mutations

MELANOMA—PATHOLOGIC FEATURES

Gross Findings

- Frequently polypoid; easily mistaken for hemorrhoids or anal tags
- Brown or black pigment suggests diagnosis, but one third amelanotic
- Size ranges from 3 mm to 3.5 cm

Microscopic Findings

- Similar to cutaneous counterpart
- In situ component with junctional nests and pagetoid intraepithelial spread is common if ulceration is not extensive
- Cell type may be epithelioid with eosinophilic granular cytoplasms and large nuclei with prominent nucleoli, monotonous spindled cells, or mixed
- Intracellular melanin may be visible in tumor cells and in melanophages
- Tumor depth or thickness is measured from the epithelial surface

Ultrastructural Findings

- Rarely necessary for diagnosis with easy availability of immunohistochemistry
- Key feature is presence of premelanosomes, membrane-bound structures with an internal lamellar pattern

Immunohistochemistry

- S-100–positive in most cases
- Melan-A–positive, sensitive, and specific
- HMB45-positive, but often very focal
- CD117/cKit may be positive

Differential Diagnosis

- Poorly differentiated carcinoma
- Lymphoma
- Small cell undifferentiated carcinoma of rectal origin

obscures the lamellar pattern, making them difficult to distinguish from lysosomes.

DIFFERENTIAL DIAGNOSIS

The "great mimicker," melanoma is considered in the differential diagnosis of many neoplasms, including poorly differentiated carcinoma, malignant lymphoma, epithelial and soft tissue spindle cell neoplasms, pleomorphic sarcomas, and small cell malignancies. The patterns of melanoma are so varied that they may even mimic signet ring cell carcinomas, clear cell neoplasms (especially the balloon cell types of melanoma), and even adenocarcinomas and papillary carcinomas (due to pseudoglandular and pseudopapillary degenerative patterns). Because the morphology of spindled melanoma can be very similar to that of gastrointestinal stromal tumors (GISTs) and because

immunoreactivity for CD117 is seen in both tumors, performing a CD34 to distinguish between the two may be necessary (70% of GISTs are positive). It is prudent to include melanoma in a differential diagnostic dilemma. As discussed previously, immunohistochemical studies are essential in the differential diagnosis of melanoma.

PROGNOSIS AND THERAPY

The prognosis for patients with anal melanoma is poor, with 5-year survival rates ranging from 6% to 22%. For patients presenting with metastatic disease, mean survival is 6 months. There is no correlation between recurrence after surgical therapy with curative intent and depth of tumor, gender, presence of perirectal nodal metastasis, or even type of surgery. No survival benefit has been shown between abdominoperineal resection and wide local excision of anal melanoma. Although the rate of local recurrence is somewhat less in patients treated with abdominoperineal resection than with wide local excision, most patients die of widely disseminated disease before local recurrence becomes an issue. For this reason,

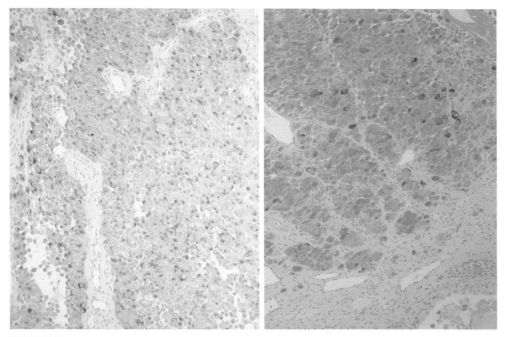

FIGURE 15-27

This melanoma with an epithelioid pattern is positive for HMB-45 (*right*) and for S-100 (*left*). A positive S-100 reaction requires nuclear staining; cytoplasmic staining alone is considered a negative result. As in this case, the S-100 staining is typically stronger and more diffuse than HMB-45 staining.

wide local excision has become the favored surgical approach to this disease. The recent identification of *C-KIT* mutations in mucosal melanomas has led to promising results with tyrosine kinase inhibitor therapy, and clinical trials are under way. As mentioned previously, *C-KIT* mutations do not correlate with immunohistochemical staining, so molecular tests to determine the specific type of mutation may be required to identify the subset of patients likely to respond to tyrosine kinase inhibitor treatment. The utility of modalities such as sentinel lymph node biopsy, traditional chemotherapy, radiation therapy, and immunotherapy in the treatment of anal melanoma has not been demonstrated.

16

Pathology of the Gallbladder and Extrahepatic Bile Ducts

■ **PEDRAM ARGANI, MD**

■ GALLBLADDER

CHOLECYSTITIS

CLINICAL FEATURES

Chronic cholecystitis due to gallstones most frequently results in intermittent right upper quadrant visceral pain that follows eating (so-called biliary colic). Acute cholecystitis typically presents with biliary colic that progressively worsens, resulting in sharp pain in the right upper quadrant, accompanied by fever and leukocytosis. Acute cholecystitis is most commonly caused by impaction of gallstones within the cystic duct, effecting obstruction and bile stasis. Most cases are sterile and secondary to mucosal damage from chemical injury; only rarely is infection the primary cause. Acalculous cholecystitis is most frequently seen in debilitated hospitalized patients with multiple medical problems. In this setting, decreased gallbladder motility and mucosal ischemia cause cholecystitis. *Cryptosporidium parvum* and cytomegalovirus may cause an acute infectious cholecystitis in immunocompromised patients.

Less common forms of cholecystitis may vary somewhat in their presentation. Xanthogranulomatous cholecystitis may be mistaken for an invasive gallbladder malignancy intraoperatively because the gallbladder adheres to and may appear to invade adjacent organs. Eosinophilic cholecystitis is three times more likely to be acalculous than usual cholecystitis and may be seen as a manifestation of eosinophilic gastroenteritis, parasitic infestation, or drug ingestion.

PATHOLOGIC FEATURES

GROSS FINDINGS

Cholecystitis causes a diffuse thickening of the normally thin gallbladder wall. In acute cholecystitis, the thickening is primarily due to edema, inflammation,

and reactive fibroblastic proliferation. The mucosa may be eroded and erythematous. In chronic cholecystitis, muscular hypertrophy and fibrosis are the main causes of the thickening. In xanthogranulomatous cholecystitis, one may see yellow nodules within the gallbladder wall and adjacent connective tissue (Fig. 16-1). The mural thickening caused by florid cholecystitis may be difficult to distinguish from an early gallbladder carcinoma, so careful gross examination and thorough sampling of such specimens are important.

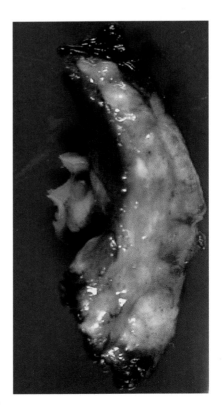

FIGURE 16-1

Gross photograph of xanthogranulomatous cholecystitis. Note the yellow nodules within the thickened gallbladder wall.

MICROSCOPIC FINDINGS

Histologically, acute cholecystitis demonstrates edema, neutrophilic infiltration, and associated reactive epithelial changes that can easily be confused with neoplasia (Fig. 16-2). Inflammatory polyps represent small protrusions of inflamed granulation tissue associated with cholecystitis. After a week or so, the acute inflammation organizes and loose fibroblastic proliferation develops. These latter changes merge with those of chronic cholecystitis.

The classic chronic cholecystitis associated with lithiasis is characterized by dense mural muscular hypertrophy and fibrosis, and only minimal chronic inflammation (Fig. 16-3). Frequently, Rokitansky-Aschoff sinuses are identified; these represent diverticuli of gallbladder mucosa into the muscular layer, associated with mild muscular hypertrophy. Rokitansky-Aschoff sinuses merge morphologically with adenomyomas,

which demonstrate greater muscular hypertrophy (Fig. 16-4). Importantly, both conditions result in displacement of benign gallbladder epithelium beyond the muscular layer of the gallbladder, a setting in which it may be confused with carcinoma. Cholecystitis is often associated with secondary papillary mucosal hyperplasia. Therefore, in the typical chronic cholecystitis associated with lithiasis, reactive epithelial changes overshadow the inflammatory ones.

Specific histopathologic variants of chronic cholecystitis are xanthogranulomatous cholecystitis, eosinophilic cholecystitis, and cholecystitis associated with primary sclerosing cholangitis (PSC). Xanthogranulomatous cholecystitis (ceroid granuloma, cholecystic granuloma) results from rupture of Rokitansky-Aschoff sinuses with bile extravasation that incites a florid histiocytic reaction. Macrophages with lightly pigmented lipofuchsin (ceroid) granules are abundant, and reactive fibroblastic cells with a storiform pattern may mimic sarcoma (Fig. 16-5). Specific histologic criteria for the diagnosis of eosinophilic cholecystitis have not been established, but a general rule is that eosinophils are out of proportion to other inflammatory cells (Fig. 16-6). Diffuse lymphoplasmacytic acalculous cholecystitis

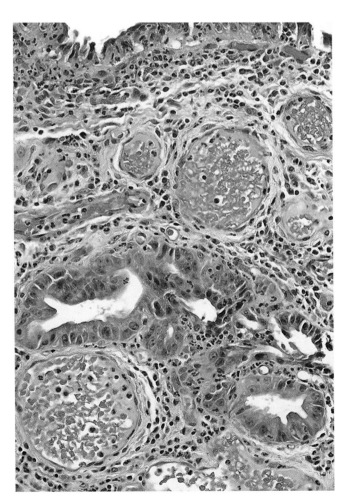

FIGURE 16-2

Acute cholecystitis. The mucosal lining cells have enlarged nuclei and an increased nuclear-to-cytoplasmic ratio. However, the uniformity of the nuclei and their relative hypochromasia and round contours, particularly in the setting of a neutrophilic infiltrate, support a benign diagnosis.

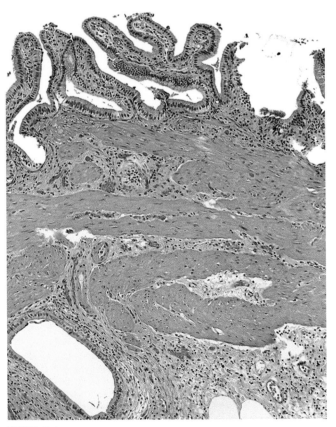

FIGURE 16-3

Mild chronic cholecystitis. This is the usual histology in patients with uncomplicated cholelithiasis. There is mural thickening and mucosal diverticuli (Rokitansky-Aschoff sinuses), but only minimal mural chronic inflammation.

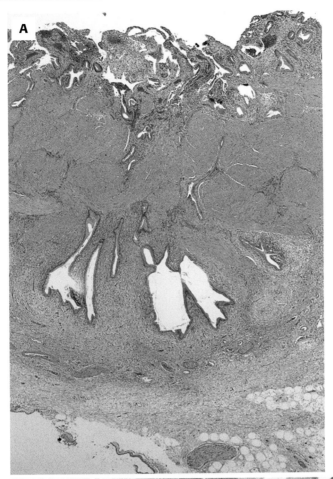

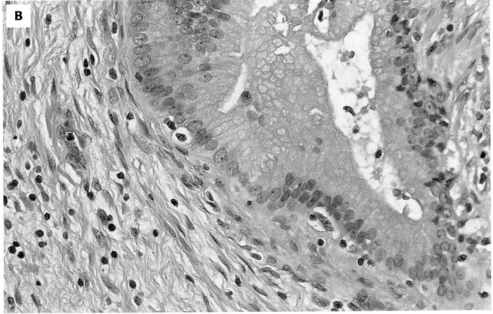

FIGURE 16-4

Adenomyoma. **A,** At low power, the presence of epithelium in the perimuscular connective tissue raises the possibility of invasive carcinoma. **B,** At high power, the benign cytology of the abnormally located epithelium is evident.

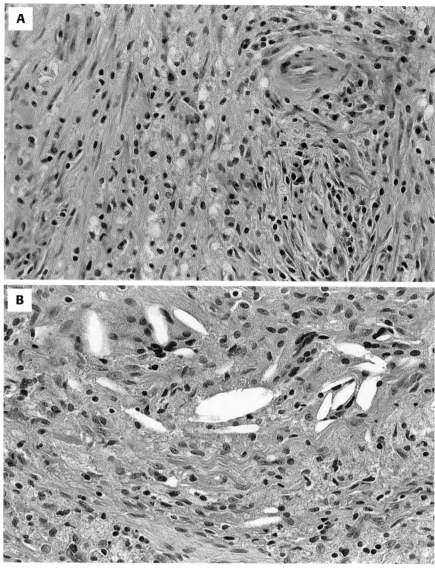

FIGURE 16-5

Xanthogranulomatous cholecystitis. **A,** Cellular areas composed of reactive fibroblasts, chronic inflammation, and macrophages raise the possibility of a neoplastic process, such as a sarcoma. **B,** Other areas contain cholesterol clefts, bile pigment, and multinucleate giant cells.

is predominantly confined to the lamina propria. Although these changes may be associated with PSC, they are not specific in that they may be found in patients with distal bile duct obstruction of any cause (such as neoplasms or choledocholithiasis; Fig. 16-7 and Table 16-1).

Metaplasia of the normal columnar absorptive epithelium of the gallbladder often accompanies cholecystitis and may represent an early, nonobligate precursor to gallbladder carcinoma. Three types of metaplasia are recognized in the gallbladder. Gastric metaplasia is seen in half of patients with cholelithiasis (Fig. 16-8). In gastric metaplasia, the normal absorptive epithelium of the gallbladder is replaced by cuboidal cells with cytoplasm composed predominantly of neutral mucin. Intestinal metaplasia is seen in approximately 50% of patients with cholelithiasis and is thought to pose a greater risk for gallbladder carcinoma.

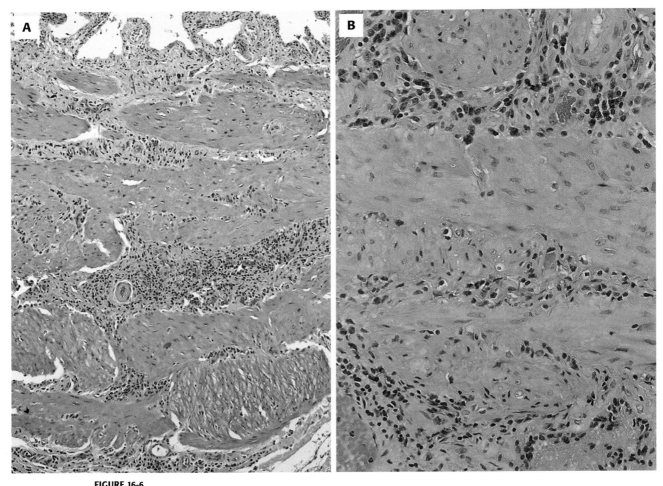

FIGURE 16-6

Eosinophilic cholecystitis. **A,** At low power, a moderate inflammatory infiltrate involves the muscularis. **B,** At higher power, the infiltrate proves to be almost exclusively eosinophils.

Histologically, one sees goblet cells with acid mucin (Fig. 16-9). Neuroendocrine cells and Paneth cells are also frequently seen. Squamous metaplasia is rare in the gallbladder but, when present, is often associated with squamous dysplasia and carcinoma.

DIFFERENTIAL DIAGNOSIS

The reactive epithelium of acute cholecystitis may be difficult to distinguish from dysplasia or carcinoma in situ. Compared with carcinoma in situ, reactive epithelial changes consist of a less monotonous, more heterogeneous cell population demonstrating less pleomorphism, more vesicular chromatin, prominent but more rounded nucleoli, and more amphophilic cytoplasm. Displaced gallbladder epithelium of adenomyomas may extend beyond the muscular layer to involve the perimuscular connective tissue or even involve perineural spaces, and thus be confused with invasive carcinoma. The absence of atypia within adenomyoma and absence of desmoplasia assures a benign diagnosis. Tangential sectioning of the papillary hyperplasia that accompanies cholecystitis may give a pseudocribriform, spongioid pattern that may mimic cribriform carcinoma. Again, the absence of significant cytologic atypia militates against neoplasia. On frozen section, the histocytes of xanthogranulomatous cholecystitis may be mistaken for signet ring cell carcinoma, especially given that malignancy is often the clinical impression of this benign disorder.

PROGNOSIS AND THERAPY

The usual acute or chronic cholecystitis associated with gallstones is cured by cholecystectomy. In contrast, approximately 40% of patients with acalculous cholecystitis die. This is likely due to underlying medical conditions that may also result in a delay in diagnosis.

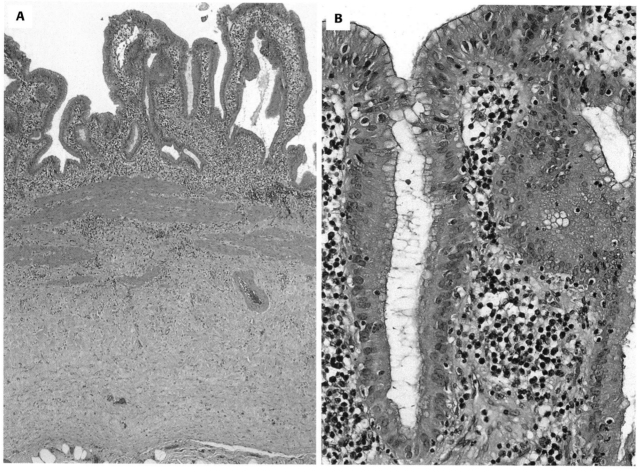

FIGURE 16-7

Diffuse acalculous lymphoplasmacytic cholecystitis secondary to bile duct obstruction. This patient had an invasive carcinoma in the head of the pancreas, causing stricture of the distal common bile duct. At low power **(A),** the gallbladder contains a superficial mucosal infiltrate of predominantly lymphocytes and plasma cells as shown in **(B).** These findings were once touted as being specific to primary sclerosing cholangitis, but, as this case shows, they are a nonspecific reflection of distal bile duct obstruction.

TABLE 16-1

Chronic Cholecystitis

Type of Cholecystitis	Histology	Associations
Usual chronic cholecystitis	Muscular hypertrophy, Rokitanky-Aschoff sinuses, minimal inflammation	Gallstones
Xanthogranulomatous cholecystitis	Xanthomatous macrophages and fibroblastic reaction	Simulates malignancy clinically
Eosinophilic cholecystitis	Eosinophils out of proportion to other inflammation	Other causes of eosinophilic gastroenteritis
Diffuse acalculous lymphoplasmacytic cholecystitis	Superficial lymphoplasmacytic infiltrate, no stones	Obstruction of distal bile ducts (i.e., primary sclerosing cholangitis, distal bile duct tumors)

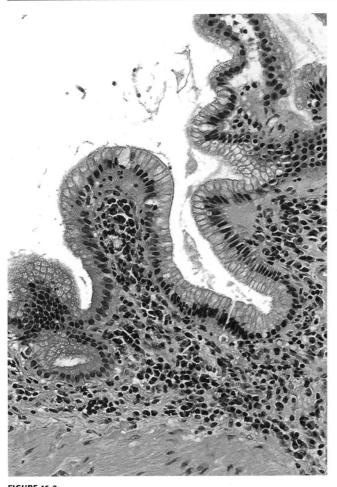

FIGURE 16-8

Gastric mucin cell metaplasia. Note the conversion of the columnar absorptive epithelium with pink cytoplasm to mucinous epithelium resembling gastric foveolar epithelium.

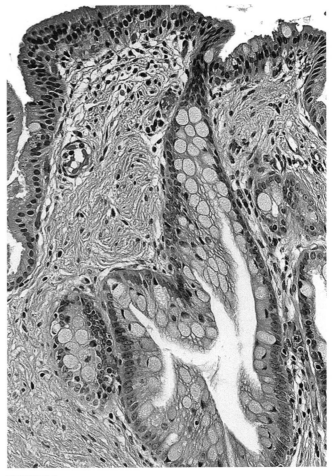

FIGURE 16-9

Intestinal metaplasia. Note the conversion of the columnar absorptive epithelium to goblet cells.

GALLBLADDER CARCINOMA

CLINICAL FEATURES

Gallbladder carcinoma is the most frequent malignancy in the biliary tract; approximately 5000 new cases are discovered each year in the United States. There is a female predominance, reflecting the female propensity to the major risk factor, cholelithiasis. The mean age at diagnosis is 72 years. The most common presentations include right upper quadrant pain, weight loss, and anorexia for advanced stage tumors, but symptoms at presentation can mimic chronic cholecystitis in early-stage tumors. Jaundice is not common at presentation because the outflow of bile via the common bile duct is not obstructed until the disease is advanced. Some series report that unsuspected gallbladder carcinoma is found in 2% of cholecystectomies, with higher frequencies in patients older than 65 years.

Risk factors for gallbladder carcinoma include genetics, cholelithiasis, and abnormal junction of the pancreatic and bile ducts (AJPBD). Genetic factors are suggested by the prevalence of the disease in American Indians and Hispanic Americans and probably reflect the tendency to form gallstones. Gallstones are found in 75% of cases of carcinoma and are thought to predispose to carcinoma by causing chronic irritation and epithelial damage, leading to increased proliferation and the opportunity for mutation. However, the low overall incidence of gallbladder carcinoma in all patients with gallstones (0.2%) renders the merits of elective cholecystectomy in patients with gallstones debatable. AJPBD refers to the union of the common bile duct and pancreatic duct outside the duodenal wall, beyond the influence of the sphincter of Oddi. This anatomic variant allows reflux of pancreatic juice into the bile duct. This condition is more common in Japan, where approximately one sixth of gallbladder carcinomas are associated with AJPBD.

GALLBLADDER CARCINOMA—FACT SHEET

Definition
- Carcinoma derived from the epithelial lining of the gallbladder

Incidence and Location
- Rare: less than 0.5% of all cancers in women in the United States
- 5000 new cases per year in the United States
- Endemic in Mexico and Chile
- Risk factors include genetics, gallstones, abnormal choledochopancreatic duct junction, and porcelain gallbladder.

Morbidity and Mortality
- Highly lethal: overall 5-year survival rate is 5% to 10%

Gender, Race, and Age Distribution
- Female predominance (M:F = 1:2)
- Incidence highest among American Indians and Hispanic Americans
- Mostly affects adults (mean age = 72 years)

Clinical Features
- Symptoms vary but include right upper quadrant pain, weight loss, and anorexia.
- Symptoms may mimic cholecystitis.
- May be asymptomatic (occult)

Prognosis and Therapy
- Generally poor
- Rare low-stage tumors have better prognosis
- Among low-stage tumors, vascular invasion and grade may have significance
- Surgical resection is the most effective treatment
- Usually CK7 positive; CK20 and CDX2 variable
- CEA positive

Differential Diagnosis
- Cholecystitis with reactive atypia
- Carcinoma in situ colonizing Rokitansky-Aschoff sinuses

GALLBLADDER CARCINOMA—PATHOLOGIC FEATURES

Gross Findings
- Firm infiltrative or polypoid mass
- May form a subtle thickening that mimics cholecystitis
- Most common in fundus or body of gallbladder

Microscopic Findings
- Usual adenocarcinoma is a gland-forming tumor with abundant desmoplastic stroma
- Cells classically have cuboidal shape and show marked cytologic atypia given degree of gland formation
- Up to 80% of invasive carcinomas are associated with carcinoma in situ
- Variants include papillary, small cell (high-grade neuroendocrine), adenosquamous, clear cell, undifferentiated

Genetics
- Complex genetic alterations
- p16 and p53 are consistently inactivated

Immunohistochemistry
- Strongly cytokeratin positive (AE1/3, Cam5.2)

PATHOLOGIC FEATURES

GROSS FINDINGS

Grossly, gallbladder carcinomas usually (70% of cases) form firm, infiltrative masses or may less frequently (30% of cases) form polyps that protrude into the lumen (Fig. 16-10). Occasional cases form subtle thickenings in the gallbladder wall that are grossly indistinguishable from chronic cholecystitis. The majority arises in the fundus (60%), followed by the body (30%) and the neck (10%), but often the epicenter of an extensive tumor cannot be definitively discerned.

AJPBD is thought to confer a 10-fold increased risk for gallbladder carcinoma. Compared with those patients with gallbladder carcinoma who do not have AJPBD, patients with gallbladder carcinoma arising in the setting of AJPBD are far less likely to have gallstones and are on average 10 years younger at presentation. Moreover, a higher percentage of their tumors carry *K-RAS* mutations, implying a different genetic pathogenesis. AJPBD is also associated with choledochal cysts, which are strongly associated with bile duct carcinoma. Other associations for gallbladder carcinoma include familial adenomatous polyposis and diffuse dystrophic calcification of the wall of the gallbladder (porcelain gallbladder). The latter is found in less than 0.5% of cholecystectomies, but approximately 20% of porcelain gallbladders are associated with gallbladder carcinoma.

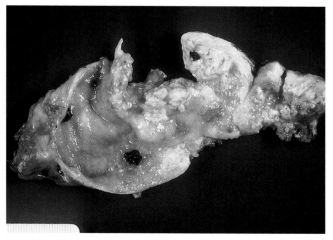

FIGURE 16-10

Gross photograph of gallbladder carcinoma. Note the thickened ulcerated mass in this gallbladder, which also contains a gallstone. *(Courtesy of David Klimstra, MD, New York.)*

MICROSCOPIC FINDINGS

The vast majority of invasive gallbladder carcinomas are adenocarcinomas composed of cuboidal or columnar cells resembling normal biliary epithelium (Fig. 16-11). Many cases contain goblet cells. The degree of cytologic atypia is often greater than one would expect for the degree of gland formation. Prominent stromal desmoplasia is characteristic. Papillary (in situ) carcinoma is the most important growth pattern to recognize, because these tumors have a better prognosis. The surface papillary component of such tumors is noninvasive and in theory metastatic incapable; when an underlying invasive component is present, it tends to be superficial. Other specific variants include mucinous (colloid) carcinoma, which is diagnosed if greater than 50% of the tumor is composed of extracellular mucin and signet ring cell carcinoma. Clear cell (glycogen-rich) carcinoma of the gallbladder must be distinguished from metastatic clear cell renal carcinoma. Adenosquamous carcinomas are characterized by dual squamous and glandular differentiation. Undifferentiated carcinomas may be composed of spindled and giant cells (similar to pancreatic anaplastic carcinoma), small signet ring cells (mimicking invasive lobular breast carcinoma), or mononuclear cells in a background of osteoclasts (similar to giant cell tumor of pancreas). Cribriform carcinomas simulate their counterparts in the breast. Small cell neuroendocrine (oat cell) carcinoma comprises 5% of gallbladder primary tumors and is morphologically identical to small cell carcinoma of lung. One may find an associated adenocarcinoma in approximately one third of cases (Fig. 16-12).

Most invasive gallbladder carcinomas arise not from the rare gallbladder adenoma but from flat dysplasia. The current model is that gallbladder carcinomas arise via genetic progression from metaplasia to dysplasia to carcinoma. Similar genetic alterations (such as in *Tp16* and *Tp53*) have been noted in all three. Dysplasia is frequently identified adjacent to the invasive carcinoma if the adjacent mucosa is well sampled. Grossly, flat dysplasia is usually inapparent. In contrast to adenomas, dysplasias are poorly delineated and arise in a background of metaplasia. Microscopically, dysplasia is graded based on cytologic atypia and loss of nuclear polarity. Low-grade dysplasia is characterized by stratified cigar-shaped nuclei, and cytologically resembles a colonic tubular adenoma (Fig. 16-13). *High-grade dysplasia* is used interchangeably with the term *carcinoma in situ* and is characterized by abnormally polarized apical nuclei, prominent nucleoli, and nuclear contour irregularities (Fig. 16-14). Dysplasia can mimic invasive carcinoma by extension into deep Rokitansky-Aschoff sinuses or extension into metaplastic pyloric glands.

In cases of pure high-grade dysplasia, the status of the cystic duct and the extent of sampling of the gallbladder are crucial. Our policy is to entirely submit any gallbladder showing high-grade dysplasia on initial representative sections, given the clinical implications of finding an occult invasive carcinoma.

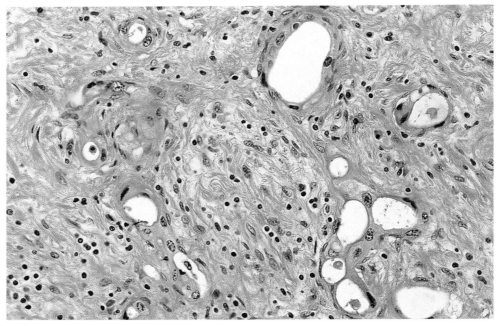

FIGURE 16-11

Gallbladder adenocarcinoma: microscopic features. The tumor cells are set in a background of dense desmoplastic stroma, have a low-cuboidal shape, and show marked cytologic atypia.

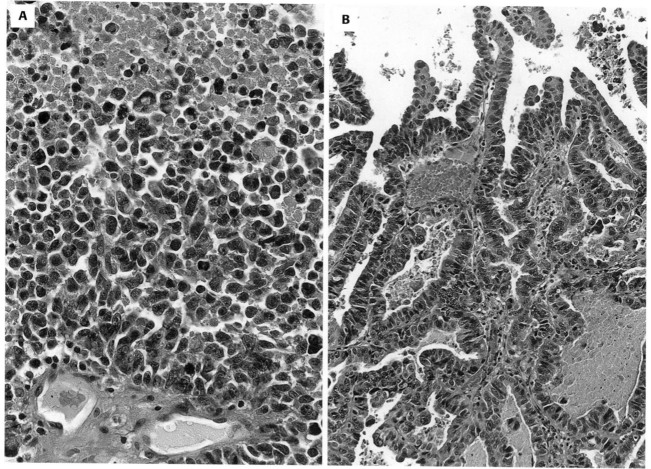

FIGURE 16-12

Mixed small cell carcinoma/adenocarcinoma of the gallbladder. **A,** The small cell carcinoma component is morphologically identical to its more common namesake in the lung. **B,** The presence of a conventional adenocarcinoma component within the gallbladder establishes that the tumor originated here.

ANCILLARY STUDIES

Gallbladder adenocarcinomas are immunoreactive for broad-spectrum cytokeratins, epithelial membrane antigen, and carcinoembryonic antigen (CEA). Similar to other pancreatobiliary carcinomas, they are consistently immunoreactive for cytokeratin (CK) 7 and variably reactive for CK20 and CDX2.

DIFFERENTIAL DIAGNOSIS

One particularly difficult challenge is distinguishing invasive carcinoma from carcinoma in situ colonizing Rokitansky-Aschoff sinuses or metaplastic pyloric glands. In general, nonrounded, irregularly placed gland contours, single cells, and the presence of desmoplasia favor invasive carcinoma (Fig. 16-15). Most typical invasive gallbladder carcinomas are not diagnostically challenging.

Several variants may pose greater problems. Clear cell carcinomas of the gallbladder may be confused with renal cell carcinoma. Unlike renal cell carcinomas, clear cell carcinomas of the gallbladder are immunoreactive for CK7 and CEA. Small cell carcinoma of the gallbladder is morphologically and immunophenotypically indistinguishable from small cell carcinomas of other primary sites. The identification of an in situ carcinoma component within the gallbladder can establish that the tumor's origin is the gallbladder.

PROGNOSIS AND THERAPY

Gallbladder carcinomas tend to present at an advanced stage; approximately 50% of patients have lymph node metastases at diagnosis. Overall prognosis is poor, with 5% to 10% survival at 5 years. Prognosis is a function of stage; stage 1 gallbladder carcinomas have a better prognosis. Papillary carcinomas may be completely in situ, which

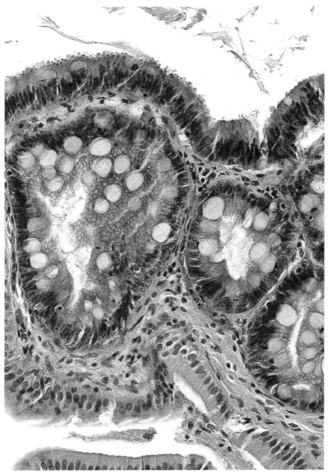

FIGURE 16-13

Low-grade dysplasia of the gallbladder. The dysplastic epithelium's cytology is identical to that of a colonic adenoma and contrasts with that of the normal epithelium at the left and bottom. Note the intestinal metaplasia in the center of the figure.

accounts for their better prognosis. Grading (based on percentage gland formation) and vascular invasion also have prognostic import for low-stage carcinomas. Currently, the only proven effective treatment is operative resection. If possible, complete resection should be performed. Unfortunately, most patients present with advanced, unresectable disease.

OTHER LESIONS OF THE GALLBLADDER

ADENOMA

Unlike the situation in the colon, adenomatous polyps are rare in the gallbladder, found in less than 0.5 % of cholecystectomies and comprising approximately 10 % of polyps. Microscopically, adenomas are well-demarcated polypoid masses that arise in normal mucosa. They can be classified by architecture as tubular or papillary. Tubular adenomas may have pyloric type or intestinal type cytology, whereas papillary adenomas may have intestinal type or biliary type cytology. The nuclei of adenomas are slightly larger and more hyperchromatic than those of the normal mucosa. They are frequently cigar shaped and are basally located. Adenomas do not share molecular alterations with gallbladder carcinomas. Specifically, inactivation of p53 and p16 are uncommon in gallbladder adenomas but found in most gallbladder carcinomas. Recently β-catenin mutations have been found in approximately 60 % of gallbladder adenomas, but in less than 5 % of gallbladder carcinomas, again supporting the view that gallbladder carcinomas do not typically arise from adenomas. Nuclear labeling for β-catenin protein by immunohistochemistry can support the diagnosis of gallbladder adenoma (Fig. 16-16).

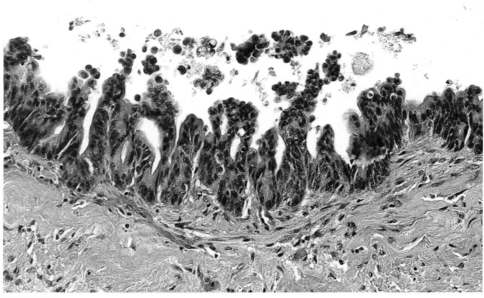

FIGURE 16-14

Carcinoma in situ of the gallbladder. The epithelium here has a micropapillary architecture and features enlarged, markedly hyperchromatic nuclei.

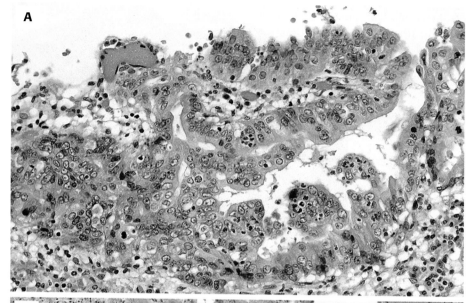

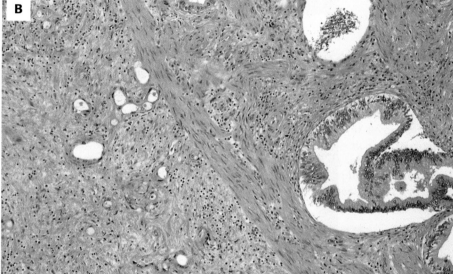

FIGURE 16-15

Invasive adenocarcinoma of the gallbladder arising in the background of extensive carcinoma in situ. **A,** The initial sections of this case revealed extensive flat carcinoma in situ. **B,** Carcinoma in situ colonized intramural Rokitansky-Aschoff sinuses, but worrisome smaller glands in desmoplastic stroma are present in the subserosal fat. **C,** At higher power, the irregular small glands show marked cytologic atypia, confirming the diagnosis of invasive carcinoma.

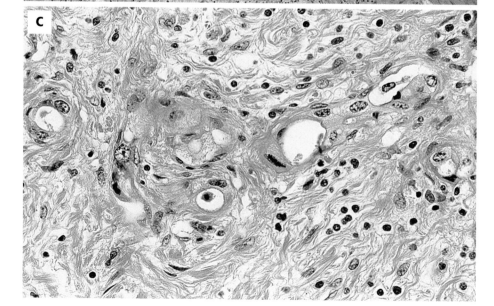

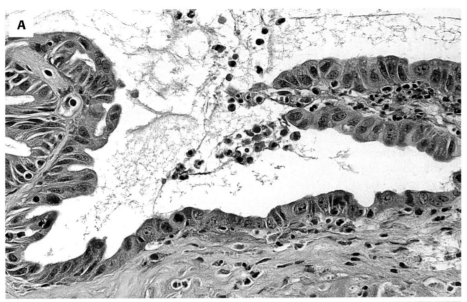

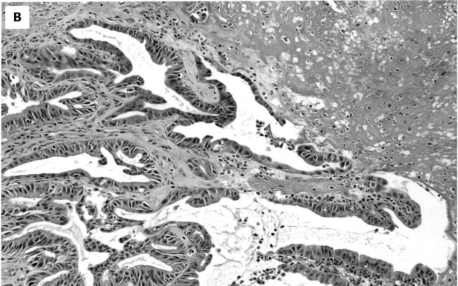

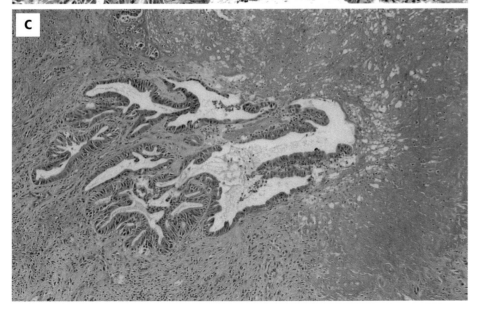

FIGURE 16-18

Ulcerated, reactive bile duct. **A,** Note the disorganized, enlarged epithelial lining cell nuclei, which suggest carcinoma on this frozen section. However, the extensive fibrin deposition and acute inflammation as seen in **B,** consistent with an ulcer, suggest the possibility of a reactive process. **C,** A lower power view of the permanent section reveals the lobular nature of the epithelium, also supporting a benign diagnosis.

carcinoma is present elsewhere (e.g., in the pancreas), knowledge of what the primary tumor looks like can be invaluable when evaluating a bile duct margin specimen.

Immunohistochemical stains offer some potential to help here, because p53 should be negative and CEA only apical in reactive processes. However, in an individual case, one should never rely exclusively on the immuno-histochemical results; the hematoxylin and eosin features must dictate the diagnosis.

■ EXTRAHEPATIC BILE DUCT CARCINOMA

CLINICAL FEATURES

There are approximately 2500 new cases of extrahe-patic bile duct carcinoma diagnosed each year in the United States. There is a slight male predominance, and the mean patient age is 68 years. Unlike gallbladder carcinoma, there are no geographic or racial variations, or association with lithiasis. Most patients present with obstructive jaundice.

Risk factors for extrahepatic bile duct carcinomas include PSC (5% to 10% of patients with PSC develop carcinoma, usually at an earlier age than sporadic cases), choledochal cyst (2.5% to 15% of patients with choledochal cysts develop cancer), and infestation with *Clonorchis sinensis* or *Opisthorchis viverrine*.

PATHOLOGIC FEATURES

GROSS FINDINGS

Bile duct carcinomas usually form ill-defined sclerotic masses that may focally show papillary exophytic growth or may concentrically surround and constrict normal bile duct mucosa.

MICROSCOPIC FINDINGS

Histologically, the same range of tumors may involve the bile ducts as affects the gallbladder. Adenocarci-noma is the most common type, typically associated with florid stromal desmoplasia (Fig. 16-19). Papillary carcinomas grow exophytically into the glandular lumen; invasion of the bile duct wall may or may not be present (Fig. 16-20). Other variants include mucinous

---

EXTRAHEPATIC BILE DUCT CARCINOMA—FACT SHEET

Definition

- Carcinoma derived from the epithelial lining of the bile ducts

Incidence and Location

- Rare: less than 0.5% of all cancers in the United States
- 2500 new cases per year in the United States
- Risk factors include PSC, choledochal cyst, and parasitic infestation (*Clonorchis sinensis, Opisthorchis viverrine*)
- Divided into upper third tumors (hepatic ducts and common hepatic duct), middle third tumors (common hepatic duct and proximal common bile duct), and lower third tumors (intrapancreatic or peripancreatic portion of the extrahepatic bile duct)

Morbidity and Mortality

- Highly lethal: overall 5-year survival rate is 5% to 10%

Gender, Race, and Age Distribution

- Slight male predominance (M:F = 1.6:1)
- No racial predilection
- Mostly affects adults (mean age = 70 years)

Clinical Features

- Usual presentation is obstructive jaundice

Prognosis and Therapy

- Generally poor
- Rare low-stage tumors have better prognosis
- Among low-stage tumors, vascular invasion and grade may have significance
- Distal bile duct tumors have slightly better prognosis (more commonly resectable)
- Surgical resection is the most effective treatment

EXTRAHEPATIC BILE DUCT CARCINOMA—PATHOLOGIC FEATURES

Gross Findings

- Firm infiltrative or polypoid mass
- May form a subtle thickening

Microscopic Findings

- Usual adenocarcinoma is a gland-forming tumor with abundant desmoplastic stroma.
- Cells classically have cuboidal shape and show marked cytologic atypia given degree of gland formation.
- Up to 75% of invasive carcinomas are associated with carcinoma in situ
- Variants include papillary, small cell (high-grade neuroendocrine), adenosquamous, and undifferentiated

Genetics

- Complex genetic alterations
- *Tp16* and *Tp53* are often inactivated.
- *K-RAS* mutations are common.

Immunohistochemistry

- Strongly cytokeratin positive (AE1/3, Cam5.2)
- Usually CK7 positive; CK20 variable
- CEA positive

Differential Diagnosis

- Reactive atypia due to a bile duct stent, stricture, PSC
- Biliary papillomatosis

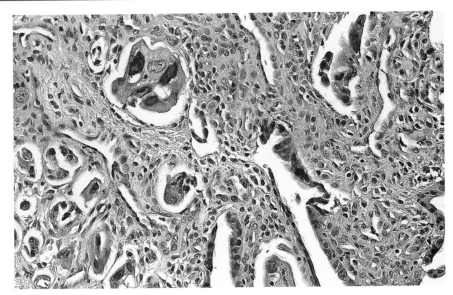

FIGURE 16-19

Invasive adenocarcinoma of the distal bile duct. In this poorly differentiated carcinoma, there are single tumor cells that feature marked cytologic atypia. Compare with the adjacent benign biliary surface epithelium.

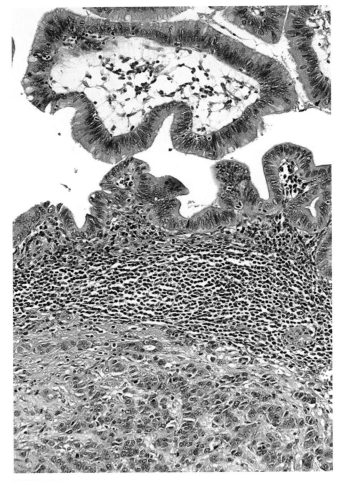

FIGURE 16-20

In situ papillary and invasive adenocarcinoma of the bile duct. The exophytic papillary component projects into the lumen, while the invasive carcinoma forms cords within the underlying stroma.

(colloid) carcinoma, clear cell adenocarcinoma, adenosquamous carcinoma, undifferentiated carcinoma, and small cell neuroendocrine (oat cell) carcinoma.

A subset of thoroughly sampled bile duct carcinomas is associated with dysplasia; many think that dysplasia is the major precursor of bile duct carcinoma but is often overrun by the invasive component. Dysplasias are generally graded as low or high depending on the degree of nuclear atypia and loss of polarity, using similar criteria to those employed in the gallbladder. A three-tiered classification system analogous to that used in the pancreas has been proposed. In this system, the three categories corresponding to increasing cytologic atypia are BilIN-1, BilIN-2, and BilIN-3.

DIFFERENTIAL DIAGNOSIS

Intramural Beale ducts are lobular aggregates of mucous glands that lie within the wall of the bile duct (Fig. 16-21). These can be distinguished from well-differentiated bile duct adenocarcinoma by their lobular architecture, lack of severe cytologic atypia, and lack of perineural invasion.

It is often extremely difficult to distinguish reactive atypia of inflamed biliary epithelium, including that of the intramural Beale ducts, from biliary carcinoma. This is particularly problematic in the setting of a bile duct stent, or in the setting of severe chronic inflammation such as PSC. Perineural invasion, along with severe cytologic atypia and loss of lobular architecture, helps in the differential diagnosis of invasive carcinoma from reactive glandular proliferations (Fig. 16-22). Reactive atypia due to stents tends to be maximal toward the

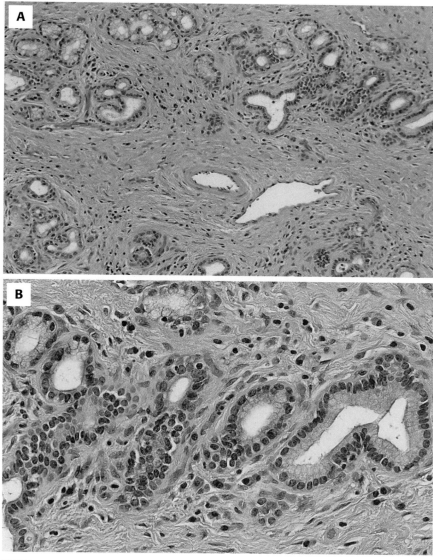

FIGURE 16-21

Benign Beale ducts. **A,** At low power, these benign intramural glands within the bile duct have a lobular architecture. **B,** At higher power, the glands have uniform nuclei and lack cytologic atypia.

lumen of the bile duct, typically in areas of stent-induced ulceration, and diminishes in severity as one moves away from the ulcer (Fig. 16-23).

PROGNOSIS AND THERAPY

Extrahepatic bile duct carcinomas are generally divided by location into upper third tumors (involving the hepatic ducts and common hepatic duct), middle third tumors (involving the common hepatic and proximal common bile duct), and lower third tumors (involving the intra- or peripancreatic portion of the distal common bile duct). Surgical therapy depends on the tumor's location; proximal tumors are treated by bile duct resection and partial hepatectomy, middle third (Klatskin) tumors by bile duct resection, and distal tumors by Whipple resection (pancreatoduodenectomy). Proximal tumors are the most common of the three, comprising more than 50% of cases. A minority of carcinomas involve the extrahepatic biliary tree and gallbladder diffusely, such that the epicenter cannot be determined. Overall, the prognosis is poor; the

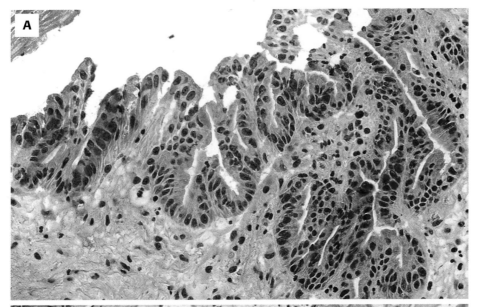

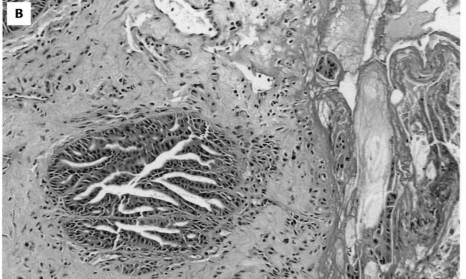

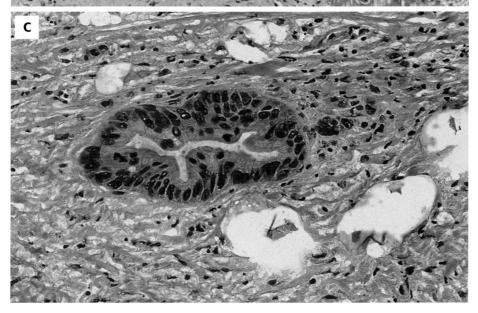

FIGURE 16-22

Stented bile duct. **A,** High-power view of the frozen section slide shows cytologic atypia at the luminal surface. **B,** Lower-power view shows the noninfiltrative nature of the epithelium and its closeness to an ulcer. **C,** The invasive pancreatic adenocarcinoma in this case showed marked nuclear hyperchromasia and irregular contours and was both grossly and microscopically separated from the bile duct.

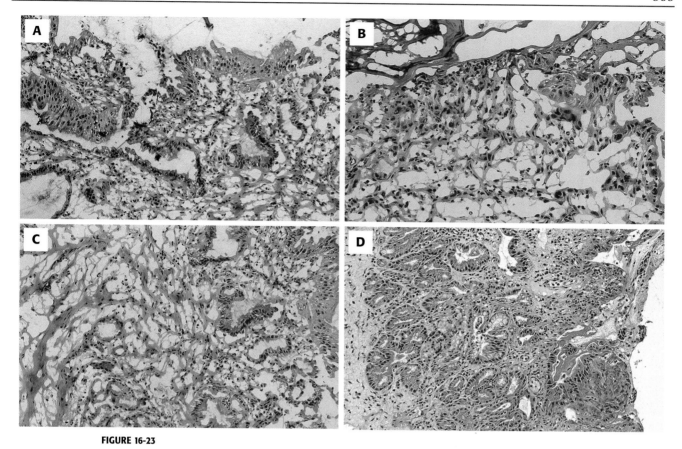

FIGURE 16-23

Stented bile duct. **A,** The frozen section of the bile duct margin shows marked atypia. **B,** Adjacent ulceration and atypical surface epithelium.
C, Lower power view of the frozen section shows that the atypia diminishes with increasing distance from the surface ulceration at the right
(maturation). **D,** Permanent section of this area shows the lobular nature of the benign epithelium.

5-year survival rate is around 10%. The prognosis for bile duct carcinomas is again a function of stage, which is related to pattern. Papillary carcinomas may be all in situ, so they have a better prognosis. Grade and vascular invasion are significant in low-stage tumors. Location is also significant: distal tumors have a better prognosis than more proximal ones, probably because they are more likely to be resectable.

■ OTHER LESIONS OF EXTRAHEPATIC BILE DUCTS

Choledochal (bile duct) cysts may be found at any age, although they are most commonly discovered in the first decade of life. They occur most frequently in Japanese females and may arise anywhere along the bile ducts. Five types are distinguished based on their anatomic location, with intraduodenal examples referred to as choledochoceles. In contrast to hepatobiliary cystadenomas, which are multilocular, choledochal cysts are unilocular dilatations of the bile ducts and microscopically are characterized by a fibrous wall with inflammation. One is more likely to see biliary epithelium in choledochal cysts arising in infants and young children; in adults, inflammation often results in complete epithelial denudation. Over 80% of choledochal cysts are associated with AJPBD outside of the sphincter of Oddi. It is thought that reflux of bile and pancreatic juice into the bile duct causes injury, leading to abnormal cystic dilatation. Hence, many choledochal cysts are not true primary congenital lesions but instead arise secondary to another structural abnormality.

Granular cell tumor of the bile ducts also causes bile duct strictures that mimic malignancy clinically and histologically can mimic carcinoma due to secondary mucosal hyperplasia. These tend to affect young females (90%), and 65% of patients are African American. All reported cases have had a benign outcome. Microscopically, these are characterized by polygonal cells with fine granular pink cytoplasm and uniform nuclei. Cytoplasmic granularity (which represents lysosomes) can be accentuated on PAS/diastase stains, while tumor cells label intensely for S-100 protein.

Hepatobiliary cystadenomas of the extrahepatic bile ducts may be viewed as the biliary analogy to mucinous cystic neoplasms of the pancreas. They are often multiloculated and occur in middle-aged females. Microscopically, they are characterized by three layers: an inner cuboidal biliary or gastric foveolar-type epithelial layer; a middle, more cellular, ovarian-like stroma that labels immunohistochemically for estrogen and progesterone receptors; and an outer, dense hyaline connective tissue (Fig. 16-24). Only rarely does dysplasia or carcinoma develop within these tumors; most are benign.

Carcinoid tumors are low-grade malignancies. Their morphology in the bile duct is entirely similar to that seen in their pulmonary and intestinal counterparts. They likely arise out of a background of intestinal metaplasia because the normal bile ducts lack endocrine cells. Histologically, these tumors demonstrate a nested growth pattern and are composed of polygonal cells with round nuclei and evenly dispersed chromatin (Fig. 16-25). The differential diagnosis includes benign diffuse islet cell proliferations, which may be present in pancreatic tissue showing chronic pancreatitis that is adjacent to the distal common bile duct; one must be sure that the lesion is outside of the pancreas before diagnosing a bile duct carcinoid.

Biliary papillomatosis of the extrahepatic and intrahepatic bile ducts may be viewed as analogous to intraductal papillary mucinous neoplasms (IPMNs) of the pancreas. Biliary papillomatosis is characterized by diffuse papillary mucinous epithelial proliferations that project into the lumen of the bile duct (Fig. 16-26). Like IPMNs, these lesions in the bile ducts demonstrate a range of cytologic atypia ranging from that of adenoma to carcinoma in situ to invasive carcinoma. However, regardless of their histology, the prognosis is poor: lesions are extensive and difficult to excise and hence frequently recur and progress. Hepatic failure may result from extensive occlusion of the biliary system (Table 16-2).

Botryoid embryonal rhabdomyosarcoma (ERMS) is the most common biliary tract tumor of childhood. Botryoid ERMS characteristically forms polypoid, grapelike masses that project into and obstruct the lumen of the bile ducts. Botryoid ERMS can be a particularly difficult diagnosis to make on a small biopsy, because hypocellular areas can be mistaken for choledochal cyst wall. The key finding is to look closely for a cambium layer, a subepithelial condensation of primitive rhabdomyoblasts that demonstrate a high nuclear-to-cytoplasmic ratio and mitotic activity (Fig. 16-27). Immunohistochemical labeling for myogenin and desmin are useful in establishing the diagnosis in limited biopsy samples.

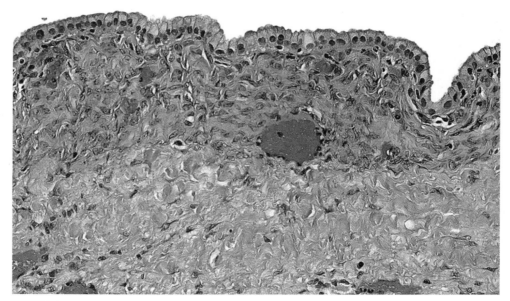

FIGURE 16-24

Hepatobiliary cystadenoma. Note the characteristic trilayered architecture: biliary-type lining, cellular stroma resembling that of the ovary, and underlying hyaline collagen.

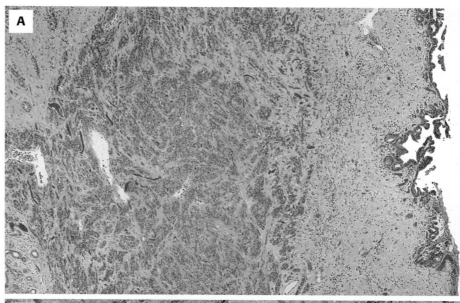

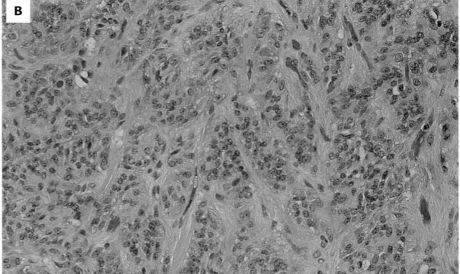

FIGURE 16-25

Bile duct carcinoid. **A,** Low-power view shows the trabecular pattern of the tumor cells within the bile duct wall. **B,** At high power, the tumor cells have uniform round nuclei. **C,** An immunohistochemical stain for chromogranin is diffusely positive, supporting the diagnosis.

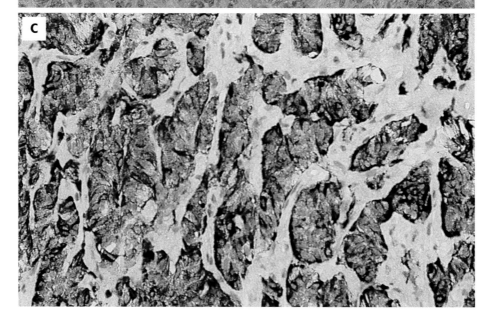

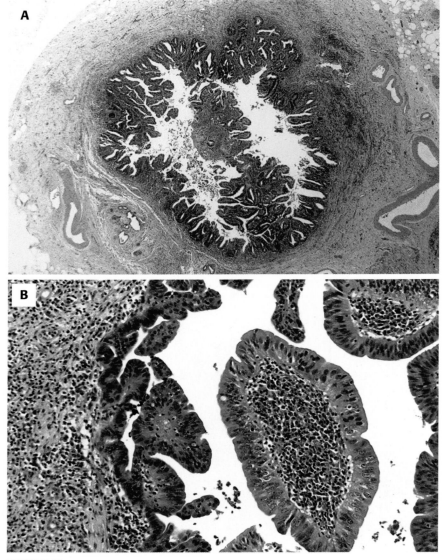

FIGURE 16-26

Biliary papillomatosis. **A,** At low power, this papillary process encircles the bile duct. Grossly, this process involved the bile duct diffusely. **B,** At higher power, the papillary epithelium features nuclear hyperchromasia and stratification consistent with carcinoma in situ.

TABLE 16-2
Biliary Neoplasms and Their Pancreatic Analogues

Histologic Features	Biliary Neoplasm	Pancreatic Neoplasm
Discrete cystic neoplasm that affects predominantly females, with ovarian-type stroma and mucinous epithelium with variable cytologic atypia	Hepatobiliary cystadenoma ± dysplasia	Mucinous cystic neoplasm
Diffuse papillary mucinous epithelial proliferation of variable cytologic atypia	Biliary papillomatosis	Intraductal papillary mucinous neoplasm

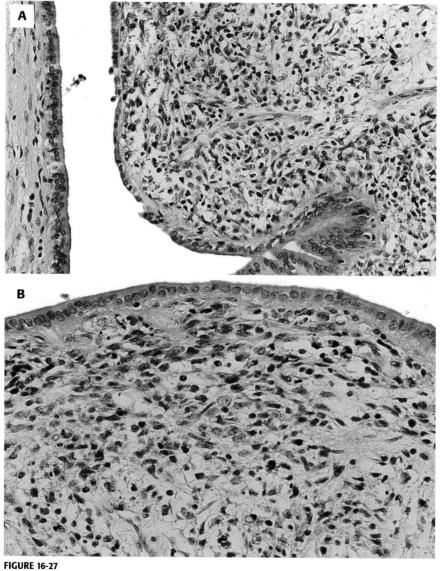

FIGURE 16-27

Botryoid embryonal rhabdomyosarcoma of the bile duct. **A,** At low power, the hypocellular stroma in the segment of bile duct to the right contrasts to the hypercellular stroma to the left. **B,** At higher power, the primitive nature of the spindled cellular stromal tumor cells is evident.

17

Non-Neoplastic and Neoplastic Pathology of the Pancreas

■ **Ralph H. Hruban, MD** ■ **Syed Z. Ali, MD**

■ NON-NEOPLASTIC DISEASES

DEVELOPMENTAL ANOMALIES

The three most commonly encountered developmental anomalies of the pancreas in routine surgical pathology practice are pancreatic divisum, annular pancreas, and ectopic pancreas.

PANCREATIC DIVISUM

CLINICAL FEATURES

Pancreatic divisum occurs in 3% to 7% of the population and is the result of failure of the duct systems of the embryonic dorsal and ventral pancreatic buds to properly fuse. As a result, the ducts produced by the two pancreatic buds remain separate. The duct of Santorini becomes the major ductal system of the pancreas, and it drains into the duodenum through the diminutive minor papilla. It is believed that the small size of the minor papilla relative to the substantial flow of pancreatic secretions passing through it impedes the flow of pancreatic secretions and, in some patients, produces pancreatitis.

RADIOLOGIC FEATURES

Endoscopic retrograde cholangiopancreatography can be used to demonstrate the abnormal ductal anatomy and to exclude other causes of the patient's symptoms.

PATHOLOGIC FEATURES

Pancreatic divisum can best be appreciated through careful gross dissection of the duct system. A probe placed in the minor papilla will pass into a pancreatic duct that drains the full length of the gland. By contrast, a probe placed into the major papilla, that is, the papilla that also drains the bile duct, will enter a short duct only 1 to 2 cm in length. Pancreatic divisum is often associated with chronic pancreatitis; the microscopic appearance of this pancreatitis is etiologically nonspecific.

ANCILLARY STUDIES

As discussed earlier, careful gross dissection of the pancreatic duct system is the best way to establish the diagnosis of pancreatic divisum in a surgically resected specimen. Imaging of a resected pancreas following the injection of a radiopaque dye into the duct system can also be used to establish the diagnosis.

DIFFERENTIAL DIAGNOSIS

The differential diagnosis includes other causes of pancreatitis (see section on Pancreatitis).

PROGNOSIS AND THERAPY

Sphincterotomy of the minor papilla has been used to treat some patients with mixed results. Some patients with longstanding pancreatic divisum develop chronic pancreatitis, and their prognosis will be determined by the severity of their pancreatitis.

ANNULAR PANCREAS

CLINICAL FEATURES

Annular pancreas is a rare malformation in which the dorsal and ventral buds of the pancreas abnormally fuse, forming a ring of pancreatic parenchyma around the

PANCREATIC DIVISUM—FACT SHEET

Definition

- A developmental anomaly characterized by an embryologic failure of the duct systems of the dorsal and ventral pancreatic buds to fuse

Incidence and Location

- Relatively common, 3% to 5% of the general population

Gender, Race, and Age Distribution

- No gender predilection, both genders equally involved
- Present at birth, but there is a wide range of age at clinical presentation from less than a year to 90 years; mean age 57 years

Clinical Features

- Mostly asymptomatic, incidental finding
- Pancreatitis

Radiologic Features

- Abnormal ductal anatomy

Prognosis and Therapy

- Sphincterotomy of the minor papilla with mixed results
- Patients may develop chronic pancreatitis.

ANNULAR PANCREAS—FACT SHEET

Definition

- A developmental anomaly of the pancreas resulting from abnormal fusion of dorsal and ventral pancreatic buds and the formation of a ring of pancreatic tissue around the duodenum, which may result in intestinal obstruction

Incidence and Location

- Rare

Gender, Race, and Age Distribution

- Younger age, mostly around 1 year

Clinical Features

- Vomiting after meals
- Abdominal distention

Radiologic Features

- "Double-bubble" sign of duodenal obstruction

Prognosis and Therapy

- Surgical resection
- Excellent prognosis

PANCREATIC DIVISUM—PATHOLOGIC FEATURES

Gross Findings

- The pancreatic duct that opens at the minor papilla drains the bulk of the gland
- The duct that drains at the major papilla goes only a short distance

Microscopic Findings

- Nonspecific, may show acute and chronic pancreatitis

Ultrastructural Findings

- Not applicable

Fine Needle Aspiration Biopsy Findings

- Not applicable

Immunohistochemistry

- Not applicable

Differential Diagnosis

- Other lesions associated with pancreatitis (see section on Pancreatitis)

ANNULAR PANCREAS—PATHOLOGIC FEATURES

Gross Findings

- A bandlike ring of pancreatic parenchyma encircling the duodenum

Microscopic Findings

- Nonspecific

Ultrastructural Findings

- Not applicable

Fine Needle Aspiration Biopsy Findings

- Not applicable

Immunohistochemistry

- Not applicable

Differential Diagnosis

- Pyloric stenosis
- Ectopic pancreas
- Duodenal atresia

distention. Abdominal radiographs sometimes reveal a classic "double-bubble" sign of intestinal obstruction.

PATHOLOGIC FEATURES

The pathology of annular pancreas is straightforward. A bandlike ring of otherwise normal pancreatic parenchyma encircles the duodenum.

duodenum. This ring can cause duodenal obstruction later in life. Most patients present clinically at a young age (about 1 year), but some patients do not develop symptoms until adulthood. Children with annular pancreas can present with vomiting after meals and even abdominal

ANCILLARY STUDIES

A careful gross dissection of resected specimens is the best way to establish the diagnosis. Clinical correlation with preoperative imaging studies and the finding at surgery are usually necessary to establish the diagnosis.

DIFFERENTIAL DIAGNOSIS

The differential diagnosis would include other causes of obstruction such as pyloric stenosis, ectopic pancreas, and duodenal atresia.

PROGNOSIS AND THERAPY

Surgery resection of the obstruction is the treatment of choice. The prognosis following successful surgery is excellent.

ECTOPIC PANCREAS

CLINICAL FEATURES

Pancreatic parenchyma located outside of the normal pancreas is referred to as ectopic pancreas. Ectopic pancreas is found in 2% of the population. Although ectopic pancreas is usually an incidental finding, it can cause bleeding, and in rare instances, intestinal obstruction.

RADIOLOGIC FEATURES

Ectopic pancreas only rarely forms a mass large enough to be detected radiographically.

PATHOLOGIC FEATURES

The duodenum is the most common location of ectopic pancreas. Other sites include the jejunum, Meckel's diverticulum, and the ileum. By light microscopy, these foci are composed of collections of normal acini and ducts and frequently islets of Langerhans.

ANCILLARY STUDIES

Ancillary studies are not necessary to establish the diagnosis.

DIFFERENTIAL DIAGNOSIS

A metastasis from a pancreatic primary tops the list for the differential diagnosis of ectopic pancreas. The absence of nuclear atypia and a mixed cell phenotype (acini, ducts, and islets) establish the diagnosis of ectopic pancreas.

PROGNOSIS AND THERAPY

Surgical resection is the treatment of choice and is usually curative.

ACUTE PANCREATITIS

CLINICAL FEATURES

Acute pancreatitis is a reversible inflammatory injury to the pancreas. It strikes approximately 20 per 100,000 population each year in Western nations. Most cases are caused by alcoholism or biliary tract disease. Patients present with epigastric pain that radiates to the back, and the diagnosis can be confirmed by demonstrating elevated serum amylase levels.

ECTOPIC PANCREAS—FACT SHEET

Definition
- A developmental anomaly characterized by pancreatic parenchyma located outside of the normal anatomic location

Incidence and Location
- 2% of the population

Clinical Features
- Usually incidental
- May cause bleeding
- May cause intestinal obstruction

Radiologic Features
- Mass lesion (rare)

Prognosis and Therapy
- Surgical resection
- Excellent prognosis

ECTOPIC PANCREAS—PATHOLOGIC FEATURES

Gross Findings
- Abnormal mass in the duodenum, jejunum, Meckel's diverticulum, or ileum

Microscopic Findings
- Collections of normal acini, ducts, and often islets of Langerhans

Ultrastructural Findings
- Not applicable

Fine Needle Aspiration Biopsy Findings
- Nonspecific

Immunohistochemistry
- Not applicable

Differential Diagnosis
- Metastases from a pancreatic primary tumor

ACUTE PANCREATITIS—FACT SHEET

Definition
- A reversible inflammatory process of the pancreas

Incidence and Location
- 20 per 100,000 people each year in Western nations

Gender, Race, and Age Distribution
- Male-to-female ratio, 2.5:1
- Mean age 52.5 years (range 9 to 100 years)

Clinical Features
- Epigastric pain that often radiates to the back
- Elevated serum amylase

Radiologic Features
- Diffuse pancreatic enlargement

Prognosis and Therapy
- Supportive care
- Prognosis varies, worse in older patients

ACUTE PANCREATITIS—PATHOLOGIC FEATURES

Gross Findings
- Enlarged and soft pancreas
- Chalky white foci of fat necrosis
- Hemorrhage in more severe cases

Microscopic Findings
- Edema
- Acute inflammation
- Fat necrosis

Ultrastructural Findings
- Not needed

Fine Needle Aspiration Biopsy Findings
- Not needed

Immunohistochemistry
- Not needed

Differential Diagnosis
- Chronic pancreatitis

RADIOLOGIC FEATURES

Ultrasonography and computed tomography (CT) reveal diffuse enlargement of the gland.

PATHOLOGIC FEATURES

The pancreas is usually enlarged and soft, and the pancreatic and peripancreatic fat contains chalky white foci of fat necrosis. In severe cases, there can be hemorrhage into the gland. Microscopic findings range from mild edema with scattered inflammatory cells, to extensive necrosis and hemorrhage (Fig. 17-1).

ANCILLARY STUDIES

Elevated serum amylase levels support the diagnosis.

DIFFERENTIAL DIAGNOSIS

The differential diagnosis for acute pancreatitis is narrow and includes chronic pancreatitis. Reversibility of the injury to the pancreas distinguishes acute pancreatitis from chronic pancreatitis. In chronic pancreatitis the injured pancreatic parenchyma has been replaced by scar tissue and therefore cannot resume normal function after the inflammatory process abates.

PROGNOSIS AND THERAPY

Ranson and colleagues have developed a list of clinical and laboratory factors that can be used to predict the prognosis of patients with pancreatitis. Adverse prognostic features include older age, elevated white blood cell count, and hyperglycemia. The treatment of acute pancreatitis primarily consists of "resting" the pancreas and supportive care.

CHRONIC PANCREATITIS

Chronic pancreatitis is defined as inflammatory injury to the pancreas associated with irreversible loss of exocrine or endocrine function. Most cases in the United States are caused by chronic alcohol abuse.

CLINICAL FEATURES

Patients present with exocrine and endocrine insufficiency, including diabetes mellitus and malabsorption with steatorrhea and weight loss.

RADIOLOGIC FEATURES

Calcifications within the pancreas can be visualized on plain abdominal radiographs. Ultrasonography demonstrates ductal dilatation; CT shows an atrophic pancreas with calcifications and small cysts.

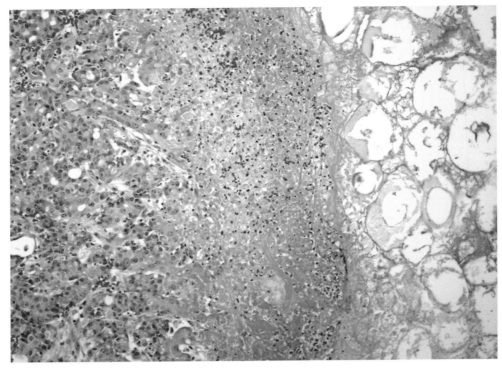

FIGURE 17-1
Acute pancreatitis with associated fat necrosis (H&E).

CHRONIC PANCREATITIS—FACT SHEET

Definition
- An inflammatory process of the pancreas characterized by an irreversible loss of exocrine and endocrine function

Incidence and Location
- Not uncommon, 4 to 6 per 100,000 population

Gender, Race, and Age Distribution
- Males > females
- Alcoholism is the most common cause in the United States

Clinical Features
- Diabetes mellitus
- Malabsorption with steatorrhea
- Weight loss

Radiologic Features
- Calcifications within the pancreas
- Ductal dilatation
- Small cysts

Prognosis and Therapy
- Mostly supportive with exocrine enzyme replacement and management of diabetes
- Steroid therapy (for lymphoplasmacytic sclerosing subtype)
- Poor long-term prognosis

CHRONIC PANCREATITIS—PATHOLOGIC FEATURES

Gross Findings
- Firm, often atrophic gland
- Calcifications
- Ductal dilatation

Microscopic Findings
- Inflammatory cell infiltrate (predominantly chronic inflammation)
- Fibrosis
- Loss of acinar tissue
- Relative sparing of the islets of Langerhans

Ultrastructural Findings
- Not needed

Fine Needle Aspiration Biopsy Findings
- Paucicellularity, mixed inflammatory cells with predominance of lymphocytes and plasma cells
- Degenerated cellular debris
- Fibroblastic cells, epithelial cells with reactive atypia

Genetics
- Can be caused by germline mutations in the cationic trypsinogen gene (PRSS1)

Immunohistochemistry
- Not needed

Differential Diagnosis
- Well-differentiated infiltrating ductal adenocarcinoma

PATHOLOGIC FEATURES

Chronic pancreatitis is characterized by an inflammatory cell infiltrate associated with replacement of the normal pancreatic parenchyma with fibrous connective tissue (Fig. 17-2). This loss of acinar tissue can be associated with dilation of the pancreatic ducts. The islets of Langerhans are relatively spared, but in severe cases there is also a substantial loss of endocrine cells. The inflammatory cell infiltrate is usually composed of a mixture of lymphocytes, plasma cells, and scattered neutrophils.

ANCILLARY STUDIES

Fine-needle aspiration (FNA) reveals paucicellular smears with mixed inflammatory cells showing a predominance of lymphocytes and plasma cells. Background may depict degenerated cellular debris and occasional discohesive fibroblastic mesenchymal cells and naked fusiform nuclei. Rarely, partially intact islets of Langerhans may be noticed. Epithelial fragments are scanty and may disclose a range of reactive cellular changes (Fig. 17-3). Quite often, the cytopathologic diagnosis in chronic pancreatitis is descriptive and not definitive on FNA.

DIFFERENTIAL DIAGNOSIS

The atrophic glands of chronic pancreatitis can mimic a well-differentiated infiltrating adenocarcinoma. Features that favor a reactive process over a neoplastic process include retention of the normal branching growth pattern of the ducts, glands with complete lumina, the absence of luminal necrosis, and only mild nuclear pleomorphism (the cross-sectional areas of the nuclei in a single gland vary by < 4:1). If present, perineural and vascular invasion would obviously strongly support the diagnosis of a carcinoma.

PROGNOSIS AND THERAPY

The prognosis for patients with chronic pancreatitis is surprisingly poor. Mortality rates of 50% at 20 years have been reported. Treatment is mostly supportive, with pancreatic exocrine enzyme replacement and careful management of diabetes. As noted below, some patients with lymphoplasmacytic sclerosing chronic pancreatitis respond to steroid therapy.

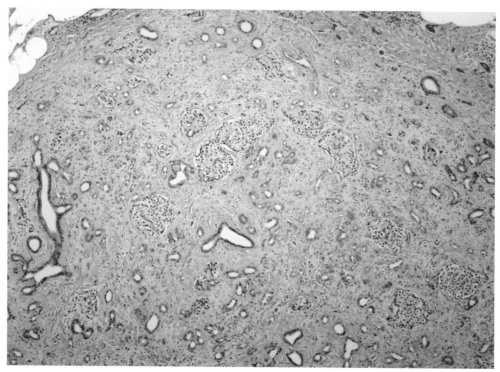

FIGURE 17-2

Chronic pancreatitis. Fibrosis, loss of exocrine parenchyma, and a relative enlargement of residual islets of Langerhans are seen (H&E).

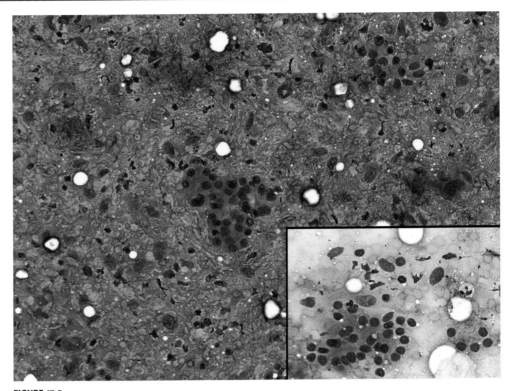

FIGURE 17-3

Chronic pancreatitis, fine-needle aspiration. Fragments of reactive ductal epithelium in a background of chronic inflammatory and fibroblastic cells. Inset shows bare spindle-shaped nuclei of fibroblasts (Diff Quik).

LYMPHOPLASMACYTIC SCLEROSING PANCREATITIS

CLINICAL FEATURES

Lymphoplasmacytic sclerosing pancreatitis, also known as autoimmune pancreatitis, is a distinctive form of pancreatitis characterized by a mixed inflammatory cell infiltrate, composed of lymphocytes and plasma cells, centered around and within the epithelium of the pancreatic ducts. A venulitis is also often present. The disease strikes men more often than women, with a male-to-female ratio of approximately 8:3. The mean age at diagnosis is 57 years, and patients typically do not have conventional risk factors for pancreatitis such as alcoholism. Some patients have other autoimmune diseases such as Sjögren's syndrome and inflammatory bowel disease.

RADIOLOGIC FEATURES

The typical finding on CT is an ill-defined mass lesion with diffuse enlargement of the gland.

PATHOLOGIC FEATURES

Three features characterize lymphoplasmacytic sclerosing pancreatitis. First, the inflammatory cell infiltrate is mixed, with lymphocytes, plasma cells, and a few polymorphonuclear leukocytes. Second, the inflammatory cell infiltrate is centered on the pancreatic ducts (Fig. 17-4). This is often best appreciated at low power. Third, there is a venulitis (see Fig. 17-4B). This venulitis is often best appreciated at the interface between diseased and normal tissues. In some, but not all, cases small aggregates of neutrophils, called granulocytic epithelial lesions (GELs), collect within the ductal epithelium. Immunolabeling for IgG4 will reveal increased numbers of IgG4 expressing plasma cells in most cases.

ANCILLARY STUDIES

Serum IgG4 levels are elevated in most patients, and this finding can be used to support a preoperative diagnosis.

DIFFERENTIAL DIAGNOSIS

The differential diagnosis includes other forms of pancreatitis.

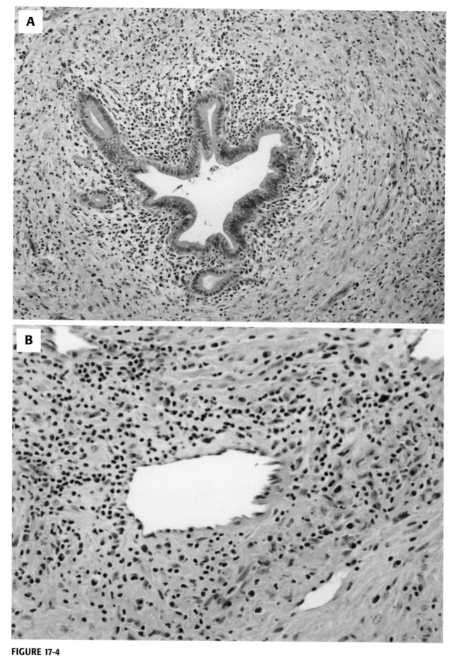

FIGURE 17-4

Lymphoplasmacytic sclerosing chronic pancreatitis. Characterized by a mixed inflammatory cell infiltrate centered around the pancreatic ducts **(A)** and a venulitis **(B)** (H&E).

LYMPHOPLASMACYTIC SCLEROSING PANCREATITIS—FACT SHEET

Definition
- A form of chronic pancreatitis characterized by a mixed inflammatory cell infiltrate centered on the pancreatic ducts, and venulitis.

Incidence and Location
- Rare, but being recognized with increasing frequency

Gender, Race, and Age Distribution
- Unlike most autoimmune diseases, lymphoplasmacytic sclerosing pancreatitis is more common in men than it is in women.
- Most patients are between the ages of 40 and 60

Clinical Features
- Can mimic pancreatic cancer with abdominal pain, weight loss, and jaundice
- Some have other autoimmune disorders such as inflammatory bowel disease and sclerosing cholangitis
- Elevated serum IgG4 levels

Radiologic Features
- Diffuse or focal enlargement of the pancreas

Prognosis and Therapy
- Although many patients respond to steroid therapy, many also undergo surgery because the disease so closely mimics pancreatic cancer
- The prognosis is excellent, but patients should be monitored for other autoimmune diseases

---

LYMPHOPLASMACYTIC SCLEROSING PANCREATITIS—PATHOLOGIC FEATURES

Gross Findings
- Diffuse or segmental enlargement of the pancreas

Microscopic Findings
- Mixed inflammatory infiltrate composed of lymphocytes, plasma cells, and eosinophils
- Inflammation centered on the pancreatic ducts and ductules
- Venulitis
- Intraepithelial collections of polymorphonuclear leukocytes (GELs) in some cases

Ultrastructural Findings
- Not applicable

Fine Needle Aspiration Biopsy Findings
- Nonspecific with a mixed inflammatory cell infiltrate

Immunohistochemistry
- Increased numbers of IgG4 expressing plasma cells

Differential Diagnosis
- Other forms of chronic pancreatitis

PROGNOSIS AND THERAPY

This form of pancreatitis is important to recognize because it can clinically mimic pancreatic cancer and because it may respond to steroid therapy.

PARADUODENAL WALL CYST

CLINICAL FEATURES

Paraduodenal wall cyst is a non-neoplastic cyst with an associated inflammatory reaction occurring in the "groove" region—the region demarcated by the superior aspect of the pancreas, the common bile duct and the minor papilla. It is thought that the cysts are caused by a small calculus obstructing a small duct associated with the minor papilla. Most patients are young males with a history of alcohol abuse.

RADIOLOGIC FEATURES

Computed tomography scanning usually reveals a thickened duodenum associated with cyst formation in the duodenal wall or subjacent pancreas.

PATHOLOGIC FEATURES

Paraduodenal wall cysts, in addition to arising in a very specific region, have a characteristic microscopic appearance. The cysts, which may contain inspissated secretions, are lined by partially denuded ductal epithelium. Often there is an associated reactive spindle cell proliferation.

ANCILLARY STUDIES

A careful gross dissection documenting the distinctive location of the lesion is critical to establishing the correct diagnosis.

DIFFERENTIAL DIAGNOSIS

The differential diagnosis includes cystic neoplasms of the pancreas (see later), as well as mesenchymal neoplasms. The characteristic location of the lesion and the presence of a partially denuded but otherwise unremarkable epithelium lining the cyst both help establish the diagnosis.

PARADUODENAL WALL CYST—FACT SHEET

Definition

- Non-neoplastic inflammatory cystic dilatation of small ducts in the "groove region"—the area demarcated by the superior aspect of the pancreatic head, the common bile duct, and the duodenum

Incidence and Location

- Rare
- By definition, located in the "groove" region

Gender, Race, and Age Distribution

- Strong male predominance
- Most patients are in their 50s

Clinical Features

- A history of alcohol abuse is common
- Common symptoms include abdominal pain and weight loss

Radiologic Features

- May produce a solid or a cystic mass lesion in the head of the pancreas/duodenum

Prognosis and Therapy

- Prognosis is excellent because these are non-neoplastic lesions

PARADUODENAL WALL CYST—PATHOLOGIC FEATURES

Gross Findings

- Cyst or a solid mass lesion located in the groove region of the pancreas

Microscopic Findings

- Cyst lined by partially denuded ductal epithelium
- Associated inflammatory cell infiltrate
- A prominent reactive spindle cell proliferation is present in some cases

Ultrastructural Findings

- Not applicable

Fine Needle Aspiration Biopsy Findings

- Not well defined

Immunohistochemistry

- Not applicable

Differential Diagnosis

- Cystic neoplasms of the pancreas
- Spindle cell neoplasms

PROGNOSIS AND THERAPY

These are entirely benign lesions.

PSEUDOCYSTS

CLINICAL FEATURES

Pseudocysts are localized collections of necrotic material rich in pancreatic enzymes. Pseudocysts lack an epithelial lining and are often extrapancreatic. Pseudocysts account for 75% of all "pancreatic" cysts. Pseudocysts usually develop after an episode of acute pancreatitis or following trauma to the pancreas. Patients often have a severe epigastric pain that radiates to the back. In the United States most patients have a history of heavy alcohol consumption.

RADIOLOGIC FEATURES

Abdominal imaging will reveal a unilocular cystic mass.

PATHOLOGIC FEATURES

Pseudocysts are usually solitary, usually extrapancreatic, and typically filled with necrotic/hemorrhagic material. Pseudocysts do not have an epithelial lining. Instead, pseudocysts are lined by granulation tissue, fibrous connective tissue, or simply by necrotic debris (Fig. 17-5).

ANCILLARY STUDIES

Two aspects of the FNA biopsy can be highly informative. First, a morphologic analysis of the cellular component can help determine if the cyst has an epithelial lining. Second, the aspirated fluid can be analyzed biochemically to determine if the cyst contents contain high concentrations of pancreatic enzymes. Aspirates of pseudocysts show abundant thin and watery, turbid fluid, which may appear hemorrhagic. The cytomorphology is often nonspecific and consists mostly of degenerated cellular debris, fibroblastic cells, macrophages, and lymphomononuclear cells (Fig. 17-6). Aspirates typically lack an epithelial component. Reactive/reparative changes in the mesenchymal cells and macrophages may raise suspicion for a neoplastic cyst. The fluid aspirated from pseudocysts is rich in lipase and amylase and has low carcinoembryonic antigen (CEA) levels. By contrast, most neoplastic cysts have low to normal amylase levels, and some have elevated CEA levels. In one study, the diagnosis of neoplastic cysts based on a CEA level greater than 10 ng/mL had a sensitivity of 100% and a specificity of 81%.

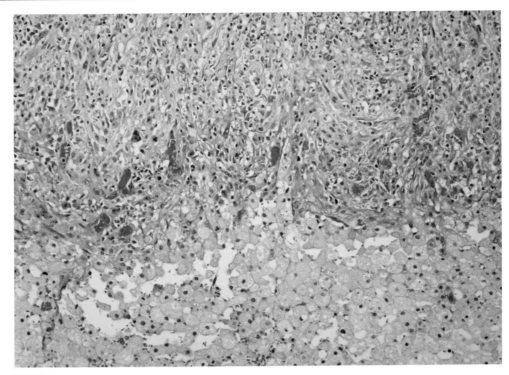

FIGURE 17-5

Pseudocysts contain necrotic material rich in pancreatic exocrine enzymes. They lack an epithelial lining and instead are usually lined by granulation or fibrous tissue (H&E).

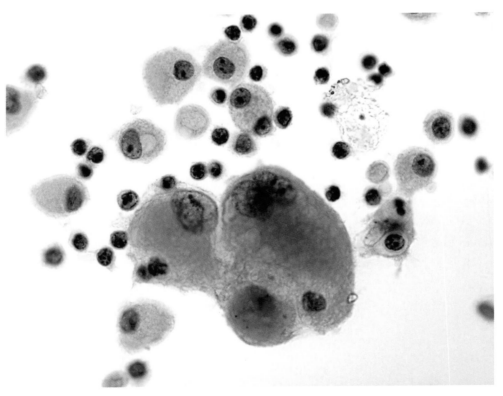

FIGURE 17-6

Pancreatic pseudocyst, fine-needle aspiration. Collection of numerous histiocytes and lymphocytes. A few large pleomorphic histiocytes with vacuolated cytoplasm are also noted. Epithelial cells are absent, and the background is clear and not mucinous (Papanicolaou).

PSEUDOCYSTS—FACT SHEET

Definition
- A localized collection of necrotic material rich in pancreatic enzymes and lacking an epithelial lining

Incidence and Location
- 75% of all pancreatic cysts
- Often extrapancreatic

Gender, Race, and Age Distribution
- Older males, especially alcoholics

Clinical Features
- Severe epigastric pain often radiating to the back

Radiologic Features
- Unilocular cystic mass

Prognosis and Therapy
- Supportive care
- Surgical drainage
- Excellent prognosis

PSEUDOCYSTS—PATHOLOGIC FEATURES

Gross Findings
- Solitary cysts, intrapancreatic or extrapancreatic
- Necrotic/hemorrhagic contents

Microscopic Findings
- Cyst without lining epithelium
- Wall composed of granulation tissue or fibrous connective tissue

Ultrastructural Findings
- Not needed

Fine Needle Aspiration Biopsy Findings
- Nonspecific findings, degenerated cystic debris, lymphomononuclear cells, and histiocytes
- Macrophages and fibroblastic cells may mimic cellular atypia
- Lack of epithelial component
- Aspirated fluid with a low CEA level and high in lipase and amylase

Immunohistochemistry
- Not applicable

Differential Diagnosis
- Retention cysts
- Serous cystadenoma
- Mucinous cystic neoplasms
- Intraductal pancreatic mucinous neoplasms
- Solid-pseudopapillary neoplasm
- Cystically degenerated carcinoma

DIFFERENTIAL DIAGNOSIS

The differential diagnosis of pancreatic cysts includes retention cysts, serous cystadenoma, mucinous cystic neoplasms, intraductal papillary mucinous neoplasms (IPMNs), the solid-pseudopapillary neoplasm, and cystic change in a usually solid pancreatic neoplasm. The absence of an epithelial lining combined with necrotic/hemorrhagic cyst contents rich in lipase and amylase establish the diagnosis of a pseudocyst.

PROGNOSIS AND THERAPY

Most pseudocysts resolve with supportive care, although some require surgical drainage. Superinfection of a pseudocyst is a serious complication.

■ EXOCRINE NEOPLASMS

SOLID NEOPLASMS

Solid neoplasms of the pancreas showing predominantly exocrine differentiation include infiltrating ductal adenocarcinoma and its variants, pancreatoblastoma, and acinar cell carcinoma.

INFILTRATING DUCTAL ADENOCARCINOMA

CLINICAL FEATURES

Infiltrating ductal adenocarcinoma ("pancreatic cancer") is a malignant invasive gland forming epithelial neoplasm. A number of variants have been described, including adenosquamous carcinoma, hepatoid carcinoma, mucinous noncystic adenocarcinoma (colloid carcinoma), signet ring cell carcinoma, undifferentiated (anaplastic) carcinoma, and undifferentiated carcinoma with osteoclast-like giant cells. Infiltrating ductal adenocarcinoma is a disease of the elderly, with most patients being older than the age of 60 years. The disease strikes men slightly more frequently than it does women, and in the United States, African Americans more than whites. Common presenting signs and symptoms include painless jaundice, unexplained weight loss, and epigastric pain radiating to the back. New-onset diabetes mellitus may be the first manifestation of the disease.

RADIOLOGIC FEATURES

CT is one of the best modalities to image the pancreas. Infiltrating ductal adenocarcinomas typically produce a hypodense mass lesion that distorts the normal architecture of the gland. The pancreatic duct is often dilated secondary to duct obstruction by the cancer.

INFILTRATING DUCTAL ADENOCARCINOMA—FACT SHEET

Definition
- A malignant invasive epithelial neoplasm with ductal differentiation

Incidence and Location
- 85% to 90% of all pancreatic neoplasms
- Pancreatic head (> 60%)

Gender, Race, and Age Distribution
- More often in men (M:F ratio, 2:1)
- Increased risk with smoking, family history of pancreatic cancer
- Older age group, usually older than 60 years

Clinical Features
- Epigastric pain, often radiating to the back
- Weight loss
- Painless jaundice
- Less often, migratory thrombophlebitis, pancreatitis, new-onset diabetes mellitus

Radiologic Features
- Poorly defined infiltrative nonenhancing pancreatic mass

Prognosis and Therapy
- Surgical resection
- Palliative bypass procedures
- Radiation and chemotherapy
- Prognosis extremely poor (slightly better for mucinous noncystic adenocarcinoma)
- 5-year survival: <2%

PATHOLOGIC FEATURES

Infiltrating ductal adenocarcinomas grossly form poorly defined, firm, white-yellow masses (Fig. 17-7). Most arise in the head of the pancreas, but they can also involve the body, tail, or even the entire gland. Focal cystic degeneration and areas of necrosis are not uncommon. As noted radiologically, the pancreatic duct is often dilated upstream of the cancer. Microscopically, varying degrees of differentiation can be seen, but all infiltrating ductal adenocarcinomas, by definition, show both epithelial and glandular differentiation (Fig. 17-8). Well-differentiated adenocarcinoma is characterized by clearly formed neoplastic glands arranged in a haphazard pattern of growth. This haphazard growth pattern, more than any other feature, helps distinguish well-differentiated adenocarcinomas from non-neoplastic reactive glands. Moderately differentiated adenocarcinomas show the same haphazard growth pattern but, in addition, are characterized by greater architectural and cytologic atypia. The neoplastic cells may form incomplete glands, cribriform structures, or papillae without fibrovascular cores. Significant nuclear pleomorphism can be appreciated, and the nuclei in a single gland

INFILTRATING DUCTAL ADENOCARCINOMA—PATHOLOGIC FEATURES

Gross Findings
- Poorly defined, firm mass with irregular boarders
- Cut surface: yellow-white microcystic areas, hemorrhage, and necrosis

Microscopic Findings
- Neoplastic glands in haphazard arrangement
- Architectural atypia with incomplete glands, luminal necrosis
- Cytologic atypia with nuclei in a single gland varying by more than 4:1
- Vascular and perineural invasion
- Glands adjacent to muscular vessels
- Mitoses and necrosis
- Solid sheets or single infiltrating cells (poorly differentiated tumors)
- Glandular and squamous differentiation (adenosquamous carcinoma)
- Hepatocellular differentiation (hepatoid carcinoma)
- Mucin-producing cells floating in pools of mucin (mucinous noncystic carcinoma)
- Individual cells with eccentric mucin vacuoles (signet ring cell carcinoma)
- Undifferentiated spindle cell component (undifferentiated/anaplastic carcinoma)
- Endocrine differentiation (mixed ductal-endocrine carcinoma)

Ultrastructural Findings
- Ductal epithelial differentiation with microvilli on the luminal surface, cell-cell junctions, and cytoplasmic mucin granules

Fine Needle Aspiration Biopsy Findings
- Hypercellularity, fragments and single neoplastic cells with ductal features, relative paucity, or total lack of acinar epithelium
- Nuclear enlargement, nuclear overlap, hyperchromasia, and irregular nuclear contours
- Pleomorphism, lack of polarity, and haphazard arrangement; "drunken honey comb" arrangement
- Bizarre neoplastic cells, multinucleation, squamoid change, mitosis, and necrosis
- Mucinous change with cytoplasmic vacuolization

Genetics
- Mutation of the KRAS oncogene
- Somatic mutations of multiple tumor suppressor genes, particularly TP53, SMAD4/DPC4, and p16/CDKN2A
- Overexpression of growth factors (epidermal growth factor, transforming growth factor α, and others)
- Familial clustering of pancreatic cancer has been observed
- Germline mutations in the STK11, BRCA2, PALB2, p16/CDKN2A, and PRSS1 genes predispose to pancreatic cancer

Immunohistochemistry
- Positive for CK7, CK8, CK18, and CK19
- Positive for CEA, CA19-9, Dupan-2, MUC1, MUC4, and MUC5AC
- Most positive for mesothelin, claudin 18, prostate stem cell antigen, and fascin
- Loss of Smad4 protein expression (55%)
- Endocrine markers (such as chromogranin) positive in mixed ductal-endocrine neoplasms

Differential Diagnosis
- Chronic pancreatitis
- Ampullary carcinoma
- Other primary and metastatic pancreatic neoplasms

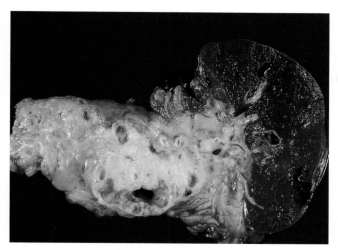

FIGURE 17-7

Infiltrating adenocarcinoma of the pancreas. An irregular firm white mass is present in the tail of the pancreas. Tongues extend out to encase arteries and toward the spleen. Note the small retention cysts formed as the tumor obstructs the pancreatic duct. The spleen is present on the right.

often vary in size by more than 4 to 1. Nucleoli may be present and may be prominent. Mitoses, including abnormal mitoses, can be seen. Poorly differentiated adenocarcinoma, as the name implies, is an infiltrating cancer in which it can be difficult to recognize the direction of differentiation of the neoplastic cells. Individual cells, cells forming solid sheets, poorly formed glands, and even single infiltrating neoplastic cells are seen. Significant pleomorphism with bizarre mitotic figures is common. Perineural and vascular invasion, when present, can help establish the diagnosis.

Several variants of ductal adenocarcinoma are worth discussing. The *adenosquamous carcinoma* is characterized by the presence of both glandular and squamous differentiation. Adenosquamous carcinomas have a particularly poor prognosis. *Hepatoid carcinoma*, as the name suggests, has prominent liver differentiation. Metastasis from a liver primary should be ruled out clinically before making this diagnosis. The *mucinous noncystic adenocarcinoma* is also known as the colloid carcinoma and is characterized by relatively well-differentiated neoplastic mucin-producing epithelial cells "floating" in large pools of extracellular mucin (Fig. 17-9). This variant is also fully malignant but may have a slightly better prognosis than infiltrating ductal adenocarcinoma. Mucinous noncystic adenocarcinoma almost always arises in association with an intraductal papillary mucinous neoplasm (IPMN). The *Signet ring cell carcinoma* is composed of noncohesive individual neoplastic cells with abundant cytoplasmic mucin that indents the nuclei pushing them toward the periphery. Metastases from a breast or gastric primary should be considered before making this diagnosis. The *undifferentiated (anaplastic) carcinoma*, as the name suggests, is an extremely aggressive neoplasm composed of highly atypical cells, with significant pleomorphism and frequent, often bizarre, mitoses. These carcinomas can have a significant spindle cell component, or they can be composed of large polygonal cells. Finally, mixed carcinomas, such as the *mixed ductal-endocrine carcinoma*, have—in addition to an infiltrating ductal adenocarcinoma—significant components with other directions of differentiation. The mixed nature of these neoplasms can usually be demonstrated with immunolabeling.

ANCILLARY STUDIES

Immunohistochemical labeling can be used to highlight epithelial and glandular differentiation of ductal adenocarcinomas, as well as to demonstrate some of the molecular alterations present in the neoplastic cells. Immunolabeling for cytokeratin (CK) 7, CK8, CK18, and CK19 is positive, as is immunolabeling for CEA, CA19-9, Dupan-2, MUC1, MUC4, and MUC5AC. The vast majority of adenocarcinomas of the pancreas also label for mesothelin, claudin 18, and fascin. Immunolabeling for the Dpc4 protein shows a complete loss of expression of Dpc4 in 55 % of the cases (see Fig. 17-8B). Mucinous noncystic adenocarcinomas label for MUC2, the squamous component of adenosquamous carcinomas with antibodies to p63, and mixed ductal-endocrine carcinoma has a significant component that strongly expresses chromogranin.

FNA is considered highly sensitive and specific for the diagnosis of ductal adenocarcinoma. Smears are usually hypercellular. Helpful cytomorphologic features are large flat sheets with subtle to prominent loss of nuclear polarity ("drunken honey comb appearance"), less often discohesive single cells, nuclear enlargement, nuclear crowding and overlap, convoluted nuclear contours ("Idaho potato" shapes), and irregular chromatin distribution. Neoplastic cells most often lack prominent nucleoli, particularly in well to moderately differentiated carcinoma, and the nuclei may appear hypochromatic. Necrosis and mitoses are often seen. Most aspirates are composed predominantly of ductal-type epithelium. Acinar epithelium and islets of Langerhans are usually not seen. Well-differentiated carcinomas may show predominantly cohesive epithelial fragments of varying sizes, minimal pleomorphism. They often lack the single neoplastic cell component (Fig. 17-10). Poorly differentiated ductal adenocarcinoma, on the other hand, is composed of predominantly discohesive pleomorphic cells. Macronucleoli may be observed (Fig. 17-11). Bizarre cells, often with multinucleation, can be seen. Squamous differentiation is not uncommon and may take the form of cells with thick opaque cytoplasm, hyperchromatic nuclei, and irregular cell shapes, often with keratinization. Mucin vacuoles may be observed and impart a clear vacuolated appearance to the cells.

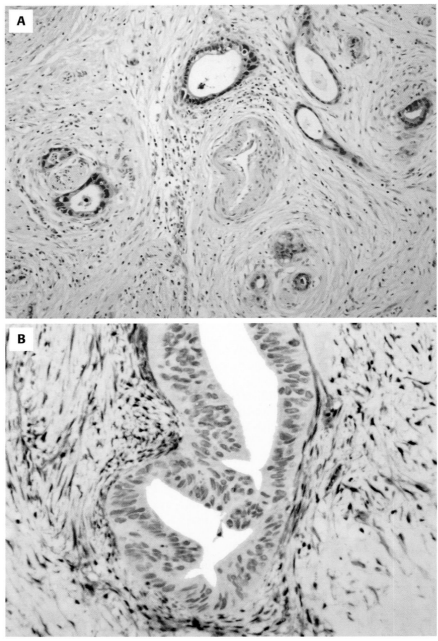

FIGURE 17-8

Infiltrating adenocarcinoma of the pancreas. **A,** Note the haphazard arrangement of glands (H&E). **B,** Immunolabeling for the SMAD4/DPC4 gene product will reveal a loss of labeling in approximately 55% of pancreatic cancer cases.

DIFFERENTIAL DIAGNOSIS

Reactive non-neoplastic glands of chronic pancreatitis top the differential diagnosis. Features useful in establishing a diagnosis of infiltrating adenocarcinomas in histologic sections are (1) haphazard pattern of growth; (2) variation in the size of nuclei by more than 4:1 in a single gland; (3) incomplete lumen formation; (4) glands adjacent to muscular vessels; (5) perineural or vascular invasion; (6) mitoses, especially abnormal mitoses; and (7) glandular luminal necrotic debris.

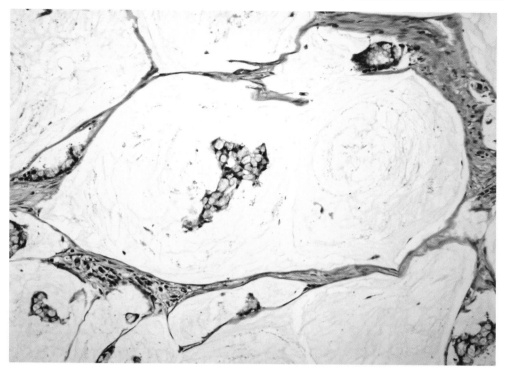

FIGURE 17-9

Infiltrating colloid adenocarcinoma. Characterized by neoplastic epithelial cells floating in pools of extracellular mucin (H&E).

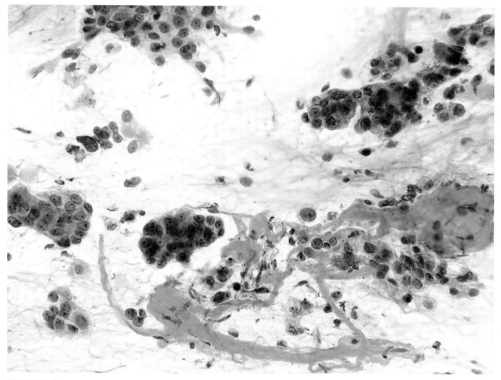

FIGURE 17-10

Well- to moderately differentiated ductal adenocarcinoma, fine-needle aspiration. Note multiple tissue fragments, as well as single discohesive pleomorphic neoplastic cells. Also noted are fragments of fibrous tissue and background mucin (Papanicolaou).

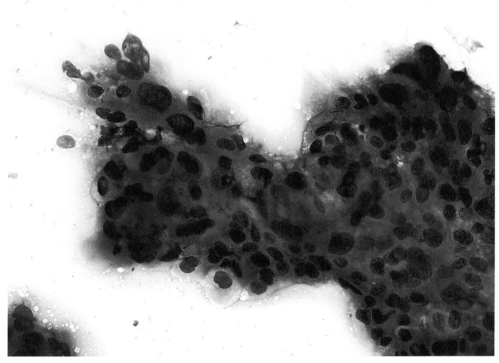

FIGURE 17-11

Poorly differentiated ductal adenocarcinoma, fine-needle aspiration. Tumor fragment composed of haphazardly placed pleomorphic tumor cells. Note the prominent anisonucleosis, occasional macronucleoli, and a total lack of glandular differentiation (Papanicolaou).

PROGNOSIS AND THERAPY

The prognosis of patients with an infiltrating adenocarcinoma of the pancreas is extremely poor. Most patients die of their disease, often within months of diagnosis. Even though surgery is the treatment of choice, most patients (about 80%) have metastatic disease at diagnosis and therefore are not candidates for surgery. Radiation and chemotherapy have a small impact on survival. The mucinous noncystic adenocarcinoma has been associated with a slightly better prognosis, whereas the adenosquamous and anaplastic variants have a worse prognosis.

UNDIFFERENTIATED CARCINOMA WITH OSTEOCLAST-LIKE GIANT CELLS

CLINICAL FEATURES

Undifferentiated carcinoma with osteoclast-like giant cells (UCOGC) is a variant of infiltrating ductal carcinoma that is worth discussing in greater detail because of the striking and unique histologic features of this neoplasm. The UCOGC is a malignant epithelial neoplasm of the pancreas characterized by a prominent component of reactive osteoclast-like giant cells.

RADIOLOGIC FEATURES

UCOGC neoplasms often attain a large size and frequently show central necrosis or hemorrhage.

PATHOLOGIC FEATURES

These neoplasms are often large, grossly hemorrhagic, and extensively necrotic. Several components can be appreciated microscopically. An in situ or invasive adenocarcinoma is frequently present. In addition, mononuclear cells, some with significant cytologic atypia, admixed with large multinucleated osteoclast-like giant cells can be appreciated (Fig. 17-12). The nuclei of the osteoclast-like giant cells are uniform. Some of the osteoclast-like giant cells are actively phagocytic.

ANCILLARY STUDIES

Molecular analyses have shown that the osteoclast-like giant cells are non-neoplastic reactive cells, whereas the atypical mononuclear cells are neoplastic and probably derived from an epithelial precursor. These distinctive neoplasms are therefore best regarded as undifferentiated carcinomas with reactive osteoclast-like giant cells, rather than true giant cell neoplasms. Immunohistochemical

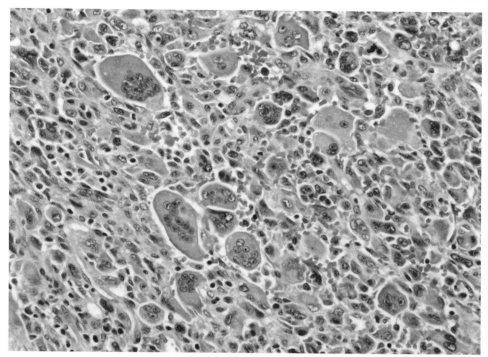

FIGURE 17-12
Undifferentiated carcinomas with osteoclast-like giant cells. They are composed of atypical mononuclear cells admixed with multinucleated giant cells. The nuclei in the giant cells are uniform (H&E).

UNDIFFERENTIATED CARCINOMA WITH OSTEOCLAST-LIKE GIANT CELLS—FACT SHEET

Definition
- A variant of infiltrating ductal carcinoma with a prominent component of reactive osteoclast-like giant cells admixed with neoplastic mononuclear cells

Incidence and Location
- Extremely rare
- Head of the pancreas

Gender, Race, and Age Distribution
- Slight female predominance
- Older age group (>60 years)

Clinical Features
- Abdominal mass
- Abdominal pain, weight loss, and jaundice

Radiologic Features
- Large mass, often with central cystic necrosis and hemorrhage

Prognosis and Therapy
- Surgical resection
- Poor prognosis (<12-month survival)

UNDIFFERENTIATED CARCINOMA WITH OSTEOCLAST-LIKE GIANT CELLS—PATHOLOGIC FEATURES

Gross Findings
- Large mass, lobulated cut surface
- Areas of necrosis or hemorrhage

Microscopic Findings
- Usually three components: in situ or invasive ductal adenocarcinoma, atypical mononuclear cells, and multinucleated osteoclast-like giant cells
- Frequent mitoses, necrosis
- Rarely osteoid formation

Ultrastructural Findings
- Mononuclear cells with epithelial differentiation (desmosomes, microvilli, and zymogen-like granules)

Fine Needle Aspiration Biopsy Findings
- Hypercellularity with discohesive round to spindled cells
- Pleomorphic nuclei, prominent nucleoli
- Second population of osteoclast-like giant cells

Immunohistochemistry
- Mononuclear cells express markers of epithelial differentiation (AE1/AE3, CAM5.2, CEA, EMA) in 50% to 70% of cases
- Vimentin positive
- Osteoclast-like giant cells express CD68, common leukocyte antigen (CD45), and α_1-chymotrypsin

Differential Diagnosis
- Other carcinomas with giant cells
- Anaplastic carcinoma

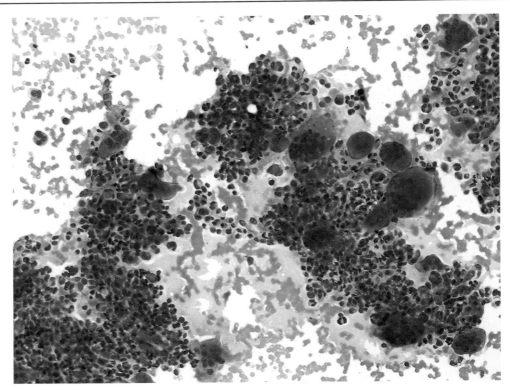

FIGURE 17-13
Undifferentiated carcinoma with osteoclast-like giant cells, fine needle aspiration. Hypercellular smear with loosely cohesive fragments of relatively small and uniform, round to spindly neoplastic cells. Note the highly characteristic multinucleated osteoclast-type giant cells (Diff Quik).

labeling often demonstrates epithelial differentiation by the atypical mononuclear cells. Almost all express vimentin and 50% to 70% express cytokeratin (Cam5.2, or AE1/AE3), CEA, or epithelial membrane antigen (EMA). The osteoclast-like giant cells express CD68 and common leukocyte antigen (CD45).

FNA yields hypercellular smears composed of isolated noncohesive round to spindled cells. These cells have pleomorphic, hyperchromatic nuclei with prominent nucleoli. Scattered among these are a variable number of highly characteristic multinucleated osteoclast-like giant cells (Fig. 17-13).

DIFFERENTIAL DIAGNOSIS

The osteoclast-like giant cells are usually so distinctive as to make diagnosis straightforward. It should be kept in mind, however, that other neoplasms of the pancreas, particularly when necrotic, can be associated with a giant cell reaction.

PROGNOSIS AND THERAPY

These are fully malignant neoplasms with a mean survival of less than 12 months. The treatment is the same as that for infiltrating adenocarcinoma of the pancreas.

PANCREATOBLASTOMA

CLINICAL FEATURES

The pancreatoblastoma is a rare neoplasm, primarily of childhood, characterized by acinar differentiation, endocrine differentiation, and distinctive squamoid nests. Although most occur in the pediatric age group, up to one third occur in adults. Patients present with symptoms related to the mass, and in some children an abdominal mass can be palpated on physical examination. Pancreatoblastomas have been reported in newborn infants with the Beckwith-Wiedemann syndrome and in an adult with familial adenomatous polyposis (FAP).

RADIOLOGIC FEATURES

Pancreatoblastomas produce large masses in the pancreas that can usually be detected on abdominal imaging. The diagnosis can be suggested if the patient is a child, but imaging cannot be used to specifically diagnose a pancreatoblastoma.

PANCREATOBLASTOMA—FACT SHEET

Definition

- A neoplasm with acinar differentiation and distinctive squamoid nests

Incidence and Location

- Extremely rare; <1.0% of all pancreatic tumors
- No predilection for a specific anatomic location

Gender, Race, and Age Distribution

- Male predominance (M:F ratio, 2:1)
- Mostly in children (mean age 4 years), up to one third in adults

Clinical Features

- Abdominal mass
- Pain, weight loss, nausea and vomiting
- Jaundice is uncommon.
- Some have elevated serum α-fetoprotein levels

Radiologic Features

- Large well-demarcated mass, often with displacement of surrounding organs

Prognosis and Therapy

- Surgical resection
- Radiation and chemotherapy
- Generally poor prognosis (45% mortality), prognosis for children better than that for adults

PANCREATOBLASTOMA—PATHOLOGIC FEATURES

Gross Findings

- Large solitary mass, often encapsulated
- Well-circumscribed with a soft fleshy cut surface
- Often lobulated, with areas of hemorrhage and necrosis

Microscopic Findings

- Large nests of uniform neoplastic cells
- Acinar (predominantly) and endocrine differentiation
- Squamoid nests in the center of the epithelial lobules, sometimes with keratinization
- Rarely, glandular or mesenchymal differentiation (chondroid or osteoid)

Ultrastructural Findings

- Zymogen-like granules and microvilli in cells with acinar differentiation
- Scattered cells with electron-dense neuroendocrine-type granules

Fine Needle Aspiration Biopsy Findings

- Oval to cuboidal neoplastic epithelial cells
- Hyperchromatic nuclei, prominent nucleoli, and granular cytoplasm
- Spindled, elongated, and triangular-shaped cells may be present
- Occasionally, smaller high nuclear-to-cytoplasmic ratio cells
- Stromal fragments with fine capillary cores surrounded by neoplastic epithelium

Genetics

- Reported in patients with Beckwith-Wiedemann syndrome and FAP

Immunohistochemistry

- Acinar component positive for cytokeratins, trypsin, chymotrypsin, and lipase
- Endocrine component positive for chromogranin and synaptophysin
- Ductal component reacts with CEA
- Biotin in squamoid nests can produce false positive nuclear labeling
- Positive for α-fetoprotein (one third of cases)

Differential Diagnosis

- Acinar cell carcinoma
- Solid-pseudopapillary neoplasm
- Endocrine neoplasm

PATHOLOGIC FEATURES

Pancreatoblastomas arise in the head and in the body and tail of the pancreas at equal frequencies. They are often large (mean 10.5 cm) and well circumscribed. On cut section they are softer and fleshier than most ductal adenocarcinomas. Microscopically, by definition, pancreatoblastomas show acinar differentiation and squamoid nests (Fig. 17-14). Neoplastic cells with endocrine differentiation are also almost always present, and in some cases cells with glandular and even mesenchymal differentiation can also be seen. The acinar component usually predominates. These cells have a granular cytoplasm, basally oriented nuclei, and are polarized around small lumina. The nuclei of cells with acinar differentiation typically contain single prominent nucleoli. Squamoid nests are, by definition, present in all cases and are usually in the center of epithelial lobules. These nests are composed of whorls of plump spindle-shaped cells. When present, endocrine cells appear as isolated single cells or as small nests or trabeculae of cells. Ductal and mesenchymal components are present in a minority of cases.

ANCILLARY STUDIES

Immunohistochemical labeling can be used to confirm the multiple directions of differentiation present in these neoplasms. The acinar component labels with antibodies to cytokeratin, trypsin, chymotrypsin, and lipase. The endocrine component labels with antibodies to chromogranin and synaptophysin, and, when present, the ductal component labels for CEA. Interestingly,

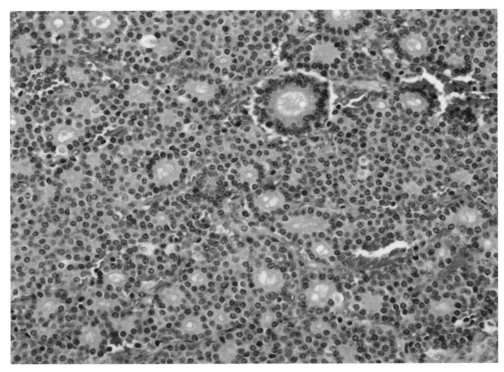

FIGURE 17-15

Acinar cell carcinoma. The neoplastic cells of acinar cell carcinoma form small lumina, have a granular cytoplasm, and often have a single prominent nucleoli (H&E).

contain mostly cohesive fragments forming acini, cellular cords, or solid nests of neoplastic epithelium. Other cell components (i.e., ductal and endocrine cells) are often absent. The latter observation is extremely helpful in well-differentiated carcinomas because the high degree of tumor differentiation makes it hard to distinguish these carcinomas from normal pancreatic acinar epithelium. In acinar cell carcinoma, the neoplastic cells do not show the compact, orderly lobular "bunch of grapes" arrangement of normal epithelium. The cells usually have eccentrically placed nuclei and granular, often basophilic cytoplasm (Fig. 17-16). The neoplastic cells often lose their fragile cytoplasm, resulting in numerous naked nuclei resembling lymphocytes in the smear background. Poorly differentiated acinar cell carcinomas depict significant anisonucleosis with occasional giant naked nuclei, prominent intranuclear inclusions, necrosis, and a characteristic single cell pattern (Fig. 17-17).

DIFFERENTIAL DIAGNOSIS

The differential diagnosis should include the well-differentiated endocrine neoplasm, pancreatoblastoma, and the solid-pseudopapillary neoplasm. Although acinar cell carcinoma can slow focal endocrine differentiation, acinar cell carcinomas can be distinguished from well-differentiated pancreatic endocrine neoplasms by acinar formation, basally oriented nuclei, cytoplasmic granulations, and single prominent nucleoli. A high mitotic rate also favors an acinar cell carcinoma, whereas a hyalinized stroma and a "salt and pepper" chromatin pattern favor a well-differentiated endocrine neoplasm. As discussed earlier, squamoid nests distinguish pancreatoblastomas from acinar cell carcinomas. Finally, solid-pseudopapillary neoplasms should also be considered in the differential diagnosis. The age and gender of the patient can help because solid-pseudopapillary neoplasms almost always arise in young women. Pseudopapillary formation, poor cohesion of the neoplastic cells, and the absence of true lumina also favor solid-pseudopapillary neoplasms. Immunolabeling can establish the diagnosis in difficult cases. Solid-pseudopapillary neoplasms express vimentin, CD10, and α_1-antitrypsin, and they show an abnormal nuclear localization of the β-catenin protein.

PROGNOSIS AND THERAPY

The overall 5-year survival rate for patients with an acinar carcinoma is only 5%. Pediatric patients may have a better prognosis than adults. Surgical resection is the treatment of choice.

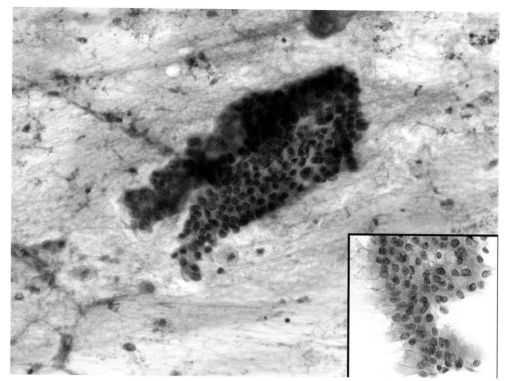

FIGURE 17-22

Mucinous cystic neoplasm, fine needle aspiration. Fragment of "atypical-appearing" ductal epithelium with folded edges in a mucinous background. Follow-up revealed carcinoma arising in a mucinous cystic neoplasm. *Inset* shows the typical mucinous appearance of the monolayered epithelium (Papanicolaou).

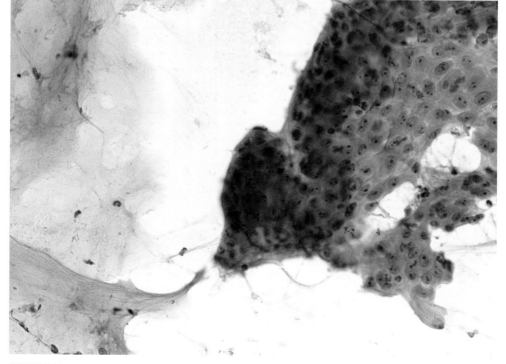

FIGURE 17-23

Invasive carcinoma arising in a mucinous cystic neoplasm, fine needle aspiration. Pleomorphic malignant cells in a large cohesive sheet are seen in a mucinous background. Note macronucleoli and anisonucleosis (Papanicolaou).

associated invasive carcinoma is almost always curative, whereas the prognosis for patients with an associated invasive carcinoma is driven by the depth of invasion of the carcinoma and by stage. Overall, the 5-year survival rate for patients with an invasive adenocarcinoma arising in association with a mucinous cystic neoplasm is about 50%.

INTRADUCTAL PAPILLARY MUCINOUS NEOPLASMS

CLINICAL FEATURES

IPMNs are usually papillary mucin-producing epithelial neoplasms that arise in the larger pancreatic ducts and lack a distinctive ovarian stroma. Patients typically present with a long history of abdominal pain, anorexia, weight loss, and recurrent episodes of pancreatitis. In some instances this history traces back many years, suggesting that these neoplasms can be present for years before they are clinically detected. More and more of these neoplasms are being discovered incidentally in asymptomatic patients imaged for another indication. The mean age at diagnosis is around 65 years, and these neoplasms occur slightly more often in men than in women, with a male-to-female ratio of 60:40.

INTRADUCTAL PAPILLARY MUCINOUS NEOPLASMS—FACT SHEET

Definition
- A mucin-producing epithelial neoplasm arising from major pancreatic ducts, lacking a distinctive ovarian-type stroma

Incidence and Location
- Rare, approximately 1% of exocrine neoplasms
- Head of the pancreas

Gender, Race, and Age Distribution
- More frequent in men (M:F ratio, 6:4)
- Mean age 64 years

Clinical Features
- Long history of abdominal pain and weight loss
- Recurrent episodes of pancreatitis
- Pancreatic insufficiency with diabetes and steatorrhea
- More and more are being discovered incidentally

Radiologic Features
- Markedly distended main pancreatic duct with polypoid intraductal lesions
- Patulous ampulla with mucin extrusion (on endoscopy)

Prognosis and Therapy
- Surgical resection
- 5-year survival rate >90% for noninvasive cases
- Prognosis significantly worse if there is an associated invasive carcinoma

---

RADIOLOGIC FEATURES

CT typically reveals a markedly distended main pancreatic duct, or a collection of cysts with a "bunch of grapes" appearance. The endoscopic finding of mucin extruding from a patulous ampulla of Vater is virtually diagnostic of an IPMN.

PATHOLOGIC FEATURES

IPMNs arise in the head of the gland more often than they do in the tail. IPMNs have a characteristic gross appearance. By definition they involve the larger pancreatic

---

INTRADUCTAL PAPILLARY MUCINOUS NEOPLASMS—PATHOLOGIC FEATURES

Gross Findings
- Dilatation of a pancreatic duct
- Papillary projections into the duct lumen
- Abundant mucin

Microscopic Findings
- Papillae lined by tall columnar mucin-producing cells
- Occasional goblet-type cells
- May have granular eosinophilic/oncocytic cytoplasm
- May have varying degrees of architectural/cytologic atypia (papillae without fibrovascular cores, cribriforming, necrosis, and mitoses)
- May harbor an associated invasive adenocarcinoma (one third of tumors)

Ultrastructural Findings
- Well-developed microvilli on apical cell surfaces
- Abundant cytoplasmic mucin vacuoles

Fine Needle Aspiration Biopsy Findings
- Cellular smears, tissue fragments with monolayered or papillary architecture
- Mucinous background
- Minimal pleomorphism, round nuclei, abundant apically clear cytoplasm
- Few goblet cells
- Epithelial atypia of varying degree, focal or confluent

Genetics
- Only rarely show loss of Dpc4 expression

Immunohistochemistry
- Positive for cytokeratins (CK7, CK8, CK18, and CK19) with variable staining with CK20
- Positive for CEA and EMA
- MUC2+/MUC1− (two thirds of tumors)

Differential Diagnosis
- Mucinous cystic neoplasms
- Retention cysts

ducts. Those that involve the main duct are designated as "main duct" type, and those that involve a side branch of the main duct are called, not too surprisingly, "branch duct" type. Many are mixed. The involved ducts are distended with copious amounts of mucin and usually lined by grossly visible papillae.

Microscopically the neoplastic epithelial cells are tall columnar mucin-producing cells (the gastrointestinal subtype), but cuboidal cells with eosinophilic cytoplasm (the pancreatobiliary subtype) can also be seen (Fig. 17-24). Some IPMNs, particularly the branch-duct type, have gastric-foveolar differentiation. Rarely, the neoplastic cells have a granular eosinophilic cytoplasm, and when this cell type predominates, these neoplasms have been designated the intraductal oncocytic papillary neoplasm (IOPN). Just as noninvasive mucinous cystic neoplasms can be divided into three groups based on the degree of cytologic and architectural atypia present, so too can IPMNs. IPMNs without cytologic or architectural atypia are called "IPMN with low-grade dysplasia." Those with a moderate degree of atypia are designated "IPMN with moderate dysplasia," and those with significant atypia, including papillae without fibrovascular cores, cribriforming, luminal necrosis, nuclear pleomorphism, and frequent mitoses, are designated "IPMN with high-grade dysplasia."

Although the percentages vary in different series, approximately one third of IPMNs have an associated invasive carcinoma. This invasive carcinoma is usually either a colloid (mucinous noncystic) carcinoma or a tubular/ductal carcinoma. When an associated invasive adenocarcinoma is present, it should be separately designated and measured. For example, a diagnosis could read "IPMN with high-grade dysplasia (4 cm) and an associated invasive well-differentiated colloid carcinoma (2 cm)."

ANCILLARY STUDIES

Mucicarmine and PAS stains confirm the presence of substantial quantities of intracellular and extracellular mucin. IPMNs express cytokeratin and label with pancytokeratin antibodies (AE1/AE3), as well as for Cam 5.2, and CK7, CK8, CK18, and CK19. Labeling for CK20 is variable. Most IPMNs also express EMA and CEA. Three patterns of MUC expression have been reported in IPMNs. Intestinal type IPMNs are MUC2+/MUC1−. These IPMNs have tall columnar mucin-containing cells typically forming papillary structures. When these MUC2+/MUC1− intestinal-type IPMNs are associated with an invasive cancer, the invasive cancer tends to be a colloid type of cancer, and colloid carcinomas are also usually MUC2+/MUC1−. Pancreatobiliary IPMNs are MUC2− and MUC1+. When pancreatobiliary type IPMNs are associated with an invasive cancer, the cancer is usually a ductal adenocarcinoma, and these ductal adenocarcinomas are usually MUC1+/MUC2−. Finally, the gastric foveolar type of IPMN is MUC1−/MUC2−.

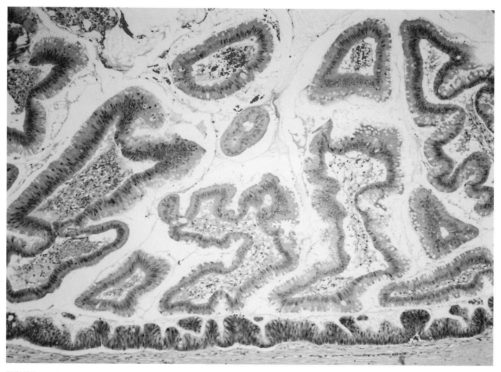

FIGURE 17-24

Intraductal papillary mucinous neoplasm. Intraductal papillary mucinous neoplasms, by definition, involve the pancreatic duct system. Most are composed of papillae lined by tall columnar mucin-producing epithelial cells (H&E).

FNA often produces grossly identifiable mucin with a thick and gelatinous quality when the smears are prepared from the aspirate. Microscopically, glandular fragments of varying size are seen, often in flat mono-layered fashion, as well as discohesive neoplastic cells. Neoplastic cells are minimally pleomorphic with uniform round nuclei and apically clear cytoplasm. Papillary architecture can be focal or extensive (Figs. 17-25 and 17-26). Goblet cells are commonly noted. Varying degrees of epithelial atypia are observed, and it is not uncommon to find overt carcinoma arising in a background of an IPMN.

DIFFERENTIAL DIAGNOSIS

The differential diagnosis for IPMNs parallels that for mucinous cystic neoplasms. The differential diagnosis includes all cystic neoplasms of the pancreas, but in reality, mucinous cystic neoplasms are the lesions most often confused with IPMNs. As noted earlier, mucinous cystic neoplasms usually arise in the body or tail of the gland in women, do not communicate with the larger pancreatic ducts, and by definition mucinous cystic neoplasms have the characteristic ovarian-type stroma. By contrast, IPMNs usually involve the head of the gland, strike men slightly more often than women, connect to the larger pancreatic ducts, and lack a distinctive stroma. The presence of a mucin-producing epithelium can be used to differentiate between mucinous cystic neoplasms and the other cystic neoplasms of the pancreas. Retention cysts should also be considered in the differential diagnosis of an IPMN. Retention cysts are localized dilatations of the pancreatic duct caused by obstruction to the duct. The lumen of retention cysts does not contain the thick tenacious mucin that is characteristic of an IPMN; the epithelium is flattened, not papillary; and, although they can contain small amounts of mucin, the epithelial cells lining retention cysts are often cuboidal with only minimal mucin. Finally, retention cysts are associated with a localized obstruction to the pancreatic duct. Careful examination of the duct system can therefore help establish the underlying etiology of the retention cyst.

PROGNOSIS AND THERAPY

Surgical resection is the treatment of choice for IPMNs. The presence or absence of an associated invasive carcinoma is the most important factor in determining patient prognosis. Surgically resected noninvasive IPMNs have a greater than 90% 5-year survival rate, whereas the 5-year survival rate for patients with an IPMN associated with an invasive carcinoma is 40%. Noninvasive IPMNs can be multifocal, and patients, even those with negative surgical margins, should be followed after surgery for metachronous disease.

FIGURE 17-25

Intraductal pancreatic mucinous neoplasm, fine needle aspiration. A papillary-like fragment of hyperchromatic and crowded columnar cells. Note the elongated palisaded nuclei and apically clear cell cytoplasm better appreciated at the periphery of the tumor fragment (Papanicolaou).

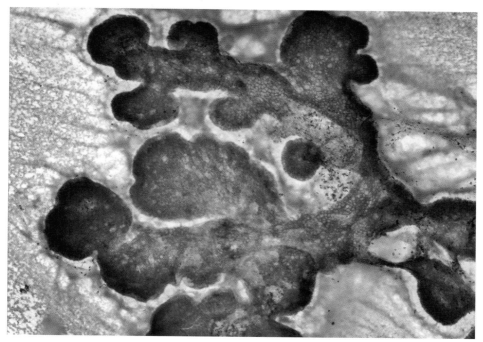

FIGURE 17-26

Intraductal papillary mucinous neoplasm, fine needle aspiration. A well-developed papillary architecture is evident with most of the neoplastic cells containing intracytoplasmic mucin (Diff Quik).

SOLID-PSEUDOPAPILLARY NEOPLASMS

CLINICAL FEATURES

The solid-pseudopapillary neoplasm is a low-grade malignant epithelial neoplasm composed of poorly cohesive cells with uniform nuclei and frequent nuclear grooves. The neoplastic cells surround delicate blood vessels and form solid masses that show cystic degeneration and intracystic hemorrhage. The vast majority of patients are women (female-to-male ratio 20:1), and most are in their 20s or 30s, with a mean age at diagnosis of about 25 years. Most patients present with nonspecific signs and symptoms related to a large intra-abdominal mass, including abdominal pain and early satiety.

RADIOLOGIC FEATURES

Solid-pseudopapillary neoplasms often appear heterogeneous on CT scan and endoscopic ultrasonography. This heterogeneity corresponds to the gross appearance of the neoplasms, which includes solid areas, pseudopapillary areas, and areas of necrosis.

PATHOLOGIC FEATURES

As suggested in the name of this neoplasm, solid-pseudopapillary neoplasms are not uniform neoplasms. Grossly solid areas intimately intermix with hemorrhagic

and necrotic cystic areas. These neoplasms are typically grossly well-demarcated from the adjacent non-neoplastic pancreas. Microscopically, the solid areas of solid-pseudopapillary neoplasms are composed of sheets of relatively uniform cells with eosinophilic slightly granular cytoplasm and uniform nuclei with nuclear grooves (Fig. 17-27A). There is a delicate background vasculature. In the necrotic/cystic areas the neoplastic cells show a loss of cohesion. Only a few remain around the delicate blood vessels. Foam cells, cells with cholesterol crystals, and red blood cells are scattered among the neoplastic cells. Some of the neoplastic cells can have a clear, almost vacuolated cytoplasm. Eosinophilic globules are often present, a feature that is diagnostically very helpful. Mitoses are rare.

ANCILLARY STUDIES

Until recently, immunolabeling has produced mixed results. The vast majority of solid-pseudopapillary neoplasms strongly and diffusely express vimentin, α_1-antitrypsin, neuron-specific enolase (NSE), and progesterone receptors. Immunolabeling for high-molecular-weight cytokeratin (AE1/AE3) and synaptophysin is variable. Recently, however, it has been demonstrated that most solid-pseudopapillary neoplasms express CD10, and that immunolabeling for β-catenin produces an abnormal nuclear labeling in greater than 90% of these neoplasms (see Fig. 17-27B). The combination of immunolabeling for CD and β-catenin is therefore diagnostically very useful. The

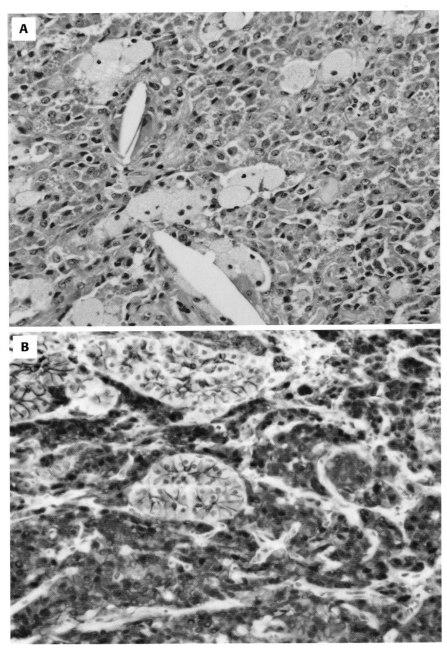

FIGURE 17-27

Solid-pseudopapillary neoplasm. **A,** These are composed of relatively uniform cells with eosinophilic slightly granular cytoplasm and uniform nuclei with nuclear grooves. Foamy macrophages, eosinophilic globules, and cholesterol clefts are often present (H&E). **B,** There is a delicate background vasculature and the neoplastic cells show a loss of cohesion. Immunolabeling will reveal an abnormal nuclear pattern of labeling (*bottom*) compared with the membranous labeling of the normal pancreas (*top*) (immunolabeling for β-catenin).

SOLID-PSEUDOPAPILLARY NEOPLASM—FACT SHEET

Definition

- A low-grade malignant epithelial neoplasm with uniform cells, delicate vessels, and a prominent discohesive pattern of growth

Incidence and Location

- Uncommon, less than 2% of exocrine pancreatic neoplasms
- No specific anatomic predilection

Gender, Race, and Age Distribution

- Predominantly women (M:F ratio, 1:20)
- Mostly in third decade (mean age approximately 25 years)

Clinical Features

- Nonspecific symptoms (abdominal pain and early satiety)
- Often incidental finding

Radiologic Features

- Sharply demarcated heterogeneous-appearing mass (solid and cystic)

Prognosis and Therapy

- Surgical resection
- Excellent prognosis

SOLID-PSEUDOPAPILLARY NEOPLASM—PATHOLOGIC FEATURES

Gross Findings

- Variably solid and cystic mass, often large
- Areas of cystic change with necrosis and hemorrhage
- Well demarcated, rarely invasive
- Variegated cut surface, solid pale brown areas admixed with cystic formations, and zones of hemorrhage and necrosis

Microscopic Findings

- Sheets of uniform cells with eosinophilic cytoplasm
- Uniform nuclei with grooves
- Delicate vasculature
- Cells with clear vacuolated cytoplasm
- Necrosis and cystic change with areas of discohesive cells
- Foam cells, cholesterol crystals
- Eosinophilic globules

Ultrastructural Findings

- Often indented nuclei, abundant mitochondria and zymogen-like granules
- Rarely neurosecretory-type granules

Fine Needle Aspiration Biopsy Findings

- Hypercellular smears, abundant fine branching capillaries surrounded by small uniform tumor cells with "Chinese character-like" appearance
- Prominent nuclear grooves or inclusions
- Globules of metachromatic myxoid material

Genetics

- β-catenin gene mutation

Immunohistochemistry

- Positive for vimentin, α_1-antitrypsin, CD10, NSE, and progesterone receptors
- Variable immuonexpression for cytokeratins (AE1/AE3) and synaptophysin
- Nuclear labeling for β-catenin (>90% of cases)

Differential Diagnosis

- Well-differentiated pancreatic endocrine neoplasms
- Ductal adenocarcinoma
- Pancreatoblastoma

hyaline globules label with antibodies to α_1-antitrypsin. Although the literature is full of discordant labeling patterns, in most cases immunolabeling for chromogranin, insulin, glucagon, somatostatin, amylase, lipase, calretinin, α-inhibin, and estrogen receptors is negative, or at most focally positive.

FNA shows a characteristic cytomorphologic appearance. The aspirates are highly cellular and are composed predominantly of tissue fragments. The neoplastic cells in these fragments are aggregated around fine branching capillary vessels, giving the fragments a "Chinese characters" appearance (Fig. 17-28). Cells are small and monomorphic with round to oval nuclei, inconspicuous nucleoli, occasional nuclear grooves, and intranuclear inclusions. Metachromatic globules are often present. Foam cells can be seen in the smears background.

DIFFERENTIAL DIAGNOSIS

The well-differentiated pancreatic endocrine neoplasm leads the list of entities to consider in the differential diagnosis for the solid-pseudopapillary neoplasm. This differential diagnosis can be particularly problematic because some well-differentiated endocrine neoplasms show cystic degeneration. Features supporting the diagnosis of a solid-pseudopapillary neoplasm include nuclear grooves, foamy macrophages, and eosinophilic globules. Immunolabeling also helps distinguish between these two neoplasms. Well-differentiated pancreatic endocrine neoplasms are strongly and diffusely positive for chromogranin and synaptophysin, whereas solid-pseudopapillary neoplasms express CD10 and show an abnormal nuclear localization of the β-catenin protein.

PROGNOSIS AND THERAPY

Surgical resection is the treatment of choice for solid-pseudopapillary neoplasms, and in most cases surgical resection is curative. A few metastasizing solid-pseudopapillary neoplasms have been reported. Remarkably, long-term survival has been reported after the surgical resection of liver metastases.

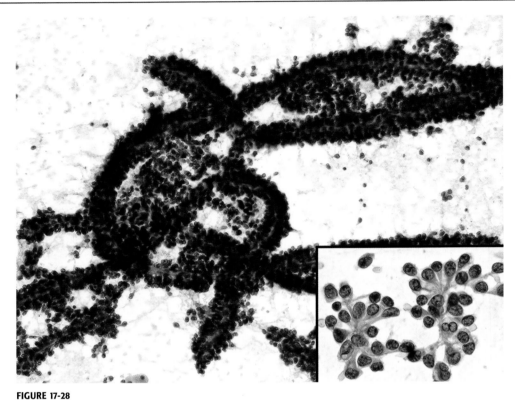

FIGURE 17-28
Solid-pseudopapillary neoplasm, fine needle aspiration. Note the characteristic branching "Chinese character-like" tumor morphology. *Inset* shows small, monomorphic cells with round nuclei and fragile wispy cytoplasm (Papanicolaou).

■ ENDOCRINE NEOPLASMS

Pancreatic endocrine neoplasms (PENs) account for only 1% of all primary pancreatic neoplasms. Undifferentiated small cell carcinomas of the pancreas are extremely rare. Most PENs are well differentiated. The well-differentiated PENs can be broadly grouped into those neoplasms associated with a clinical syndrome caused by excess hormone production by the neoplasm (the syndromic PENs) and those without such an association (the nonsyndromic PENs).

SYNDROMIC ENDOCRINE NEOPLASMS

CLINICAL FEATURES

As noted earlier, syndromic PENs are, by definition, associated with a clinical syndrome caused by the excessive release of hormones by the neoplasm. The clinical syndrome produced depends on the hormone produced. Approximately 40% of all syndromic PENs are insulinomas. Almost all insulinomas are benign (90% to 95%), and patients with an insulinoma develop significant hypoglycemia (blood glucose often

<40 mg/dL), particularly after fasting. In severe cases the patients may present with seizures, unconsciousness, and even coma.

Twenty percent of syndromic PENs are gastrinomas. Most gastrinomas are malignant (85%), and the unregulated production of gastrin leads to the Zollinger-Ellison syndrome with multiple and recurrent ulcers. These ulcers can develop in unusual locations, and in some cases the overproduction of gastrin also produces diarrhea.

Although only 5% to 10% of PENs produce excess quantities of glucagon, glucagonomas are important because they are usually malignant (70%), and they produce a dramatic syndrome with weight loss, necrolytic migratory erythema, diabetes mellitus, cheilosis or stomatitis, and diarrhea. Necrolytic migratory erythema is a symmetric skin rash with an eczematous appearance, most often seen on the buttocks, thighs, groin, and perineum.

Somatostatinomas and VIPomas are significantly less common. Most syndromic somatostatinomas are malignant (75%). Somatostatin inhibits the release of other hormones, and syndromic somatostatinomas can produce diabetes mellitus, diarrhea, steatorrhea, cholelithiasis, anemia, and weight loss. VIPomas produce vasoactive intestinal polypeptide (VIP), causing the syndrome of severe watery diarrhea, hypokalemia, and achlorhydria, also known as the Verner-Morrison syndrome.

Syndromic PENs can be a manifestation of multiple endocrine neoplasia type 1 (MEN1). For example, 10% of insulinomas and 20% of gastrinomas arise in the setting of MEN1.

Most syndromic PENs arise between the ages of 30 and 60 years old; however, they can develop in children and in the aged. The male-to-female ratio varies depending on the syndrome. Insulinomas and glucagonomas are more common in women, whereas gastrinomas are more common in men.

RADIOLOGIC FEATURES

CT and endoscopic ultrasonography usually reveal a well-demarcated mass. Syndromic PENs can arise in the head, body, or tail of the gland. Most glucagonomas and insulinomas arise in the body or tail of the gland, whereas most gastrinomas arise in the head of the pancreas. Gastrinomas are often multifocal and can also arise in extrapancreatic locations, including the duodenum, the liver, and the extrapancreatic lymph nodes.

PATHOLOGIC FEATURES

Most syndromic PENs are relatively small (<2 cm), single, well-circumscribed, soft lesions. On cut section they are partially encapsulated and have a yellow to reddish pink cut surface. Some cases are cystic.

Microscopic examination reveals a variety of different patterns. Syndromic PENs can have a solid/diffuse, lobular, or trabecular/gyriform appearance (Fig. 17-29). The deposition of amyloid in the fibrovascular stroma may suggest an insulinoma, and psammoma bodies suggest a somatostatinoma, but the light microscopic appearance of these neoplasms cannot be used to establish the production of a specific hormone. Immunolabeling and correlation with the patient's clinical features are necessary. At higher magnification, these neoplasms have a slightly granular eosinophilic cytoplasm and uniform round nuclei with a "salt and pepper" chromatin. Mitoses and pleomorphism are both uncommon.

ANCILLARY STUDIES

Ultrastructural examination is rarely performed in the current era of sensitive and specific immunomarkers for endocrine differentiation. When performed, ultrastructural examination reveals numerous intracytoplasmic neurosecretory granules. These granules with dense cores are smaller than the zymogen granules of acinar cells, measuring 100 to 400 nm. In some instances the structure of the neurosecretory granules can be used to suggest the production of a specific hormone. For example, the granules of insulinomas often have a crystalline structure.

Syndromic PENs label with antibodies to NSE, chromogranin, and synaptophysin. They can express cytokeratin, but in contrast to infiltrating ductal adenocarcinomas of the pancreas, syndromic PENs usually do not express CK7. Most are argyrophilic with the Grimelius silver reaction. Immunolabeling can also be used to confirm the production of a specific endocrine hormone by the neoplasm, although it should be noted that the antigenic component of the hormone and the functional component of the hormone often differ. In occasional cases there can therefore be a discrepancy between the clinical syndrome and the pattern of immunolabeling.

FNA shows hypercellular smears with a predominantly noncohesive cell pattern (Fig. 17-30). The neoplastic cells are uniform and small- to medium-sized with monomorphic nuclei showing finely dispersed chromatin (endocrine chromatin). Occasional punctuate chromatin distribution gives the nuclei a "checkerboard" appearance (Fig. 17-31). Mitoses are rare. Cells have scant to moderate basophilic cytoplasm, and often a lymphocyte-like appearance. Occasionally, a prominent "plasmacytoid" morphology is observed with eccentrically placed nuclei and granular basophilic cytoplasm (Fig. 17-32). Binucleation and multinucleation can be seen. Rarely a well-formed acinar or glandular pattern may be present. Poorly differentiated PENs may show pleomorphism with mitoses/karyorrhexis and necrosis.

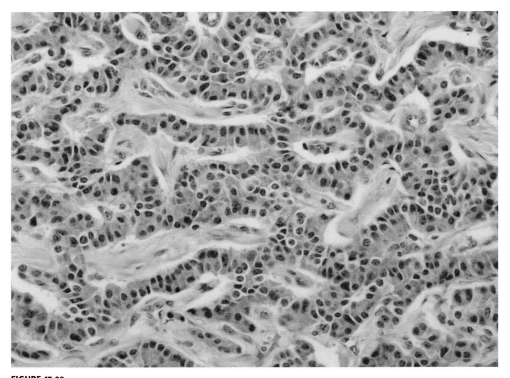

FIGURE 17-29

Well-differentiated pancreatic endocrine neoplasm. Note the trabecular growth pattern and the typical "salt and pepper" chromatin (H&E).

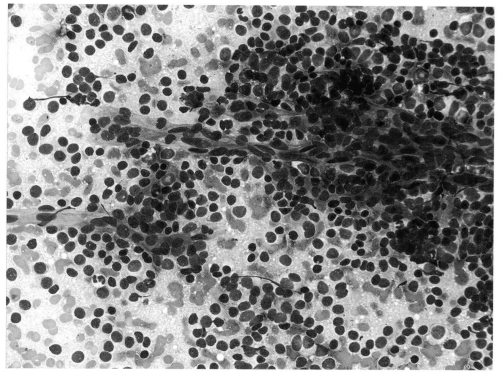

FIGURE 17-30

Pancreatic endocrine neoplasm, fine needle aspiration. Hypercellular smear with discohesive single tumor cells resembling lymphocytes. Cells have round uniform nuclei, mostly devoid of cytoplasm with a finely granular chromatin, lacking nucleoli. Also noted are few fine capillary vessels (Diff Quik).

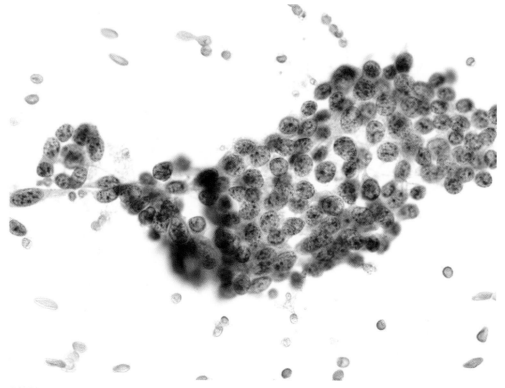

FIGURE 17-31

Well-differentiated endocrine neoplasm, fine needle aspiration. Extremely monotonous neoplastic cells with barely discernible cytoplasm displaying the characteristic speckled "check board" chromatin (Papanicolaou).

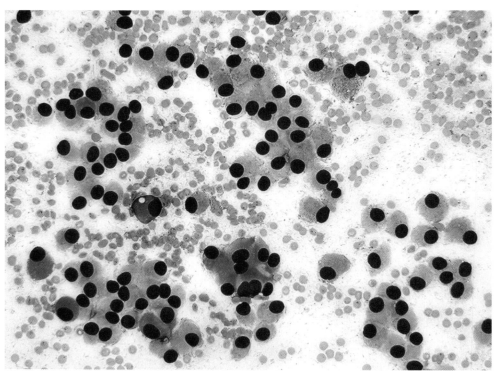

FIGURE 17-32

Pancreatic endocrine neoplasm, fine needle aspiration. Loosely aggregated neoplastic cells with eccentrically placed nuclei and finely granular cytoplasm depicting a "plasmacytoid" appearance (Diff Quik).

DIFFERENTIAL DIAGNOSIS

The diagnosis of a syndromic PEN is usually straightforward because of the associated clinical syndrome. It should be remembered, however, that rarely extrapancreatic neoplasms produce pancreatic endocrine hormones.

PROGNOSIS AND THERAPY

As is true for most endocrine neoplasms, it can be extremely difficult to determine the malignant potential of a syndromic PEN. Well-differentiated PENs less than 0.5 cm, so-called microadenomas, can be considered benign. Larger PENs should be considered malignant. As is true for nonfunctioning endocrine neoplasms of the pancreas, three features can be used to prognosticate. These are large vessel invasion, invasion into other organs, and metastases.

Surgical resection is the treatment of choice. For neoplasms that are unresectable (such as the ones with metastases), additional approaches are used such as antihormonal (diazoxide) or chemotherapeutic agents (streptozotocin, 5-fluorouracil, and Adriamycin) and radiation treatment.

NONSYNDROMIC ENDOCRINE NEOPLASMS

CLINICAL FEATURES

Nonsyndromic endocrine neoplasms of the pancreas are well-differentiated epithelial neoplasms with morphologic and immunohistochemical evidence of endocrine differentiation, but they do not produce a clinical syndrome related to hormone production. These patients present with nonspecific signs and symptoms related to the presence of an intra-abdominal mass. Some present with a palpable pancreatic mass, whereas others develop weight loss and abdominal pain. Neoplasms arising in the head of the pancreas can obstruct the bile duct and produce jaundice. Nonsyndromic endocrine neoplasms strike men and women equally, and the average age at diagnosis is approximately 60 years.

RADIOLOGIC FEATURES

As was true for syndromic endocrine neoplasms of the pancreas, most nonsyndromic PENs appear as enhancing well-demarcated masses by CT.

PATHOLOGIC FEATURES

Most nonfunctioning PENs arise in the head of the pancreas. They are usually larger (from 1 cm to >15 cm) than the syndromic endocrine neoplasms, presumably because they do not cause clinical signs and symptoms until they reach a larger size. They are pink/red on cross-section and often are clearly demarcated from the surrounding normal pancreatic tissue. This contrasts with the infiltrative growth of infiltrating ductal adenocarcinoma. Large vessel invasion, gross invasion into adjacent structures, and metastases are all features of aggressive behavior and should be noted at gross examination. Size can also have prognostic significance, and it too should be carefully documented. An occasional nonfunctioning PEN is cystic.

As is true for syndromic PENs, microscopic examination of the nonsyndromic PENs reveals a variety of different patterns of growth, including solid/diffuse, lobular, and trabecular/gyriform architectures (see Fig. 17-29). The neoplastic cells have an eosinophilic, slightly granular cytoplasm and uniform round nuclei with a "salt and pepper" chromatin. Mitoses and pleomorphism are both uncommon.

ANCILLARY STUDIES

Ultrastructural examination is only rarely utilized to establish the diagnosis. When performed, it reveals characteristic small (100 to 400 nm), dense core neurosecretory granules in the neoplastic cells.

The immunolabeling of nonsyndromic PENs parallels that of syndromic PENs. The neoplastic cells label with antibodies to NSE, chromogranin, and synaptophysin. They can express cytokeratin, but in contrast to ductal adenocarcinomas of the pancreas, they usually do not express CK7. Most are argyrophilic with the Grimelius silver reaction. Immunolabeling for specific endocrine hormones is also often, but not necessarily, positive. It is important to note that the immunohistochemical demonstration of hormone production by a neoplasm does not mean that the hormones produced by the neoplasm will cause a clinical syndrome. Quite the opposite; most do not. FNA biopsy findings are identical to those seen with syndromic endocrine neoplasms (see Figs. 17-31 and 17-32).

DIFFERENTIAL DIAGNOSIS

As discussed earlier, solid-pseudopapillary neoplasms can closely mimic a well-differentiated endocrine neoplasm. This differential diagnosis can be particularly problematic because some well-differentiated endocrine neoplasms show cystic degeneration. Features supporting the diagnosis of a solid-pseudopapillary neoplasm include nuclear grooves, foamy macrophages, and eosinophilic globules. Immunolabeling is often necessary to distinguish between these two neoplasms. Well-differentiated pancreatic endocrine neoplasms are strongly and diffusely positive for chromogranin and synaptophysin, while solid-pseudopapillary neoplasms express CD10 and show an abnormal nuclear localization of β-catenin. A well-differentiated adenocarcinoma should also be considered in the differential diagnosis. A nested pattern of growth, the absence of true lumen formation, uniform nuclei, and a "salt and pepper" chromatin pattern all suggest the diagnosis of a well-differentiated pancreatic endocrine neoplasm. Immunolabeling can be used to definitively establish the diagnosis in difficult cases. In contrast to well-differentiated ductal adenocarcinomas, endocrine neoplasms express chromogranin but not CK7.

An enlarged non-neoplastic islet may sometimes mimic a PEN. A non-neoplastic islet is characterized by the presence (at least focally) of the four main endocrine cell types. If the enlarged islet were seen in the context of chronic pancreatitis, it would show a close topographic relationship with atrophic acinar tissue. The problem can be further compounded by a pseudoinfiltrative pattern produced by entrapment of the non-neoplastic islet tissue in fibrotic stroma, often with close proximity to the nerves, mimicking perineural invasion.

Most undifferentiated small cell carcinomas in the pancreas are metastases from other organs; however, rare undifferentiated small cell carcinomas of the pancreas have been reported and they should be considered in the differential diagnosis of well-differentiated pancreatic endocrine neoplasms. A solid growth pattern, numerous mitoses, nuclear molding, high nuclear to cytoplasmic ratio, hyperchromatic nuclei, inconspicuous nucleoli, and finely granular, evenly dispersed chromatin all support the diagnosis of a small cell carcinoma. Confluent areas of necrosis and numerous karyorrhectic nuclei are usually present.

PROGNOSIS AND THERAPY

Surgical resection is the treatment of choice for well-differentiated endocrine neoplasms, and it can prolong survival even when metastases are present. As is true in other organs, it is, however, very difficult to predict the behavior of a surgically resected endocrine neoplasm of the pancreas. Poor prognostic features include metastases, large vessel invasion, and invasion into adjacent organs. Other factors associated with a poorer prognosis, include larger tumor size (<2 cm vs. ≥ 2 cm), high mitotic rate (≤ 2 mitoses per 10 high-power fields vs. >2), and an elevated ki-67 labeling index ($\leq 2\%$ vs. $>2\%$). For example, most nonsyndromic well-differentiated pancreatic endocrine neoplasms smaller than 2 cm are curable after surgical resection, whereas those larger than 2 cm have a significant risk for recurrence. As noted earlier, only those less than 0.5 cm should be considered absolutely benign.

■ OTHER NEOPLASMS

Although significantly rarer than the neoplasms discussed up to this point, a variety of mesenchymal and hematopoietic neoplasms can involve the pancreas. The diagnostic criteria and prognoses for these neoplasms parallel those of other organs.

Finally, although it is much more common for pancreatic cancer to metastasize to other organs, rarely carcinomas primary to other sites can metastasize to the pancreas.

18

Metabolic and Toxic Conditions of the Liver

■ **Roger Klein Moreira, MD** ■ **Kay Washington, MD, PhD**

■ ACCUMULATION OF METALS

IRON ACCUMULATION

Hemochromatosis is defined as excessive accumulation of iron in the liver and other organs, and may be a manifestation of a primary disease process (hereditary hemochromatosis) or secondary to other acquired or genetic disorders such as chronic anemias and alcoholic liver disease.

HEREDITARY HEMOCHROMATOSIS

CLINICAL FEATURES

Hereditary hemochromatosis (HH) is a group of inherited disorder that results in excess iron storage. HH is the most common genetic disorder in whites, with a prevalence of approximately 1 in 200. Up to 85% of clinically recognized cases in patients of northern and western European origin are homozygotes for the *C282Y* mutation, but this mutation is rare in southern European populations and is not found in African and Asian populations. The distribution of the mutation suggests a Celtic origin, and a competitive advantage for heterozygotes by making iron deficiency less likely is postulated.

Several forms of the disease are recognized: HFE hemochromatosis accounts for more than 90% of cases. Three *HFE* mutations are described; the most common is a missense mutation designated C282Y, which prevents formation of a disulfide bond necessary for binding of HFE protein to β_2-microglobulin. Other less common mutations are designated H63D and S65C. Juvenile hemochromatosis is caused by mutations of the hemojuvelin (HJV) and hepcidin antimicrobial peptide (HAMP) genes. Transferrin receptor 2 (TFR2) hemochromatosis is related to *TFR2* gene mutations, and type B ferroportin disease is caused by SLC40A1 mutation of the membrane iron-regulated transporter ferroportin. All forms of the disease are transmitted as an autosomal recessive disorder, except the type B ferroportin disease, which has an autosomal dominant inheritance. Hepcidin, a peptide hormone encoded by the *HAMP* gene in hepatocytes, plays a central role in iron metabolism, analogous to that of insulin in glucose metabolism. All currently known forms of HH are due to an abnormal production, regulation, or activity of hepcidin.

Clinical manifestations of HH are varied. The process of iron accumulation to toxic levels may take decades, with most patients presenting between ages 40 and 60 years. Clinical manifestations occur earlier in juvenile hemochromatosis. Women present later than men beause of the protective effects of menstruation. Common presenting symptoms are lethargy, hepatomegaly, arthropathy, hypogonadism, abdominal pain, and skin pigmentation. Cardiac failure may occur due to iron deposition in myocardial fibers. Diabetes mellitus and cirrhosis are late manifestations. Endocrine gland compromise is typically the predominant clinical manifestation in juvenile hemochromatosis, although hepatic iron overload also occurs.

RADIOLOGIC FEATURES

Severe iron overload can be detected by computed tomography scan and magnetic resonance imaging. The latter is considered more accurate in estimating hepatic iron stores.

PATHOLOGIC FEATURES

GROSS FINDINGS

In early stages of HH, the liver may appear grossly normal or slightly darker in color. As iron accumulates, the liver and other organs such as the pancreas become rust colored. Cirrhosis due to HH is initially micronodular, evolving into macronodular cirrhosis (Fig. 18-1). Nodules of hepatocellular carcinoma often contain less iron and so appear lighter than cirrhotic nodules.

HEREDITARY HEMOCHROMATOSIS—FACT SHEET

Definition

- Group of inherited disorders of iron overload leading to cirrhosis and damage to other organs

Incidence and Location

- The most common identified genetic disorder in whites
- Prevalence of homozygous state is 1 in 200 in whites; gene frequency is 1 in 10 to 1 in 20
- Rare in patients of non-European descent

Morbidity and Mortality

- Deposition of iron in liver, pancreas, heart, and endocrine tissues leads to organ damage and dysfunction (cirrhosis, diabetes mellitus, congestive heart failure, hypogonadism)
- Up to 70% of patients have cirrhosis at diagnosis
- High risk for hepatocellular carcinoma

Gender, Race, and Age Distribution

- Both sexes affected, but men present earlier than women
- White race; rare in other races
- Most patients present between 40 and 60 years of age
- Earlier onset of disease in juvenile hemochromatosis

Clinical Features

- Common presenting symptoms are arthralgias, skin pigmentation, signs of diabetes mellitus, and hepatomegaly
- Endocrine and cardiac manifestations may be presenting symptoms in younger patients (juvenile hemochromatosis)
- Many patients diagnosed in precirrhotic stages, by follow-up of incidental high serum ferritin level

Prognosis and Therapy

- Phlebotomy; chelating agents are less effective
- 10-year survival rate of cirrhotic patients is 60%
- Hepatocellular carcinoma occurs as a late complication in approximately 30% of cirrhotic patients with HH

HEREDITARY HEMOCHROMATOSIS—PATHOLOGIC FEATURES

Gross Findings

- Early cirrhosis is micronodular, evolving into macronodular cirrhosis
- Deposition of iron in liver results in rusty color
- Pancreas, spleen, and other organs are similarly discolored

Microscopic Findings

- Deposition of iron in periportal hepatocytes, with later accumulation in zone 2 and zone 3 hepatocytes
- Lesser degree of iron deposition in Kupffer cells
- Periportal and bridging fibrosis progress to cirrhosis

Ultrastructural Findings

- Ferritin and hemosiderin accumulate within secondary lysosomes (siderosomes)

Genetics

- Autosomal recessive inheritance (except juvenile hemochromatosis—autosomal dominant)
- Approximately 80% of HH is due to single G to A mutation at position 282 of *HFE* gene (C282Y)
- Non-C282Y mutations result in less severe iron overload, and clinical manifestation of disease does not occur
- Non-HFE HH include juvenile hemochromatosis (*HJV* and *HAMP* gene mutations), transferrin receptor 2 hemochromatosis (*TRF2* gene mutations), and type B ferroportin disease (*SLC40A1* mutation)

Differential Diagnosis

- Secondary iron overload
- Hemolytic anemias and other hematologic disorders
- Blood transfusions
- Hemosiderosis in alcoholic liver disease, hepatitis C, hemodialysis, and metabolic syndrome

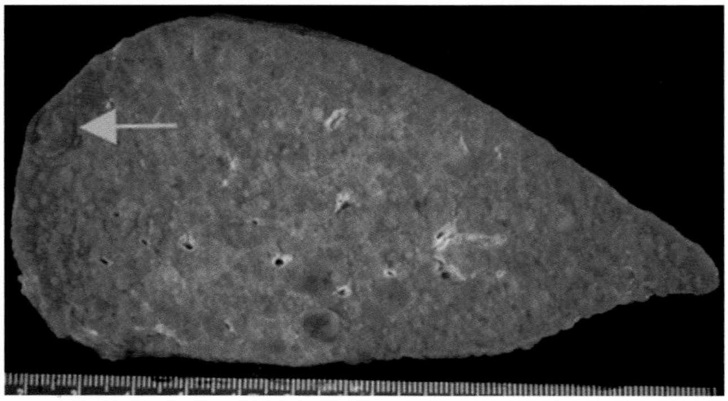

FIGURE 18-1

Cirrhosis due to hereditary hemochromatosis is initially micronodular. The liver is rust colored because of accumulation of excess iron. Note nodule of hepatocellular carcinoma (*arrow*).

MICROSCOPIC FINDINGS

Iron deposits in HH first appear in periportal hepatocytes as finely granular yellow-brown pigment most easily recognized on iron stain and concentrated in a pericanalicular location in the cell. No increase in fibrosis is seen in early stages, and there is little or no inflammation. As iron continues to accumulate, the deposits become coarser, and while the periportal accentuation is maintained (Fig. 18-2A), hepatocytes throughout the lobule exhibit excess iron stores. Hemosiderin granules are also seen in Kupffer cells and bile duct epithelial cells in these later stages. Fibrosis is initially periportal, and expands to form portal-portal bridging septa and cirrhotic nodules with disease progression.

ANCILLARY STUDIES

Special stains for iron such as Prussian blue stain are helpful in confirming accumulation of iron in hepatocytes (see Fig. 18-2B) and differentiation of iron from other brown pigments such as bile and lipofuscin. Immunohistochemistry and electron microscopy are not useful.

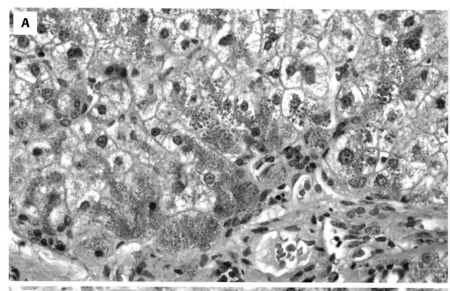

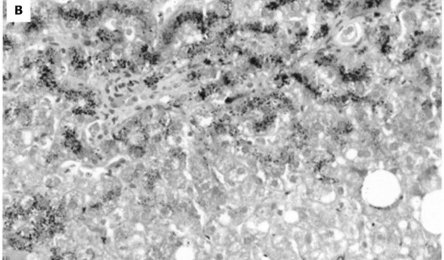

FIGURE 18-2

A, In hereditary hemochromatosis, iron accumulates in hepatocytes before spilling over to Kupffer cells. The iron deposition is in a zonal distribution, with accumulation predominantly in periportal hepatocytes in early stages of the disease. **B,** Prussian blue stain for iron is helpful in highlighting the zone 1 distribution in HH. **C,** In late stages of secondary hemochromatosis due to iron overload, heavy iron deposition may be seen in both Kupffer cells (*arrow*) and hepatocytes.

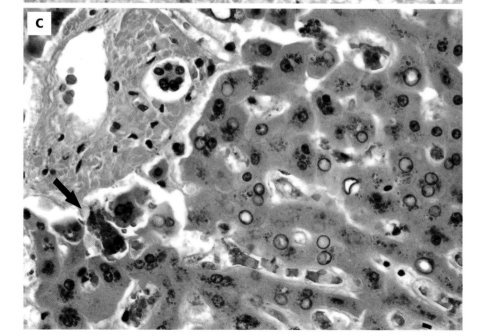

DIFFERENTIAL DIAGNOSIS

HH must be distinguished from secondary iron overload seen most commonly in various forms of chronic anemia such as sickle cell disease and in hepatic siderosis associated with alcoholic liver disease. Whereas iron accumulation in hepatocytes as compared with Kupffer cells is more pronounced in HH, considerable overlap in the pathologic features is seen with secondary hemochromatosis, and quantitative iron determination by chemical techniques or atomic absorption spectrophotometry is more accurate. The hepatic iron index, obtained by dividing the weight of iron in the biopsy by the patient's age, is usually greater than 1.9 in patients with HH but less than 1.9 in heterozygotes and in patients with alcoholic siderosis. HH due to common HFE gene mutations can be established easily using polymerase chain reaction–based techniques.

PROGNOSIS AND THERAPY

Prognosis is related to the presence of organ damage, which correlates with severity of iron overload. Patients without cirrhosis or diabetes who undergo treatment have survivals similar to those of age- and sex-matched normal subjects. The 10-year survival rate in cirrhotic patients who undergo treatment is roughly 70%; hepatocellular carcinoma is an important late complication and may occur years after iron depletion.

Treatment is aimed at reducing iron burden; the most commonly used strategy is phlebotomy at regular intervals until the serum ferritin level falls below 50 ng/mL. Iron chelation agents are not often used to treat HH but are more commonly used to treat secondary iron overload, for which phlebotomy may not be a practical option.

SECONDARY IRON OVERLOAD

CLINICAL FEATURES

Secondary iron overload is most commonly associated with chronic anemias such thalassemia, sideroblastic anemia, anemias associated with defective heme synthesis, and sickle cell disease. Other causes include transfusion-related iron overload in aplastic anemia, hemosiderosis associated with alcoholic liver disease, hemodialysis, hepatitis C, porphyrias, and nonalcoholic fatty liver disease/metabolic syndrome. Dietary iron overload (Bantu siderosis or African iron overload) in sub-Saharan Africans is related to consumption of home-brewed alcohol; recent studies suggest a non-C282Y genetic influence in this population. As in HH, many forms of acquired iron-overload syndromes are

now believed to be related to downregulation of hepcidin. Clinical features in secondary iron overload vary according to disease severity but may be similar to those of HH.

PATHOLOGIC FEATURES

GROSS FINDINGS

Gross findings in secondary iron overload are similar to those of HH. Cirrhosis appears to be less common in hemochromatosis related to chronic anemia compared with HH.

MICROSCOPIC FINDINGS

Iron accumulation in secondary hemochromatosis is initially seen in Kupffer cells rather than hepatocytes. In late stages of iron overload, spillover into hepatocytes occurs (see Fig. 18-2C), and quantitative iron determination or genetic testing may be needed to exclude HH. In alcoholic siderosis, other features of alcoholic liver disease such as steatosis, centrilobular pericellular fibrosis, and Mallory's hyaline may be found.

DIFFERENTIAL DIAGNOSIS

Heavy deposition in iron in Kupffer cells as compared with hepatocytes favors secondary hemochromatosis over HH. Clinical history is usually helpful, but genetic testing for HFE mutations and quantitative iron determination may be necessary.

PROGNOSIS AND THERAPY

Therapy in secondary iron load is aimed at treating the underlying disease. Iron chelation therapy is the only effective treatment for iron overload due to refractory anemias. Prognosis is usually related to the underlying disease.

COPPER ACCUMULATION (WILSON'S DISEASE)

CLINICAL FEATURES

Wilson's disease is an autosomal recessive disorder of copper metabolism; the defect has been identified as mutation in a cation-transporting ATPase ATP7B, the protein responsible for transporting copper into hepatocyte secretory pathways for excretion into bile. A large number of different mutations, mostly missense mutations, have been identified. The majority of affected individuals are compound heterozygotes; no

WILSON'S DISEASE—FACT SHEET

Definition
- Inherited disorder of copper metabolism due to decreased copper excretion through the biliary tract

Incidence and Location
- Carrier frequency estimated between 1 in 90 and 1 in 400
- Disease prevalence of 1 in 30,000
- Occurs in all ethnic groups, but particular mutations and clinical presentations are more common in some populations

Morbidity and Mortality
- Progressive disorder, leading to cirrhosis if untreated
- Copper deposition in brain, particularly in thalamus, putamen, and cerebral cortex, leads to extrapyramidal motor disorders
- Fulminant hepatitis with nonimmune hemolytic anemia and massive release of copper by the liver may be seen in teenagers

Gender, Race, and Age Distribution
- Occurs equally in males and females
- Reported in all races
- Most patients present between ages 3 and 40 years

Clinical Features
- Liver disease and neurologic manifestations are most frequent presenting features
- Kayser-Fleischer rings are always present in those with neurologic disease
- Serum ceruloplasmin is decreased; serum copper and urinary copper are increased
- Most homozygotes have hepatic copper levels of greater than 250 μg/g (normal, <50 μg/g).

Prognosis and Therapy
- Lifelong treatment with metal chelating agents such as penicillamine prevents disease progression
- Liver transplantation for patients with end-stage liver disease or fulminant hepatic failure
- Excellent prognosis for patients compliant with medical therapy

WILSON'S DISEASE—PATHOLOGIC FEATURES

Gross Findings
- Early: liver may be grossly normal or mildly enlarged
- Massive hepatic necrosis in some cases
- Late: macronodular cirrhosis

Microscopic Findings
- Early: nonspecific chronic hepatitis pattern of injury
- Glycogen nuclei in hepatocytes and steatosis are common
- Mallory's hyaline may be seen
- Progressive hepatocyte necrosis and fibrosis lead to cirrhosis
- Copper accumulation in liver, primarily in hepatocyte cytoplasm, may be visualized with special stains (rhodanine, rubeanic acid)

Ultrastructural Findings
- Mitochondrial changes include heterogeneity in size and shape, increased matrix density, and crystalline inclusions
- Increase in peroxisomes and lipofuscin granules

Genetics
- Autosomal recessive disorder
- *ATP7B* gene on 13q14.3 is mutated
- Numerous mutations reported
- Gene product transports copper across hepatocyte membrane into bile canaliculus

Differential Diagnosis
- Chronic viral hepatitis
- Autoimmune hepatitis
- Nonalcoholic fatty liver disease
- Pathologic findings are relatively nonspecific

consistent correlation between genotype and clinical manifestations has been observed. Elevated copper is believed to induce cell damage by stimulating the production of reactive oxygen species.

Most patients with Wilson's disease present with hepatic or neuropsychiatric manifestations, due to accumulation of copper to toxic levels in liver or basal ganglia, respectively. Presentation with hepatic disease is most common in children 10 to 13 years of age but may be seen late in life. Serum transaminase levels are commonly elevated, and patients may present with cirrhosis. Some patients present with massive hepatic necrosis and fulminant liver failure, usually accompanied by hemolytic anemia due to abrupt release of massive amounts of copper from the liver. Initial presentation with neurologic symptoms, most commonly parkinsonian symptoms, occurs roughly 10 years later than presentation with hepatic findings. Kayser-Fleischer rings are due to the deposition of copper in the limbus of the cornea and may be detected on slit-lamp examination.

Laboratory findings in Wilson's disease include low serum ceruloplasmin and elevated urinary copper concentrations. Hepatic copper concentration is elevated (more than 250 μg/g dry weight).

PATHOLOGIC FEATURES

GROSS FINDINGS

The liver may be grossly normal or mildly steatotic in early stages of Wilson's disease. In later stages, progressive fibrosis leads to predominantly macronodular cirrhosis (Fig. 18-3).

MICROSCOPIC FINDINGS

Morphologic changes in early Wilson's disease may be mild (Fig. 18-4A), and a high index of suspicion is needed on the part of the pathologist. Mild to moderate

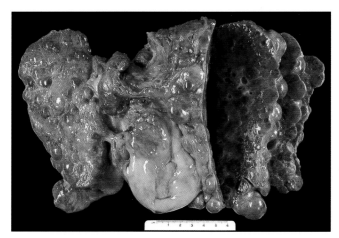

FIGURE 18-3

Cirrhosis due to Wilson's disease is coarsely macronodular with variation in nodule size.

steatosis is common and may be microvesicular or macrovesicular. Glycogenated nuclei (see Fig. 18-4B) are also found. A mild chronic hepatitis pattern of injury with increased lymphocytes in portal tracts and spotty hepatocyte necrosis is relatively common. Mallory's hyaline may also be seen in Wilson's disease. As the disease progresses, periportal fibrosis (see Fig. 18-4C) progresses to bridging fibrosis and cirrhosis. Copper is not visible on routine hematoxylin and eosin stains but may be visualized with special stains such as rhodanine or rubeanic acid. Victoria blue or Shikata stains such as orcein and aldehyde fuchsin stain copper binding protein and may show a granular cytoplasmic pattern of staining in hepatocytes. Distribution of copper within the liver is irregular, especially in cirrhotic nodules. Copper and copper binding protein may be found in Kupffer cells in patients presenting with fulminant liver failure (see Fig. 18-4D).

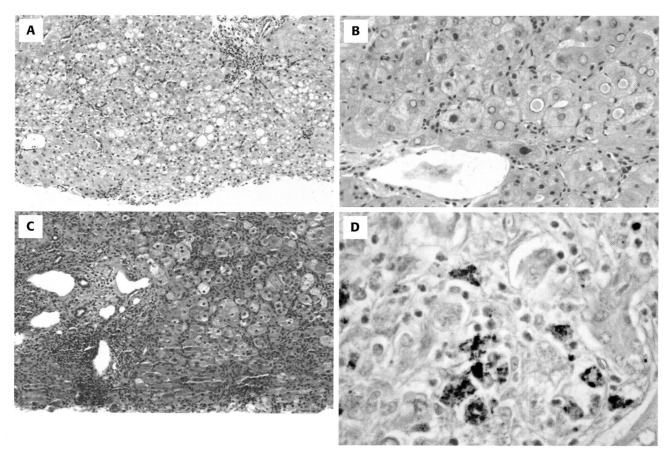

FIGURE 18-4

A, Early-stage Wilson's disease often shows a nonspecific chronic hepatitis pattern of injury, with portal chronic inflammation and focal interface hepatitis. **B,** Glycogenated nuclei are a common but nonspecific finding in Wilson's disease. **C,** In more advanced disease, extensive fibrosis and chronic inflammation is seen and hepatocytes may show ballooning degeneration. **D,** Victoria blue stain (*shown*) and Shikata stains highlight increased copper binding protein in Wilson's disease. In this case of fulminant liver failure, copper binding protein was present in both hepatocytes and Kupffer cells.

DIFFERENTIAL DIAGNOSIS

The histologic differential diagnosis of Wilson's disease depends on the pattern of injury manifested in the liver biopsy. Other common causes of a chronic hepatitis pattern of injury in young patients include chronic viral hepatitis and autoimmune hepatitis and must be excluded by appropriate clinical testing. The combination of low serum ceruloplasmin and high urinary copper excretion should suggest Wilson's disease. The diagnosis is usually confirmed by quantitative copper analysis of hepatic tissue. Other childhood syndromes associated with increased hepatic copper content include Indian childhood cirrhosis, which has been linked to consumption of foods cooked in copper pots. It most likely has a genetic component and is seen only in India. Similar rare disorders include idiopathic copper toxicosis, endemic Tyrolean cirrhosis, and non-Indian childhood cirrhosis.

PROGNOSIS AND THERAPY

The copper-chelating agent D-penicillamine, accompanied by dietary restriction of copper, is the treatment of choice and in most cases halts disease progression. Patients with fulminant hepatic failure or decompensated cirrhosis are candidates for hepatic transplantation.

Prognosis depends on compliance with therapy and with stage of disease at diagnosis. Rarely, hepatocellular carcinoma occurs in the setting of cirrhosis in Wilson's disease. Hepatic onset may be associated with a poorer prognosis.

■ α₁-ANTITRYPSIN DEFICIENCY

CLINICAL FEATURES

α_1-Antitrypsin (α_1AT), a plasma serine protease inhibitor, plays a key role in controlling tissue degradation by complexing with proteases, such as elastase, trypsin, chymotrypsin, and thrombin. This function is particularly critical in the lung, where α_1AT inhibits leukocyte elastase and prevents degradation of alveolar walls by this enzyme. More than 100 genetic variants of α_1AT have been identified; most are associated with normal levels and function of the protein. The deficiency state is most commonly caused by homozygosity for the PI*Z allele, in which alanine is substituted for leucine at amino acid 213, causing self-aggregation of the protein, which is trapped within the endoplasmic reticulum of hepatocytes. The PI*Z protein migrates more slowly on isoelectric focusing than the normal PI*M protein.

The most common clinical disorder associated with α_1AT deficiency is pulmonary disease, specifically emphysema, which preferentially affects basal regions of the lung. Roughly 17% of patients with α_1AT present with liver disease in infancy, manifested as neonatal cholestasis, with 25% of these patients developing cirrhosis in childhood. Liver disease associated with α_1AT deficiency may be clinically silent in early life and present in late adulthood as cirrhosis, usually in male patients.

PATHOLOGIC FEATURES

GROSS FINDINGS

Cirrhosis due to α_1AT deficiency is typically macronodular, with variation in nodule size.

MICROSCOPIC FINDINGS

The most characteristic histologic feature of α_1AT is the presence of globular eosinophilic period acid-Schiff (PAS)-positive, diastase-resistant cytoplasmic inclusions found predominantly in periportal hepatocytes (Fig. 18-5A and B). The inclusions are variable in size, increasing in number and size with age, and may be inconspicuous in biopsy samples from children. In infants presenting with cholestatic liver disease, morphologic changes of neonatal hepatitis such as canalicular cholestasis, giant cell transformation of hepatocytes, and hepatocyte ballooning degeneration (see Fig. 18-5C) are seen. In these cases, interlobular bile ducts may be reduced in number. Biopsies from adults presenting with liver disease typically show a nondescript cirrhosis with mild to moderate necroinflammatory activity.

ANCILLARY STUDIES

ULTRASTRUCTURAL FINDINGS

By electron microscopy, α_1AT inclusions appear as electron-dense material within the endoplasmic reticulum.

SPECIAL STAINS

α_1AT cytoplasmic inclusions are strongly positive on PAS stain and resistant to diastase digestion. Immunohistochemistry is more specific and is particularly helpful in highlighting accumulation of the protein in liver biopsy samples from children, in which the globules may be small and inconspicuous. A finely granular cytoplasmic

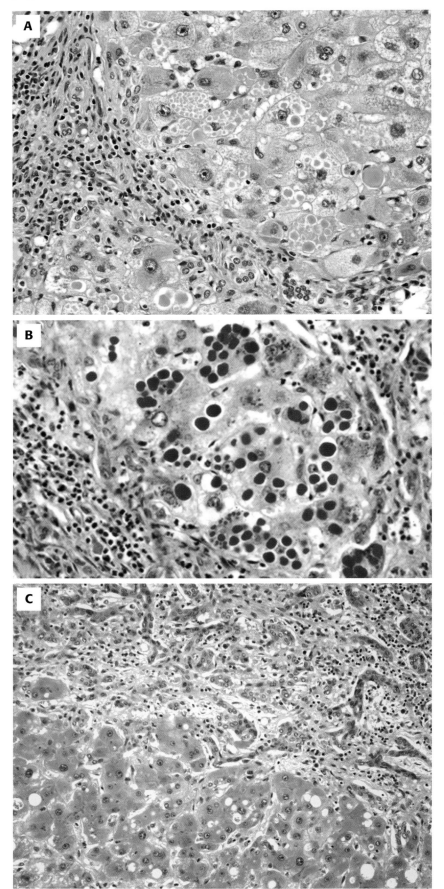

FIGURE 18-5

A, Rounded eosinophilic cytoplasmic inclusions in periportal hepatocytes represent accumulation of α_1AT in endoplasmic reticulum in α_1AT deficiency. **B,** The inclusions are PAS-positive, diastase resistant. **C,** In infants with α_1AT deficiency who present with neonatal cholestasis, the cytoplasmic inclusions are inconspicuous; portal fibrosis and bile ductular reaction with associated prominent cholestasis may lead to an erroneous diagnosis of biliary disease.

α_1-ANTITRYPSIN DEFICIENCY—FACT SHEET

Definition

- Autosomal recessive disorder leading to accumulation of α_1AT in hepatocytes, with decrease in circulating α_1AT

Incidence and Location

- Homozygous state occurs in 1 in 6700 to 1 in 2000 births in North America
- Geographic variation, with highest incidence in Northern Europe, particularly Scandinavia

Morbidity and Mortality

- Symptomatic liver disease in 11% of infants
- Increased risk for emphysema, hepatocellular carcinoma, and glomerulonephritis
- Increased risk for cirrhosis (roughly 20% older than age 50 years)

Gender, Race, and Age Distribution

- Equal distribution in males and females
- More common among whites of northern European ancestry
- Rarely found in individuals of Asian or African descent
- May be diagnosed at any age

Clinical Features

- Persistent jaundice in neonate
- Hepatosplenomegaly or ascites in late childhood
- Presents with cryptogenic cirrhosis and portal hypertension in adults
- Low (10% to 14% of normal) serum α_1AT levels
- Abnormal protein identified by serum electrophoresis

Prognosis and Therapy

- Most important treatment is avoidance of cigarette smoking.
- No specific therapy
- Liver transplantation for end-stage disease

α_1-ANTITRYPSIN DEFICIENCY—PATHOLOGIC FEATURES

Gross Findings

- Hepatomegaly with bile staining in young children
- Cirrhosis in late stages

Microscopic Findings

- PAS-positive, diastase-resistant eosinophilic cytoplasmic globules in hepatocytes
- Globules are more prominent in periportal hepatocytes and represent accumulation of α_1AT in endoplasmic reticulum
- In neonates, bile ducts may be decreased in number
- Chronic hepatitis pattern of injury with cirrhosis in adults

Ultrastructural Findings

- Amorphous proteinaceous material in endoplasmic reticulum

Genetics

- Autosomal recessive disorder
- Gene is located on chromosome 14q
- α_1AT is a single-chain protease inhibitor in the Serpin family
- Most common normal protein is M form; Z form is due to single base substitution

Immunohistochemistry

- α_1AT accumulation is more pronounced in periportal hepatocytes
- Granular accumulation in neonates, without globule formation

Differential Diagnosis

- Neonatal hepatitis
- Biliary atresia
- Paucity of intrahepatic bile ducts
- Chronic viral hepatitis
- Cryptogenic cirrhosis

staining pattern with accentuation in periportal hepatocytes is typical in biopsy specimens from young children (Fig. 18-6).

DIFFERENTIAL DIAGNOSIS

In children presenting with neonatal cholestasis, the histologic differential diagnosis is broad and includes other causes of a neonatal hepatitis pattern of injury, as well as paucity of intrahepatic bile ducts. Immunohistochemical stains for α_1AT show granular accumulation of the protein in periportal hepatocytes and help suggest the diagnosis, which should be confirmed by protein electrophoretic testing. In adults with cirrhosis, the differential diagnosis includes chronic viral hepatitis and nonalcoholic steatohepatitis (NASH). Identification of characteristic cytoplasmic inclusions is highly suggestive but not pathognomonic of α_1AT deficiency; accumulation of the protein is also seen in end-stage liver disease associated with other causes and in livers with metastases.

PROGNOSIS AND THERAPY

Most children with α_1AT deficiency who present with liver disease show recovery of liver function. Elevated serum transaminase levels are adverse prognostic factors. Men older than 50 years (usually without a history of neonatal hepatitis) with α_1AT deficiency are at higher risk for cirrhosis. Liver disease in adults presenting with cirrhosis appears to show rapid progression, with death occurring within 2 years of the diagnosis of cirrhosis. A small increased risk for hepatocellular carcinoma in male patients with or without cirrhosis has been reported.

Therapy for liver disease associated with α_1AT deficiency is supportive, and there is no rationale for replacement therapy with α_1AT, because the liver injury is likely due to accumulation of the protein within hepatocytes. Augmentation of serum levels by the infusion of purified human α_1AT is approved for treatment of pulmonary disease.

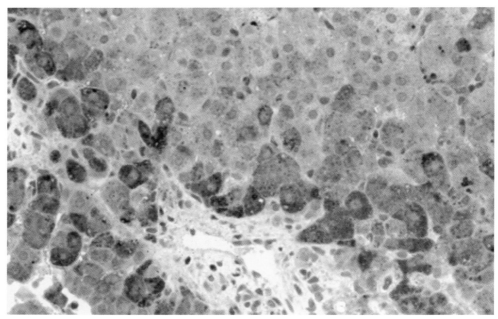

FIGURE 18-6

In biopsy samples from children, immunohistochemistry for α_1AT may be helpful and shows granular cytoplasmic accumulation, more prominent in periportal hepatocytes.

■ GLYCOGEN STORAGE DISEASES

CLINICAL FEATURES

The glycogen storage diseases (GSDs) are inherited disorders of glycogen metabolism; specific enzymatic defects in glycogen metabolism pathways result in accumulation of excess or structurally abnormal glycogen in the liver and other organs such as the heart, kidney, and skeletal muscle, depending on the metabolic defect. Because the liver and skeletal muscle normally has abundant glycogen, they are the most commonly affected tissues. GSD types I, II, III, IV, VI, and IX produce morphologic changes in liver; the most common form is GSD I. Most GSDs involving the liver present with hepatomegaly and hypoglycemia. All are autosomal recessive with the exception of some subtypes of GSD IX, which are X-linked.

PATHOLOGIC FEATURES

GROSS FINDINGS

The liver in glycogen storage disease is enlarged and pale. Increased fibrosis in some types of GSD imparts a firm texture to the parenchyma.

MICROSCOPIC FINDINGS

Hepatocytes in glycogen storage disease are swollen with excess free cytoplasmic accumulation of glycogen, which imparts a pale appearance (Fig. 18-7A and B).

The sinusoidal compression and prominent hepatocyte cell membranes result in a mosaic appearance. Excess nuclear glycogen is seen in some but not all GSDs (Table 18-1). The excess glycogen may be demonstrated by PAS stain, with removal of glycogen by diastase (see Fig. 18-7C). The exception is GSD II, a lysosomal storage disorder; a mosaic pattern is not seen (see Fig. 18-7D), hepatocytes demonstrate cytoplasmic lipid accumulation, and glycogen is found in lysosomes as beta particles. Hepatocellular adenomas develop in the setting of GSD I.

ANCILLARY STUDIES

ULTRASTRUCTURAL FINDINGS

By electron microscopy, monoparticulate glycogen is seen in the cytoplasm and displacing organelles. Intranuclear glycogen may also be identified in some types of GSD (see Table 18-1). In GSD IV, fibrillar aggregates characteristic of amylopectin are present.

DIFFERENTIAL DIAGNOSIS

For GSDs without hepatic fibrosis, the main differential diagnosis is normal liver, in which glycogen accumulation can be substantial. Diabetes mellitus is also associated with accumulation of hepatic glycogen. The GSDs may show considerable morphologic overlap with each other, and definitive diagnosis relies on

GLYCOGEN STORAGE DISEASE—FACT SHEET

Definition

- Inherited disorders of glycogen metabolism leading to abnormal accumulation of glycogen in the liver
- Multiple types are described; types I, II, III, IV, VI, and IX have hepatic manifestations

Incidence and Location

- Type I: 1 in 100,000
- Type II: less than 1 in 100,000 live births
- Other types: very rare

Morbidity and Mortality

- Depends on type; many patients display growth retardation
- Patients with type I survive into adulthood but may suffer from focal segmental glomerulosclerosis and hepatic adenomas
- Type II is variable in severity
- Patients with type IV often die in early perinatal period
- Type VI is relatively benign; adults are asymptomatic

Gender, Race, and Age Distribution

- Males and females equally affected, except for some subtypes of type IX, which are X-linked
- No known race predilection
- Age at presentation is variable and depends on type

Clinical Features

- Definitive diagnosis requires biochemical determination of enzyme defect
- Patients present with variable hepatomegaly
- Hypoglycemia is seen in types I, IV, and VI
- Failure to thrive is common
- Hepatic adenomas develop in patients with type I

Prognosis and Therapy

- Treatment is dietary supplementation with glucose drip feedings and uncooked cornstarch in type I, high-protein diets in types II and III, and uncooked cornstarch in type VI
- Prognosis depends on type: good for type VI, poor for type IV, and intermediate for other types

GLYCOGEN STORAGE DISEASE—PATHOLOGIC FEATURES

Gross Findings

- Hepatomegaly
- Liver is paler than normal
- Fine fibrosis in types III and IV, with development of cirrhosis

Microscopic Findings

- Hepatocytes are enlarged by glycogen accumulation, with pale watery cytoplasm
- Mosaic pattern due to compression of sinusoids and accentuation of hepatocyte cell membranes (type II lacks mosaic pattern)
- In type IV, hepatocytes contain rounded basophilic cytoplasmic inclusions
- Fibrosis leading to cirrhosis may be found in types III, IV, and VI

Ultrastructural Findings

- Large pools of glycogen displace cytoplasmic organelles
- In type I, double-contoured vesicles are seen in the endoplasmic reticulum
- In type II, glycogen accumulates in lysosomes
- In type IV, non–membrane-bound inclusions are seen

Genetics

- Autosomal recessive inheritance, except for some subtypes of type IX, which are X-linked
- Type Ia: chromosome 17; G6P gene
- Type Ib: chromosome 11q23; transmembrane transport protein (G6P receptor)
- Type II: chromosome 17q25; acid maltase gene
- Type III: chromosome 1p21; 1,2 amylo-1,6-glucosidase gene
- Type IV: chromosome 3; branching enzyme gene
- Type VI: chromosome 14; gene for subunit of liver phosphorylase isoform
- Type IX: gene for subunit of phosphorylase kinase; genetically complex

Differential Diagnosis

- Normal liver
- Type IV: Lafora's disease

and promotes normal growth in GSD I. Liver transplantation may be considered in cases with cirrhosis.

■ LYSOSOMAL STORAGE DISORDERS

CLINICAL FEATURES

The lysosomal storage disorders (LSDs) most commonly involve glycolipid, phospholipid, or mucopolysaccharide metabolism and are characterized by accumulation of storage products in membrane-bound vesicles. The liver is affected in a number of these disorders, and storage product usually accumulates in both Kupffer cells and hepatocytes. Most LSDs are rare and exhibit an autosomal recessive inheritance pattern (Table 18-2). Clinical progression varies widely, depending on the disorder.

biochemical testing of fresh or frozen liver tissue or other target tissue.

PROGNOSIS AND THERAPY

Prognosis depends on the biochemical defect. Many of the GSDs show clinical heterogeneity in presentation and outcome; severely affected patients often die in childhood, for instance, in GSD II, whereas other patients present as older adults with only skeletal muscle involvement.

For most GSDs, no specific treatment is available. Dietary manipulation in milder cases may be helpful; nocturnal nasogastric glucose drip feedings or ingestion of uncooked cornstarch prevents hypoglycemia

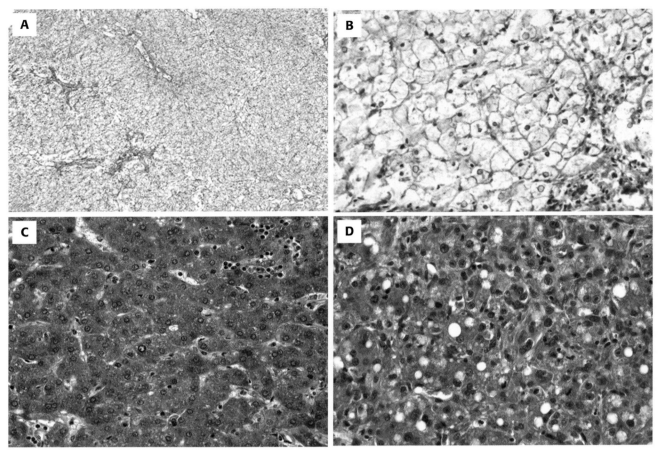

FIGURE 18-7

A, On low power, most of the glycogen storage diseases show a mosaic pattern. **B,** Cytoplasmic accumulation of glycogen in hepatocytes leads to a clear appearance on hematoxylin and eosin stain. **C,** PAS stain highlights the glycogen accumulation (shown), with removal of glycogen with diastase digestion. **D,** Type II GSD, a lysosomal storage disorder, does not show a mosaic pattern; hepatocytes contain lipid vacuoles.

PATHOLOGIC FEATURES

GROSS FINDINGS

Most of the LSDs produce hepatomegaly. In Wolman's disease, the liver is yellow to orange on gross examination because of lipid accumulation.

MICROSCOPIC FINDINGS

The characteristic finding in most LSDs is accumulation of foamy material in hepatocytes and Kupffer cells (Table 18-3; Fig. 18-8). Hepatic fibrosis with progression to cirrhosis is a feature of many of the LSDs with hepatic involvement.

ANCILLARY STUDIES

ULTRASTRUCTURAL FINDINGS

Electron microscopy shows lysosomal inclusions, usually granular or fibrillar. In Niemann-Pick disease, the inclusions resemble myelin. Lipid droplets and cholesterol clefts are seen in Wolman's disease and cholesterol ester storage disease.

DIFFERENTIAL DIAGNOSIS

Although some of the LSDs have characteristic liver findings, definitive diagnosis is based on demonstration of decreased enzyme activity in appropriate tissues, or on molecular testing.

PROGNOSIS AND THERAPY

Prognosis varies widely, depending on the specific LSD (see Table 18-2). Whereas some LSDs are fatal in early childhood, milder forms are compatible with a normal life span. Bone marrow transplantation is performed as therapy for some of the LSDs; enzyme replacement therapy is under active development for a number of these conditions.

TABLE 18-1

Glycogen Storage Diseases with Hepatic Manifestations

Glycogen Storage Disease	Clinical Presentation	Enzyme Deficiency	Histopathologic Findings
Type Ia (von Gierke's disease)	Growth retardation, hepatomegaly, lactic academia, hyperlipidemia	Glycose-6-phosphatase in liver, kidney, intestine	Uniform mosaic pattern; excess glycogen and fat in hepatocytes; nuclear hyperglycogenation; hepatic adenomas
Type Ib	As for Ia; neutropenia and impaired PMN function	Transmembrane protein (translocase A1)	As for Ib, except mosaic pattern is nonuniform
Type II (Pompe's disease)	Variable; cardiomegaly, hypotonia, hepatomegaly; adult presentation with only skeletal muscle involvement	Lysosomal acid α-glucosidase (acid maltase)	Nonmosaic pattern; intralysosomal glycogen accumulation; vesicular hepatocytes
Type III (Cori's disease)	Similar to type I but less severe	Amylo-1, 6-glucosidase debranching enzyme	Uniform mosaic pattern; nuclear hyperglycogenation; may have portal septal fibrosis with progression to cirrhosis
Type IV (Andersen's disease)	Hepatosplenomegaly and failure to thrive; hypoglycemia is rare	Branching enzyme	Cirrhosis before age 5; nonprogressive disease also exists; basophilic diastase-resistant cytoplasmic inclusions in hepatocytes
Type VI (Hers' disease)	Hepatomegaly, growth retardation; variable hypoglycemia and hyperlipidemia, usually mild	Liver phosphorylase system; heterogeneous group of disorders	Nonuniform mosaic pattern; may have portal septal fibrosis
Type IX	As for type VI	Defect in one of four subunits of phosphorylase kinase	Nonuniform mosaic pattern; may have portal septal fibrosis or cirrhosis; low-grade necroinflammatory activity

PMN, polymorphonuclear.

TABLE 18-2

Clinical Features of Selected Lysosomal Storage Diseases

Disorder	Inheritance	Clinical Features	Clinical Outcome
Mucopolysaccharidoses (MPS) (7 distinct types)	Autosomal recessive (6 types); X-linked for MPS II	Multisystem involvement; organomegaly; abnormal facies; mental retardation in some types	Chronic progressive course; survival depends upon specific disease type and severity and ranges from early childhood to old age
Sphingolipidoses			
Gaucher disease types 1, 2, and 3	Autosomal recessive	Hepatosplenomegaly, all types; CNS degeneration, types 2 and 3	Type 1: 6-80 yr Type 2: <2 yr Type 3: 2nd to 4th decades of life
Niemann-Pick disease types A, B, and C	Autosomal recessive	Type A: failure to thrive; hepatosplenomegaly; neurologic degeneration Type B: variable presentation, no neurologic involvement Type C: progressive neurologic degeneration, hepatosplenomegaly	Type A: fatal by age 3 Types B and C: survival into adulthood
Acid lipase deficiency (Wolman's disease)	Autosomal recessive	Hepatosplenomegaly; steatorrhea, adrenal calcification	Wolman's disease is fatal by 1 year
Metachromatic leukodystrophy	Autosomal recessive	Gait disturbances, mental regression, dementia, seizures	Variable; may be slowly progressive over decades
Mucolipidoses (I cell disease and pseudo-Hurler polydystrophy)	Autosomal recessive	Severe psychomotor retardation; abnormal facies, hepatomegaly in I-cell disease; joint abnormalities and growth retardation in pseudo-Hurler polydystrophy	Death in first decade for I-cell disease; survival into adulthood for pseudo-Hurler polydystrophy

LYSOSOMAL STORAGE DISORDERS—FACT SHEET

Definition
- Inherited disorder of degradation of substances normally broken down in lysosomes
- Examples
  - Sphingolipidoses (e.g., Gaucher's disease, Niemann-Pick disease)
  - Mucopolysaccharidoses (e.g., Hurler's disease, Hunter's disease)
  - Mucolipidoses
  - Oligosaccharidoses
  - Acid lipase deficiency (Wolman's disease, cholesterol ester storage disease)

Incidence and Location
- All are rare disorders
- Gaucher's disease is most common
- No reported geographic predilection

Morbidity and Mortality
- Depends on biochemical defect

Gender, Race, and Age Distribution
- For most of these disorders, males and females are affected equally
- No reported racial predilection for most LSDs
- Most are diagnosed in infancy or childhood, but some may present in late adulthood (type I Gaucher's disease)

Clinical Features
- Hepatomegaly is common
- Clinical liver disease is variable
- Many of these disorders are associated with progressive neurologic degeneration

Prognosis and Therapy
- Bone marrow transplantation has been performed for some of the lysosomal storage disorders
- Liver transplantation is rarely indicated and is not curative
- Prognosis is variable, depending on genetic defect

■ GALACTOSEMIA

CLINICAL FEATURES

Galactosemia is an autosomal recessive disorder due to mutation in the gene encoding galactose-1-phosphate uridyltransferase (GALT), located on the short arm of chromosome 9 in the p13 region. Severe GALT deficiency (classic galactosemia) presents in early infancy with failure to thrive, vomiting, diarrhea, cataracts, and liver dysfunction. Patients may also present in early infancy with *Escherichia coli* septicemia.

PATHOLOGIC FEATURES

GROSS FINDINGS

The liver exhibits macronodular cirrhosis in late-stage galactosemia.

LYSOSOMAL STORAGE DISORDERS—PATHOLOGIC FEATURES

Gross Findings
- Hepatomegaly
- Steatosis in some LSDs

Microscopic Findings
- Kupffer cells are enlarged and may appear vacuolated, foamy, or exhibit striated cytoplasm
- Steatosis is present in cholesteryl ester storage disease

Ultrastructural Findings
- Lysosomal or lamellar inclusions
- Membrane-bound vacuoles containing granular or fibrillar material in some disorders

Genetics
- Most are autosomal recessive
- Some exhibit X-linked pattern of inheritance

Differential Diagnosis
- Specific diagnosis is established by biochemical or genetic testing

MICROSCOPIC FINDINGS

The initial finding is severe panlobular macrovesicular steatosis. Canalicular cholestasis and giant cell transformation of hepatocytes is often prominent, and bile ductular reaction/proliferation is seen (Fig. 18-9). Periportal fibrosis progresses to cirrhosis in early childhood, usually by 6 months of age in untreated children.

DIFFERENTIAL DIAGNOSIS

The differential diagnosis for galactosemia includes other metabolic disorders producing steatosis, cholestasis, and fibrosis, such as hereditary fructose intolerance and tyrosinemia. Diagnosis is made on the basis of a fluorescent spot test for GALT activity in blood, followed by further biochemical or molecular testing for confirmation.

PROGNOSIS AND THERAPY

Dietary restriction of galactose is the only effective long-term treatment for galactosemia. Long-term complications such as cataracts and mental retardation may not be prevented, however, due to the impossibility of complete elimination of galactose from the diet; endogenous galactose production may also be a factor. Ovarian failure is a late complication.

TABLE 18-3

Liver Histopathologic Features in Selected Lysosomal Storage Disorders

Disorder	Microscopic Features
Mucopolysaccharidoses (liver involvement in types I, II, III, VI, and VII)	Vacuolization of Kupffer cells and hepatocytes, well demonstrated on colloidal iron stain; liver fibrosis and cirrhosis may develop
Sphingolipidoses	
Gaucher disease	Accumulation of storage material in Kupffer cells; striated or wrinkled cytoplasm more obvious on PAS stain; progressive fibrosis in some cases; hepatocytes not affected.
Niemann-Pick disease	Progressive increase in lipid-laden foam cells in hepatic sinusoids; hepatocyte and Kupffer cell vacuolization; progressive portal fibrosis; cholestasis.
Acid lipase deficiency (Wolman's disease)	Hepatomegaly; vacuolated, swollen, pale-staining Kupffer cells and hepatocytes; needle-shaped birefringent crystals in hepatocytes; fibrosis and cirrhosis may develop
Metachromatic leukodystrophy	Light brown granules in Kupffer cells, portal macrophages, and biliary epithelium; metachromatic with cresyl violet staining of frozen sections.
Mucolipidoses	Vacuolated hepatocytes, Kupffer cells, and portal fibroblasts.

PAS, periodic acid-Schiff.

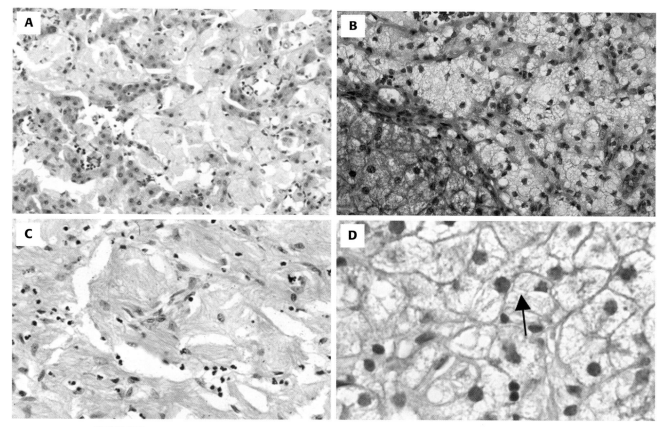

FIGURE 18-8

Lysosomal storage diseases. **A,** In Gaucher's disease, Kupffer cells are markedly distended and accumulate in hepatic sinusoids; hepatoctyes do not accumulate glucosylceramide and are thus uninvolved, although they may show atrophic changes. **B,** The Gaucher cells are characterized by striated or wrinkled cytoplasm. **C,** In Niemann-Pick disease, both Kupffer cells (*top*) and hepatocytes develop cytoplasmic vacuoles. Fibrosis is typically not prominent. **D,** In Wolman's disease, both hepatocytes and Kupffer cells are swollen and pale staining. Lipid droplets may be seen in hepatocytes. Needle-shaped birefringent crystals of cholesterol may be inconspicuous (*arrow*).

GALACTOSEMIA—FACT SHEET

Definition

- Inherited disorder of galactose metabolism leading to increased serum levels of galactose

Incidence and Location

- 1 in 40,000 births in the United States
- No reported geographic predilection

Morbidity and Mortality

- Sepsis due to *E. coli* is common in newborn period
- Long-term neurologic sequelae may not be prevented by dietary restrictions

Gender, Race, and Age Distribution

- Males and females equally affected
- No race predilection
- Identified by screening of newborns or presentation early in life

Clinical Features

- Common presentations include failure to thrive, jaundice, and cataracts
- Hemolytic anemia may occur
- Neurologic effects include ataxia and delayed development
- Ovarian failure may occur in girls

Prognosis and Therapy

- Therapy is exclusion of galactose from diet
- Patients identified by neonatal screening and treated appropriately may survive into adulthood

GALACTOSEMIA—PATHOLOGIC FEATURES

Gross Findings

- Liver may be bile stained
- Texture is firmer than normal due to increased fibrosis
- Cirrhosis in older infants

Microscopic Findings

- Steatosis
- Bile ductular proliferation, with cholangiolar bile plugs
- Pseudoacinar rosette formation by hepatocytes
- Cirrhosis develops by 6 months
- Macroregenerative nodules may be seen

Genetics

- Chromosome 9q13, gene for galactose-1-phosphate uridyl transferase
- Autosomal recessive

Differential Diagnosis

- Tyrosinemia
- Hereditary fructose intolerance

■ TYROSINEMIA

CLINICAL FEATURES

Hepatorenal tyrosinemia, also known as tyrosinemia type I and hereditary tyrosinemia, is a clinically severe autosomal recessive disorder caused by deficiency of fumarylacetoacetate hydrolase. The human *FAH* gene has been mapped to chromosome 15 q23-q25, and at least 34 different mutations have been described, with founder mutations in the high incidence areas of Quebec and Finland. The liver, kidney, and peripheral nerve are the principal organs affected; the mechanisms of hepatic and

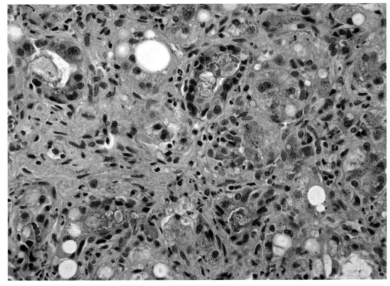

FIGURE 18-9

Steatosis, marked cholestasis, bile ductular reaction, and rapidly developing fibrosis are characteristic of untreated galactosemia.

renal injury are unclear. Presenting symptoms are variable and include acute liver failure, cirrhosis, hepatocellular carcinoma, renal Fanconi's syndrome, hypophosphatemic rickets, glomerulosclerosis, and peripheral neuropathy. Hepatic synthetic and clotting functions are typically severely affected. Transaminase levels may be normal or only slightly elevated. A "boiled cabbage" odor due to accumulation of methionine and other amino acids may be noted in acute hepatic crisis.

PATHOLOGIC FEATURES

GROSS FINDINGS

The liver is usually enlarged in hepatorenal tyrosinemia. In most cases, macronodular cirrhosis is present. Hepatocellular carcinoma is a frequent complication.

MICROSCOPIC FINDINGS

Cirrhosis develops rapidly in untreated patients and may be seen within the first few weeks of life. Regenerative nodules are variable in size and often prominent, even in young patients. Large cell change or small cell change is commonly found, and the hepatocellular carcinomas arising in hepatorenal tyrosinemia may be multifocal.

TYROSINEMIA—FACT SHEET

Definition
- Inherited disorder of tyrosine metabolism, characterized by progressive liver injury

Incidence and Location
- Incidence of up to 1 in about 17,000 live births in high-incidence areas; approximately 1 in 120,000 live births elsewhere
- Worldwide distribution, but most common in province of Quebec, traced to founder effect

Morbidity and Mortality
- Hepatocellular carcinoma develops in up to one third of cases
- Clinical course has improved with early diagnosis and treatment; survival into adulthood is common

Gender, Race, and Age Distribution
- Occurs equally in males and females
- No race predilection, except more common in those of French-Canadian descent
- Patients present in early childhood

Clinical Features
- Patients present in early childhood with signs of liver disease, including ascites, peripheral edema, and coagulopathy
- Neurologic crisis with paralysis may be preceded by infection
- 80% have renal tubular defects

Prognosis and Therapy
- Treatment is dietary restrictions and NTBC, which prevents accumulation of toxic metabolites
- Liver transplantation if medical treatment fails
- Risk for hepatocellular carcinoma

Nonspecific steatosis, a variable chronic inflammatory infiltrate, and cholestasis are often seen. In acute hepatic crisis presenting in early infancy, liver biopsy samples show marked canalicular cholestasis with cholestatic rosettes and giant cell transformation.

DIFFERENTIAL DIAGNOSIS

Histologically, hepatorenal tyrosinemia may show overlap with neonatal hepatitis and with other metabolic disorders (such as galactosemia) that produce a rapidly progressive cirrhotic pattern of injury. Metabolic or molecular testing of blood or liver tissue is necessary for definitive diagnosis. Demonstration of increased succinylacetone in blood, plasma, or urine assays is virtually pathognomonic of the disease.

PROGNOSIS AND THERAPY

Age of onset of symptoms may be an important prognostic indicator in patients who are not identified by newborn screening programs. Onset of symptoms prior to 2 months of age is associated with a 1-year mortality rate of 60%, compared with 4% in children presenting after 6 months of age. Treatment is with 2-(2-nitro-4-trifluoromethy-benzoyl)-1, 3-cyclohexanedione (NTBC), an inhibitor of 4HPPD, an enzyme involved in metabolism of tyrosine, combined with dietary restriction of tyrosine and phenylalanine. Dietary restriction alone slows disease progression but does not eliminate the complications of the disease. Liver transplantation cures the hepatic disease and prevents development of further neurologic crises.

TYROSINEMIA—PATHOLOGIC FEATURES

Gross Findings
- Cirrhotic liver at autopsy is enlarged, yellow, and strikingly nodular
- Cirrhosis may be micronodular, macronodular, or mixed
- Nodules may be variegated and are described as yellow, tan, or green

Microscopic Findings
- Fatty change
- Liver cell dysplasia, both large and small cell change, may be seen
- Marked cholestasis may be present

Genetics
- Autosomal recessive
- Type I is caused by deficiency of fumarylacetoacetate hydrolase; gene is located on chromosome 15q22-25

Differential Diagnosis
- Neonatal hepatitis
- Galactosemia

■ HEREDITARY FRUCTOSE INTOLERANCE

CLINICAL FEATURES

Hereditary fructose intolerance, an autosomal recessive disorder, is caused by mutation of the aldolase B gene, leading to deficiency of fructaldolase B of liver, kidney cortex, and small intestine. The disease is characterized by severe hypoglycemia and vomiting following ingestion of fructose, with affected patients developing a strong aversion for fructose- and sucrose-containing food. In infants, prolonged fructose ingestion, usually given as in a cow's milk formula, leads to failure to thrive, vomiting, hepatomegaly, jaundice, and proximal renal tubular syndrome. If ingestion of fructose continues, severe liver injury with hepatic failure and death may ensue. Patients remain healthy on a fructose- and sucrose-free diet. Undiagnosed hereditary fructose intolerance in adult patients is sometimes suspected by dentists who note the complete absence of caries in these individuals.

PATHOLOGIC FEATURES

GROSS FINDINGS

The liver is yellow and enlarged due to steatosis. Cirrhosis rarely occurs.

MICROSCOPIC FINDINGS

Diffuse macrovesicular steatosis, spotty hepatocyte necrosis, and periportal and pericellular fibrosis are described (Fig. 18-10). Canalicular cholestasis and bile ductular proliferation may also be seen.

DIFFERENTIAL DIAGNOSIS

The differential diagnosis of hereditary fructose intolerance includes other metabolic diseases, such as galactosemia, characterized by a steatotic pattern of injury. Diagnosis is made by clinical history and confirmed by DNA analysis or assay of fructaldolase in liver tissue.

PROGNOSIS AND THERAPY

Hereditary fructose intolerance is compatible with good health and normal life span, as long as fructose and sucrose intake is avoided. Undiagnosed patients may die following routine surgical procedures, however, if given intravenous infusions containing fructose, sorbitol, or invert sugar. No specific therapy, other than avoidance of the offending agent, is indicated.

■ PORPHYRIAS

CLINICAL FEATURES

The porphyrias are a group of inherited metabolic disorders associated with decreased activities of specific enzymes in the heme biosynthesis. Significant liver pathology is found in three of the porphyrias: acute intermittent porphyria (AIP), porphyria cutanea tarda (PCT), and erythropoietic protoporphyria (EPP). Clinical severity of the hepatic porphyrias is

---

HEREDITARY FRUCTOSE INTOLERANCE—FACT SHEET

Definition
- Inherited disorder of fructose metabolism

Incidence and Location
- Incidence of 1 in 18,000 births
- Cases reported worldwide

Gender, Race, and Age Distribution
- Occurs equally in males and females
- Patients present in early childhood, on introduction of fructose into diet
- No known racial predilection

Clinical Features
- Patients present with poor feeding and failure to thrive
- Hepatomegaly and signs of liver disease may be seen
- Older patients have an aversion to sweets
- Serum fructose levels are elevated

Prognosis and Therapy
- Treatment is dietary, with restriction of fructose, sucrose, and sorbitol
- Normal survival if offending foods are avoided

HEREDITARY FRUCTOSE INTOLERANCE—PATHOLOGIC FEATURES

Gross Findings
- Steatosis is common
- Cirrhosis rarely occurs

Microscopic Findings
- A neonatal hepatitis pattern of injury may be seen
- Steatosis
- Canalicular cholestasis
- Fibrosis; cirrhosis may develop

Ultrastructural Findings
- Concentric irregular membranous arrays in the cytoplasm of hepatocytes

Genetics
- Mutation in aldolase B gene, located on chromosome 9q22
- Autosomal recessive inheritance pattern

Differential Diagnosis
- Neonatal hepatitis
- Galactosemia

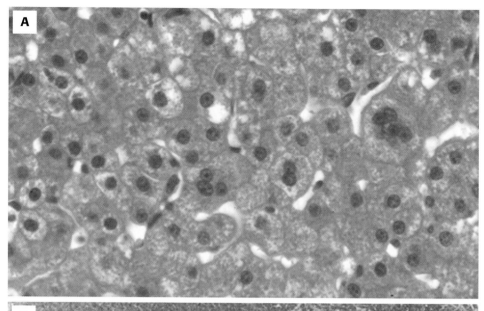

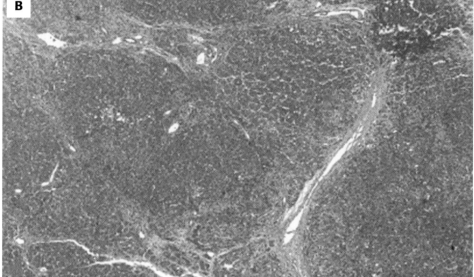

FIGURE 18-10

A, A variable degree of fatty change is seen in hereditary fructose intolerance. Other reported changes include cholestasis and bile ductular reaction. **B,** Periportal fibrosis may develop in children with hereditary fructose intolerance who are given formulas containing the offending agent (Masson trichrome). **C,** Delicate pericellular fibrosis is present in this case (Masson trichrome).

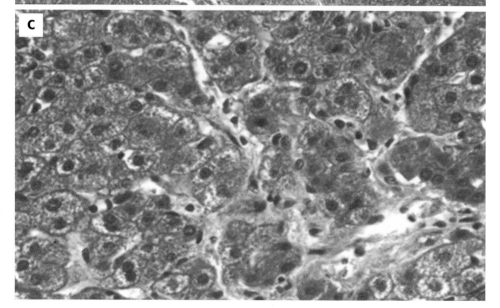

PORPHYRIAS—FACT SHEET

Definition

- Disorders of biosynthesis of porphyrins and heme
- PCT and EPP affect the liver; AIP produces nonspecific hepatic changes

Incidence and Location

- Incidence of AIP is 1 in 20,000; may be more common in northern Europe
- PCT is most common porphyria in the United States; common among Bantu of South Africa
- Incidence of EPP is 1 in 75,000 to 1 in 200,000 worldwide

Morbidity and Mortality

- Most patients with AIP have normal life; risk for death with acute attack
- PCT is associated with systemic lupus erythematosus, rheumatoid arthritis, Sjögren's syndrome, acquired immunodeficiency syndrome (AIDS), and hepatitis B and C
- EPP: 10% develop cirrhosis

Gender, Race, and Age Distribution

- AIP: Clinical symptoms are more common in women; usually manifested by fourth decade
- PCT: Sporadic PCT (80%) occurs in male patients; familial PCT is equally common in males and females
- EPP: Males affected twice as often as females
- Sporadic PCT occurs between ages 40 and 50 years
- EPP: Most patients are older than 30 years

Clinical Features

- AIP: Patients present with intermittent neurologic symptoms and visceral pain
- PCT presents with bullous lesions on sun-exposed skin
- Patients with PCT usually have liver damage manifested by elevated serum transaminases
- EPP: Patients present with photosensitivity; may develop right upper quadrant pain

Prognosis and Therapy

- AIP is treated with intravenous heme; good prognosis
- PCT: Approximately 65% develop cirrhosis; approximately 50% develop hepatocellular carcinoma
- Treatment for PCT is avoidance of sun exposure and alcohol; phlebotomy to decrease iron stores if increased; chloroquine is effective in some cases
- EPP: Hematin is effective treatment; liver transplantation for patients with cirrhosis

PORPHYRIAS—PATHOLOGIC FEATURES

Gross Findings

- AIP: No specific findings
- In PCT, the liver may exhibit patchy gray discoloration
- In EPP, the liver is discolored black

Microscopic Findings

- AIP: Nonspecific steatosis, increased iron deposition in Kupffer cells and hepatocytes
- In PCT, needle-shaped cytoplasmic inclusions of uroporphyrin are birefringent, best seen in unstained paraffin sections
- Other findings in PCT are hepatic steatosis, iron deposition, and fibrosis
- EPP: focal accumulation of dense brown autofluorescent pigment in canaliculi, biliary epithelium, Kupffer cells; cirrhosis in 10%

Ultrastructural Findings

- PCT: crystalline inclusions
- EPP: protoporphyrin crystals have a "starburst" pattern

Genetics

- AIP: autosomal dominant
- PCT: familial PCT (20% of cases) is inherited as autosomal dominant pattern; gene is located on chromosome 1p34
- EPP: mutation in ferrochelatase gene on chromosome 18; most cases show autosomal dominant inheritance

Differential Diagnosis

- AIP: drug reaction, chronic viral hepatitis
- PCT: chronic viral hepatitis, iron overload
- EPP: cholestatic disorders, including extrahepatic biliary obstruction

autosomal dominant disorder due to decreased activity of ferrochelatase, is occasionally associated with severe liver damage; the major manifestation is cutaneous photosensitivity.

PATHOLOGIC FEATURES

GROSS FINDINGS

Gross findings are for the most part nonspecific. Excess accumulation of uroporphyrin in PCT results in red fluorescence from fresh liver tissue on exposure to long-wave ultraviolet light.

MICROSCOPIC FINDINGS

Microscopic changes in the liver in AIP are nonspecific and include steatosis and accumulation of iron in Kupffer cells and hepatocytes. Hepatocellular carcinoma may develop in histologically normal liver in AIP. In PCT, distinctive cytoplasmic uroporphyrins may be identified. These inclusions are yellow-brown and birefringent and exhibit red autofluorescence, but they may be difficult to identify in routinely processed sections. Nonspecific histologic findings in PCT include spotty hepatocyte necrosis, mild portal inflammation, and steatosis (Fig. 18-11).

influenced by environmental and host factors, such as drugs, hormones, and diet. Patients with AIP, an autosomal dominant disorder, usually present after puberty with episodes of severe abdominal pain. Peripheral neuropathy may also be present. Patients with PCT, usually an autosomal dominant disorder, present with chronic blistering of sun-exposed skin and usually have abnormal liver test results. Precipitating factors include increased hepatic iron stores, hepatitis C or human immunodeficiency virus (HIV) infection, ethanol use, and estrogen administration. EPP, an

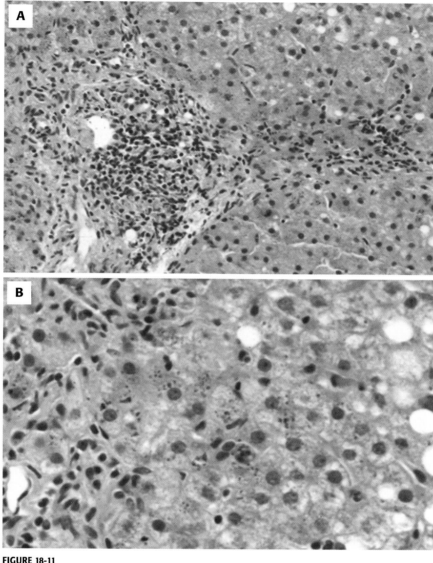

FIGURE 18-11

A, The liver in porphyria cutanea tarda (PCT) may exhibit nonspecific changes such as portal chronic inflammation and mild interface hepatitis. **B,** Iron accumulation in periportal hepatocytes is a common feature.

Increased iron deposition in hepatocytes is a common finding in PTC and is at least in part due to down regulation of hepcidin expression. Cirrhosis occurs in up to one third of cases and may be complicated by the development of hepatocellular carcinoma. In EPP, dark brown protoporphyrin pigment is deposited in hepatocytes, Kupffer cells, and occasionally within bile duct epithelium. Pericellular and portal fibrosis may develop.

ANCILLARY STUDIES

Deposits of uroporphyrin in PCT and protoporphyrin in EPP exhibit red autofluorescence in sections examined under ultraviolet light.

DIFFERENTIAL DIAGNOSIS

Microscopic findings of AIP and PCT are largely nonspecific, with a broad differential diagnosis; demonstration of characteristic inclusions in PCT and in EPP may be helpful, but diagnosis relies on testing for porphyrin precursors in urine and enzyme and DNA analyses.

PROGNOSIS AND THERAPY

Infusion of intravenous heme is used to treat acute crises in AIP; other therapies are largely supportive. Over the past 30 years, outlook for patients with acute attacks of AIP has improved from a mortality rate as high as 80% to approximately 75% of patients reporting normal lives. PCT is treated with phlebotomy to reduce hepatic iron stores and chloroquine; the mechanism of action of the latter has not been established. Disease course often depends on the presence of other diseases, such as hepatitis C or HIV infection. EPP is treated with β-carotene and avoidance of sunlight. Long-term outlook is generally good, with most patients having a stable course for many years.

■ CYSTIC FIBROSIS

CLINICAL FEATURES

Cystic fibrosis (CF) is an autosomal recessive disease caused by mutation in the gene encoding the cystic fibrosis transmembrane conductance receptor (CFTR), which functions as a cell membrane chloride channel. Disruption of CFTR function leads to defective electrolyte transport across the cell membrane; organs most severely affected are the lung and pancreas. The prevalence of

---

CYSTIC FIBROSIS—FACT SHEET

Definition
- Inherited disorder of chloride transport due to mutations in CF transmembrane receptor protein, manifested by lung, pancreas, and liver disease

Incidence and Location
- Incidence is 1 in 2500 live births
- More common in whites of northern European descent

Morbidity and Mortality
- Mortality rate from lung disease is approximately 80%
- Incidence of liver disease approximately 17%, clinically important in approximately 3%
- Up to 10% develop diabetes mellitus
- Median survival 33 years

Gender, Race, and Age Distribution
- Males and females affected equally, but male predominance for liver disease
- Predominantly seen in whites
- Most patients are diagnosed in childhood

Clinical Features
- Most patients present with sinopulmonary disease
- Pancreatic exocrine insufficiency is common
- Rarely present with liver disease
- Diagnosis is by sweat chloride test or genetic testing

Prognosis and Therapy
- Prognosis for liver disease is usually good; liver disease usually overshadowed by pulmonary disease
- Portosystemic shunts may be used to treat portal hypertension
- Liver transplantation is performed in some cases, usually in conjunction with lung transplantation

---

clinically significant hepatobiliary disease in patients with CF is difficult to quantify, but cirrhosis has been reported in up to about 9% of older patients with CF. Liver disease may be manifested as neonatal cholestasis, occurring in 5% of newborns with CF. Up to 50% of these infants also have meconium ileus. Asymptomatic elevations in hepatic enzymes are common in CF patients. The most serious hepatic manifestation, biliary cirrhosis, usually presents as asymptomatic hepatomegaly; portal hypertension and hypersplenism are late occurrences in the course of the liver disease.

PATHOLOGIC FEATURES

GROSS FINDINGS

The liver in CF may appear grossly steatotic. So-called focal biliary cirrhosis associated with CF results in irregular scarring, which may progress to generalized cirrhosis.

MICROSCOPIC FINDINGS

In focal biliary cirrhosis, bile ducts and proliferating bile ductules contain inspissated eosinophilic concretions. Portal tracts in these areas are expanded by fibrosis, and there is a variable inflammatory infiltrate (Fig. 18-12). The fibrous scarring is slowly progressive, eventually resulting in cirrhosis. Bile duct strictures can produce changes of large duct obstruction and may mimic sclerosing cholangitis. In neonatal cholestasis associated with CF, a neonatal hepatitis pattern of injury with

---

CYSTIC FIBROSIS—PATHOLOGIC FEATURES

Gross Findings
- Multiple stellate gray-white scars, irregularly distributed (focal biliary cirrhosis)
- Steatosis in some cases

Microscopic Findings
- Concentrations of inspissated mucus in cholangioles or interlobular bile ducts
- Periportal fibrosis and bile ductular reaction
- Lesions may coalesce to form large irregular scars

Ultrastructural Findings
- Filamentous material in lumen of bile ducts and ductules

Genetics
- Autosomal recessive
- Genetic defect is mutation in *CFTR* gene on chromosome 7q31.2
- No correlation between specific mutations and development of liver disease

Differential Diagnosis
- Large duct obstruction
- Sepsis

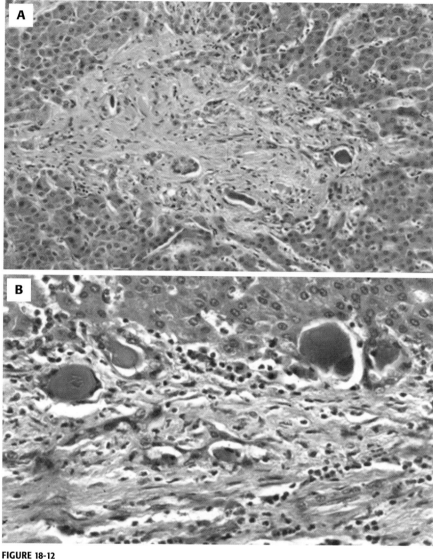

FIGURE 18-12

A, Portal tracts in affected areas of the liver in cystic fibrosis (CF) are enlarged by fibrous tissue. **B,** Inspissated bile plugs lead to localized obstruction and scarring in CF.

marked canalicular cholestasis and giant cell transformation of hepatocytes is seen; additionally, steatosis and inspissated material in bile ducts may be present.

DIFFERENTIAL DIAGNOSIS

The differential diagnosis of CF presenting as neonatal cholestasis includes biliary atresia, α_1AT deficiency, and other causes of neonatal hepatitis. The presence of inspissated eosinophilic material in bile ducts and ductules should suggest the diagnosis. Clinical diagnosis of CF is based on characteristic clinical findings and documentation of CFTR dysfunction, either by elevated sweat chloride concentration or genetic testing.

PROGNOSIS AND THERAPY

Therapy in CF is aimed at reducing complications of the disease. Aggressive nutritional management has reduced the incidence of hepatic steatosis. Combined liver and lung transplantation is sometimes offered to patients with severe pulmonary and hepatic disease. Overall prognosis generally depends on the severity of the pulmonary disease. Median cumulative survival is approximately 33 years.

■ TOXIC INJURY

Liver injury from drugs is a common cause of liver disease and often goes unrecognized; indeed, more than half the cases of fulminant hepatic failure are due to drug toxicity, with acetaminophen the single most common offender. Patterns of injury caused by drugs and other hepatoxins may mimic other types of liver disease, and a high index of suspicion is necessary to make the diagnosis.

CLINICAL FEATURES

Clinical presentation is highly variable and encompasses many of the features of acute and chronic liver disease. Liver injury from exposure to toxins or hepatotoxic drugs may present with fulminant acute hepatic failure or may be clinically silent and manifested only by elevated serum liver tests. Jaundice is a common presenting sign. Systemic signs of hypersensitivity reaction such as fever, rash, and peripheral eosinophilia may be seen. Presumptive diagnosis of drug-induced hepatic injury depends on exclusion of other causes of liver disease and a history of a temporal relationship between drug administration and onset of liver dysfunction. Recovery, even after withdrawal of the offending agent, may be protracted.

PATHOLOGIC FEATURES

GROSS FINDINGS

Gross findings depend on the pattern and severity of injury and range from normal to massive hepatocyte necrosis. In cholestatic injury, the liver is bile stained. Neoplasms such as hepatic adenoma, hepatocellular carcinoma, and angiosarcoma that arise in the setting of drug-induced injury are morphologically identical to their sporadic counterparts.

MICROSCOPIC FINDINGS

Histologic patterns in drug-induced injury may mimic any form of liver disease (Table 18-4). Common patterns of liver injury include bland cholestasis, with bile accumulation in centrilobular hepatocytes and Kupffer cells, little portal inflammation, and no bile ductular reaction to suggest large duct obstruction (Fig. 18-13A). This pattern of injury is usually associated with estrogens or anabolic steroids. Cholestatic drug reactions (see Fig. 18-13B), which may have a component of bile duct injury and destruction (see Fig. 18-13C), are associated with a wide

---

TOXIC INJURY—FACT SHEET

Definition

- Hepatic injury secondary to exposure to injurious chemical agent or drug

Incidence and Location

- 10% of cases of "hepatitis" may be due to drug reaction
- 25% of cases of fulminant hepatic failure are drug related
- No geographic predilection

Morbidity and Mortality

- Depends on severity of injury and offending agent
- Low mortality for mild reactions and prompt withdrawal of injurious agent
- High mortality for agents acting as direct hepatotoxins

Gender, Race, and Age Distribution

- Both males and females affected
- Racial distribution is largely unknown; certain genotypes associated with variations in drug metabolism may be more prevalent in some racial groups than others
- All ages affected

Clinical Features

- Depend on injurious agent and exposure
- May present as mild hepatitis, cholestasis, hepatomegaly
- Severe liver injury is manifested as fulminant hepatic failure

Prognosis and Therapy

- Treatment is withdrawal of injurious agent
- Supportive measures
- Prognosis depends on severity of injury

TOXIC INJURY—PATHOLOGIC FEATURES

Gross Findings

- Variable; dependent on severity of injury
- Hepatomegaly is common
- Steatosis is common
- Massive hepatic necrosis produces a shrunken, flaccid liver with islands of regenerating hepatocytes

Microscopic Findings

- Variable; common patterns of injury include
  - Acute or chronic hepatitis
  - Confluent necrosis, with zonal or multilobular distribution
  - Cholestasis, often with interlobular bile duct injury
  - Steatosis, macro- or microvesicular
  - Granulomas
  - Fibrosis
  - Vascular disorders, such as veno-occlusive disease
  - Neoplasms, such as hepatic adenoma, hepatocellular carcinoma, angiosarcoma, cholangiocarcinoma

Differential Diagnosis

- Viral hepatitis
- Autoimmune hepatitis
- Biliary disorders, such as primary biliary cirrhosis or large duct obstruction
- Sarcoidosis
- Nonalcoholic fatty liver disease

TABLE 18-4

Patterns of Injury in Drug- and Toxin-Induced Hepatic Injury

Pattern of Injury	Morphologic Findings	Examples of Associated Agents
Cholestatic	Bland hepatocellular cholestasis, without Inflammation	Contraceptive and anabolic steroids; estrogen replacement therapy
Cholestatic hepatitis	Cholestasis with lobular necroinflammatory activity; may show bile duct destruction	Numerous antibiotics; phenothiazines
Hepatocellular necrosis	Spotty hepatocyte necrosis Submassive necrosis, zone 3 Massive necrosis	Methyldopa, phenytoin Acetaminophen, halothane Isoniazid, phenytoin
Steatosis	Macrovesicular	EtOH, methotrexate, corticosteroids, total parenteral nutrition
	Microvesicular	Valproic acid, tetracycline
Steatohepatitis	Similar to alcoholic liver disease	Amiodarone
Fibrosis and cirrhosis	Periportal and pericellular fibrosis	Methotrexate, isoniazid, enalapril
Granulomas	Noncaseating epithelioid granulomas	Sulfonamides, numerous other agents
Vascular lesions	Veno-occlusive disease: obliteration of central veins Budd-Chiari syndrome Sinusoidal dilatation	High-dose chemotherapy, bush teas Oral contraceptives Oral contraceptives, numerous other agents
	Peliosis hepatis: blood-filled cavities, not lined by endothelial cells	Anabolic steroids, tamoxifen
Neoplasms	Hepatic adenoma Hepatocellular carcinoma Cholangiocarcinoma Angiosarcoma	Oral contraceptives, anabolic steroids Thorotrast Thorotrast Thorotrast, vinyl chloride

variety of drugs and vary in severity from mild spotty hepatocyte necrosis to fulminant hepatic failure requiring urgent liver transplantation (see Fig. 18-13D). Macrovesicular steatosis (see Fig. 18-13E) is commonly associated with corticosteroid use but is a common pattern of hepatic injury associated with numerous drugs. Microvesicular steatosis is less common (see Fig. 18-13F) but is seen in Reye's syndrome (fortunately rare) and is associated with tetracycline or valproic acid treatment. Non-necrotizing granulomas, sometimes accompanied by numerous eosinophils, are a common finding often attributed to hepatotoxic agents (see Fig. 18-13G). Vascular injury is an uncommon pattern of injury; veno-occlusive disease (see Fig. 18-13H) has been associated with high-dose chemotherapy and ingestion of Jamaican bush teas. A zonal pattern of hepatocyte necrosis (see Fig. 18-13I) is associated with halothane toxicity, acetaminophen, and exposure to hydrocarbons such as carbon tetrachloride.

DIFFERENTIAL DIAGNOSIS

The differential diagnosis for drug-related hepatic injury depends on the pattern of injury. Because drug and toxic reactions can mimic other liver diseases, other causes of hepatic injury must be excluded on clinical grounds, and temporal relationship of the injury to the drug in question must be established. Algorithms for causality assessment, with clinical diagnostic scales, are widely used.

PROGNOSIS AND THERAPY

Therapy, after withdrawal of the offending agent, is largely supportive. Prognosis depends on the severity of the liver injury. For mild liver injury, the prognosis is excellent and full recovery is the rule. More severe liver injuries, such as massive hepatic necrosis, may be rapidly fatal unless liver transplantation is performed. Drug-induced prolonged cholestasis with bile duct injury and destruction may be associated with a prolonged recovery phase.

■ ALCOHOLIC LIVER DISEASE

CLINICAL FEATURES

Excess alcohol consumption is a leading cause of liver disease worldwide. Risk for severe hepatic injury correlates with daily intake, with intake of at least 80 g of alcohol per day being a risk factor for severe hepatic injury. However, only 10% to 15% of alcoholics develop cirrhosis. Three forms of alcoholic liver disease are recognized: hepatic steatosis, alcoholic hepatitis, and cirrhosis; even though progression from milder to more severe forms occurs, these patterns of disease do not necessarily represent a continuum. Hepatic steatosis, the mildest form of alcoholic liver disease, presents with hepatomegaly and

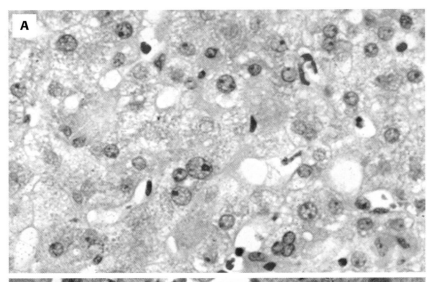

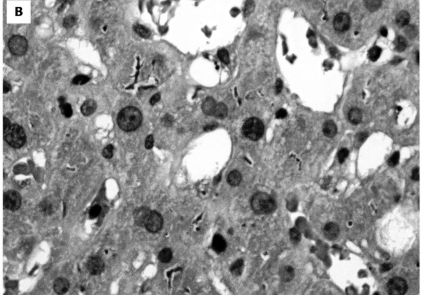

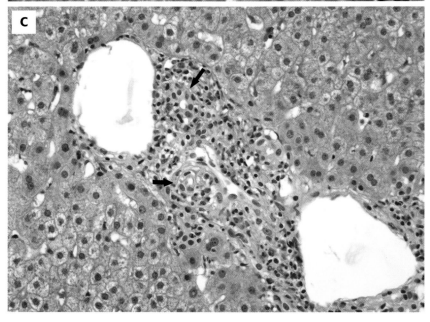

FIGURE 18-13

Toxic injuries. **A,** Bland cholestasis, with accumulation of bile in canaliculi and hepatocytes without significant portal inflammation, is a pattern of injury sometimes associated with estrogen administration. **B,** Canalicular cholestasis is usually more prominent in zone 3 in drug-related hepatic injury. **C,** Bile duct injury and destruction (*arrow*) result in prolonged cholestasis in some cases of drug reaction. Also note the markedly increased number of eosinophils in this example.

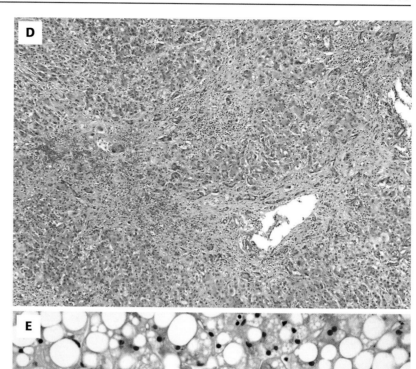

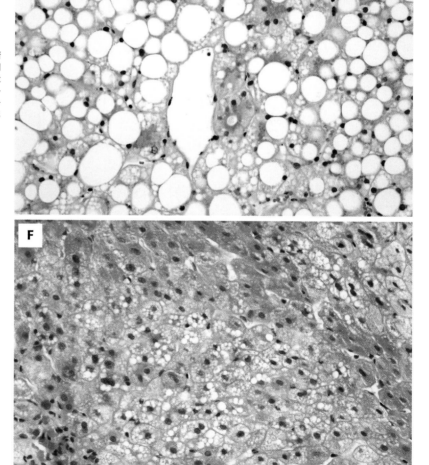

FIGURE 18-13, cont'd

D, Massive hepatic necrosis has led to parenchymal collapse in this case of hepatic injury due to isoniazid; nests of regenerating hepatocytes are separated by collapsed stroma. **E,** Macrovesicular steatosis is a common but nonspecific pattern of toxic injury. **F,** Microvesicular steatosis is less common than macrovesicular fatty change. This pattern is classically seen in Reye's syndrome, associated with aspirin use in children, or in valproic acid and tetracycline toxicity.

Continued

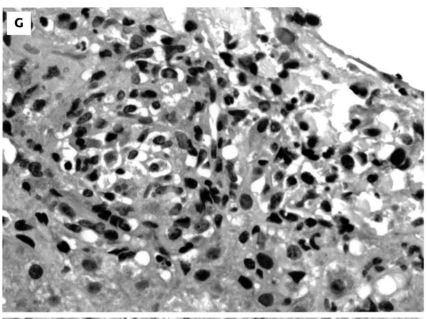

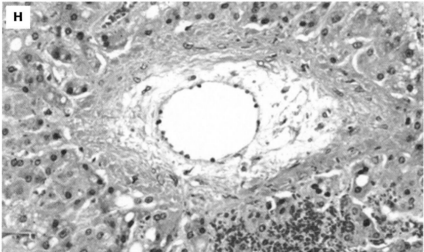

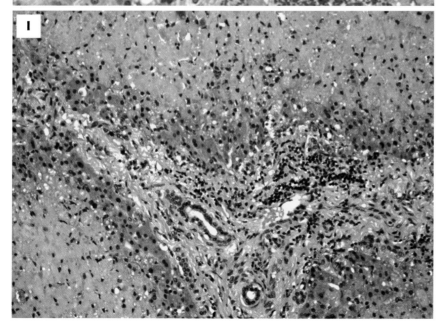

FIGURE 18-13, cont'd

G, Granulomas are a common pattern of injury due to drugs and may feature a prominent eosinophilic infiltrate. **H,** Veno-occlusive disease, or sinusoidal obstruction syndrome, affects central veins and is associated with high-dose chemotherapy used in bone marrow transplantation. The lumen of the central vein is narrowed by edematous fibrous tissue. **I,** Some injurious agents, such as halothane, carbon tetrachloride, and acetaminophen, may cause prominent zonal necrosis without significant inflammation.

ALCOHOLIC LIVER DISEASE—FACT SHEET

Definition

- Liver disease due to excessive consumption of ethanol
- Three patterns of injury occur
  - Steatosis
  - Alcoholic hepatitis
  - Cirrhosis

Incidence and Location

- Prevalence of alcohol abuse is approximately 7% in U.S. population older than 18 years
- 10% to 15% of chronic alcoholics develop cirrhosis; true incidence of milder forms of alcoholic liver disease is unknown
- Worldwide distribution

Morbidity and Mortality

- For hepatic steatosis, full recovery is expected with cessation of alcohol intake
- For alcoholic hepatitis, 10% to 20% risk for death with each episode of hepatitis; may progress to cirrhosis or occur in the setting of cirrhosis
- For alcoholic cirrhosis, 5-year survival rate is approximately 50% for those who continue to consume ethanol; hepatocellular carcinoma is common complication

Gender, Race, and Age Distribution

- More common in men (men are more likely to abuse alcohol)
- Common in all races
- Alcoholic cirrhosis is more common in older adults
- Hepatic steatosis and alcoholic hepatitis may be seen in younger adults
- Steatosis may occur at any age

Clinical Features

- Steatosis presents with hepatomegaly; mild elevation of liver test results
- Alcoholic hepatitis usually follows an episode of binge drinking and is associated with systemic symptoms, such as malaise or anorexia, with or without fever; liver tests are more markedly elevated than for steatosis
- Alcoholic cirrhosis presents with typical signs of cirrhosis; presentation with portal hypertension and bleeding esophageal varices is common

Prognosis and Therapy

- Steatosis has excellent prognosis, with full resolution of abnormalities on cessation of ethanol consumption
- Alcoholic hepatitis may slowly resolve or may progress to cirrhosis; treatment is cessation of ethanol consumption and supportive therapy
- Alcoholic cirrhosis has a poor prognosis in patients who continue to drink, with a 5-year survival rate of 50%; treatment is supportive or liver transplantation

ALCOHOLIC LIVER DISEASE—PATHOLOGIC FEATURES

Gross Findings

- Steatosis: liver is enlarged, yellow, and greasy due to lipid accumulation; texture is soft
- Alcoholic hepatitis: liver may be enlarged; yellow due to fatty change; increased fibrosis imparts a firm texture
- Alcoholic cirrhosis: enlarged liver with micronodular cirrhosis in early stages, with finely granular texture; evolution to small shrunken liver with mixed macronodular and micronodular pattern; often shows broad expanses of fibrous scar

Microscopic Findings

- Steatosis: large droplet fat (macrovesicular steatosis) in hepatocytes
  - Hepatocyte nucleus is displaced to the periphery
  - Usually more pronounced in zone 3, but may be panlobular
- Alcoholic hepatitis
  - Hepatocyte ballooning degeneration
  - Mallory's hyaline, eosinophilic ropey perinuclear cytoplasmic inclusions in ballooned hepatocytes
  - Variable degree of steatosis
  - Neutrophilic inflammation, accumulating around degenerating hepatocytes containing Mallory's hyaline
  - Zone 3 pericellular and sinusoidal fibrosis, progressing to central-portal bridging fibrosis
- Alcoholic cirrhosis
  - Delicate central-portal fibrous septa in early stages form micronodules, which lack internal portal tracts or central veins
  - Hepatocyte regeneration and continued fibrosis lead to remodeling to mixed macronodular and micronodular cirrhosis pattern
  - Steatosis and Mallory's hyaline usually not apparent unless superimposed alcoholic hepatitis is present

Differential Diagnosis

- Nonalcoholic fatty liver disease
- Drug-induced hepatic injury
- Chronic cholestatic conditions such as primary biliary cirrhosis and primary sclerosing cholangitis

PATHOLOGIC FEATURES

GROSS FINDINGS

The liver in steatosis is enlarged, yellow, soft, and greasy. Fat may be irregularly distributed (Fig. 18-14A). Gross findings in alcoholic hepatitis are variable; the liver is often enlarged and steatotic. In alcoholic cirrhosis, the liver is enlarged in early stages, with a finely granular capsular and cut surface (see Fig. 18-14B). The texture is firmer than normal. As the cirrhosis progresses, a mixed macronodular and micronodular pattern may be seen. Broad expanses of fibrous scar are common.

MICROSCOPIC FINDINGS

In steatosis, the hepatocytes contain large clear vacuoles that displace the nucleus to one side. The accumulation of lipid is usually more pronounced in zone 3 but may be panlobular. No inflammation or fibrosis is present.

mild elevation of serum liver test results. Complete resolution after cessation of alcohol intake is the rule. In contrast, alcoholic hepatitis may be life threatening and presents with malaise, anorexia, weight loss, and sometimes fever or jaundice. Liver test results are elevated to a greater degree, and hyperbilirubinemia may be seen. Clinical presentation of alcoholic cirrhosis is similar to other forms of cirrhosis; signs of portal hypertension such as esophageal varices are common initial presenting symptoms.

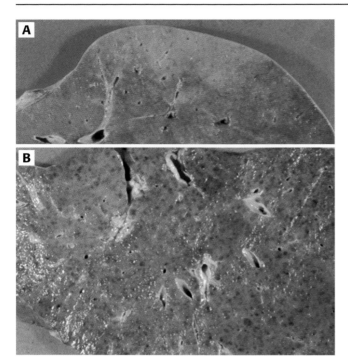

FIGURE 18-14

A, The liver with steatosis is enlarged, soft, and yellow. The fat may be irregularly distributed. **B,** Cirrhosis due to excess alcohol consumption is micronodular, with a uniform cut surface.

Alcoholic hepatitis has four characteristic features:

1. Hepatocyte necrosis and ballooning degeneration. Hepatocytes are swollen, with pale-staining, finely granular or clumped cytoplasm; apoptotic bodies may be present but are less conspicuous.
2. Mallory's hyaline consists of tangled intermediate filaments and appears as eosinophilic ropey cytoplasmic inclusions, usually in a perinuclear location, in hepatocytes undergoing ballooning degeneration.
3. Neutrophilic infiltrate. Polymorphonuclear cells (PMNs) are present in small clusters in the lobule and are commonly found surrounding ballooned hepatocytes containing Mallory's hyaline. A portal lymphocytic infiltrate may be seen but is not a prominent feature (Fig. 18-15A and B).
4. Zone 3 pericellular and sinusoidal fibrosis. Delicate strands of collagen surround centrilobular hepatocytes in a "chicken wire" pattern (see Fig. 18-15C). As fibrosis progresses, central-portal fibrous bridges form, eventually resulting in micronodular cirrhosis.

The degree of steatosis is variable.

Because the micronodules of alcoholic cirrhosis are formed by portal-central bridging, they lack internal structures such as portal tracts or central veins. In later stages, alcoholic cirrhosis is nondescript and generally lacks significant steatosis. Mallory's hyaline is usually not seen.

DIFFERENTIAL DIAGNOSIS

Nonalcoholic fatty liver disease is the major differential diagnosis for alcoholic steatosis and alcoholic hepatitis. In general, PMN infiltrate is less conspicuous in NASH, and Mallory's hyaline is found in only scant quantities. However, NASH and alcoholic hepatitis cannot always be reliably distinguished by morphology, and clinical history is of utmost importance. Therapy with amiodarone, an antiarrhythmic agent, causes hepatic injury that exactly mimics the histopathologic changes of alcoholic liver disease, including alcoholic hepatitis. Again, clinical history is key to making the distinction between alcoholic liver disease and drug reaction. Alcoholic cirrhosis in its early stages is micronodular, but later stages are relatively nondescript, and the differential diagnosis includes other causes of end-stage liver disease, such as chronic viral hepatitis.

PROGNOSIS AND THERAPY

Prognosis depends on the severity of liver injury and abstinence from further intake of alcohol. Steatosis resolves without morphologic sequelae, but alcoholic hepatitis frequently progresses to cirrhosis. Therapy is supportive; liver transplantation may be offered to selected patients who abstain from alcohol.

■ DIABETES MELLITUS

CLINICAL FEATURES

Diabetes mellitus (DM) is a metabolic disorder characterized by chronic hyperglycemia and associated disturbances of carbohydrate, fat, and protein metabolism. Other than nonalcoholic fatty liver disease (see Chapter 19), the two main liver diseases described in association with DM are glycogenic hepatopathy (GH) and diabetic hepatosclerosis (DH). GH is a disease seen in patients with poorly controlled type 1 diabetes, both adults and children, in whom hepatomegaly, abdominal pain, and sometimes markedly elevated transaminases typically develop while the patient is on insulin therapy. Mauriac's syndrome, originally described in children with type 1 diabetes, consists of hepatic glycogenosis with associated growth retardation, dwarfism, and delayed puberty, among other features. This syndrome may represent the full spectrum of abnormalities that can occur in association with GH at an early age. DH, on the other hand, is often clinically silent and occurs in patients with either type 1 or type 2 diabetes. Patients with DH are typically adults with long-standing DM and evidence of microvascular disease (especially diabetic nephropathy). DH may represent a hepatic form of diabetic microangiopathy.

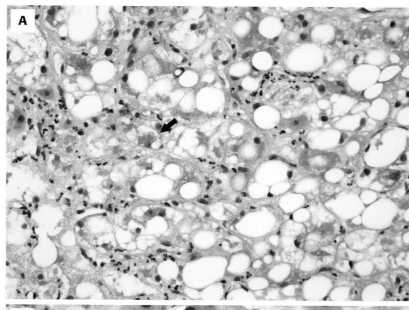

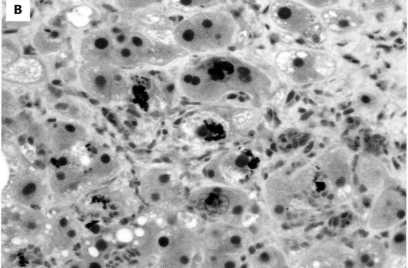

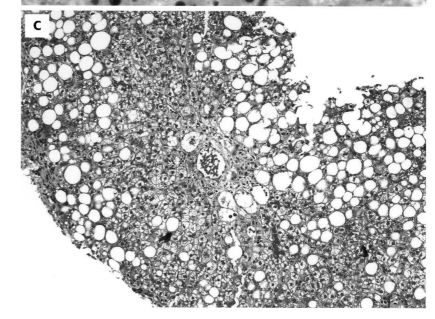

FIGURE 18-15

A, In alcoholic steatohepatitis, the amount of steatosis is variable; hepatocyte injury, Mallory's hyaline accumulation (*arrow*), and a neutrophilic infiltrate are key diagnostic features. **B,** Ubiquitin immunohistochemistry highlighting conglomerates of intermediate filaments in Mallory's hyaline. **C,** Pericellular fibrosis in alcoholic hepatitis has a chicken-wire appearance and is most prominent in the centrilobular region, where ballooned hepatocytes are frequently present.

LIVER DISEASE IN DIABETES MELLITUS—FACT SHEET

Definition

- Liver disease seen in patients with type 1 or 2 diabetes mellitus (DM)
- Two forms of disease are seen (excluding non-alcoholic fatty liver disease)
  - Glycogenic hepatopathy (GH)
  - Diabetic hepatosclerosis (DH)

Incidence and Location

- GH: uncommon, only case series reported in literature; liver is primarily affected
- DH: prevalence of 12% in diabetic patients without NAFLD (large autopsy series); often associated with end-stage renal disease

Gender, Race, and Age Distribution

- GH: affects both males and females, children and young adults
- DH: both males and females, usually middle age and older (mean age 56)
- No reported specific racial distribution for either GH or DH

Clinical Features

- GH
  - Hepatomegaly, abdominal pain, elevated transaminases (up to 10 times greater than upper limits of normal), modest elevation of alkaline phosphatase
  - Ascites is present in some cases
  - Other abnormalities include dwarfism/growth retardation, delayed puberty, cushingoid features, and hypercholesterolemia (Mauriac's syndrome, as originally reported in pediatric patients)
  - Patients often present with findings of poorly controlled type 1 DM, such as marked hyperglycemia, elevated hemoglobin A1c, and diabetic ketoacidosis
- DH
  - Elevated alkaline phosphatase and mild transaminase elevation common in patients undergoing biopsy
  - More often subclinical in autopsy series
  - Significant association with diabetes-related end-organ damage (especially end-stage renal disease)

Prognosis and Therapy

- GH: liver dysfunction and symptoms gradually improve upon normalization of glycemia
- DH: prognosis unclear; may represent a form of end-organ damage—a manifestation of microvascular disease in the liver

PATHOLOGIC FEATURES

MICROSCOPIC FINDINGS

In GH, the most striking feature is the prominent cytoplasmic clearing of hepatocytes, which appear enlarged and swollen, compressing adjacent sinusoids. Hepatocyte cell membranes are often distinct due to the pronounced cytoplasmic rarefaction. Nuclear glycogenation is also common. Megamitochondria, seen as eosinophilic cytoplasmic globules, may also be present. Otherwise, the liver architecture is preserved and no other consistent abnormalities are seen. Specifically, changes such as steatosis, inflammation, acidophil bodies, and fibrosis are either absent or minimal. PAS stain is useful to highlight the presence of abundant cytoplasmic glycogen (Fig. 18-16).

LIVER DISEASE IN DIABETES MELLITUS—PATHOLOGIC FEATURES

Gross Findings

- Gross findings not well described. Advanced fibrosis and steatosis are not features of either GH or DH
- Hepatomegaly is a common clinical finding in GH

Microscopic Findings

- GH
  - Marked glycogen accumulation in the cytoplasm of hepatocytes, leading to a diffusely pale, swollen appearance
  - Overall preserved liver architecture, with no significant fibrosis
  - Minimal or no inflammation, steatosis, or acidophil bodies
  - Special stains (PAS) and electron microscopy can confirm the presence of cytoplasmic glycogen
- DH
  - Prominent, dense perisinusoidal (pericellular) fibrosis, typically involving the centrilobular (zone 3) region, often extending to zone 2
  - Azonal distribution of perisinusoidal fibrosis is seen in a minority of cases
  - Immunohistochemically, the presence of basement membrane components (laminin and type IV collagen) can be demonstrated in a perisinusoidal distribution (not seen in normal livers)

Differential Diagnosis

- GH: glycogen storage diseases, microvesicular steatosis, hepatocyte ballooning degeneration, cholate stasis (feathery degeneration), drug-induced hepatocyte cytoplasmic changes
- DH: other cases of perisinusoidal fibrosis: steatohepatitis (alcoholic and nonalcoholic), chronic venous outflow obstruction

In DH, the main histologic finding is a conspicuous, dense perisinusoidal fibrosis without associated features of steatohepatitis. The perisinusoidal fibrosis usually involves zone 3 (centrilobular) hepatocytes, but zone 2 is also commonly affected. In a minority of cases, the fibrosis is azonal. Additional features seen in most cases include eccentric central perivenular fibrosis, thickening of the hepatic artery wall, and portal lipogranulomas (Fig. 18-17).

DIFFERENTIAL DIAGNOSIS

The differential diagnosis of GH includes glycogen storage diseases, as well as other genetic disorders. The clinical setting in which these occur should make the diagnosis clear in most cases. Microvesicular steatosis occurs in a very limited number of clinical situations (i.e., acute fatty liver of pregnancy, Reye syndrome, and as a side effect of certain anticonvulsant drugs and antibiotics) and should not be confused with glycogen accumulation. Hepatocyte ballooning, seen in steatohepatitis and other forms of liver cell injury, is not

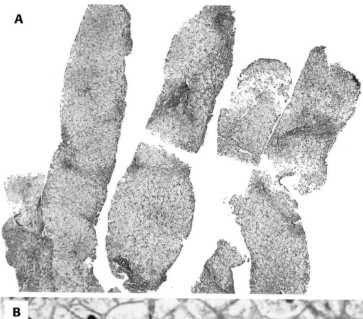

FIGURE 18-16

Glycogenic hepatopathy. **A,** Prominent cytoplasmic clearing is present throughout this biopsy sample from a 14-year-old patient with poorly controlled type 1 diabetes and elevated transaminases. **B,** Hepatocytes show uniform cytoplasmic distention and glycogenated nuclei. **C,** PAS stain demonstrating intracytoplasmic glycogen.

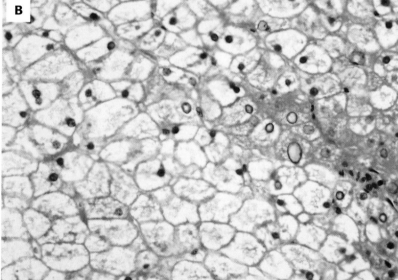

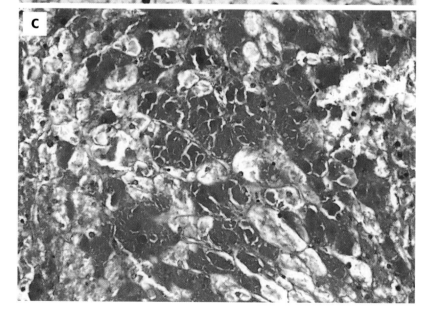

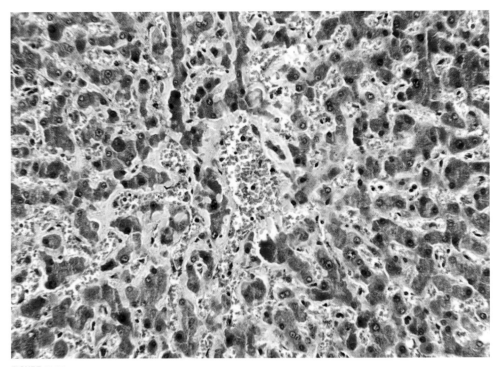

FIGURE 18-17
Diabetic hepatosclerosis (DH). Marked sinusoidal/pericellular fibrosis, often in a centrilobular distribution, is characteristic of DH.

typically as diffuse as the cytoplasmic glycogenation seen in GH and is usually accompanied by other changes, such as inflammation, Mallory hyalin, and fibrosis. Periportal hepatocyte cytoplasmic clearing can be seen in chronic cholestatic diseases (e.g., cholate stasis, feathery degeneration). Special stains can be used to highlight copper or copper-binding protein present in these cases. Cholestasis and other features of biliary disease may also be present. Cytoplasmic clearing can sometimes be seen in the setting of multiple medications and reflects adaptive hyperplasia of the endoplasmic reticulum. PAS stain is helpful and confirms the presence of cytoplasmic glycogen.

The differential diagnosis of DH includes alcoholic and nonalcoholic fatty liver disease. Perisinusoidal fibrosis with a predominant centrilobular distribution is the characteristic pattern of fibrosis seen in steatohepatitis. In these cases, however, one or more additional changes such as steatosis, hepatocyte ballooning, lobular inflammation, or Mallory hyalin are usually present. Perisinusoidal fibrosis may also be seen in chronic venous outflow obstruction. Centrilobular sinusoidal congestion, central vein thrombosis or obliteration, as well as zone 3 hepatocyte changes are often present in these cases. Right-sided heart failure, hepatic vein thrombosis, or other processes causing venous obstruction are often clinically apparent.

PROGNOSIS AND THERAPY

Symptoms and laboratory abnormalities seen in GH gradually improve with adequate glycemic control. The clinical significance of DH is unclear; however, it is postulated to represent a form of microvascular disease, and a significant association with end-stage renal disease is reported.

19

Inflammatory and Infectious Diseases of the Liver

■ **Roger Klein Moreira, MD** ■ **Kay Washington, MD, PhD**

■ NONHEPATOTROPIC INFECTIONS

BACTERIAL INFECTIONS

CLINICAL FEATURES

Bacterial infections in the liver may be manifested by pyogenic abscess, scattered microabscesses with small granulomas (tularemia and listeriosis), noncaseating granulomas (brucellosis), or necrotizing granulomas (tuberculosis). In addition, the liver in sepsis may show a wide spectrum of hepatic injury, such as predominantly neutrophilic inflammation (both portal and lobular) with microabscesses, centrilobular canalicular cholestasis, and ductular cholestasis with ductular proliferation and inspissated bile. Only pyogenic abscess will be considered further here.

Pyogenic abscess usually occurs in older adults; presenting symptoms are nonspecific and include abdominal pain, hepatomegaly, malaise, fever, and, rarely, jaundice. Transaminases and alkaline phosphatase are usually elevated.

In general, pyogenic abscesses are secondary infections seeded from other sites, particularly biliary tree, and gastrointestinal tract. More than one microorganism, most commonly gram-negative aerobes, *Escherichia coli*, and *Klebsiella* species, is isolated in most cases. Underlying or predisposing conditions include hepatobiliary or pancreatic malignancy (approximately 40% of patients), diabetes mellitus (10%), cholangitis, idiopathic inflammatory bowel disease, appendicitis, and diverticulosis. Tumors, cysts, and infarctions may also become secondarily infected, leading to abscess formation.

PATHOLOGIC FEATURES

GROSS FINDINGS

Hepatic abscesses may be multiple or solitary and are more common in the right lobe. They are similar in appearance to abscesses in other sites and are usually filled with purulent debris. Size is variable, ranging up to 10 cm.

MICROSCOPIC FINDINGS

Pyogenic abscesses consist of central necrotic purulent debris surrounded by a fibrous rind containing inflammatory cells, predominantly neutrophils (Fig. 19-1). The adjacent liver often shows nonspecific reactive changes due to mass effect, including cholestasis, portal inflammation, and bile ductular reaction. Bacteria are occasionally detectable with special stains. In sepsis, inspissated bile may be seen in periportal cholangioles (Fig. 19-2).

ANCILLARY STUDIES

Culture of aspirated abscess contents is useful but may not be necessary if blood cultures are positive.

DIFFERENTIAL DIAGNOSIS

The differential diagnosis of bacterial hepatic abscess primarily includes other causes of hepatic abscess, including amebas, hydatid disease, and necrotic tumors. Amebic abscess is distinguished by finding amebas in the cyst contents. Hydatid disease has a characteristic gross appearance, and scolices are identified histologically. Necrotic tumors may require further biopsy material for diagnosis if only necrotic tissue is received.

PROGNOSIS AND THERAPY

Outcome for hepatic abscesses is highly dependent on underlying comorbid conditions. Traditional treatment of hepatic abscess has been open surgical drainage, although percutaneous drainage or intermittent needle aspiration followed by antibiotic therapy is now widely used. Risk

PYOGENIC ABSCESS—FACT SHEET

Definition

- Bacterial infections spreading to the liver via the portal vein, hepatic artery, or biliary tree; may manifest as hepatic pyogenic abscess

Incidence and Location

- Common in sepsis; pyogenic abscess occurs in approximately 10 per 100,000 hospital admissions; more common in right lobe

Morbidity and Mortality

- Appreciable; depends on organism; for pyogenic abscess, approximately 10% mortality

Gender, Race, and Age Distribution

- For pyogenic abscess, male and female equally affected; no race predilection; any age, mostly older

Clinical Features

- For pyogenic abscess, presenting complaints of constitutional symptoms, sometimes right upper quadrant pain

Radiologic Features

- For pyogenic abscess, decreased attenuation on computed tomography (CT)

Prognosis and Therapy

- Prognosis is dependent on underlying medical conditions. Treatment is of underlying bacterial infection in disseminated cases; for pyogenic abscess, medical therapy, percutaneous drainage in some cases; surgery sometimes required

PYOGENIC ABSCESS—PATHOLOGIC FEATURES

Gross Findings

- Single or multiple abscesses of variable size containing pus

Microscopic Findings

- Exudate contains necrotic liver tissue and numerous neutrophils
- Fibrous capsule in many cases

Fine-Needle Aspiration Biopsy Findings

- Numerous neutrophils in a background of debris
- Organisms rarely identified on Gram stain

Differential Diagnosis

- Amebic abscess
- Secondarily infected tumor, cyst, or infarct

factors for poor outcome include multiple abscesses, malignant etiology, septic shock, hyperbilirubinemia, and fungal infection. Mortality is roughly 14% for patients treated with surgical drainage, followed by antibiotic therapy.

VIRAL INFECTIONS

A wide variety of viruses other than hepatitis A, B, and C may affect the liver, with the results ranging from mild, transient transaminase elevations to dramatic and fatal hepatic necrosis. These viruses are often seen in neonates or immunocompromised persons as a part of disseminated infection.

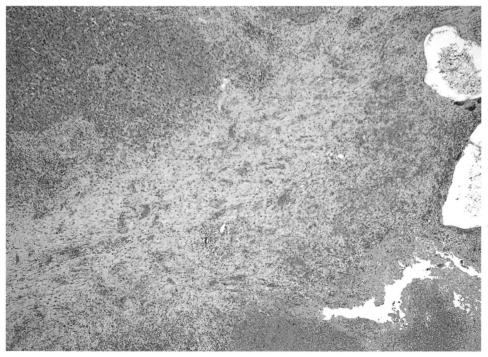

FIGURE 19-1

Pyogenic abscesses in the liver often have thick fibrous rinds; the abscess cavity is filled with purulent exudate and necrotic debris.

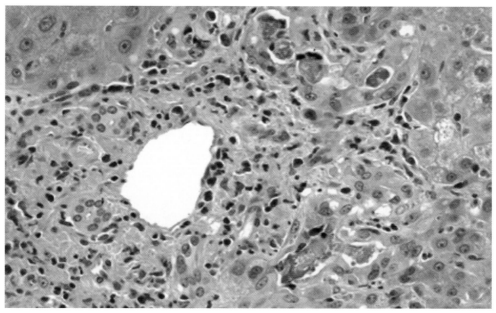

FIGURE 19-2
The most characteristic finding in the liver in sepsis is inspissated bile in periportal cholangioles. Microabscesses may also be seen in the parenchyma.

EPSTEIN-BARR VIRUS

CLINICAL FEATURES

The liver is affected in more than 90% of cases of Epstein-Barr virus (EBV)-related mononucleosis. Hepatic involvement is indicated by elevated aminotransferases, often accompanied by the other symptoms of mononucleosis. Jaundice occurs in only a minority of patients. Fulminant liver failure secondary to EBV infection has been described, particularly in immunocompromised children but also in healthy ones. Fulminant hepatic failure due to EBV may not be accompanied by the typical features of mononucleosis.

PATHOLOGIC FEATURES

MICROSCOPIC FINDINGS

The most characteristic histologic feature in healthy patients is a diffuse lymphocytic sinusoidal infiltrate in a single-file, "string-of-beads" pattern, occasionally containing atypical lymphocytes. Focal apoptotic hepatocytes and steatosis may be seen; cholestasis is not typical. Small Kupffer cell clusters and non-necrotizing granulomas can be seen. EBV hepatitis may also develop after solid organ transplantation, most often in children (Fig. 19-3). The histologic picture may be more severe in this context, with a marked portal and periportal inflammatory infiltrate containing numerous atypical lymphocytes, immunoblasts, and plasma cells, and mild bile duct damage.

ANCILLARY STUDIES

Confirmatory tests include serologic, immunohistochemical, and in situ hybridization studies. Infiltrating lymphocytes are positive by immunohistochemistry for EBV viral antigens.

DIFFERENTIAL DIAGNOSIS

The differential diagnosis predominantly includes other viruses, most importantly cytomegalovirus (CMV) infection. Hepatic involvement by leukemia or lymphoma must also be excluded when atypical lymphocytes are numerous. Human herpesvirus-6 has been implicated in a similar mononucleosis-like illness with hepatic involvement.

PROGNOSIS AND THERAPY

Most patients recover within 4 to 6 weeks without specific therapy; treatment is generally supportive. Rarely, death occurs secondary to overwhelming infection. Reduction of immunosuppression in transplant patients may be indicated.

NONHEPATOTROPIC VIRAL INFECTIONS—FACT SHEET

Definition

- Hepatic involvement by viruses other than hepatitis A, B, C, D, and E

Incidence and Location

- EBV: clinically evident liver involvement in approximately 10% infectious mononucleosis cases; worldwide distribution
- CMV: low incidence of clinically evident disease; worldwide distribution
- HSV: low incidence; worldwide distribution

Morbidity and Mortality

- EBV: low
- CMV: low in immunocompetent patients
- HSV: high mortality

Gender, Race, and Age Distribution

- EBV: adolescents and young adults; males equal to female
- CMV: clinically apparent CMV hepatitis more common in early childhood; transplant and other immunosuppressed patients; males equal to female
- HSV: neonates; transplant patients; males equal to female

Clinical Features

- EBV: usually subclinical; lymphadenopathy; constitutional symptoms; hepatosplenomegaly, jaundice
- CMV: usually subclinical; hepatosplenomegaly; neonates with neonatal hepatitis have hepatomegaly and jaundice
- HSV: severe hepatitis, with liver failure

Prognosis and Therapy

- Variable prognosis, depending on underlying conditions and patient population
- Good prognosis in immunocompetent patients for hepatic CMV and EBV
- Poor prognosis in all groups for hepatic HSV
- Treatment is supportive therapy and antivirals: ganciclovir for CMV, acyclovir for HSV

NONHEPATOTROPIC VIRAL INFECTIONS—PATHOLOGIC FEATURES

Gross Findings

- Hepatomegaly
- HSV: geographic areas of necrosis with hyperemic borders

Microscopic Findings

- EBV: sinusoidal lymphocytosis with "string of pearls" pattern of lymphocytes in sinusoids
- CMV: nuclear inclusions in enlarged cells
- Involves biliary epithelium, endothelium, and less commonly, hepatocytes
- Hepatic microabscesses in transplant patients
- HSV: randomly distributed areas of coagulative necrosis; multinucleated hepatocytes with ground-glass nuclear inclusions

Ultrastructural Findings

- Demonstration of viral particles in infected cells

Immunohistochemistry

- EBV: positive staining in lymphocytes for EBV
- CMV: positive nuclear staining in infected cells
- HSV: positive nuclear staining in infected cells

Differential Diagnosis

- EBV: other causes of hepatitis
- CMV: other causes of hepatitis, especially in immunocompetent host
- HSV: varicella zoster infection

CYTOMEGALOVIRUS

CLINICAL FEATURES

The clinical and histologic features of CMV hepatitis depend on the immune status and age of the host. Liver involvement is a common feature of neonatal/

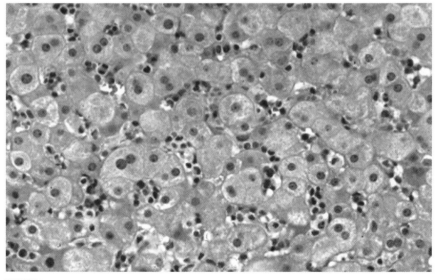

FIGURE 19-3
Prominent sinusoidal lymphocytosis with minimal hepatocellular injury is characteristic of Epstein-Barr virus (EBV) hepatitis.

perinatal CMV infection, with affected infants usually demonstrating marked hepatosplenomegaly and jaundice. CMV hepatitis in immunocompetent persons is often part of a multiorgan infectious process and is usually self-limited. Rare cases of fulminant liver failure have been described, but chronic liver disease does not develop in this population. Patients with CMV hepatitis may show an increase in transaminases and/or a cholestatic pattern of enzyme elevation.

Clinically significant CMV infection of the liver is more commonly seen in immunocompromised persons, and CMV is the single most important pathogen in solid organ transplant patients of all types. CMV infection may be acquired through primary infection, reactivation, or superinfection by a new strain in a previously seropositive patient. Infection occurs approximately 2 to 16 weeks following solid organ transplantation, and symptoms range from mild to life threatening. Although any organ may be involved in these patients, hepatic involvement may predominate; in liver transplant patients particularly, the allograft is the most common site of involvement.

PATHOLOGIC FEATURES

MICROSCOPIC FINDINGS

In immunocompromised patients, CMV-infected cells are markedly enlarged and contain the characteristic "owl's eye" inclusions (Fig. 19-4). Inclusions may be seen in any cell type within the liver, including hepatocytes, bile duct cells, and endothelial cells. Infected cells are often surrounded by neutrophilic microabscesses, with or without admixed mononuclear cells, but may have only minimal accompanying inflammation. Other associated features include hepatocyte apoptosis and focal necrosis; a portal and lobular mononuclear cell infiltrate; and rarely granulomas. In immunocompetent patients, liver biopsy resembles EBV infection histologically. Viral inclusions are not seen on routine stains or immunohistochemical studies in these patients. In the neonate, CMV infection may cause a neonatal hepatitis pattern of injury, with marked cholestasis, giant cell transformation, focal necrosis, and prominent extramedullary hematopoiesis. Viral inclusions are variable in number. Bile duct damage may lead to nonsyndromic paucity of intrahepatic bile ducts.

ANCILLARY STUDIES

Viral inclusions may be demonstrated by immunohistochemical stains for CMV, most commonly in immunocompromised hosts. Other useful diagnostic aids include viral culture, polymerase chain reaction assays, in situ hybridization, and CMV serologic studies/antigen tests.

DIFFERENTIAL DIAGNOSIS

Other viral infections, particularly EBV, should be considered in the differential diagnosis in healthy persons. In immunocompromised patients, the differential diagnosis is broader and includes herpes virus and adenovirus; in most cases, characteristic viral inclusions

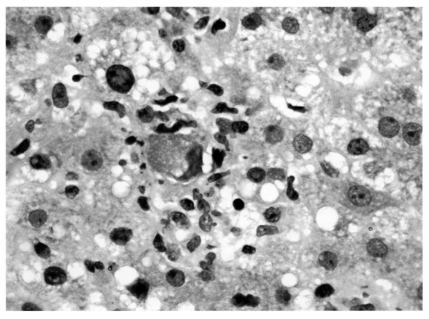

FIGURE 19-4

In immunocompromised hosts, enlarged cells with intranuclear inclusions are found in variable numbers. Associated microabscesses are often seen in liver transplant cases, but are not specific for cytomegalovirus (CMV) infection.

or immunohistochemical staining is diagnostic. Other causes of microabscesses, such as sepsis, should be considered, particularly in transplant patients. In the neonate, the differential diagnosis includes other causes of neonatal hepatitis and paucity of interlobular bile ducts, depending on the pattern of injury.

PROGNOSIS AND THERAPY

Treatment for immunocompromised patients and neonates is with ganciclovir. In most immunocompetent patients, CMV hepatitis is mild and self-limited. CMV infection in early childhood may result in hepatomegaly and chronic low-grade liver dysfunction. In the first year after liver transplantation, CMV infection is associated with a fourfold increase in the relative risk for death.

HERPES SIMPLEX VIRUS

CLINICAL FEATURES

Herpes simplex virus (HSV) hepatitis is usually seen in immunocompromised patients or neonates as part of disseminated infection, although it can be seen in otherwise healthy persons. Patients present with fever and may have concomitant oral or mucosal herpetic lesions, as well as nonspecific constitutional symptoms. Transaminases are markedly elevated, and hepatomegaly is frequently present. HSV hepatitis is rapidly progressive and usually fatal.

PATHOLOGIC FEATURES

GROSS FINDINGS

Grossly, the liver is enlarged, mottled, and shows multiple foci of geographic necrosis, often surrounded by a hyperemic zone (Fig. 19-5).

MICROSCOPIC FINDINGS

Randomly distributed zones of coagulative necrosis surrounded by congested parenchyma are typical of HSV hepatitis. Infected hepatocytes contain nuclear ground-glass inclusions and are often multinucleated (Fig. 19-6). Cowdry A-type inclusions are also seen. Inflammatory response is generally minimal.

ANCILLARY STUDIES

Even though HSV inclusions are readily visualized in liver biopsy material, viral culture is a valuable confirmatory tool. Immunohistochemistry is commonly used, and in situ hybridization is available in some centers.

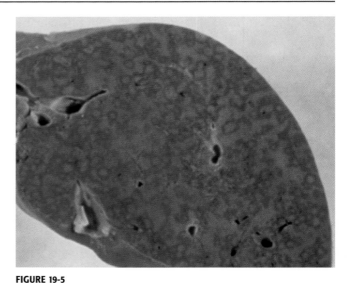

FIGURE 19-5
Areas of geographic necrosis with hyperemic borders are seen in herpes simplex hepatitis.

DIFFERENTIAL DIAGNOSIS

The differential diagnosis predominantly includes other viral infections, including CMV and adenovirus. Herpesvirus and varicella-zoster virus may produce an identical histologic lesion, and viral cultures may be needed to make the distinction. Coagulative necrosis in ischemia or toxic injury is usually zonal in distribution, and viral inclusions are not seen.

PROGNOSIS AND THERAPY

Treatment is with acyclovir. Outcome is poor, with rapid progression to hepatic failure and death. Many cases are recognized only at autopsy.

PARASITIC INFECTIONS

SCHISTOSOMIASIS

CLINICAL FEATURES

Schistosomiasis is a trematode fluke infection common in tropical areas. Infecting more than 200 million people, it is the most common cause of portal hypertension in the world. Most hepatobiliary disease is caused by *Schistosoma mansoni*, *S. japonicum*, and *S. mekongi*, which prefer the mesenteric vascular bed. Adult worms lodge in species-specific target vessels, where they may live for decades. Liver disease is the result of entrapment of eggs that lodge in small portal vein radicals; hypersensitivity reaction to the eggs results in inflammation, leading to fibrosis and

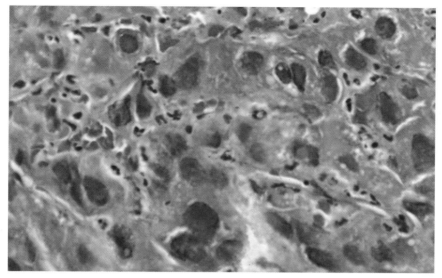

FIGURE 19-6

Herpes simplex hepatitis: Infected cells contain ground-glass nuclear inclusions; multinucleated cells may be seen.

obstructive hepatobiliary disease. Presinusoidal portal hypertension leads to hepatosplenomegaly and esophageal and gastric varices. Hepatic function is usually preserved.

PATHOLOGIC FEATURES

GROSS FINDINGS

Grossly, the liver is enlarged and nodular. Thick fibrosis surrounding large portal areas, known as pipestem or Symmers fibrosis, is noted on examination of the cut surface.

MICROSCOPIC FINDINGS

In early schistosomiasis, eosinophilic abscesses may be seen surrounding ova newly lodged in small portal vein radicals. In chronic disease, epithelioid granulomas and fibrous scar tissue develop around the eggs. Calcified shells of dead ova are seen in long-standing lesions (Fig. 19-7). Whereas the eggs of various species differ in morphology, speciation of schistosomes within the liver may be difficult.

Progressive fibrosis leads to enlarged, sclerotic portal tracts. Although portal-portal bridging fibrous septa develop, the hepatic parenchyma remains largely unaffected, and cirrhosis does not develop. Portal hypertension is the result of the inflammatory process and fibrosis in the

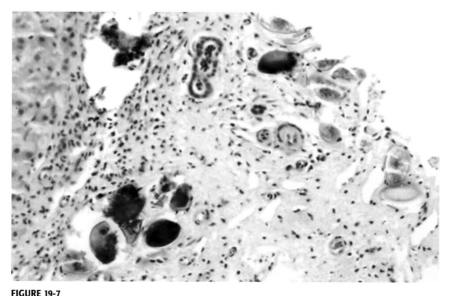

FIGURE 19-7

Calcified schistosomal eggs may be found in portal tracts; earlier, a granulomatous response to the eggs may be seen.

PARASITIC INFECTIONS—FACT SHEET

Definition

- Hepatic infection by parasitic pathogens, most commonly *Schistosoma* species and other biliary trematodes, various helminths, liver flukes, and *Echinococcus* species, as well as protozoal pathogens, most commonly *Entamoeba histolytica*

Incidence and Location

- Schistosomiasis is common in parts of Asia, Africa, the Middle East, and Central and South America; more than 200 million are infected worldwide
- Liver flukes are common in Southeast Asia; 10% of population has symptomatic infection in Thailand
- *E. granulosus* is found worldwide, whereas *E. multilocularis* is found mainly in Arctic regions, central Europe, and central Asia
- Amebic abscess is widespread; approximately 10% of world population may be asymptomatic carriers of *E. histolytica*; hepatic abscess is less common

Morbidity and Mortality

- Morbidity of schistosomiasis is related to development of portal hypertension
- Mortality of liver flukes is related to development of cholangiocarcinoma
- Mortality for *E. granulosus* infection is low with modern therapies; higher for *E. multilocularis*

Gender, Race, and Age Distribution

- Males and females equally susceptible; exposure may vary by occupation
- All races affected
- Wide age range

Clinical Features

- Patients with schistosomiasis may present with splenomegaly and gastrointestinal bleeding from portal hypertension
- Patients with hydatid cyst may present with symptoms of a space-occupying lesion
- Patients with liver fluke infection are frequently asymptomatic, and clinical disease is insidious
- Amebic abscess usually presents with hepatomegaly and fever; serologic tests are diagnostic

Prognosis and Therapy

- Praziquantel is used to treat schistosomiasis
- Surgery is often indicated for resectable hidatid cysts
- Albendazole is used to treat cysts, followed by percutaneous injection of the cyst with hypertonic saline to kill scolices
- Liver fluke infection is treated with praziquantel

PARASITIC INFECTIONS—PATHOLOGIC FEATURES

Gross Findings

- Schistosomiasis exhibits characteristic thick periportal fibrosis (Symmers clay pipestem fibrosis)
- Hydatid cysts contain daughter cysts surrounded by white membranes. Infiltrative lesions may occur in *E. multilocularis* infection
- Biliary strictures and calculi are frequent in liver fluke infection; the liver is enlarged but not cirrhotic; worms may be identified in the bile duct lumen

Microscopic Findings

- Schistosomal eggs are surrounded by epithelioid granulomas; the eggs may be obliterated by fibrous tissue or calcified and are usually located in portal tracts
- Hydatid cysts are surrounded by a multi-layered cyst wall; protoscolices bud from the inner germinal membrane; shed hooklets are found within the cyst
- Liver flukes are found in the distal bile ducts; associated biliary epithelium is hyperplastic; ascending cholangitis may be seen

Fine-Needle Aspiration Biopsy Findings

- For hydatid cyst, scolices with hooklets, positive with modified acid-fast stain. Scolices rarely present in *E. multilocularis* infection

Differential Diagnosis

- Pyogenic abscess
- Amebic abscess
- Sarcoidosis and other causes of hepatic granulomas
- Recurrent pyogenic cholangitis

DIFFERENTIAL DIAGNOSIS

The differential diagnosis includes other trematodes infecting the liver and biliary tree, such as the flukes, *Clonorchis sinensis* and *Opisthorchis* species, and *Fasciola hepatica*, which may cause calculi, cholangitis, obstructive jaundice, and a granulomatous hepatitis. Identification of schistosomal eggs within the liver is diagnostic; stool tests may also aid in the diagnosis.

PROGNOSIS AND THERAPY

Effective oral drugs include praziquantel and oxamniquine; cure rate is up to 90%. Surgical intervention, such as shunt operation, for control of portal hypertension may be indicated.

ECHINOCOCCUS GRANULOSUS AND RELATED SPECIES

CLINICAL FEATURES

Hydatid disease, caused by larval stages of the cestodes of the genus *Echinococcus*, is often subclinical, but some patients develop hepatomegaly, marked abdominal

portal tracts with resulting obliteration of portal vein branches. Schistosomal pigment, brown pigment derived from hemoglobin metabolism by the adult worms, accumulates within Kupffer cells and macrophages.

ANCILLARY STUDIES

Stool examination for eggs is the diagnostic method of choice in active infection; rectal biopsy may be necessary to demonstrate eggs in some cases. An enzyme-linked immunosorbent assay (ELISA) is also available.

enlargement and distension, and ascites. In cystic echinoc-cocosis (*E. granulosus*), the most common form of the disease, eggs are transmitted to humans from infected dog feces, whereas sheep represent the main intermediate host in the natural cycle. A more aggressive form of the disease—alveolar echinococcosis (*E. multilocularis*)—is transmitted to humans through infected feces of wild foxes (rarely other canids), whereas rodents serve as the natural intermediate host. The majority of cases of hydatid cysts involve the liver, but pulmonary disease is also common. Brain, bones, and other sites may also be involved.

RADIOLOGIC FEATURES

Hepatic cysts with internal septations and calcification are characteristic of echinococcal infection.

PATHOLOGIC FEATURES

GROSS FINDINGS

Grossly, hydatid cysts in cystic echinoccocosis are large (up to 35 cm), unilocular, and rounded, with a predilection for the right lobe. Multiple daughter cysts are usually present within the cyst, which has a fibrous rim (Fig. 19-8). In alveolar echinoccocosis, numerous small vesicles are present, often forming an infiltrative mass in a pattern reminiscent of a malignant neoplasm. "Metastatic" spread is a well-described phenomenon in this form of the disease.

MICROSCOPIC FINDINGS

The endocyst consists of an internal cellular layer (germinal membrane), from which scolices, or immature heads of adult worms, develop, and an outer layer, composed of hyalinized, laminated, periodic acid-Schiff (PAS)-positive material (Fig. 19-9). Scolices, however,

are rarely present in *E. multilocularis* infection. As the endocyst expands, reactive fibrosis occurs and a connective tissue layer (the pericyst) is formed.

ANCILLARY STUDIES

Aspiration of cyst fluid is not indicated because of risk for spread of infection and anaphylaxis. Serology (indirect hemaglutination test or ELISA) or detection of circulating antigens to hydatid infection is the preferred form of diagnosis.

DIFFERENTIAL DIAGNOSIS

The differential diagnosis includes other cystic lesions. The scolex of the worm distinguishes hydatid disease from amebic abscess, pyogenic abscess, or noninfectious processes such as fibropolycystic liver disease. Grossly, alveolar echinoccocosis may be confused with infiltrating malignant tumors.

PROGNOSIS AND THERAPY

Treatment is largely surgical, with complete excision of the cysts being the preferred therapy. The cyst fluid is strikingly antigenic and may lead to anaphylaxis if spilled during operation. Intraperitoneal spread of infective material can also occur during surgery. Albendazole may prove effective in inoperable cases and is an effective treatment for small, incidentally discovered cysts. Ultimately, some patients develop liver failure, portal hypertension, involvement of adjacent organs, and death. Because of its infiltrative growth pattern and potential for distant spread, alveolar echinoccocosis is usually fatal if left untreated.

■ VIRAL HEPATITIS

ACUTE VIRAL HEPATITIS

Viral hepatitis may be defined as hepatocyte necrosis and hepatic inflammation resulting from systemic viral infection and leading to a characteristic constellation of clinical and morphologic features. Most cases are caused by one of four well-known hepatotropic viruses (hepatitis A, B, C, or E); hepatitis B infection may be further complicated by coinfection or superinfection with hepatitis D. Other agents of viral hepatitis are postulated, based in part on the continued, albeit rare, occurrence of hepatitis following transfusion, despite screening of blood donors for known infectious agents.

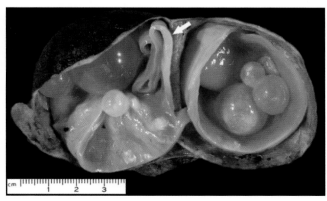

FIGURE 19-8

Echinococcal infection: Hydatid cysts have a characteristic multiloculated appearance due to the presence of numerous daughter cysts. The yellow, gelatinous wall represents the acellular, laminated layer of the endocyst (*arrow*). Also note the outer, white, reactive connective tissue capsule surrounding the endocyst (pericyst).

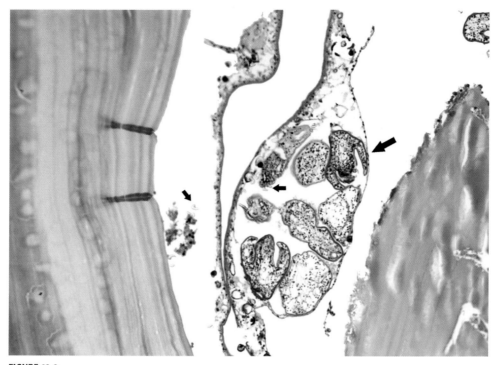

FIGURE 19-9

Echinococcal infection: The outer, acellular laminated layer forms the outer layer of the endocyst (*left*). The cellular (germinal) layer containing protoscoleces (*larger arrow*) and scattered refractile hooklets (*small arrows*) are seen at the center of the image.

Viral hepatitis is divided into acute and chronic forms, based on evidence of chronicity (Fig. 19-10). The term *chronic hepatitis* is used when hepatic necrosis and inflammation are present for at least 6 months (Figs. 19-11 and 19-12).

CLINICAL FEATURES

Acute viral hepatitis is often asymptomatic and undiagnosed and recognized only in retrospect when serologic testing reveals past infection. In many patients, symptoms are mild and nonspecific and include malaise, fatigue, low-grade fever, and flulike complaints. Asymptomatic or mild inapparent cases of acute viral hepatitis are more common in children; adults are more likely to be symptomatic.

Symptomatic acute viral hepatitis is generally preceded by a prodrome phase lasting from a few days to several weeks and characterized by nonspecific symptoms such as nausea and vomiting, myalgias, anorexia, and malaise. Once jaundice appears, the constitutional symptoms typically begin to wane. Physical examination is notable only for jaundice and hepatomegaly; the liver may be tender to palpation in some patients. Serum transaminases are elevated, usually in the range of five- to 10-fold above normal. Alkaline phosphatase is only mildly elevated; conjugated hyperbilirubinemia is present in some but not all patients. Full recovery usually occurs within weeks, but in some cases convalescence may be

prolonged. In a small minority of cases of acute viral hepatitis (<1%), fulminant hepatic failure may develop, as evidenced by the rapid development of liver failure. The clinical course is characterized by coagulopathy and encephalopathy; the mortality rate may exceed 80% without liver transplantation.

Hepatitis A and E are transmitted by fecal-oral routes or ingestion of contaminated water. Hepatitis B and C are transmitted parenterally (Table 19-1), although in a significant number of hepatitis C cases, the route of transmission is unknown.

PATHOLOGIC FEATURES

GROSS FINDINGS

The liver may be swollen in acute hepatitis and may be discolored yellow or green due to jaundice. In massive hepatic necrosis, the liver is soft and flaccid, with a wrinkled capsule. Islands of regenerating hepatocytes may be randomly scattered throughout the parenchyma or may cluster in one lobe.

MICROSCOPIC FINDINGS

On low power, the necroinflammatory process involves all areas of the lobule and is not confined to portal regions. The combination of hepatocyte loss and regeneration and a mononuclear inflammatory infiltrate leads to lobular disarray, reflecting the disruption of the normal

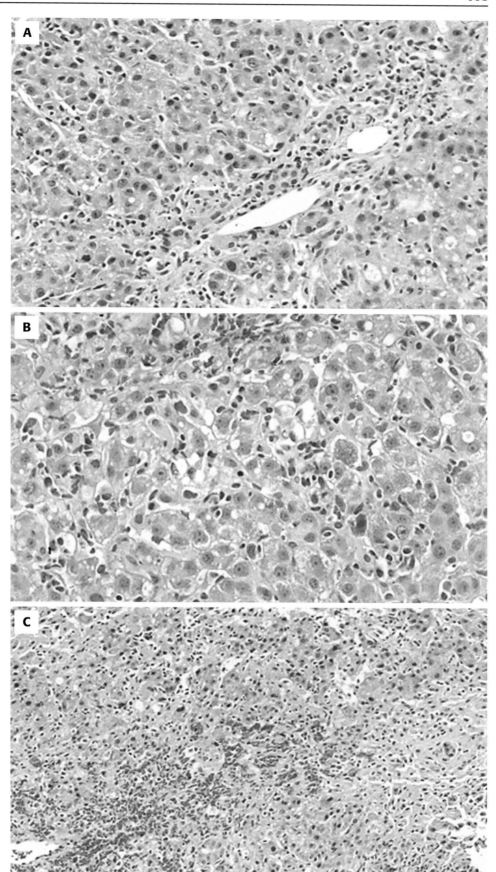

FIGURE 19-10

A, Both portal and lobular inflammation is seen in acute hepatitis; the inflammatory infiltrate is mixed, but mononuclear cells predominate. **B,** Hepatocyte necrosis and regeneration, inflammation, and Kupffer cell hyperplasia contribute to the busy appearance of the lobule (lobular disarray). **C,** Portal-central bridging may be seen in more severe cases and may be an adverse prognostic feature in older patients.

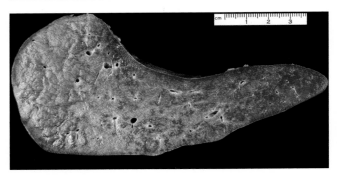

FIGURE 19-11
Massive hepatic necrosis in acute viral hepatitis. The liver is shrunken and soft; islands of regenerating hepatocytes (*right*) may be localized to one area and mimic a neoplasm.

orderly architecture of the liver cell plates. Nonspecific steatosis may also be seen.

Hepatocellular changes include ballooning degeneration, in which the affected cells are swollen and pale-staining, with clumping of cytoplasm around the nucleus and various forms of hepatocyte necrosis. Ballooned hepatocytes often undergo lytic necrosis, marked by small clusters of mononuclear inflammatory cells. Hepatocytes may also undergo acidophilic changes, in which the cell becomes shrunken, angular, and hypereosinophilic, with a densely staining pyknotic nucleus. Such cells may develop into acidophilic bodies (apoptotic bodies) and small mummified rounded cell remnants, and they may extrude nuclear fragments. Individual or small clusters of necrotic hepatocytes are collectively referred to as *spotty hepatocyte necrosis*.

The inflammatory infiltrate in acute hepatitis is primarily mononuclear and is composed of lymphocytes, macrophages, scattered eosinophils, and occasional plasma cells and neutrophils. In contrast to chronic hepatitis, in which portal inflammation usually predominates, in acute hepatitis the inflammatory infiltrate is generally not concentrated in portal tracts but is spread throughout the lobule. Sinusoidal mononuclear cells are often prominent. Although the necroinflammatory process is panlobular, inflammation and necrosis may be more pronounced in centrilobular areas in acute hepatitis. Bridging necrosis may be seen in more severe cases, with a zone of necrosis extending from portal tract to central vein, and may be associated with a more protracted clinical course.

In severe cases of acute hepatitis, portions of lobules (submassive necrosis) or entire contiguous lobules (massive necrosis) may undergo necrosis. Proliferating bile ductules with associated neutrophils are prominent in periportal areas.

ANCILLARY STUDIES

Special studies such as immunohistochemistry for viral antigens are generally not useful in the evaluation of acute hepatitis, even in massive hepatic necrosis, because virus is rapidly eliminated from liver cells and is not detectable using immunostains. Serologic studies are generally readily available and are more reliable.

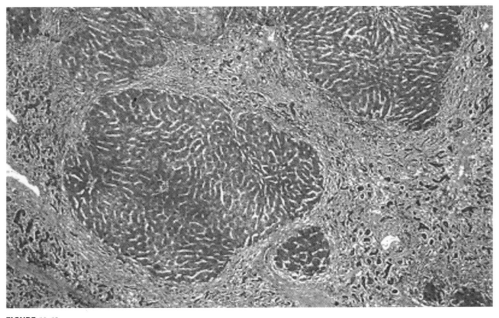

FIGURE 19-12
Massive hepatic necrosis in acute viral hepatitis. Collapse of the parenchymal framework may be mistaken for cirrhosis. Bile ductular reaction is common.

TABLE 19-1

Hepatitis Viruses

Virus	Hepatitis A	Hepatitis B	Hepatitis C	Hepatitis D	Hepatitis E
Type of virus	Single-stranded RNA	Partially double-stranded DNA	Single-stranded RNA	Single-stranded circular defective RNA	Single-stranded RNA
Viral family	Hepatovirus; related to Picornavirus	Hepadnavirus	Flaviridae	Subviral particle in Deltaviridae family	Calicivirus
Route of transmission	Fecal-oral (contaminated food or water)	Parenteral (IV drug use), sexual contact, perinatal	Parenteral; intranasal cocaine use is a risk factor	Parenteral	Fecal-oral
Mean incubation period	2 to 4 weeks	1 to 4 months	7 to 8 weeks	Same as HBV	4 to 5 weeks
Frequency of chronic liver disease	Never	10%	>85%	Never	5% (coinfection); up to 70% for superinfection
Diagnosis	Detection of serum IgM antibodies	Detection of HBsAg or antibody to HBcAg	PCR for HCV RNA; third-generation ELISA for antibody detection	Detection of IgM and IgG antibodies; HDV RNA in serum; HDAg in liver	PCR for HEV RNA; detection of serum IgM and IgG antibodies
Treatment	Supportive	α-interferon, lamivudine	α-interferon, ribavirin	α-interferon	Supportive

ELISA, Enzyme-linked immunosorbent assay; *HBcAg,* hepatitis B core antigen; *HBsAg,* hepatitis B surface antigen; *HBV,* hepatitis B virus; *HCV,* hepatitis C virus; *HDAg,* hepatitis D antigen; *HEV,* hepatitis E virus; *IV,* intravenous; *PCR,* polymerase chain reaction.

DIFFERENTIAL DIAGNOSIS

Major entities that may be confused with acute viral hepatitis are chronic hepatitis, autoimmune hepatitis (AIH), and drug-induced hepatitis. Serologic tests are useful in definitive diagnosis of acute viral hepatitis. If the lobular inflammatory component is prominent, chronic hepatitis may be confused with acute hepatitis, but concentration of the inflammatory infiltrate in portal areas, with formation of dense lymphoid aggregates, and periportal fibrosis favor chronic hepatitis. AIH may have a prominent lobular component and prove difficult to distinguish from acute viral hepatitis; autoimmune markers such as antinuclear antibody (ANA) are helpful but are not always positive early in the course of AIH.

The histologic features of submassive and massive hepatic necrosis are not specific for acute viral hepatitis but may be the result of a variety of insults, such as toxic injury, severe drug reactions, and Wilson's disease. Trichrome stain for connective tissue is useful in distinguishing massive hepatic necrosis from cirrhosis, by demonstrating the lack of dense collagen deposition in massive necrosis. Reticulin stain is also helpful in demonstrating the collapsed reticulin framework of the liver.

Although drug reaction and acute viral hepatitis may have considerable morphologic overlap, prominent eosinophils, granulomas, sinusoidal dilatation, and fatty change suggest drug reaction.

PROGNOSIS AND THERAPY

Full recovery from acute viral hepatitis usually occurs within weeks, but in some cases convalescence may be prolonged. Treatment is generally supportive. In a small minority of cases of acute viral hepatitis (<1%), fulminant hepatic failure may develop, as evidenced by the rapid development of liver failure. Mortality is more common in older patients and in those with chronic liver disease. The clinical course is characterized by coagulopathy and encephalopathy; mortality may exceed 80% without liver transplantation.

Histopathologic features generally are not predictive of progression of acute hepatitis to chronicity. For instance, interface hepatitis is not a reliable predictive feature because it may be seen in cases of acute hepatitis A, which does not progress to chronic hepatitis. Bridging necrosis is predictive of progression to chronic hepatitis in some but not all studies. In patients with massive hepatic necrosis, liver biopsy may not be representative of the overall status of the liver, given the heterogeneity of regeneration and necrosis from region to region.

ACUTE VIRAL HEPATITIS—FACT SHEET

Definition

- Infection by the liver by hepatitis A, B, C, or E lasting 6 months or less

Incidence and Location

- Incidence difficult to measure because many cases are subclinical
- Hepatitis A, B, and C are common worldwide, with hepatitis B more common in Southeast Asia and sub-Saharan Africa
- Hepatitis E is more common in India and Mexico

Morbidity and Mortality

- Mortality rate for acute hepatitis A is low, but up to 22% with clinical apparent hepatitis require hospitalization; mortality rate is higher (approximately 1.8%) in patients older than 50 years
- Hepatitis C commonly (more than 90%) progresses to chronic hepatitis
- Hepatitis B progresses to chronic disease in approximately 10% of cases
- Mortality for hepatitis E is greater in pregnant women; case fatality rate ranges up to 4%

Gender, Race, and Age Distribution

- Occurs equally in males and females
- Occurs in all races
- All ages are affected

Clinical Features

- Common presenting features are jaundice, malaise, nausea and vomiting, and low-grade fever
- Transaminase levels are usually 1000 to 2000 IU/L

Prognosis and Therapy

- Treatment of acute hepatitis is generally supportive
- Hepatitis A virus and E virus never progress to chronic liver disease
- HBV progresses to chronic liver disease in approximately 10% of cases
- HCV progresses to chronic liver disease in greater than 85% of cases

ACUTE VIRAL HEPATITIS—PATHOLOGIC FEATURES

Gross Findings

- Liver is swollen and congested
- May be discolored yellow or green due to cholestasis
- In fulminant hepatitis, the liver is shrunken, with a wrinkled capsular surface and soft texture; islands of regenerating hepatocytes may be seen

Microscopic Findings

- Panlobular inflammatory infiltrate composed of primarily mononuclear cells
- Lobular disarray due to hepatocyte necrosis, regeneration, and Kupffer cell hyperplasia
- Hepatocyte ballooning degeneration and acidophilic degeneration
- Cholestasis is common
- Bridging necrosis is seen in severe cases, with portal-central bridging more common than portal-portal bridging
- Massive hepatic necrosis with panlobular necrosis is the most severe form

Fine-Needle Aspiration Biopsy Findings

- Mononuclear cell infiltrate
- Acidophilic bodies
- Reactive hepatocytes characterized by:
  - Cohesive fragments with irregular, jagged edges
  - Cellular and nuclear enlargement with preservation of low nuclear-to-cytoplasmic (N:C) ratio
  - Binucleation
  - Prominent nucleoli

Differential Diagnosis

- Drug reaction
- AIH
- Other nonhepatotropic viral hepatitides

CHRONIC VIRAL HEPATITIS

CLINICAL FEATURES

Chronic hepatitis is generally defined as liver disease with persistent necroinflammatory activity lasting more than 6 months. As with acute hepatitis, chronic hepatitis has a wide spectrum of clinical manifestations, ranging from asymptomatic infection to decompensated cirrhosis. Many patients are asymptomatic or have only mild nonspecific complaints such as fatigue. Findings on physical examination are few but include hepatomegaly and stigmata of chronic liver disease such as palmar erythema. Patients with advanced cirrhosis may also have ascites and varices. Serum transaminase levels are usually elevated in the two- to 10-fold range, although patients with mild chronic hepatitis C may have persistently normal transaminase levels. Alkaline phosphatase and bilirubin levels are usually normal to mildly elevated, unless hepatic decompensation occurs. Fibrosing cholestatic hepatitis (FCH) is a severe, rapidly progressive form of hepatitis that occurs in immunosuppressed patients in a variety of clinical settings. Although most commonly seen after liver transplantation, FCH has also been reported in patients with chronic viral hepatitis after other solid organ transplants, new HCV infection post solid organ transplant, and in patients with HIV coinfection.

PATHOLOGIC FEATURES

GROSS FINDINGS

The liver may appear grossly normal in early stages of chronic hepatitis. In later stages, the hepatic parenchyma is firm because of increased fibrosis. Cirrhosis due to viral hepatitis is generally macronodular.

CHRONIC VIRAL HEPATITIS—FACT SHEET

Definition

- Chronic infection of the liver by hepatitis B (with or without hepatitis D) or hepatitis C, with clinical symptoms or elevated liver tests persisting for more than 6 months

Incidence and Location

- Common worldwide
- Approximately 3% of world population (approximately 100,000,000) has chronic hepatitis C infection
- Approximately 15% in high-incidence areas have chronic hepatitis B infection
- Rarer in western countries
- 300,000,000 hepatitis B carriers worldwide; approximately 1 million carriers in United States

Morbidity and Mortality

- Lifetime risk for liver-related death is up to 50% in Chinese men with chronic hepatitis B, less in women
- Hepatitis B survival is related to severity of liver disease at presentation: 5-year survival rate is 97% with minimal activity, 86% for chronic active hepatitis, 55% with cirrhosis
- Morbidity is related to progression to cirrhosis, which ranges from 2 to greater than 20 years for hepatitis C
- Liver-related mortality for chronic hepatitis C infection is approximately 11%
- Risk for hepatocellular carcinoma is high in chronic viral hepatitis, particularly for hepatitis B

Gender, Race, and Age Distribution

- Both sexes and all races are affected
- Wide age range for both hepatitis B and hepatitis C; hepatitis B is commonly acquired perinatally in high-incidence areas

Clinical Features

- Chronic hepatitis may be clinically silent
- Patients may present with fatigue and signs of chronic liver disease

Prognosis and Therapy

- Treatment for hepatitis B is α-interferon and lamivudine
- Treatment for hepatitis C is α-interferon and ribavirin
- Prognosis for hepatitis B is related to severity of liver disease at presentation
- Prognosis for hepatitis C is variable; risk factors for progression include presence of fibrosis in liver biopsy, immune status, alcohol use, viral genotype, age older than 50 years at infection, and male gender

CHRONIC VIRAL HEPATITIS—PATHOLOGIC FEATURES

Gross Findings

- Liver may be firmer than normal due to fibrosis
- Nodularity in cases with advanced fibrosis or cirrhosis
- In late stage, decompensated cirrhosis, bile staining may be seen

Microscopic Findings

- Portal inflammatory infiltrate with predominantly lymphocytes; scattered eosinophils, plasma cells, neutrophils may be present
- Interface hepatitis is variable
- Lobular activity is manifested by acidophilic bodies, spotty hepatocyte necrosis, and sinusoidal lymphocytosis
- In severe cases, bridging necrosis linking portal tracts or portal tracts to central veins may be seen
- Fibrosis is primarily portal or periportal, with eventual portal-portal and portal-central bridging and progression to cirrhosis

Immunohistochemistry

- Positive nuclear staining for HBcAg in cases with active viral replication
- Positive cytoplasmic accumulation of HBsAg in hepatitis B corresponds to ground-glass inclusions

Differential Diagnosis

- AIH
- Drug reaction
- Early PBC
- Early PSC
- Lymphoma or leukemic infiltrate

MICROSCOPIC FINDINGS

Regardless of etiology, chronic hepatitis is characterized by a combination of portal inflammation, interface hepatitis, parenchymal inflammation, and necrosis, and, in many cases, fibrosis (Fig. 19-13).

PORTAL INFLAMMATION

In most cases of chronic hepatitis, a prominent inflammatory infiltrate consisting of lymphocytes with a variable number of plasma cells involves the portal tracts. Scattered macrophages, neutrophils, and eosinophils are typically a minor component of the infiltrate. Lymphoid follicles and germinal centers may be seen (see Fig. 19-13A). Bile ductular reaction may be present at the periphery of the portal tracts but is typically not prominent.

Interface hepatitis, also known as piecemeal necrosis or periportal necrosis, is an important feature of chronic hepatitis, although it is focal or not present in cases with minimal necroinflammatory activity. The lymphocytes and plasma cells of the inflammatory periportal infiltrate are closely associated with degenerating hepatocytes at the limiting plate (see Fig. 19-13B). Hepatocytes in areas of piecemeal necrosis often undergo ballooning degeneration and appear pale and swollen, with clumping of cytoplasm. Oncocytic change is also seen in the setting of chronic hepatitis (see Fig. 19-13C). Apoptotic bodies may also be seen in areas of active interface hepatitis. The periportal parenchyma is gradually destroyed and replaced by fibrosis, and this irregular expansion of the portal tracts and periportal regions by fibrous tissue leads to entrapment of single hepatocytes and small clusters of hepatocytes.

LOBULAR NECROINFLAMMATORY ACTIVITY

Hepatocyte necrosis in chronic hepatitis is variable in severity but usually spotty. Apoptotic hepatocytes (acidophil bodies) are scattered throughout the lobule.

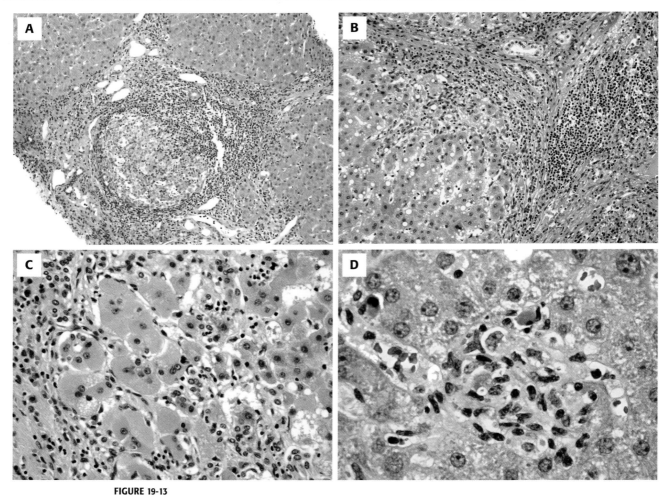

FIGURE 19-13

A, Portal tracts are expanded by an exuberant inflammatory infiltrate with prominent germinal center in this case of chronic viral hepatitis. Interlobular bile ducts show no significant injury. **B,** Lymphocytic inflammation extending into the lobular region (interface hepatitis), causing focal hepatocyte injury. **C,** Oncocytic change of periportal hepatocytes is present in this case of chronic hepatitis C, resembling ground-glass hepatocytes. **D,** Lobular activity is variable; small collections of mononuclear inflammatory cells mark sites of lytic necrosis of hepatocytes.

Mononuclear inflammatory cells cluster around injured hepatocytes and may obscure focal hepatocyte necrosis (see Fig. 19-13D). Kupffer cells in these areas of spotty hepatocyte necrosis may contain phagocytosed cellular debris. Ballooning degeneration of hepatocytes may be seen in exacerbations of chronic viral hepatitis and may be associated with zone 3 cholestasis. Regeneration of hepatocytes is recognizable by the formation of liver cell plates that are two cells thick and by the formation of regenerating rosettes of hepatocytes.

FIBROSIS

Progressive fibrosis at the limiting plate as a result of continued necroinflammatory activity leads to stellate enlargement of the portal tract. Portal-portal fibrous septa are the result of linkage of adjacent fibrotic portal tracts. Portal-central fibrous bridges can also develop, generally from superimposed episodes of severe lobular necroinflammatory activity involving zone 3. The end

result of bridging fibrosis, if periseptal activity continues, is cirrhosis, which is usually macronodular or mixed micro- and macronodular.

ANCILLARY STUDIES

Chronic Hepatitis B

Ground-glass cells containing abundant hepatitis B surface antigen in smooth endoplasmic reticulum are more likely to be numerous in biopsy samples with little necroinflammatory activity. Hepatitis B core antigen (HBcAg) accumulation in hepatocyte nuclei produces a "sanded" appearance, but such changes are difficult to recognize on routine stains. Identification of cytoplasmic hepatitis B surface antigen may be facilitated by use of one of the Shikata stains, such as Victoria blue, orcein, or aldehyde fuchsin, or by immunohistochemical stain. HBcAg accumulation may be identified using immunohistochemical stains, and cytoplasmic or membranous expression of this antigen correlates with high necroinflammatory activity (Fig. 19-14). The FCH variant is characterized by prominent sinusoidal/pericellular fibrosis extending from portal tracts into the lobular region, ductular reaction, hepatocellular changes (including ballooning and ground-glass inclusions), and prominent intracellular and canalicular cholestasis, whereas inflammatory infiltrate tends to be minimal (Fig. 19-15A and B).

Delta Virus

Sanded hepatocyte nuclei may be seen in hepatitis B with delta virus infection. Delta antigen may be demonstrated within nuclei of hepatocytes by immunohistochemical stains. Overall, the histopathology resembles hepatitis B without delta infection, but the necroinflammatory activity is often more severe.

Hepatitis C

Histologically, chronic hepatitis caused by hepatitis C tends to be mild. Characteristic features are portal lymphoid aggregates and follicles, bile duct infiltration by lymphocytes, and steatosis. Dense aggregates of lymphocytes in portal tracts are a distinctive but not pathognomonic feature of hepatitis C. The bile duct injury in hepatitis C is rarely severe, and duct loss is not a feature. The biliary epithelium of affected ducts may be focally disrupted and in addition to infiltration by lymphocytes shows reactive changes such as vacuolation of epithelium and nuclear crowding and enlargement. In addition to bile duct damage, portal eosinophils and endotheliitis

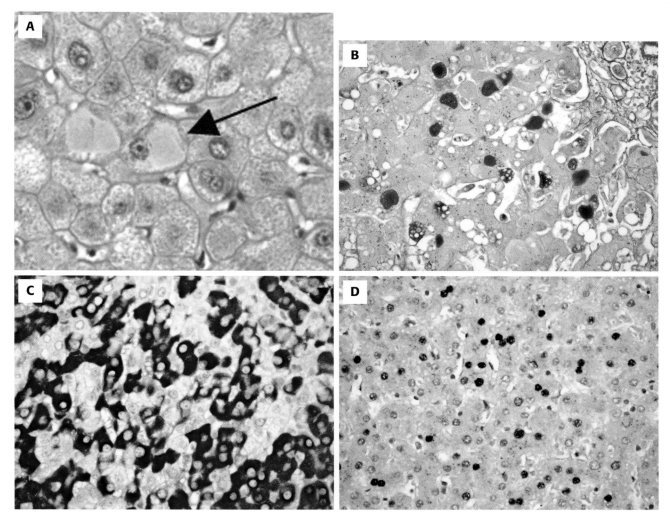

FIGURE 19-14

Chronic hepatitis B. **A,** Hepatocytes with accumulation of hepatitis B surface antigen (HBsAg) have a ground-glass appearance *(arrow).* **B,** Cytoplasmic HBsAg in ground-glass hepatocytes is highlighted by orcein stain. **C,** Immunohistochemistry for hepatitis B surface antigen shows accumulation of HBsAg in hepatocytes. **D,** Core antigen (HBcAg) immunohistochemistry showing nuclear positivity in approximately half of the nuclei in this biopsy, with only trace amounts of core antigen seen in the cytoplasm. Cytoplasmic HBcAg staining correlates with high necroinflammatory activity.

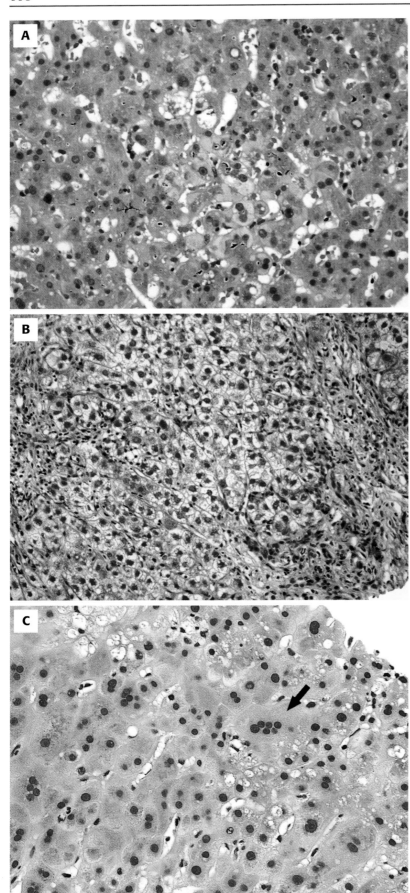

FIGURE 19-15

A, Canalicular cholestasis and hepatocyte injury are present in this case of fibrosing cholestatic hepatitis C. **B,** Prominent pericellular fibrosis extending from portal tracts with associated ductular proliferation are features of fibrosing cholestatic hepatitis C. This lung transplant patient had extremely high hepatitis C viral load. **C,** Giant cell transformation (*arrow*) may be seen in chronic hepatitis C, especially in the setting of HIV coinfection.

can also occur in chronic hepatitis C. Awareness of these "rejection-like" features is important in the posttransplantation setting. Steatosis seen in hepatitis C is usually macrovesicular, may be associated with more severe necroinflammatory activity, and is often particularly prominent in patients with HCV genotype 3. Portal and lobular granulomas may be seen in a small minority of patients with no associated conditions. Granulomas have also been reported as an uncommon feature of recurrent hepatitis C after liver transplantation. Another unusual feature described in chronic hepatitis C is the presence of centrilobular syncytial giant cells. This finding is seen more frequently in the setting of HCV-HIV coinfection but is also seen in HCV monoinfection (see Fig. 19-15C). In contrast to cases in adults, the degree of inflammation is often minimal and steatosis is frequently lacking in children. Fibrosing cholestatic hepatitis C shows similar histologic features to those seen in the setting of hepatitis B (see earlier discussion). Portal inflammation tends to be more pronounced in FCH C than in FCH B, and no ground-glass cell hepatocytes are seen. Reliable immunoperoxidase stains for HCV are not commercially available.

DIFFERENTIAL DIAGNOSIS

The morphologic pattern of chronic hepatitis may be seen in a variety of conditions and is not specific for viral hepatitis. The portal lymphocytic inflammation of early-stage primary biliary cirrhosis (PBC) and primary sclerosing cholangitis (PSC) may resemble chronic viral hepatitis. Loss of interlobular bile ducts is the most helpful distinguishing feature because bile duct loss occurs in PBC and PSC but not in chronic hepatitis. Portal granulomas should suggest PBC in the appropriate clinical setting. Knowledge of viral serologic studies and the antimitochondrial antibody status may be necessary to make the distinction. Cholangiography is usually necessary to establish the diagnosis of PSC. In patients with ulcerative colitis and liver biopsy with a pattern of inflammation suggesting chronic hepatitis, the possibility of PSC should be strongly considered.

Cytoplasmic inclusion mimicking the ground-glass hepatocytes seen in hepatitis B have been described in a variety of conditions, including Lafora's disease (familial myoclonus epilepsy), glycogen and fibrinogen storage diseases, uremia, and after cyanamide treatment. Similar cellular changes can also occur in drug-induced hypertrophy of the endoplasmic reticulum, oncocytic change in the setting of chronic hepatitis, and glycogen pseudoground glass change (most commonly seen in immunosuppressed patients).

Chronic viral hepatitis may be indistinguishable from AIH on morphologic grounds. The presence of numerous plasma cells in the portal inflammation infiltrate and plasma cells in the lobule is suggestive of AIH. Wilson's disease also has a chronic hepatitis pattern of injury on liver biopsy and should be considered in biopsy samples from young patients with negative viral serologies. Serum ceruloplasmin and quantitative copper studies on liver tissue are necessary for definitive diagnosis. α_1-Antitrypsin deficiency may also have a chronic hepatitis pattern of injury; accumulation of PAS-positive, diastase-resistant cytoplasmic globules in hepatocytes is generally evident in liver biopsy samples from adults.

Classic cases of fibrosing cholestatic hepatitis show a characteristic combination of histologic features (see earlier discussion). Individual features, however, are relatively nonspecific and must be evaluated carefully. Pericellular fibrosis may be seen in alcoholic and nonalcoholic steatohepatitis. In this setting, the fibrosis is predominantly centrilobular, rather than periportal, and severe cholestasis is generally lacking. Cholestasis and ductular reaction may be seen in large duct obstruction (LDO), which must be included in the differential diagnosis of FCH in the posttransplantation setting. Periductal edema is often seen in obstructive processes but is not a feature of FCH, whereas prominent hepatocyte damage and pericellular fibrosis are not features of LDO. Other causes of cholestasis in the posttransplantation period such as chronic ductopenic rejection and drug reaction must also be considered.

PROGNOSIS AND THERAPY

Fibrosis on index biopsy is a predictor of progressive disease in hepatitis B. Current treatment strategies include α-interferon and lamivudine, as well as other antiviral drugs. High pretreatment alanine aminotransferase (ALT) and low serum hepatitis B virus (HBV) DNA are predictive of good response to interferon therapy.

Viral genotype may be important in progression in hepatitis C infection, with genotype 1b being associated with more severe disease. Males, older individuals, and patients with other chronic liver diseases are more likely to have progression of fibrosis. Alcohol consumption increases replication of hepatitis C and is associated with more severe disease. In general, grade of hepatic necroinflammatory activity in the liver biopsy correlates with serum hepatitis C virus (HCV) RNA levels, and rate of progression to cirrhosis correlates with high-grade activity and advanced stage in initial biopsies. Hepatic steatosis is associated with increased disease severity, increased risk of fibrosis progression, and lower rates of sustained viral response to HCV antiviral therapy. Conflicting evidence exists regarding the role of hepatic iron accumulation in disease progression and response to therapy. FCH is usually associated with rapid progression of fibrosis, liver failure, and poor prognosis. Early recognition of this variant is essential because prompt initiation of specific antiviral treatment and reduction of immunosuppression may improve the otherwise dismal outcome associated with FCH. Current treatment strategies for hepatitis C are pegylated interferon and ribavirin.

AUTOIMMUNE HEPATITIS

CLINICAL FEATURES

AIH is more common in young women and is associated with other autoimmune disorders, such as thyroiditis and arthritis. Clinical onset is often acute, but liver biopsy often reveals evidence of chronic disease, suggesting acute exacerbation of a chronic process. Patients present with evidence of liver dysfunction, such as fatigue and elevated liver test results; jaundice may be seen in more severe cases.

AUTOIMMUNE HEPATITIS—FACT SHEET

Definition
- Autoimmune liver disease producing hepatitis pattern of injury

Incidence and Location
- Prevalence is approximately 50 to 200 cases per million in Northern Europe and North American white populations
- Rare in Asia and Africa

Morbidity and Mortality
- High rate of progression to cirrhosis if untreated
- 65% 5-year mortality rate if untreated

Gender, Race, and Age Distribution
- Approximately 70% are female
- More common in patients of European white background
- All ages affected: more common between 10 and 30 years and after age 50

Clinical Features
- Often presents abruptly, similar to acute viral hepatitis
- Anorexia, jaundice, hepatomegaly, abdominal pain
- May present with arthralgia and skin rash
- Serologic abnormalities include
  - Hypergammaglobulinemia
  - Positive ANA
  - Positive liver-kidney microsomal antibodies
  - Positive smooth muscle antibodies

Prognosis and Therapy
- Variable clinical course
- Corticosteroids and other immunosuppressants significantly improve survival

---

PATHOLOGIC FEATURES

GROSS FINDINGS

The gross appearance of the liver in AIH depends on the activity and stage of the disease. In severe cases, massive hepatic necrosis or cirrhosis may be seen.

MICROSCOPIC FINDINGS

The histopathology of AIH is relatively nonspecific and variable, ranging from mildly active chronic hepatitis to massive hepatic necrosis to cirrhosis. The necroinflammatory activity is often severe, with marked interface hepatitis and hepatocytic rosettes. Sometimes it is associated with bridging necrosis (Fig. 19-16). Plasma cells in the portal and lobular infiltrate may be prominent, but their absence does exclude AIH. Several nonclassic phenotypes have been described and are now accepted as part of the histopathologic spectrum of AIH. Centrilobular necrosis is seen in patients with acute onset of the disease and may occur in the absence of other classic features of AIH. This feature is thought to represent an early histologic manifestation of the disease. Bile duct changes are seen in up to 24% of cases, most often in the form of nondestructive cholangitis. Whereas destructive cholangitis has typically been considered a feature of primary biliary disease, this finding has been reported in rare cases of AIH that responded appropriately to steroid treatment and that were negative for several molecular markers of PBC.

AUTOIMMUNE HEPATITIS—PATHOLOGIC FEATURES

Gross Findings
- In severe cases, may produce massive hepatic necrosis, with shrunken liver with wrinkled capsule
- In late stages, fibrous scarring produces firm liver, with progression to cirrhosis

Microscopic Findings
- Chronic hepatitis pattern of injury, with portal chronic inflammation
- Interface hepatitis
- Marked lobular hepatitis
- Plasma cells may be prominent in inflammatory infiltrate
- Fibrosis, with portal-portal and portal-central bridging as disease progresses

Genetics
- Genetic predisposition associated with HLA-A1-B8-DR haplotype

Differential Diagnosis
- Other causes of acute and chronic hepatitis, especially viral hepatitis
- Other forms of autoimmune liver disease, especially PBC
- Drug reaction

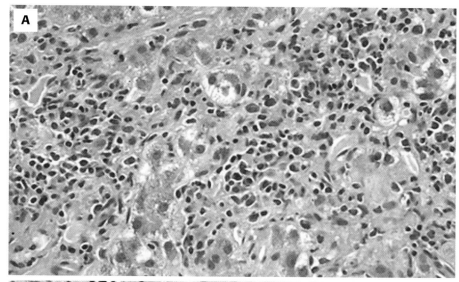

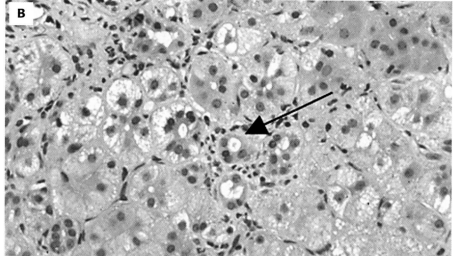

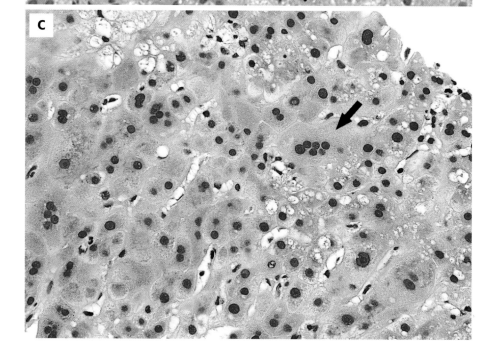

FIGURE 19-16

A, Interface hepatitis and lobular activity are often pronounced in autoimmune hepatitis; plasma cells in clusters in the inflammatory infiltrate are a helpful but relatively nonspecific feature of AIH. **B,** Hepatocyte regeneration may lead to formation of hepatocyte rosettes (*arrow*). **C,** Significant fibrosis, such as bridging fibrosis shown here on Masson stain, is often present on index biopsy in autoimmune hepatitis and is indicative of the chronic nature of the disease.

ANCILLARY STUDIES

Serum immunoglobulin G (IgG) levels are generally elevated. Autoantibodies associated with AIH include ANA, anti–liver/kidney microsomal antibodies, and anti–smooth muscle antibodies. Some cases may be associated with "atypical" serologic markers such as perinuclear antineutrophil antibodies (pANCA). Autoantibodies are absent in approximately 13 % of adult cases of AIH in North America that are otherwise typical cases. Anti mitochondrial (AMA) positivity has been detected in a small minority of AIH patients.

DIFFERENTIAL DIAGNOSIS

The differential diagnosis for AIH includes other causes of chronic hepatitis such as viral hepatitis and drug reaction, as well as other autoimmune conditions affecting the liver. AIH is distinguished from PBC and PSC by preservation of bile ducts in the majority of cases of AIH (Table 19-2). Clinically, PBC and PSC usually present as a cholestatic syndrome, as opposed to a hepatic syndrome generally seen in AIH. Appropriate serologic testing (positive ANA; negative HCV and HBV serologies) aids in distinguishing AIH from chronic viral hepatitis.

PROGNOSIS AND THERAPY

Immunosuppressive therapy is the mainstay of treatment and is effective in many cases, preventing further hepatic damage and prolonging survival. Relapse is common upon withdrawal of immunosuppression, but AIH usually responds rapidly to retreatment. Patients with severe activity have decreased survival.

Liver transplantation is used for treatment of end-stage disease; recurrence in the transplanted liver occurs in some instances.

■ DISORDERS OF THE BILE DUCTS

LARGE DUCT OBSTRUCTION

CLINICAL FEATURES

Mechanical blockage of extrahepatic or large intrahepatic ducts is usually manifested by abdominal pain and elevated alkaline phosphatase and serum bilirubin levels. If bacterial cholangitis is superimposed, fever is generally present.

RADIOLOGIC FEATURES

Ultrasonography may demonstrate dilated intrahepatic ducts but cholangiography, either by endoscopic retrograde or percutaneous transhepatic routes, is considered the gold standard for demonstrating biliary obstruction.

PATHOLOGIC FEATURES

GROSS FINDINGS

Prolonged obstruction can lead to biliary cirrhosis; the liver in such cases is nodular and bile stained. Biliary sludge or stone material may be seen in the obstructed biliary tree, and areas of extravasated bile may form bile lakes or bile infarcts.

TABLE 19-2
Clinicopathologic Features of Primary Biliary Cirrhosis and Primary Sclerosing Cholangitis

	Primary Biliary Cirrhosis	Primary Sclerosing Cholangitis
Age	Median age 50 years (30 to 70)	Median age 30 years
Gender	90% female	70% male
Clinical course	Progressive	Unpredictable but progressive
Associated conditions	Sjögren's syndrome (70%) Scleroderma (5%) Rheumatoid arthritis Thyroid disease (20%)	Inflammatory bowel disease Pancreatitis (up to 25%) Idiopathic fibrosing diseases (retroperitoneal fibrosis)
Serology incidence	95% AMA positive 20% ANA positive 60% ANCA positive	0% to 5% AMA positive (low titer) 6% ANA positive 82% ANCA positive
Radiology	Normal	Strictures and beading of large bile ducts; "pruning" of smaller ducts
Duct lesion	Florid duct lesion; loss of small ducts	Concentric periductal fibrosis; loss of small ducts

AMA, Antimitochondrial antibody; *ANA*, antinuclear antibody; *ANCA*, antineutrophil cytoplasmic antibody.

LARGE DUCT OBSTRUCTION—FACT SHEET

Definition
- Obstruction of large bile ducts by biliary stones, fibrosis, impingement by external structures, or intrinsic biliary lesions

Incidence and Location
- Common; liver biopsy is rarely obtained
- Worldwide distribution

Morbidity and Mortality
- Severe secondary bacterial cholangitis can lead to abscesses and strictures.
- Many hepatic changes are reversible with relief of obstruction
- Biliary obstruction may progress to cirrhosis in cases with long-standing obstruction

Gender, Race, and Age Distribution
- Males and females equally affected; obstruction secondary to gallstones more common in females
- All races affected; gallstones more common in some populations
- Wide age range, depending on etiology of obstruction

Clinical Features
- Persistent jaundice with elevation of alkaline phosphatase
- Colicky abdominal pain suggests biliary obstruction from stones
- Painless jaundice suggests obstruction from malignancy
- Fever may be seen with superimposed bacterial cholangitis

Radiologic Features
- Ultrasonography may show dilated intrahepatic ducts
- Endoscopic or percutaneous cholangiography can demonstrate site of obstruction

Prognosis and Therapy
- Treatment is relief of obstruction, either by surgery, endoscopic or percutaneous drain or stent placement, endoscopic removal of stones, or endoscopic dilatation of stricture
- Prognosis depends on underlying etiology but is generally good for nonmalignant causes of obstruction

LARGE DUCT OBSTRUCTION—PATHOLOGIC FEATURES

Gross Findings
- Liver is bile stained
- Bile lakes may be seen in long-standing severe obstruction
- Strictures of large bile ducts with intrabiliary stones in some cases

Microscopic Findings
- Centrilobular cholestasis is an early change
- Portal tract edema, more pronounced around interlobular bile ducts
- Variable portal inflammatory infiltrate
- Bile ductular reaction, accompanied by neutrophils
- Late changes include bile infarcts
- Neutrophils are present in the lumens of interlobular bile ducts in bacterial cholangitis

Differential Diagnosis
- PSC
- Drug reaction
- Sepsis
- Acute or chronic hepatitis

DIFFERENTIAL DIAGNOSIS

PSC may exhibit features of biliary obstruction because of the presence of large duct strictures. Bile duct loss with an obstructive pattern of injury should suggest PSC. Drug reaction may mimic large duct obstruction. In sepsis, bile plugs in dilated periportal cholangioles may suggest obstruction, but periductal edema is usually not seen.

PROGNOSIS AND THERAPY

If biliary obstruction is relieved, the liver can revert to normal. Prolonged obstruction leads to portal fibrosis and ultimately to biliary cirrhosis.

PRIMARY BILIARY CIRRHOSIS

CLINICAL FEATURES

PBC, a chronic progressive disorder characterized by inflammatory destruction of small interlobular bile ducts, has distinctive clinical features, being found primarily in women (90% of patients), mostly in the fifth to seventh decades of life. PBC is probably autoimmune in etiology, judging by its association with other autoimmune disorders such as Sjögren's disease and keratoconjunctivitis sicca, and may in some patients represent a generalized disorder of lacrimal, salivary, and pancreaticobiliary small duct epithelia. Large

MICROSCOPIC FINDINGS

Portal tract abnormalities appear after 1 to 2 weeks of obstruction. Early in large duct obstruction, portal tracts are edematous and periductal edema may be evident. The portal inflammatory infiltrate contains lymphocytes and neutrophils and is generally modest, increasing with duration of biliary obstruction. Mild periductal fibrosis may be seen, but bile duct loss is not a feature of biliary obstruction. Proliferating bile ductules may be prominent. Cholestasis from large duct obstruction starts in zone 3, where canalicular bile plugs may be seen. With evolution to a chronic cholestatic process, accumulation of bile salts in the cytoplasm of hepatocytes imparts a rarefied feathery appearance to the cells, most noticeably in periportal areas. Fibrosis may develop if obstruction is unrelieved; biliary cirrhosis has a characteristic low-power appearance of irregular "jigsaw puzzle piece" nodules (Fig. 19-17).

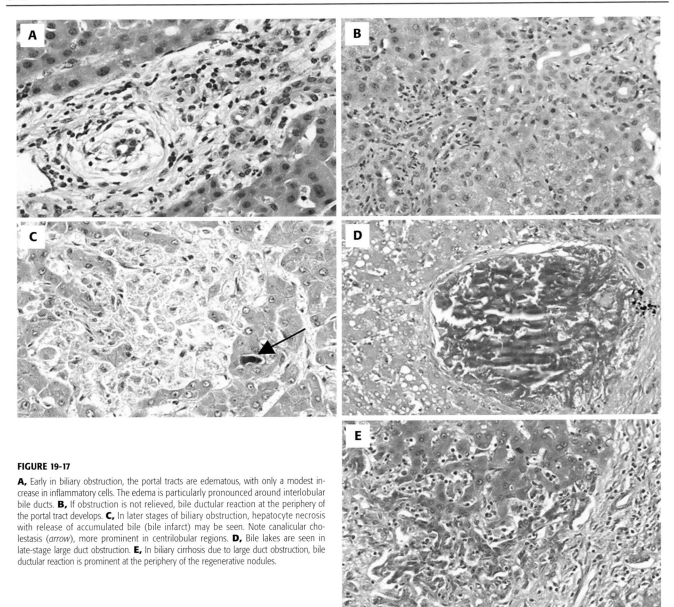

FIGURE 19-17

A, Early in biliary obstruction, the portal tracts are edematous, with only a modest increase in inflammatory cells. The edema is particularly pronounced around interlobular bile ducts. **B,** If obstruction is not relieved, bile ductular reaction at the periphery of the portal tract develops. **C,** In later stages of biliary obstruction, hepatocyte necrosis with release of accumulated bile (bile infarct) may be seen. Note canalicular cholestasis (*arrow*), more prominent in centrilobular regions. **D,** Bile lakes are seen in late-stage large duct obstruction. **E,** In biliary cirrhosis due to large duct obstruction, bile ductular reaction is prominent at the periphery of the regenerative nodules.

intrahepatic and extrahepatic bile ducts are not affected. Most patients with PBC present with fatigue (21%) and pruritus (19%), the latter due to the accumulation of bile salts. Many asymptomatic patients are now identified after screening tests show elevation of serum alkaline phosphatase.

PATHOLOGIC FEATURES

GROSS FINDINGS

In late-stage PBC, the liver is grossly cirrhotic and bile stained. Early-stage PBC may have few gross findings, although nodular regenerative hyperplasia is occasionally seen (Fig. 19-18).

MICROSCOPIC FINDINGS

The characteristic lesion of PBC is the so-called florid duct lesion, involving interlobular bile ducts 40 to 80 μm in diameter. The three components of the florid duct lesion are inflammation, injury to bile duct epithelial cells, and disruption of the bile duct basement membrane. The inflammatory infiltrate is composed of lymphocytes, scattered eosinophils, macrophages, and a variable number of plasma cells and is intimately associated with the bile duct (Fig. 19-19). The macrophages may be dispersed throughout the portal inflammatory infiltrate or may be aggregated into loose clusters or occasionally into well-formed granulomas. Granulomas and Kupffer cell aggregates may be present in the lobule. The biliary

PRIMARY BILIARY CIRRHOSIS—FACT SHEET

Definition

- Progressive chronic cholestatic liver disease characterized by destruction of intrahepatic bile ducts and antimitochondrial antibodies

Incidence and Location

- Variable prevalence reported, from 3.7 to 65 per 100,000
- More common in Western countries

Morbidity and Mortality

- Progressive disease leading to cirrhosis
- Morbidity is related to cirrhosis and chronic cholestasis
- Median survival for asymptomatic patients is 16 years, 7.5 for symptomatic
- Slight increased risk for hepatocellular carcinoma

Gender, Race, and Age Distribution

- 90% are female
- More common in whites
- Most patients are 40 to 60 years old at diagnosis
- Does not occur in children

Clinical Features

- Strongly associated with antimitochondrial antibodies and with other autoimmune diseases
- Asymptomatic in early stages; may be detected by elevated alkaline phosphatase
- Late symptoms related to chronic cholestasis include osteoporosis and pruritus

Prognosis and Therapy

- Ursodeoxycholic acid improves serum biochemical liver tests and may decrease rate of progression to cirrhosis
- Liver transplantation for patients with decompensated cirrhosis
- PBC can recur after liver transplantation but does not generally affect graft survival

PRIMARY BILIARY CIRRHOSIS—PATHOLOGIC FEATURES

Gross Findings

- Macronodular cirrhosis in late stages, with bile staining
- No large duct strictures

Microscopic Findings

- Florid duct lesion, with granulomatous destruction of small bile ducts
- Infiltration of bile ducts by lymphocytes, with associated epithelial degenerative changes
- Variable portal inflammatory infiltrate with eosinophils and interface hepatitis
- Variable bile ductular proliferation in early stage
- End stage is ductopenic biliary cirrhosis with bile stasis

Genetics

- Increased prevalence among first-degree relatives; variety of reported HLA haplotypes

Differential Diagnosis

- PSC
- AIH
- Chronic viral hepatitis, especially hepatitis C

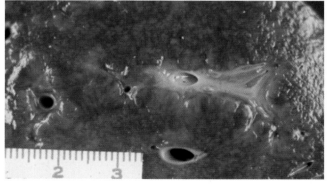

FIGURE 19-18
The liver is bile stained and finely nodular in late-stage primary biliary cirrhosis (PBC).

epithelial cells of injured bile ducts are swollen and focally stratified and may be vacuolated. Lymphocytes commonly infiltrate bile duct epithelium. In small portal tracts, bile ducts are often absent and seem to have vanished without a trace. Canalicular cholestasis is not a feature of early-stage PBC.

As the duct destruction progresses, bile ductular proliferation accompanied by fibrosis develops at the periphery of portal triads, and portal tracts enlarge by this process of biliary piecemeal necrosis. In some cases the inflammatory infiltrate spills over into the adjacent parenchyma, and lymphocytic piecemeal necrosis may mimic chronic hepatitis. At this stage the changes of chronic cholestasis begin to appear, with swollen and rarefied periportal hepatocytes and accumulation of copper. As periportal fibrosis progresses, portal-portal fibrous bridges are formed. Bile ductular proliferation often subsides in late-stage PBC, and in the cirrhotic stage little ductular or ductal epithelium can be identified. The cirrhosis has a typical biliary pattern, in which the nodules have an irregularly shaped jigsaw puzzle piece profile.

ANCILLARY STUDIES

The most specific feature of PBC is the presence of anti-mitochondrial antibodies in the serum of 90% of patients affected. Antibodies directed to the PDC-E2 antigen, a

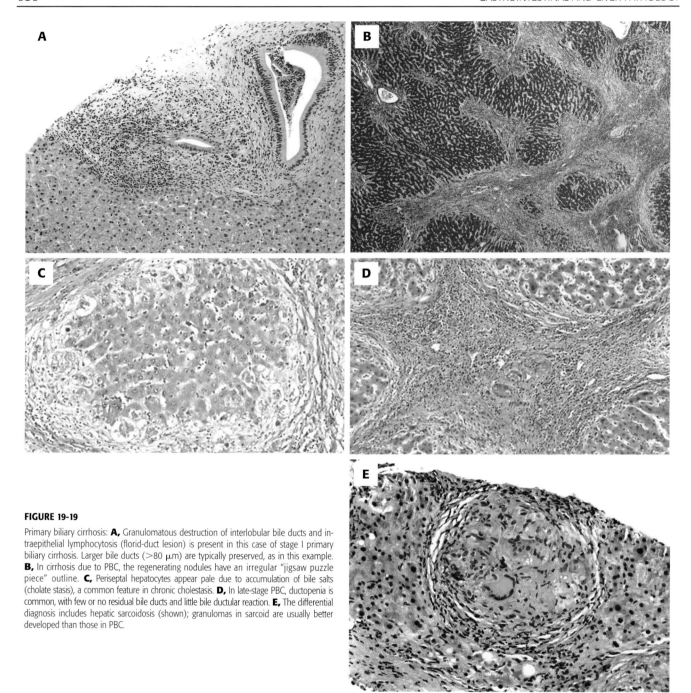

FIGURE 19-19

Primary biliary cirrhosis: **A,** Granulomatous destruction of interlobular bile ducts and intraepithelial lymphocytosis (florid-duct lesion) is present in this case of stage I primary biliary cirrhosis. Larger bile ducts (>80 μm) are typically preserved, as in this example. **B,** In cirrhosis due to PBC, the regenerating nodules have an irregular "jigsaw puzzle piece" outline. **C,** Periseptal hepatocytes appear pale due to accumulation of bile salts (cholate stasis), a common feature in chronic cholestasis. **D,** In late-stage PBC, ductopenia is common, with few or no residual bile ducts and little bile ductular reaction. **E,** The differential diagnosis includes hepatic sarcoidosis (shown); granulomas in sarcoid are usually better developed than those in PBC.

component of the pyruvate dehydrogenase enzyme complex present on the inner mitochondrial membrane, are highly specific (96%) for PBC. Hypergammaglobulinemia with a selective elevation of IgM is often seen.

DIFFERENTIAL DIAGNOSIS

The differential diagnosis for PBC depends on the stage of the disease. In stage 1 and 2 disease, portal inflammation, piecemeal necrosis, and bile ductular proliferation may mimic chronic hepatitis, particularly hepatitis C.

Bile duct damage is less prominent in chronic hepatitis and bile duct loss is rarely seen, but lymphocytic infiltration of bile duct epithelium is often a feature of hepatitis C. Clinical information such as antimitochondrial antibody status and serologic markers for viral hepatitis is helpful in most cases.

Distinction of AIH from PBC may prove impossible on histologic grounds. Difficulties arise because the portal inflammatory infiltrate of PBC often contains numerous plasma cells, and infiltration of bile duct epithelium by lymphocytes is not uncommon in AIH. Although nondestructive bile duct lesions are quite common in AIH, duct loss is generally not a feature and granulomatous bile duct destruction is not seen. Serum alkaline phosphatase, cholesterol, and IgM levels are elevated to higher levels in PBC.

Distinction of PBC from those cases of sarcoidosis with destruction of bile ducts by granulomas may be difficult. The granulomas of sarcoidosis tend to be better formed and more numerous than those of PBC (see Fig. 19-19E). The lack of antimitochondrial antibody positivity and the presence of pulmonary involvement also favor a diagnosis of hepatic sarcoidosis.

PROGNOSIS AND THERAPY

Primary biliary cirrhosis follows a progressive clinical course in most untreated patients, and most but not all asymptomatic patients develop significant liver disease. Survival is variable, ranging from 6 to 12 years after presentation for symptomatic patients to several decades for asymptomatic patients. Ursodeoxycholic acid is an effective treatment, especially when started early in the course of the disease and has been shown to decrease the rate of progression to late histologic stages. Liver transplantation is the only effective therapy for late stage disease.

PRIMARY SCLEROSING CHOLANGITIS

CLINICAL FEATURES

PSC is a chronic progressive disease resulting in strictures of large intra- and extrahepatic bile ducts and loss of interlobular ducts. In contrast to PBC, PSC is a disease of men, with a male predominance of 2:1. The median age of onset is young (30 years), but there is an extraordinarily wide age range of 1 to 90 years. PSC was previously thought to be rarer than PBC but is probably about equal in prevalence. The prevalence of PSC in the United States is estimated at 2 to 7 cases per 100,000 population, but this is likely to be an underestimate.

The association of PSC with ulcerative colitis remains an enigma. Approximately 70% of patients with PSC have ulcerative colitis. Conversely, 3% to 7.5% of patients with ulcerative colitis have PSC. The ulcerative colitis typically involves a majority of the colon but often has a relatively mild clinical course. Patients with PSC and ulcerative colitis may be at even higher risk for adenocarcinoma of the colon than the usual patient with ulcerative colitis, and patients with PSC may be at higher risk for pancreatic carcinoma. Like PBC, PSC is considered to be a disease of autoimmunity, and a marked increase in prevalence of HLA antigens B8 and DR3 has been found in patients with PSC.

RADIOGRAPHIC FEATURES

Diagnosis of PSC is established on cholangiography, usually endoscopic retrograde cholangiopancreatography, by the appearance of multifocal beading and structuring and irregularity of the intra- and extrahepatic biliary system (Fig. 19-20). Magnetic resonance cholangiopancreatography (MRCP) is also used.

PATHOLOGIC FEATURES

GROSS FINDINGS

In late-stage PSC, the liver is grossly cirrhotic and bile stained. Hilar fibrosis may be prominent, as are extrahepatic biliary strictures. Dense hilar scarring may obscure cholangiocarcinoma (Fig. 19-21).

MICROSCOPIC FINDINGS

A wide variety of morphologic changes that reflect the varying levels of duct involvement is seen in PSC. The classic lesion of periductal concentric "onion-skinning" fibrosis, rarely seen in needle biopsy specimens, has only a sparse inflammatory infiltrate. The bile duct epithelium is atrophic and epithelial cells are shrunken, with pyknotic nuclei. A rounded scar often marks the site of a

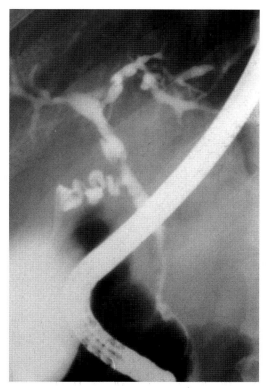

FIGURE 19-20

Primary sclerosing cholangitis. Extrahepatic and large intrahepatic bile ducts show alternating areas of beading and structuring.

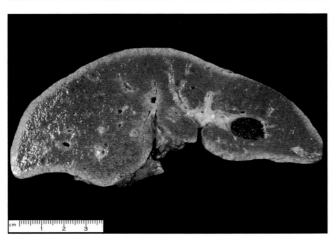

FIGURE 19-21

In late-stage primary sclerosing cholangitis (PSC), the liver is bile stained and variably nodular. Note area of biliary dilatation containing dark-colored calculi.

PRIMARY SCLEROSING CHOLANGITIS—FACT SHEET

Definition
- Chronic condition characterized by inflammation and fibrosis of biliary tree, involving both intra- and extrahepatic bile ducts

Incidence and Location
- Up to 7.5% prevalence in patients with ulcerative colitis
- Prevalence in U.S. population approximately 7 per 100,000

Morbidity and Mortality
- Progressive disease, with median survival from diagnosis approximately 12 years
- Complications include bacterial cholangitis and biliary stones
- Cholangiocarcinoma develops in more than 15% of patients

Gender, Race, and Age Distribution
- More common in young men ($\approx$70%)
- More common in patients of northern European descent; rare in Asia
- Mean age at diagnosis approximately 40 years
- Also occurs in children

Clinical Features
- Strongly associated with ulcerative colitis and other autoimmune diseases
- Presentation ranges from asymptomatic to liver failure from cirrhosis
- Fluctuating jaundice, fevers, fatigue, and weight loss are common presenting symptoms
- Elevated alkaline phosphatase

Radiologic Features
- Endoscopic retrograde cholangiography or magnetic resonance cholangiopancreatography (MRCP) is method of choice
- Multifocal strictures and beading involving extra- and intrahepatic biliary tree

Prognosis and Therapy
- No effective medical treatment
- Dominant bile duct strictures may be treated with balloon dilatation, stent placement, or surgery
- Liver transplantation for end-stage disease results in 85% 3-year survival rate

destroyed bile duct. Alternatively the smaller interlobular bile ducts may vanish without a trace, especially in pediatric cases, and residual scars are not identified. The bile duct epithelium may be vacuolated and focally infiltrated by lymphocytes. The portal inflammatory infiltrate is usually sparse and primarily made up of mononuclear inflammatory cells, with scattered eosinophils. Early in the disease portal eosinophils may be unusually prominent. Portal granulomas are distinctly unusual, although a granulomatous response to leakage of bile products does occur in 3% to 4% of biopsies. Lobular changes early in the disease are generally minor; late in the disease, changes of chronic cholestasis are common. The pattern of fibrosis is similar to that seen in PBC (Fig. 19-22).

Changes of large duct obstruction are often superimposed on small duct changes of PSC. Bile ductular proliferation is common, and periductal edema and acute cholangitis may also be seen, especially in the setting of bacterial cholangitis. Canalicular bile plugs may be present.

In the liver explant, larger intrahepatic bile ducts are often dilated and contain inspissated bile plugs and sludge. The walls of large bile ducts are fibrotic and contain chronic inflammatory cells. Cholangiocarcinoma may be difficult to distinguish from reactive change in peribiliary glands. Clues to malignancy are unequivocal perineural invasion, cribriform glandular structures, and pronounced nuclear pleomorphism and atypia.

DIFFERENTIAL DIAGNOSIS

The differential diagnosis for PSC changes with disease stage. Histologic overlap with PBC is occasionally a problem, although knowledge of the clinical setting,

PRIMARY SCLEROSING CHOLANGITIS—PATHOLOGIC FEATURES

Gross Findings
- Macronodular cirrhosis in late stages, with bile staining
- Large intrahepatic and extrahepatic ducts may demonstrate strictures

Microscopic Findings
- Concentric periductal fibrosis
- Large ducts show fibrotic thickening with mixed inflammatory infiltrate
- Loss of interlobular bile ducts and variable portal inflammatory infiltrate
- Progressive portal fibrosis with bile ductular proliferation
- End-stage is biliary cirrhosis

Genetics
- Strong association with HLA haplotypes B8 and DR3

Differential Diagnosis
- Large duct obstruction
- PBC
- AIH
- Idiopathic adulthood ductopenia

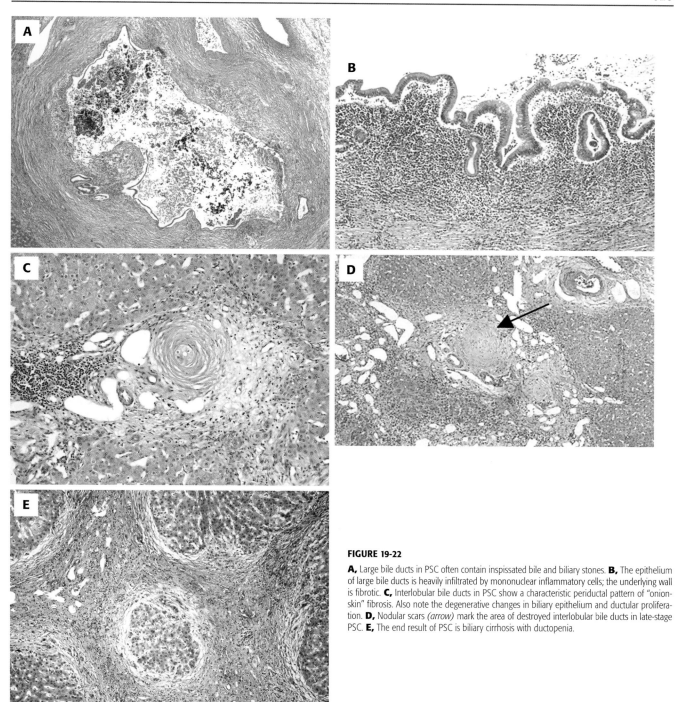

FIGURE 19-22

A, Large bile ducts in PSC often contain inspissated bile and biliary stones. **B,** The epithelium of large bile ducts is heavily infiltrated by mononuclear inflammatory cells; the underlying wall is fibrotic. **C,** Interlobular bile ducts in PSC show a characteristic periductal pattern of "onion-skin" fibrosis. Also note the degenerative changes in biliary epithelium and ductular proliferation. **D,** Nodular scars *(arrow)* mark the area of destroyed interlobular bile ducts in late-stage PSC. **E,** The end result of PSC is biliary cirrhosis with ductopenia.

serologic tests, and radiographic appearance generally results in resolution. The portal inflammatory infiltrate in PSC is usually sparser than that seen in PBC, and florid duct lesions are not seen.

Chronic large duct obstruction may be difficult to distinguish from PSC because extrahepatic obstruction from bile duct strictures is part of the pathologic process in this disease. Periductal fibrosis, bile ductular proliferation, and cholestasis are seen in both obstruction and PSC. However, in large duct obstruction from other causes, loss of interlobular bile ducts does not generally occur. The presence of numerous eosinophils in the portal inflammatory infiltrate also favors PSC.

Other causes of biliary strictures that may mimic PSC are recurrent pyogenic cholangitis, intrahepatic artery chemotherapy, immunodeficiency syndromes, and Langerhans cell histiocytosis. Hepatic artery infusion of floxuridine for treatment of hepatic metastases from colorectal carcinoma has been associated with a sclerosing cholangitis-like lesion resulting in hepatic failure. Langerhans cell histiocytosis may present with isolated hepatic involvement or with involvement of other organ systems, most commonly lymph node and skin. Small and medium intrahepatic bile ducts may be injured by infiltrating Langerhans' cells, and concentric periductal fibrosis similar to that of PSC may be seen. Langerhans cells may be undetectable in the liver, and the diagnosis may be established by biopsy of extrahepatic sites.

Autoimmune pancreatitis-associated sclerosing cholangitis is believed to be a different clinicopathologic entity than PSC. Histopathologically, fibro-obliterative lesions were more common in PSC, while IgG4-positive plasma cell infiltration was significantly more prominent in autoimmune pancreatitis-associated sclerosing cholangitis. As opposed to PSC, significant improvement of strictures is seen in cases of autoimmune pancreatitis-associated sclerosing cholangitis with steroid therapy.

PROGNOSIS AND THERAPY

The natural history of PSC is more variable than that of PBC. For the most part, PSC is a progressive disease. Because of the presence of bile duct strictures and the formation of biliary stones and sludge, PSC is commonly complicated by bacterial cholangitis. The development of cholangiocarcinoma is a major complication, seen in up to 16% of PSC patients. Elevated CA19-9 levels, if greatly elevated, may be of utility, although considerable overlap with PSC without cancer is seen. Immunosuppression is ineffective, and liver transplantation is the treatment of choice for late-stage disease. Mean survival (without transplantation) is approximately 17 years from time of diagnosis.

NONALCOHOLIC FATTY LIVER DISEASE

CLINICAL FEATURES

Nonalcoholic fatty liver disease (NAFLD) is becoming more common in developing countries because of its association with obesity, glucose intolerance and diabetes, and hyperlipidemia and accounts for up to 10% of referrals to hepatologists in some U.S. practices. Most patients have insulin resistance. The liver disease is usually asymptomatic and is discovered because of mildly elevated transaminase levels, but some patients present with cirrhosis. NAFLD has also been recognized as an emerging health problem in the children.

PATHOLOGIC FEATURES

GROSS FINDINGS

The liver is grossly enlarged, yellow, and greasy when markedly steatotic. In late stages, micronodular cirrhosis may be evident (Fig. 19-23).

MICROSCOPIC FINDINGS

Microscopic findings are variable in NAFLD and range from macrovesicular steatosis without necroinflammatory activity or fibrosis to end-stage cirrhosis. Key histologic features of nonalcoholic steatohepatitis (NASH) are macrovesicular steatosis, spotty hepatocyte necrosis with small collections of lymphocytes in the lobule, ballooning degeneration of hepatocytes, and delicate pericellular fibrosis surrounding centrilobular hepatocytes. Mallory's hyaline is usually inconspicuous, and collections of neutrophils in the lobule are relatively rare. As fibrosis progresses, fibrous septa bridge central veins and adjacent portal tracts, resulting in cirrhosis in long-standing cases (Fig. 19-24). Morbidly obese patients may have steatosis associated with centrilobular or periportal fibrosis without other features of steatohepatitis. In addition, "burned-out" steatohepatitis presenting in the cirrhotic stage often shows only focal residual features and may be difficult to recognize. Ubiquitin immunohistochemistry can be useful in this setting.

In children, an unusual pattern of NAFLD consisting of moderate to severe steatosis, periportal rather than centrilobular fibrosis, lymphocytic portal inflammation, and virtually no lobular inflammation, hepatocyte ballooning, or Mallory hyalin has been described (referred to as type 2 NASH). This pattern seems to be the most common pattern of NASH in childhood. Only a minority of pediatric patients present with classic adult-type NASH.

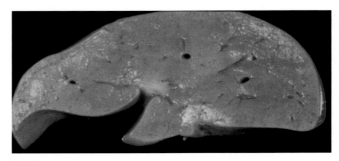

FIGURE 19-23

Accumulation of fat leads to an enlarged yellow liver in nonalcoholic fatty liver disease (NAFLD).

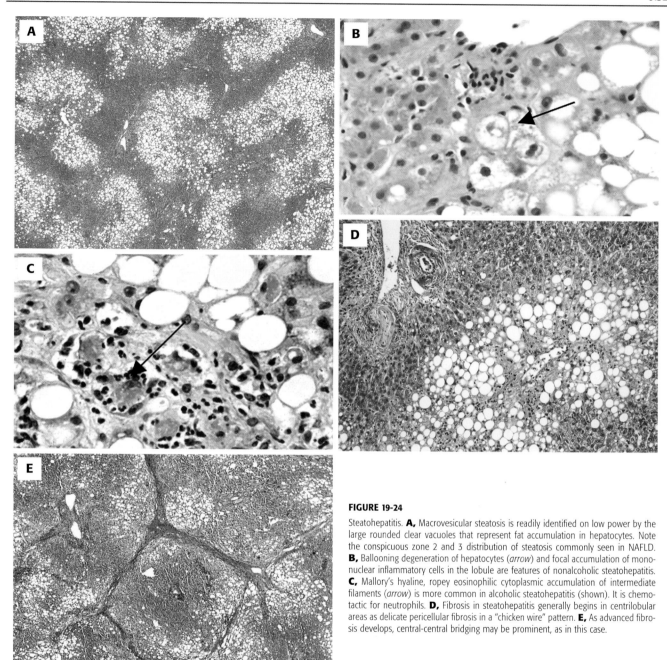

FIGURE 19-24

Steatohepatitis. **A,** Macrovesicular steatosis is readily identified on low power by the large rounded clear vacuoles that represent fat accumulation in hepatocytes. Note the conspicuous zone 2 and 3 distribution of steatosis commonly seen in NAFLD. **B,** Ballooning degeneration of hepatocytes (*arrow*) and focal accumulation of mononuclear inflammatory cells in the lobule are features of nonalcoholic steatohepatitis. **C,** Mallory's hyaline, ropey eosinophilic cytoplasmic accumulation of intermediate filaments (*arrow*) is more common in alcoholic steatohepatitis (shown). It is chemotactic for neutrophils. **D,** Fibrosis in steatohepatitis generally begins in centrilobular areas as delicate pericellular fibrosis in a "chicken wire" pattern. **E,** As advanced fibrosis develops, central-central bridging may be prominent, as in this case.

DIFFERENTIAL DIAGNOSIS

The principal differential diagnosis is alcoholic steatohepatitis, which tends to have a more pronounced neutrophilic infiltrate and more prominent Mallory's hyaline. However, significant overlap between nonalcoholic NAFLD and alcoholic liver disease occurs, and these entities cannot be reliably distinguished on morphologic grounds alone. Drug reaction should also be considered because amiodarone causes a pattern of

injury indistinguishable from alcoholic steatohepatitis. Estrogens, tamoxifen, and glucocorticoids have also been reported as causing a NASH-like pattern of injury.

PROGNOSIS AND THERAPY

NAFLD has been classified in four categories based on the different diagnostic features: type 1, simple steatosis; type 2, steatosis plus inflammation; type 3, steatosis plus

NONALCOHOLIC FATTY LIVER DISEASE—FACT SHEET

Definition

- Hepatic steatosis with or without inflammation and fibrosis, associated with obesity, glucose intolerance, and hypertriglyceridemia
- Underlying cause is probably metabolic, with increased oxidative stress as a mechanism for recruitment of inflammatory cells

Incidence and Location

- Very common chronic liver disease in U.S. population; exact prevalence is unclear
- More common in developed countries because of association with obesity

Morbidity and Mortality

- May progress to cirrhosis
- Overall survival of patients with cirrhosis due to NAFLD is 84% at 10 years

Gender, Race, and Age Distribution

- Common in both males and females, but more common in women
- All races affected
- NAFLD may be seen in obese children (reported in children age 4 to 18 years)

Clinical Features

- Most cases are asymptomatic, discovered because of abnormal liver tests (ALT greater than AST) or hepatomegaly
- Associated with obesity
- Glucose intolerance and insulin resistance
- Hypertriglyceridemia and other dyslipidemias

Radiologic Features

- Fatty liver may be demonstrated on ultrasonography as hyperechoic
- Fat may be irregularly distributed in the liver on CT or magnetic resonance imaging

Prognosis and Therapy

- Fibrosis on index biopsy is associated with progressive disease, which may lead to cirrhosis
- Treatment is aimed at weight reduction and control of blood glucose; oral hypoglycemic agents may have beneficial effect
- May recur after liver transplantation

NONALCOHOLIC FATTY LIVER DISEASE—PATHOLOGIC FEATURES

Gross Findings

- Liver is enlarged and soft
- Yellow with greasy texture due to lipid accumulation
- Fat may be decreased in late stages, especially in cirrhosis due to NAFLD

Microscopic Findings

- Variable degree of predominantly macrovesicular steatosis
- Delicate pericellular centrilobular fibrosis surrounds individual hepatocytes
- Ballooning degeneration of hepatocytes
- Spotty hepatocyte necrosis in lobule, with associated lymphocytes or neutrophils
- Mallory's hyaline may be inconspicuous

Fine-Needle Aspiration Biopsy Findings

- Large single or multiple small vacuoles in hepatocytes

Differential Diagnosis

- Alcoholic liver disease
- Drug reaction
- Hepatitis C
- Metabolic disorders

■ CIRRHOSIS

CLINICAL FEATURES

Cirrhosis represents end-stage chronic liver disease and is associated with a variety of etiologies. The most common cause in Western countries is alcoholic liver disease, followed by chronic viral hepatitis, AIH, PSC, PBC, and metabolic disorders. The clinical manifestations are similar, regardless of etiology, and are dominated by consequences of portal hypertension and diminished hepatic synthetic function. Ascites, esophageal varices (Fig. 19-25), splenomegaly with sequestration of platelets, and hepatic encephalopathy are common complications mainly attributed to portal hypertension and portosystemic shunting. Decreased synthetic function may be manifested by clotting abnormalities and hypoalbuminemia.

PATHOLOGIC FEATURES

GROSS FINDINGS

The cirrhotic liver is diffusely nodular, firm, and variable in size; even though it is usually smaller than normal, in early cirrhosis hepatomegaly is not uncommon. The capsular surface is nodular or may have a pig-skin texture. Cirrhosis is classified as micronodular (nodules <3 mm) and macronodular (nodules >3 mm), based on the nodule size, but many cases show a mixture of nodule sizes (Fig. 19-26).

hepatocyte ballooning and inflammation; and type 4, all previous features plus Mallory hyalin and centrilobular/pericellular fibrosis. NASH types 3 and 4 are associated with higher risk of progression with cirrhosis and higher liver-related mortality compared with types 1 and 2. Approximately 15% of patients with NASH and early fibrosis develop cirrhosis within 8 to 13 years. Many cases labeled "cryptogenic cirrhosis" in the past undoubtedly represent end-stage NASH. Recurrence of NASH in the transplanted liver has been reported. Treatment is aimed at weight reduction and control of serum glucose and lipid levels.

CIRRHOSIS—FACT SHEET

Definition

- Chronic end-stage liver disease characterized by diffuse architectural distortion with fibrosis and parenchymal nodular regeneration

Incidence and Location

- Overall prevalence of approximately 0.5%
- Annual incidence approximately 150 to 250 per million
- Common worldwide; etiologies vary

Morbidity and Mortality

- Morbidity is related to liver failure and consequences of portal hypertension
- High risk for hepatocellular carcinoma
- 5-year survival rate is roughly 66%

Gender, Race, and Age Distribution

- More common in men
- No race predilection
- More common in older adults, but may be seen in children as well

Clinical Features

- Clinical manifestations range from asymptomatic to hepatic failure
- Ascites, hypersplenism, and esophageal varices are manifestations of portal hypertension
- Hepatic encephalopathy and hepatorenal syndrome are late features

Prognosis and Therapy

- Treatment is aimed at underlying cause of cirrhosis
- Management of esophageal varices and encephalopathy has impact on survival
- Outcome depends on cause, severity, and treatment options
- Liver transplantation is indicated in many cases

CIRRHOSIS—PATHOLOGIC FEATURES

Gross Findings

- Hepatic size is variable—liver may be normal, enlarged, or shrunken.
- Liver is firmer than normal because of fibrosis and diffusely nodular
- Cirrhosis is subdivided into macronodular (nodules >3 mm, usually variable) or micronodular (nodules <3 mm)

Microscopic Findings

- Fibrous scars bridge portal tracts to each other or to central veins
- Variable inflammatory infiltrate and bile ductular reaction in fibrous septa
- Fibrosis surrounds regenerating nodules of hepatocytes; liver cell plates are thickened

Fine-Needle Aspiration Biopsy Findings

- Fibrosis
- Reactive hepatocytes characterized by
  - Cohesive fragments with irregular, jagged edges
  - Cellular and nuclear enlargement with preservation of low N/C ratio
  - Binucleation
  - Prominent nucleoli

Differential Diagnosis

- Focal nodular hyperplasia
- Nodular regenerative hyperplasia
- Congenital hepatic fibrosis
- Massive hepatic necrosis

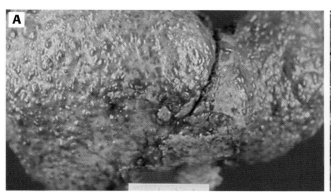

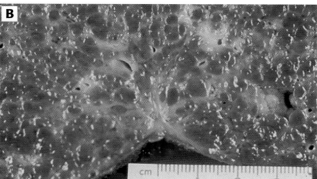

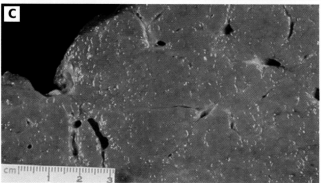

FIGURE 19-25

A, The capsular surface of the liver is nodular in established cirrhosis. **B,** On cut surface, the cirrhotic liver displays fibrous scars and nodularity; macronodular cirrhosis is characterized by nodule size greater than 3 mm. **C,** In micronodular cirrhosis, the nodule size is 3 mm or less.

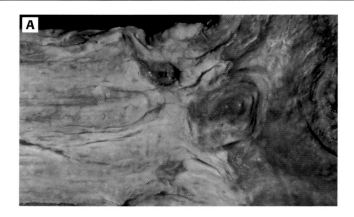

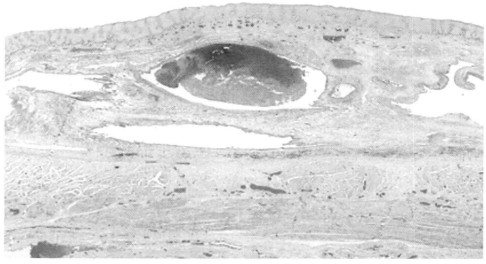

FIGURE 19-26

A, Ruptured esophageal varices secondary to portal hypertension are a common cause of increased morbidity and mortality in cirrhosis.
B, Microscopically, the varices are dilated thin-walled veins just beneath the esophageal mucosa.

MICROSCOPIC FINDINGS

Fibrous bands surround the regenerative nodules, which contain thickened liver cell plates. The fibrous septa contain a variable number of inflammatory cells, with predominance of lymphocytes. Interface hepatitis may be seen, particularly in cirrhosis due to chronic viral hepatitis. Bile ductular reaction is often prominent, and neutrophils may be prominently associated with the proliferating ductules. Continued lobular necroinflammatory activity is seen in many cases, especially in viral hepatitis. In biliary cirrhosis due to PBC or PSC, interlobular bile ducts are often diminished or absent (Fig. 19-27).

In micronodular cirrhosis, fibrous septa bridge portal tracts and central veins, resulting in a small nodule without central structures. The nodules of macronodular cirrhosis are more variable in composition and are often composed of multiple acini. Nodules in biliary cirrhosis display irregular outlines and a jigsaw puzzle piece profile. Hepatocyte inclusions such as Mallory's hyaline may be seen, especially in chronic cholestatic disorders; bile may not be evident at this stage, but accumulation of bile salts imparts a rarefied appearance to the hepatocyte cytoplasm.

DIFFERENTIAL DIAGNOSIS

Nodular regenerative hyperplasia, a cause of noncirrhotic portal hypertension, is characterized by diffuse nodularity of the liver due to hepatocyte regeneration, without significant fibrous bridging as is seen in cirrhosis. Hepatic function is generally preserved in nodular regenerative hyperplasia. Although focal nodular hyperplasia (FNH) resembles cirrhosis microscopically, FNH is a circumscribed nodular mass, and the changes are not diffusely distributed throughout the liver as in cirrhosis. Congenital

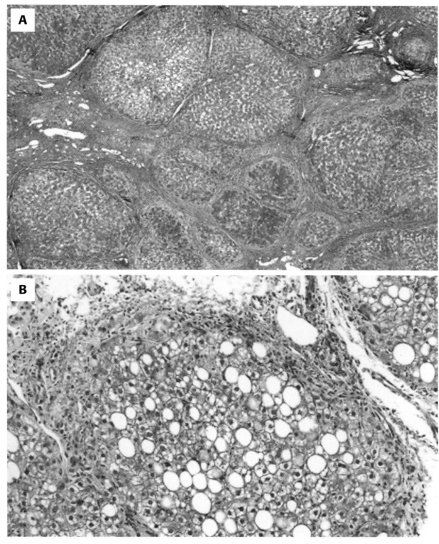

FIGURE 19-27

A, Masson stain highlights the broad fibrous scars separating regenerating nodules of hepatocytes in cirrhosis. **B,** Nodularity may also be appreciated on needle biopsy with Masson stain.

hepatic fibrosis is distinguished from cirrhosis by its lack of nodular regeneration and the characteristic distribution of biliary channels at the periphery of the fibrous scars. Massive hepatic necrosis is an acute process, but the presence of islands of regenerating hepatocytes and the resemblance of the collapsed parenchyma to fibrous scar can mimic cirrhosis both grossly and microscopically. On Masson stain, areas of parenchymal collapse do not stain as darkly as the dense collagen of cirrhosis. Grossly, the liver in massive hepatic necrosis is soft, not diffusely firm as in cirrhosis.

PROGNOSIS AND THERAPY

The prognosis of cirrhosis depends on the underlying etiology, availability of effective treatment, and severity of liver injury. If the offending agent is removed, hepatic regeneration and remodeling of scar tissue may lead to improvement in liver function. However, progressive clinical deterioration may be expected in most cases, and liver transplantation is the only definitive treatment. Overall mortality from cirrhosis remains high, estimated at approximately 10 per 100,000 in the United States.

20

Liver Neoplasms

■ **Roger Klein Moreira, MD** ■ **Kay Washington, MD, PhD**

Primary tumors of the liver are divided into epithelial and mesenchymal lesions and further classified as benign or malignant (Table 20-1). Overall, metastatic tumors are more common than primary hepatic neoplasms. Clinical history, such as age of the patient and the involvement of the non-neoplastic liver by disease processes such as cirrhosis, can be helpful in the evaluation of hepatic masses.

■ EPITHELIAL TUMORS

HEPATOCELLULAR TUMORS

FOCAL NODULAR HYPERPLASIA

Focal nodular hyperplasia (FNH) is a localized hyperplastic overgrowth of hepatocytes around a vascular anomaly, particularly an arterial malformation, and may coexist with hepatic cavernous hemangiomas in about 20% of cases. Patients with multiple FNHs who have one or more other lesions, including hepatic hemangioma, berry aneurysms, and brain tumors (astrocytoma and meningioma), are considered to have the multiple FNH syndrome. Although FNH is generally considered non-neoplastic, some lesions appear to be monoclonal.

CLINICAL FEATURES

FNH is found mainly in women of reproductive age (80% to 95%). Oral contraceptive use is implicated in promotion of FNH growth but is generally not considered a causative factor. Up to 15% of cases occur in children and may be associated with glycogen storage disease type Ia. FNH is usually an incidental finding; nonspecific abdominal pain is the most common complaint in symptomatic patients. FNH may increase in size over time. The serum α-fetoprotein (AFP) level is normal.

RADIOLOGIC FEATURES

FNH is suggested when computed tomography (CT) or magnetic resonance imaging (MRI) shows a mass with a central scar, when angiography or Doppler ultrasonography discloses centrifugal hypervascularity, or when technetium 99 sulfur colloid scan shows normal or increased uptake. Sensitivity is around 70% for a preoperative diagnosis of FNH, and false-positive results are rare.

TABLE 20-1

World Health Organization Classification of Primary Liver Mass Lesions

Epithelial Mass Lesions	Nonepithelial Mass Lesions
Benign	Benign
Large regenerative nodule (macroregenerative nodule)	Hemangioma
Low-grade dysplastic nodule	Angiomyolipoma
High-grade dysplastic nodule	Infantile hemangioendothelioma
Hepatic adenoma	Mesenchymal hamartoma
Focal nodular hyperplasia	Localized fibrous tumor
Bile duct adenoma	Solitary necrotic nodule
Bile duct hamartoma	Inflammatory pseudotumor
Biliary cystadenoma	Malignant
Intraductal biliary papillomatosis	Epithelioid hemangioendothelioma
Congenital biliary cyst	Angiosarcoma
Focal fatty change	Undifferentiated (embryonal) sarcoma
Malignant	Lymphoma
Hepatocellular carcinoma	Kaposi's sarcoma
Hepatoblastoma	Other rare sarcomas
Cholangiocarcinoma	
Biliary cystadenocarcinoma	
Intraductal papillary adenocarcinoma	

FOCAL NODULAR HYPERPLASIA—FACT SHEET

Definition

- Non-neoplastic mass lesion caused by nodular overgrowth of hepatocytes in region of altered hepatic blood flow

Incidence and Location

- Up to 0.6% in autopsy series
- 2% of hepatic tumors in children
- No geographic predilection

Morbidity and Mortality

- Low morbidity
- Rupture is rare
- No increase in mortality

Gender, Race, and Age Distribution

- More common in women than men, 9:1
- Occurs in all age groups
- No race predilection

Clinical Features

- Usually incidental finding
- Associated with oral contraceptive use in 50% to 60% of cases
- Rarely associated with abdominal pain, hepatomegaly, or tenderness
- Associated with extrahepatic vascular lesions

Radiologic Features

- Central scar by ultrasonography, CT, MRI
- Doppler imaging may detect feeding artery
- Hypodense lesion on CT with enhancement during arterial phase

Prognosis and Therapy

- Prognosis is excellent; most patients remain asymptomatic
- Treatment for asymptomatic lesions: observation
- Surgical resection for symptomatic or enlarging lesions

FOCAL NODULAR HYPERPLASIA—PATHOLOGIC FEATURES

Gross Findings

- Single subcapsular lesion in right lobe
- Average size less than 5 cm to 10 cm
- Central stellate scar with radiating septa

Microscopic Findings

- Nodular overgrowth of normal-appearing hepatocytes
- Large caliber vessels in central stellate scar
- Bile ductular proliferation in scar

Fine-Needle Aspiration Biopsy Findings

- Normal hepatocytes
- Large flat sheets of hepatocytes have irregular edges
- Fibrous tissue and bile duct epithelium helpful if present

Genetics

- Clonality is reported in some cases

Differential Diagnosis

- Cirrhosis
- HA

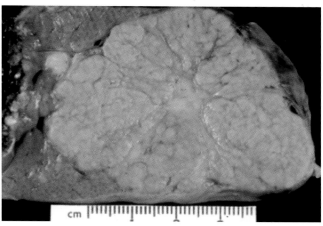

FIGURE 20-1

Focal nodular hyperplasia (FNH) is a sharply circumscribed nodular mass often appearing lighter than the surrounding liver. The central stellate scar is characteristic.

PATHOLOGIC FEATURES

GROSS FINDINGS

FNH is usually a subcapsular, well-circumscribed, bulging, tan, nodular mass. Most measure less than 5 cm in diameter, but larger lesions occur. The surrounding liver is normal. The most characteristic finding is the presence of a central stellate scar with radiating fibrous septa that subdivide the mass into multiple smaller nodules (Fig. 20-1). The central scar may be inconspicuous in smaller lesions. Hemorrhage, necrosis, and bile staining are rare.

MICROSCOPIC FINDINGS

FNH is composed of nodules of hepatocytes surrounded by fibrous septa that contain artery branches, bile ductules (a variable but key feature), a variable chronic and/or acute inflammatory infiltrate, and decreased or absent interlobular bile ducts and portal vein branches. The central scar is composed of dense collagen (Fig. 20-2A) and contains numerous thick-walled arteries and bile ductules (see Fig. 20-2B). In the telangiectatic variant, numerous small, dilated vessels (resembling hemangioma) are seen centrally, and the adjacent sinusoids are markedly dilated. The histologic features overall resemble a biliary type of cirrhosis with ductopenia.

The hepatocytes in FNH lesions are similar to those in the surrounding liver, although they may be somewhat larger and paler and may incorporate variable quantities of fat or glycogen. Nuclear pleomorphism, prominent nucleoli, and mitotic figures are not found in classic FNH, but cytologic atypia may be seen in variant forms. The variant formerly referred to as "telangiectatic FNH" has been shown to be a form of hepatic adenoma by genetic and molecular studies.

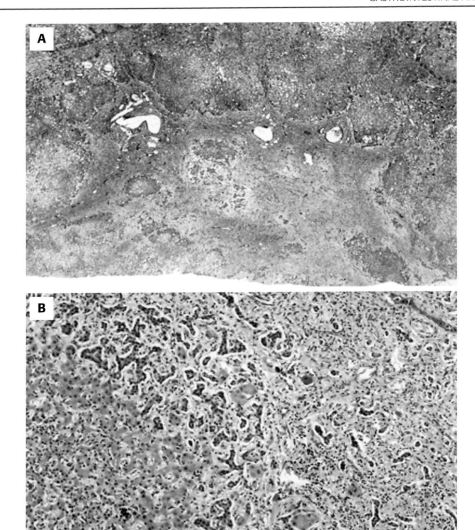

FIGURE 20-2

Focal nodular hyperplasia. **A,** The central stellate scar is composed of dense collagen. **B,** A variable degree of bile ductular proliferation is present at the interface of the scar with the parenchyma.

ANCILLARY STUDIES

FINE-NEEDLE ASPIRATION BIOPSY

Fine-needle aspiration (FNA) biopsies are generally not useful for definitive diagnosis because the central stellate scar is usually not represented. The hepatocytes of FNH are cytologically indistinguishable from normal.

DIFFERENTIAL DIAGNOSIS

FNH may be confused on biopsy with cirrhosis, hepatic adenoma (HA) (especially the telangectatic variant), and well-differentiated hepatocellular carcinoma (HCC). The presence of biliary epithelium distinguishes FNH from HA. The localized nature of the lesion and its origin in normal liver exclude cirrhosis. Well-differentiated HCC generally displays more pronounced cellular atypia and may demonstrate vascular invasion. Glipican-3 immunohistochemistry (which may be used in combination with CD-34) can be useful in this setting, being positive in at least half of well-differentiated HCCs and negative in benign hepatocytic lesions.

PROGNOSIS AND THERAPY

Most FNHs are not progressive lesions, and they do not undergo malignant degeneration. Unlike hepatic adenomas, FNHs rarely rupture or cause intraperitoneal bleeding. Due to the low risk for complications and negligible risk for malignant transformation associated with these lesions, surgery may not be indicated. However, if imaging studies are not considered diagnostic, or if the patient has persistent symptoms, surgical management may be necessary.

HEPATIC ADENOMA

CLINICAL FEATURES

HA is a benign hepatocellular neoplasm arising in a normal liver. The overwhelming majority of cases (95%) develop in women in their childbearing years, and long-term oral contraceptive steroid (OCS) use is a common risk factor. In men, HA is seen in the context of the use of anabolic/androgenic steroids and antiestrogens, as well as in Klinefelter's syndrome. HAs are rarely found in children and are usually associated with metabolic disorders such as glycogen storage disease, diabetes mellitus, and Hurler's disease.

HEPATIC ADENOMA—FACT SHEET

Definition
- Benign neoplasm of hepatocytes

Incidence and Location
- 3.4 per 100,000 in long-term users of oral contraceptives
- Approximately 1.3 per million in women who have never used oral contraceptives
- No geographic predilection

Morbidity and Mortality
- Hemorrhage in approximately 40% of patients
- Mortality rate of 6% to 20% in patients with hemorrhage

Gender, Race, and Age Distribution
- More common in young to middle-aged women (average age 30 years)
- Rare in men
- In children, seen mainly in setting of glycogen storage disease types I and III, where they occur before age 20 (males to females, 2:1)
- No race predilection

Clinical Features
- More than 90% of patients have history of OCP use for more than 5 years
- Most common complaint is right upper quadrant abdominal pain
- Occasionally seen in patients taking anabolic steroids

Radiologic Features
- Vascular lesion on CT scan, with irregular enhancement
- MRI shows well-defined mass, low signal to slightly hyperintense on T1-weighted images

Prognosis and Therapy
- Surgical resection if technically possible
- Withdrawal of estrogens may be indicated to reduce tumor size
- Liver transplantation is considered for multiple lesions
- Malignant transformation to HCC is rare

Patients with HA often present with acute abdominal pain secondary to hemorrhage within the tumor. Intraperitoneal rupture produces hemoperitoneum and may lead to shock. Only one third of patients have an abdominal mass. Serum AFP levels are normal.

RADIOLOGIC FEATURES

HA is visualized as a vascular lesion on CT scan, with irregular enhancement. MRI shows a well-defined mass with low to slightly hyperintense signal on T1-weighted images.

PATHOLOGIC FEATURES

GROSS FINDINGS

HA is a well-circumscribed, often subcapsular mass in the right lobe of an otherwise normal liver. Most are larger than 10 cm. Ruptured HAs may be obscured by blood clot and difficult to recognize, but the tumor is usually paler or more yellow than the adjacent liver (Fig. 20-3). The cut surface has a variegated appearance, generally due to the presence of blood clot. Fibrous septa are usually a result of previous infarct.

MICROSCOPIC FINDINGS

On first glance, most HAs resemble normal liver microscopically, being composed of virtually normal hepatocytes in cords that are one to two cells thick and separated by sinusoids lined by inconspicuous Kupffer cells. However, no normal portal tracts are present, and there is a notable lack of any biliary epithelium. The third key feature of HA

HEPATIC ADENOMA—PATHOLOGIC FEATURES

Gross Findings
- Yellow, tan, or red-brown solitary nodule in noncirrhotic liver
- Most measure 5 to 15 cm
- May be hemorrhagic

Microscopic Findings
- Benign hepatocytes without acinar architecture or portal tracts
- Tumor cells often contain glycogen or fat
- Thin-walled vascular channels scattered throughout tumor
- No biliary epithelium

Fine-Needle Aspiration Biopsy Findings
- Single population of benign hepatocytes
- Absence of other cellular elements (bile duct epithelium, fibrous tissue)

Differential Diagnosis
- FNH
- Well-differentiated HCC
- Normal liver (needle biopsy)

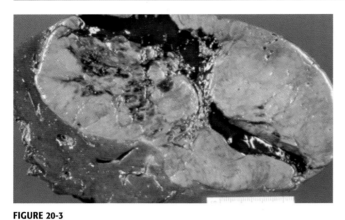

FIGURE 20-3
Hepatic adenomas are sharply circumscribed lesions. Intrahepatic hemorrhage is common in resected specimens.

is the presence of haphazardly distributed arteries and thin-walled veins (Fig. 20-4). Hepatocellular rosettes (pseudoglands) should not be confused with bile ducts.

The hepatocytes of HA frequently display clear or vacuolated cytoplasm due to accumulation of glycogen or fat. Cytoplasmic inclusions representing α_1-antitrypsin, megamitochondria, and Mallory's hyalin is occasionally found. Focal cellular pleomorphism and prominent nucleoli may occasionally be seen, especially in tumors associated with androgenic steroid use. Mitoses, vascular invasion, and stromal invasion are not seen in HA and are suggestive of malignancy. Various degenerative changes in HA include dilated sinusoids and larger blood-filled (pelioid) spaces, a myxoid stroma, and areas of necrosis, infarct, and hematoma.

A new classification of HAs has been proposed based on genotype-phenotype correlation. Based on two molecular criteria (presence of HNF1α or β-catenin mutation) and one histologic criterion (presence or absence

of an inflammatory infiltrate), HAs can be subclassified into four categories: (1) HAs with mutations of the *HNF1α* gene, (2) HAs with β-catenin gene mutation, (3) tumors without β-catenin or HNF1α mutations with inflammatory features, and (4) lesions showing no mutation and no inflammatory component. Tumors in group 1 are the most common (30% to 50% of adenomas) and histologically show prominent steatosis without cellular atypia or inflammation. Type 2 tumors are more common in males, tend to show cytologic abnormalities and acinar growth pattern, and may show areas of either borderline lesion between HA and HCC or unequivocal HCC. Type 3 tumors are characterized by presence of inflammatory infiltrates (especially around portal tractlike structures) and telangiectatic areas (Fig. 20-5). Most lesions previously classified as "telangiectatic FNHs" are now classified as inflammatory/telangiectatic adenoma, in that their molecular features and clinical behavior (propensity to bleed if not resected) mimic those of adenomas rather than FNHs. Finally, type 4 lesions comprise a minority of lesions and lack distinctive features.

The term *adenomatosis* is sometimes used for those cases with multiple (usually more than 10) adenomas. Because the etiologic associations appear to be similar for multiple and solitary adenomas, distinction between these two groups is probably not warranted on clinicopathologic grounds.

ANCILLARY STUDIES

FINE-NEEDLE ASPIRATION BIOPSY

FNA biopsy shows a single population of benign hepatocytes and absence of other cellular elements such as bile duct epithelium and fibrous tissue.

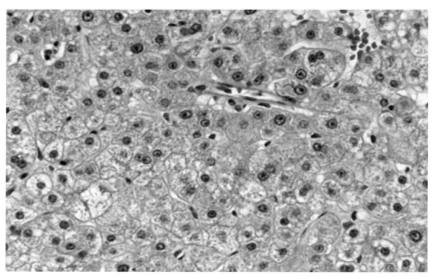

FIGURE 20-4
Hepatic adenoma. Normal portal structures are lacking, and there is no biliary epithelium. The hepatocytes are bland. Haphazardly arranged parenchymal vessels are characteristic.

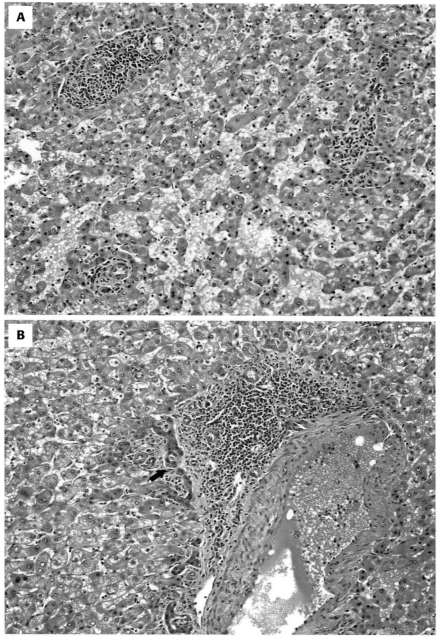

FIGURE 20-5

A, Portal tractlike structures with chronic inflammatory infiltrate and dilated (telangectatic) sinusoids are characteristic of telangectatic adenomas. **B,** Portal tract like structures may contain poorly formed ductules (*arrow*) but lack normal, well-formed bile ducts.

DIFFERENTIAL DIAGNOSIS

On biopsy, distinguishing HA from FNH, well-differentiated HCC, and normal liver may be difficult. Fibrous scars in HA are rare and lack the large vessels seen in the fibrous septa of FNH. As noted, HA lacks vascular invasion and significant mitotic activity, distinguishing it from well-differentiated HCC. The absence of an aberrant trabecular pattern in HA and the relatively low nuclear-to-cytoplasmic (N:C) ratio are also helpful features discriminating features. HA is distinguished from normal liver by the lack of normal portal tracts and the total absence of biliary epithelium.

PROGNOSIS AND THERAPY

Rupture with subsequent massive bleeding into the peritoneal cavity is the most common cause of death related to HA. Because of this risk, HAs are completely excised when technically possible. Liver transplantation is occasionally performed for very large or multiple lesions. There is a low, incompletely defined risk for transformation to HCC.

MACROREGENERATIVE AND DYSPLASTIC (BORDERLINE) NODULES

Numerous terms have been applied to large hepatocellular nodules arising in the setting of cirrhosis, but the following nomenclature is widely accepted. Macroregenerative nodules (MRNs) are larger than surrounding nodules but do not display other atypical features. Dysplastic or "borderline," nodules (DNs) exhibit atypical architectural or cytologic features, but do not meet histologic criteria for HCC.

PATHOLOGIC FEATURES

GROSS FINDINGS

Macroregenerative and dysplastic nodules are usually similar to other cirrhotic nodules, although they may be paler or more bile stained. A thick fibrous capsule or variegated appearance is more suggestive of small HCC. MRNs are larger than other cirrhotic nodules and may measure up to 5 cm or more in diameter (Fig. 20-6). High-grade DNs resemble MRNs grossly but may appear less well circumscribed.

MICROSCOPIC FINDINGS

Most of the MRNs in cirrhosis are multiacinar, containing more than one portal tract scattered throughout the nodule. The hepatocytes within these nodules are identical to those in the surrounding liver. The hepatocellular plates are one or two cells thick. Prominent bile ductular reaction may be seen in the adjacent fibrous scar. The reticulin framework is intact, as in a typical cirrhotic nodule.

In DNs, the hepatocytes typically display nuclear density more than twice normal. Occasional foci of small cell change (small cell dysplasia; Fig. 20-7A), characterized

---

MACROREGENERATIVE NODULES AND DYSPLASTIC NODULES—FACT SHEET

Definition
- MRN: large dominant nodule in cirrhotic liver
- DN: putative precursor lesion to HCC; does not meet definite histologic criteria of malignancy

Incidence and Location
- Reflect the etiology of the underlying cirrhosis

Morbidity and Mortality
- Related to the risk for development of HCC

Gender, Race, and Age Distribution
- Reflects etiology of underlying cirrhosis

Clinical Features
- Arise in setting of cirrhosis
- Asymptomatic

Radiologic Features
- Indistinguishable from cirrhotic nodules

Prognosis and Therapy
- Treatment of DNs is excision when possible, which also facilitates further pathologic classification

Prognosis depends on status of underlying cirrhosis
- High risk for development of HCC

MACROREGENERATIVE NODULES AND DYSPLASTIC NODULES—PATHOLOGIC FEATURES

Gross Findings
- MRNs are larger than other nodules in cirrhotic liver; no difference in color or texture
- DNs may be of any size; may be paler than other cirrhotic nodules and bile stained

Microscopic Findings
- MRNs are similar to other nodules in the cirrhotic liver
- Low-grade DNs show minimal nuclear atypia and only slight architectural abnormalities; large cell change may be seen
- High-grade DNs may show nodule-within-nodule architecture
- Trabeculae are two cells thick; pseudoglands may be present
- Increased mitotic activity
- Focal liver cell atypia, with either small cell or large cell change

Fine-Needle Aspiration Biopsy Findings
- Reactive hepatocytes in groups with irregular edges
- Fibrous tissue
- Abscess of endothelial cells wrapping around hepatocyte groups
- Irregular distribution of dysplastic hepatocytes

Genetics
- MRNs are polyclonal
- Low- and high-grade DNs may be monoclonal or polyclonal

Differential Diagnosis
- Liver cell adenoma
- HCC

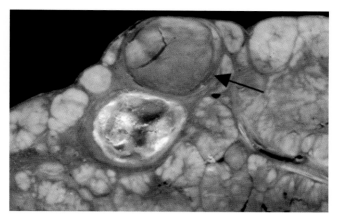

FIGURE 20-6

The macroregenerative nodule in this cirrhotic liver (*arrow*) is distinguishable from the background cirrhosis only by its larger size. The variegated nodule of similar size is a small hepatocellular carcinoma.

by smaller size and a greater N:C ratio than the surrounding hepatocytes, are seen. Other focal architectural and cytologic abnormalities include pseudoglands, large cell change (see Fig. 20-7B), rare mitoses, and isolated liver plates that are three cells thick. Portal tracts may be structurally abnormal. Increased iron deposition is sometimes noted.

PROGNOSIS AND THERAPY

DNs are considered an important precursor to HCC. Ablation or resection of the lesion is recommended because of the potential to develop into HCC. MRNs cannot always be reliably distinguished from low-grade DNs, and patients with apparent MRNs on imaging studies should be followed at frequent intervals.

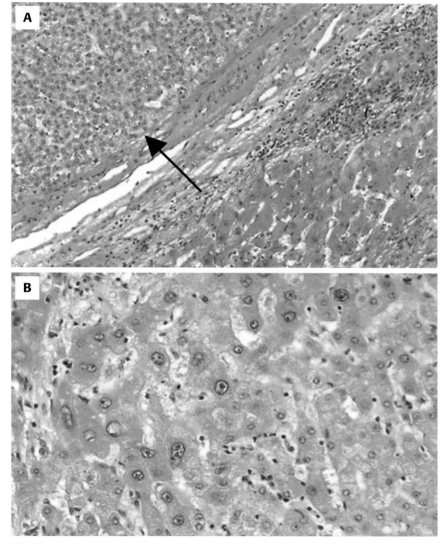

FIGURE 20-7

A, Dysplastic nodules often exhibit small cell change (*arrow*), a dysplastic change that is recognized by the presence of densely packed hepatocytes smaller than those of the surrounding liver. **B,** In large cell change, the hepatocytes are enlarged, with atypical, irregular nuclei and large nucleoli. Aberrant architecture of hepatocellular carcinoma is absent.

DIFFERENTIAL DIAGNOSIS

Separation of low-grade DNs from MRNs, as well as high-grade DNs from HCC, may be impossible on histologic grounds. Features more often seen in HCC are a moderate number of mitotic figures, hepatocyte plates more than three cells thick, marked reduction in the reticulin framework, and the absence of portal tracts. Vascular invasion is diagnostic of HCC, but it is rarely seen in these early lesions.

HEPATOCELLULAR CARCINOMA

CLINICAL FEATURES

Hepatocellular carcinoma is the single most common histologic type of epithelial primary liver tumor. Although relatively uncommon in Western countries, HCC is one of the most prevalent malignant tumors worldwide, responsible for 20% to 40% of cancer deaths in regions of high incidence, such as sub-Saharan Africa and Southeast Asia. In low-incidence areas, HCC is a tumor of elderly men. In areas of higher incidence, HCC occurs at earlier ages (20s to 30s) due to the high prevalence of perinatally acquired hepatitis B.

Virtually any chronic liver disease may predispose toward HCC. The most common predisposing condition is cirrhosis from any cause, with hepatitis B, hepatitis C, and alcoholic liver disease the most common causes. Obesity-related liver disease is increasingly recognized as a risk factor for HCC, and genetic hemochromatosis carries a particularly high risk. The annual risk for HCC developing in a cirrhotic liver is estimated at 1% to 6%.

Patients may present with abdominal pain, fullness or a mass, or clinical signs and symptoms of cirrhosis. HCC rarely presents with metastases. The most useful serum marker is elevation of AFP, which may be highly elevated in patients with large tumors. Of note, serum AFP levels may also be elevated viral hepatitis and cirrhosis. High AFP levels are also seen in hepatoid gastric adenocarcinomas and germ cell tumors containing a yolk sac component.

RADIOLOGIC FEATURES

Advanced HCC is generally easily detected by ultrasonography, CT, or MRI. HCC on CT is usually low attenuation and may have daughter nodules. Ultrasonography is the most useful modality in screening for HCC in cirrhotic livers; a mosaic pattern with peripheral sonolucency is typical.

PATHOLOGIC FEATURES

GROSS FINDINGS

Several macroscopic patterns of HCC are reported. HCC arising in a noncirrhotic liver usually grows as a single large mass, with or without satellite nodules, and may also exhibit this pattern in the setting of cirrhosis (Fig. 20-8A). However, tumors arising in cirrhosis often grow as numerous smaller nodules (diffuse type) that may be difficult to distinguish from the background liver (see Fig. 20-8B). Tumor nodules are soft, bile stained, or yellow to tan; they often appear variegated due to foci of hemorrhage and necrosis (see Fig. 20-6). Separate tumor nodules may represent multicentric growth or may represent tumor spread via intrahepatic vascular routes. Macroscopic portal vein, hepatic vein, and bile duct invasion are present in some cases (see Fig. 20-8C). Involvement of the inferior vena cava, sometimes with extension into the right atrium, may be found.

MICROSCOPIC FINDINGS

Hepatocellular carcinoma typically displays obvious hepatocellular differentiation, with arrangement of cells resembling hepatocytes in a trabecular pattern outlined by sinusoids. Most HCCs have scant stroma. Bile production by neoplastic cells is pathognomonic of HCC but should not be confused with bile production by trapped non-neoplastic hepatocytes. The presence of bile canaliculi is also diagnostic. Cytoplasmic inclusions such as Mallory's hyalin, α_1-antitrypsin inclusions, and fat are frequently present, often in focal areas of the tumor or in individual tumor nodules. Vascular lakes may simulate peliosis hepatis. The World Health Organization classification divides tumors into well-, moderately, poorly, and undifferentiated grades. Although most tumors are moderately differentiated, more than one histologic grade is often present within a given tumor.

Four major histologic patterns are described and are frequently found together in the same tumor. Only the fibrolamellar type (FL-HCC) appears to have prognostic significance. The trabecular pattern consists of trabeculae that vary in thickness and are surrounded by sinusoids lined by flattened endothelial cells and Kupffer cells (Fig. 20-9A). In the compact or solid pattern, compression of broad trabeculae forms sheets with inconspicuous sinusoids (see Fig. 20-9B). The pseudoglandular (acinar) variant, with dilated rounded spaces rounded by cytologically malignant hepatocytes, may be mistaken for adenocarcinoma (see Fig. 20-9C). The lumen may contain bile. The rare scirrhous variant displays prominent desmoplastic stroma (see Fig. 20-9D). Pleomorphic (giant cell), clear cell, and sarcomatoid variants are rare subtypes (see Figs. 20-9E and F).

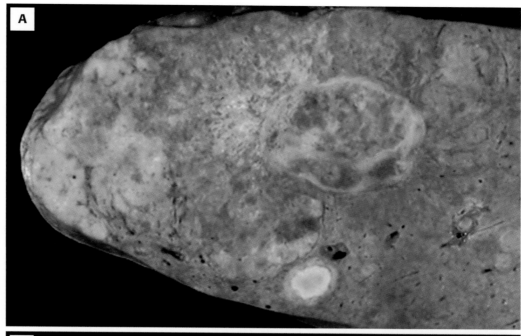

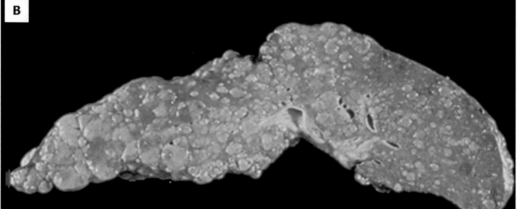

FIGURE 20-8

A, Variegated appearance and greenish color (due to the presence of bile) are characteristic of hepatocellular carcinoma (HCC). Satellite nodules are often present. **B,** In the cirrhotic liver, nodules of HCC may be difficult to distinguish from cirrhosis. **C,** Invasion of large veins is common.

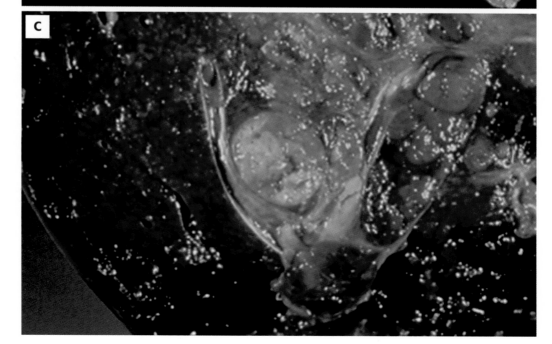

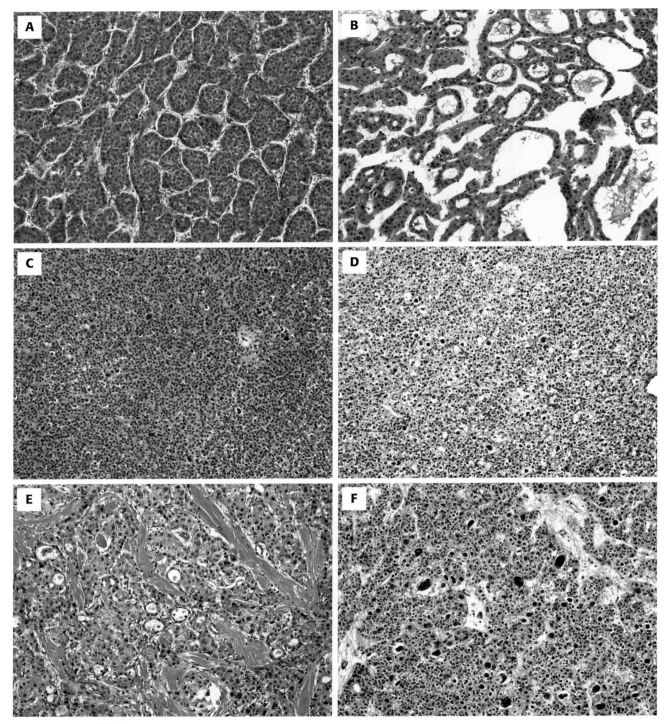

FIGURE 20-9

A, Trabecular architecture, with markedly thickened cell plates lined by endothelial cells, is the most common microscopic pattern in HCC. **B,** Pseudoglandular pattern may be prominent in HCC and may lead to an erroneous diagnosis of adenocarcinoma. Note the absence of a desmoplastic background. **C,** Solid (compact) pattern. **D,** Cytoplasmic clearing of neoplastic hepatocytes due to glycogen accumulation (clear cell pattern). **E,** Prominent bands of collagen are seen in the rare scirrhous pattern. Note that the cytologic features of fibrolamellar-hepatocellular carcinoma (FL-HCC) are not present. **F,** Pleomorphic pattern of HCC showing markedly enlarged, hyperchromatic nuclei, which were present throughout this lesion.

HEPATOCELLULAR CARCINOMA—FACT SHEET

Definition
- Malignant neoplasm showing hepatocellular differentiation

Incidence and Location
- Most common primary liver malignancy in adults
- In United States, incidence is 4 per 100,000
- Wide geographic variation in incidence, with high incidence in Southeast Asia and sub-Saharan Africa, low incidence in Western countries

Morbidity and Mortality
- High mortality
- Median survival for resectable tumors is up to 45 months; for unresectable tumors, less than 6 months
- Patients with cirrhosis are at risk for development of new tumors

Gender, Race, and Age Distribution
- Male predominance 2:1 to 5:1
- Predilection for Asian and African population probably due to chronic viral hepatitis and aflatoxin exposure
- Incidence increases with age in Western countries (peak incidence seventh decade), but mean age in South Africa is 35 years

Clinical Features
- Associated with chronic hepatitis C and hepatitis B infections and exposure to aflatoxins
- Commonly arises with a background of cirrhosis
- Presentation is variable, ranging from decompensated liver disease to malaise, weight loss, and hepatomegaly
- Serum AFP is elevated in approximately 50% of cases

Radiologic Features
- Ultrasonography is method of choice for screening in setting of cirrhosis
- CT shows low-attenuation nodules

Prognosis and Therapy
- Prognosis is heavily dependent on status of liver disease
- Treatment is surgical excision when feasible
- Liver transplantation may be indicated when tumors are small and low stage
- Palliative treatments include ethanol injection, cryoablation, and chemoembolization
- Chemotherapy has limited benefit

HEPATOCELLULAR CARCINOMA—PATHOLOGIC FEATURES

Gross Findings
- Single large mass, with or without satellite nodules, or multiple nodules diffusely involving the liver
- Tumor is soft, often variegated, and bile stained
- Vascular invasion is common, with involvement of portal or hepatic veins

Microscopic Findings
- Wide range of differentiation
- Most tumors have trabecular growth pattern; pseudoglandular pattern is also common
- Stroma is sparse in most tumors
- Bile production, fat droplets, Mallory's hyalin, and other cytoplasmic inclusions may be seen

Ultrastructural Findings
- Bile canaliculi may be demonstrated

Fine-Needle Aspiration Biopsy Findings
- Highly cellular smears with cohesive nests and thick trabeculae of atypical hepatocytes
- Cellular atypia may be minimal in well-differentiated tumors, with slight pleomorphism and increase in N:C ratio
- Endothelial cells wrap around periphery of cell clusters

Genetics
- TP53 mutations associated with progression from early to advanced stage
- Frequent allelic losses on multiple chromosomes

Immunohistochemistry
- Tumor cells are positive for HepPar-1 (hepatocyte), with a granular cytoplasmic pattern
- Less than 50% of tumors are positive for AFP
- Polyclonal CEA demonstrates a canalicular staining pattern; monoclonal CEA is negative

Differential Diagnosis
- HA
- DN in cirrhosis
- Metastatic tumors, especially neuroendocrine tumors
- CC

ANCILLARY STUDIES

ULTRASTRUCTURAL FINDINGS

Electron microscopy is rarely indicated, but demonstration of canaliculi or bile may be useful.

FINE-NEEDLE ASPIRATION BIOPSY

Aspirates of HCC are generally highly cellular, and the tumor cells are polygonal with centrally placed hyperchromatic nuclei and variably prominent nucleoli. The N:C ratio is typically increased, varying with the degree of differentiation. Naked tumor cell nuclei are common and should not be confused with lymphoma. Intranuclear cytoplasmic invaginations and the various cytoplasmic deposits (bile, hyaline globules, Mallory's hyalin), described in the section on histologic features, can be identified in cytologic preparations. Peripheral rimming of the tumor cell clusters by endothelial cells (Fig. 20-10) is a helpful feature.

IMMUNOHISTOCHEMISTRY

The most useful immunohistochemical markers for HCC are canalicular staining pattern with antibodies to CD-10 and certain antibodies to carcinoembryonic antigen (CEA), as well as positivity for hepatocyte (HepPar-1). Immunostaining with polyclonal anti-CEA antiserum or certain monoclonal CEA (m-CEA) antibodies that

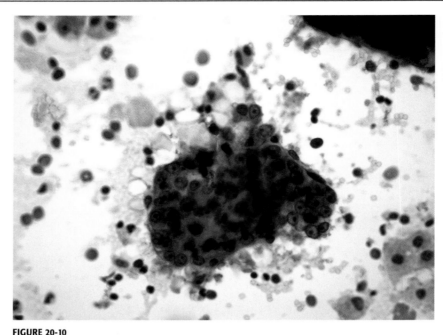

FIGURE 20-10

Hepatocellular carcinoma. Aspirates are hypercellular; large clusters of neoplastic hepatocytes rimmed by endothelial cells are common.

cross-react with canalicular biliary glycoprotein 1 demonstrates a canalicular pattern in up to 80% of HCCs (Fig. 20-11A). Positive staining with antisera to AFP is very suggestive of HCC (see Fig. 20-11B). HepPar-1, a relatively hepatocyte-specific monoclonal antibody that reacts with a hepatocyte epitope that is resistant to formalin fixation and tissue processing, produces a granular cytoplasmic staining pattern in HCC and normal hepatocytes (see Fig. 20-11C). Positive staining for α_1-antitrypsin and alpha-1-antichymotrypsin is nonspecific.

Glypican-3 (an oncofetal protein) immunohistochemistry has also been shown to be a useful marker. Glypican-3 has a high sensitivity for poorly differentiated HCCs and can be used in this situation to differentiate the latter from cholangiocarcinomas and metastatic lesions (see Fig. 20-11D). This marker is also expressed by most well-differentiated HCCs (although sensitivity may be lower than in poorly differentiated lesions). Positive staining is not seen in benign hepatocytic neoplasms.

Cytokeratin (CK) profiles are not particularly useful in diagnosis of HCC. In situ hybridization for albumin messenger RNA appears to be highly sensitive but is not widely used. In practice, many investigators currently use a panel of p-CEA or CD10 (canalicular pattern), m-CEA, HepPar-1, and AFP antibodies for diagnosis of HCC.

DIFFERENTIAL DIAGNOSIS

Neuroendocrine tumors metastatic to the liver may be difficult to distinguish from HCC because of their trabecular architecture. However, the cells usually display the characteristic finely stippled chromatin pattern and lack prominent nucleoli. The presence of a delicate fibrovascular stroma surrounding groups of tumor cells favors neuroendocrine tumor, and diffuse positivity for neuroendocrine markers such as synaptophysin and chromogranin is helpful.

Hepatocellular carcinoma is distinguished from adenocarcinoma and cholangiocarcinoma (CC) by its trabecular growth pattern, lack of a fibrous stroma, and immunohistochemical profile, with canalicular staining pattern with p-CEA and CD10 and cytoplasmic positivity for HepPar-1 and AFP.

PROGNOSIS AND THERAPY

Hepatocellular carcinoma generally carries a very poor prognosis, with survival after diagnosis measured in months. The prognosis is determined primarily by HCC stage and the functional status of the liver. Nonoperative palliative therapies include percutaneous ethanol injection, cryoablation, and transcatheter arterial chemoembolization; chemotherapy has largely proven ineffective. At autopsy, metastases, most commonly to lung and porta hepatis lymph nodes, are found in up to 75% of patients. Bone, adrenal gland, and virtually any site in the body can be involved by metastatic disease. Tumor size, number and location (one or both lobes) of tumor nodules, presence of gross or microscopic vascular invasion, and disease status of the uninvolved liver are the most important prognostic variables. In carefully selected patients,

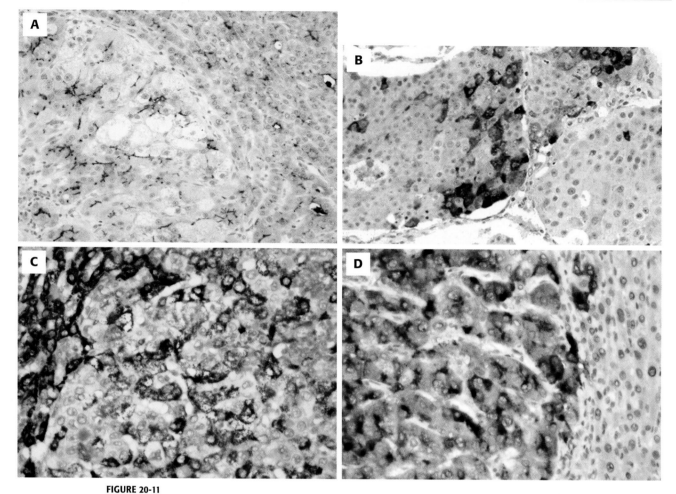

FIGURE 20-11

A, A canalicular staining pattern with cross-reactive (polyclonal) antibodies to carcinoembryonic antigen (shown) and CD10 is characteristic of HCC. Note that both normal liver (*upper right*) and HCC (*lower left*) show the typical canalicular pattern. **B,** Immunohistochemistry for α-fetoprotein is patchy; only approximately 50% of HCC will stain for this marker. **C,** Hepatocyte antibody (HepPar-1) has a granular cytoplasmic staining pattern in HCC. Normal liver (*upper left*) shows similar pattern. **D,** Cytoplasmic and membranous pattern of glipican-3 reactivity in HCC. No staining is seen in normal liver (*right*).

hepatic resection and/or liver transplantation may be performed with success. Small, low-stage, incidentally discovered HCCs in a cirrhotic liver at transplantation do not adversely affect outcome.

FIBROLAMELLAR CARCINOMA

CLINICAL FEATURES

Fibrolamellar-hepatocellular carcinoma (FL-HCC) is a rare HCC variant arising in noncirrhotic liver in young patients. It is associated with a better prognosis than typical HCC, perhaps because of the younger age of the patients and their lack of significant underlying liver disease. Clinical presentation is similar to typical HCC. In most cases serum AFP levels are normal or only modestly elevated.

PATHOLOGIC FEATURES

GROSS FINDINGS

Most FL-HCCs arise in the left lobe, but large tumors may affect both lobes. The tumors are usually solitary, firm, and well circumscribed and may be bile stained, necrotic, or hemorrhagic. They are typically large, measuring up to 25 cm. A central stellate scar similar to that seen in FNH may be present (Fig. 20-12). The adjacent non-neoplastic liver is unremarkable.

MICROSCOPIC FINDINGS

The tumor cells of FL-HCC are very large, display abundant granular eosinophilic cytoplasm (due to large numbers of mitochondria) and distinct cell borders, and have a distinctive oncocytic appearance (Fig. 20-13A). A defining feature of FL-HCC is the presence of parallel

FIBROLAMELLAR CARCINOMA—FACT SHEET

Definition

- Rare variant of HCC with characteristic pathologic findings and distinctive clinical features

Incidence and Location

- Rare in Asian and African countries
- Age-adjusted incidence rate approximately 0.02 per 100,000

Morbidity and Mortality

- More indolent course than typical HCC

Gender, Race, and Age Distribution

- Male to female ratio 3:4
- No race predilection in U.S. population
- Mean age 23 years

Clinical Features

- Symptoms are nonspecific: nausea, weight loss, abdominal pain, malaise
- Not associated with chronic viral hepatitis or cirrhosis
- Normal serum AFP

Radiologic Features

- Well-demarcated hypodense tumor on CT scan
- Central scar may mimic FNH

Prognosis and Therapy

- Approximately 60% are surgically resectable
- Chemotherapy is reserved for patients with unresectable disease and is not curative
- Liver transplantation may be considered if tumor is confined to the liver
- Most significant determinant of survival is tumor stage
- 5-year survival rate is approximately 60%

FIBROLAMELLAR CARCINOMA—PATHOLOGIC FEATURES

Gross Findings

- Two thirds are located in left lobe
- Single mass in 56% of cases
- Firm tan or green circumscribed mass
- Central scar in many cases
- Surrounding liver is noncirrhotic

Microscopic Findings

- Lamellar fibrous stroma
- Large polygonal, granular oncocytic tumor cells
- Cytoplasmic inclusions contain pale bodies (accumulated fibrinogen), Mallory's hyalin, α_1-antitrypsin

Ultrastructural Findings

- Numerous densely packed mitochondria

Fine Needle Aspiration Biopsy Findings

- Aspirate often paucicellular
- Discohesive large hepatocytes with granular cytoplasm
- Intranuclear pseudoinclusions and macronucleoli

Genetics

- 4q+, 9p−, 16p−, and Xq− have been reported

Immunohistochemistry

- Positive for HepPar-1 (hepatocyte)
- Polyclonal CEA positive with a canalicular distribution
- AFP negative

Differential Diagnosis

- FNH
- Ordinary HCC
- CC

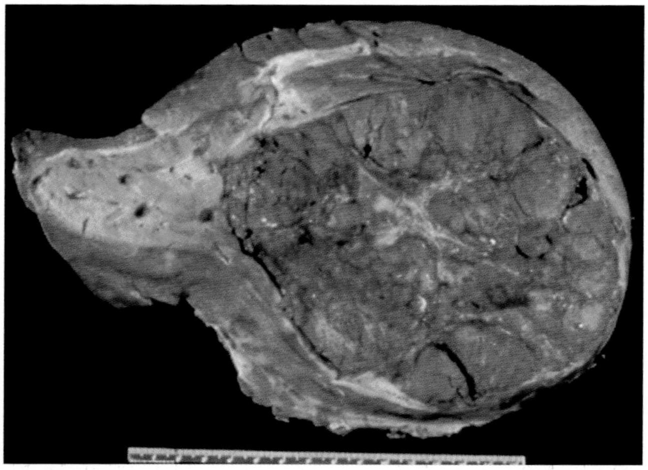

FIGURE 20-12

Fibrolamellar carcinoma (FL-HCC) is usually a single mass; note the noncirrhotic adjacent liver and the central stellate scar.

bands of hyalinized fibrous tissue separating the tumor cells into nests (see Fig. 20-13B). Cytoplasmic eosinophilic hyaline globules, which may be periodic acid-Schiff (PAS) positive diastase resistant, may represent α_1-antitrypsin. Cytoplasmic pale bodies contain fibrinogen and are present in about 50% of cases.

ANCILLARY STUDIES

ULTRASTRUCTURAL FINDINGS

The cytoplasm contains numerous mitochondria, as expected from the oncocytic appearance of the tumor cells. Dense core neuroendocrine-like granules may also be found.

DIFFERENTIAL DIAGNOSIS

The most common lesions in the differential diagnosis for FL-HCC are FNH, typical HCC, and metastatic tumors with extensive fibrosis. Although FNH and FL-HCC may have central stellate scars, microscopically the lack of

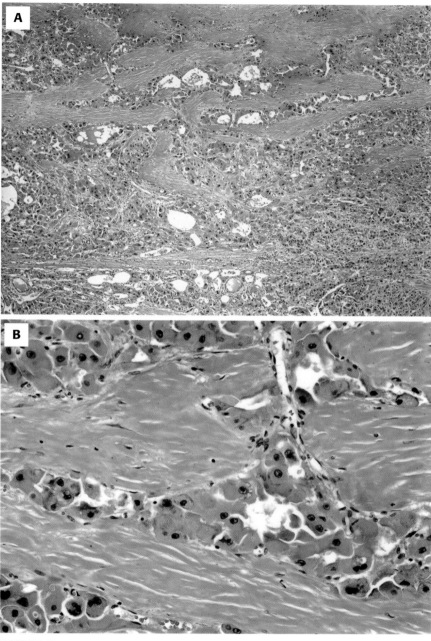

FIGURE 20-13

A, The cells of FL-HCC are very large and polygonal, with abundant granular pink cytoplasm (oncocytes). Central nucleus with prominent nucleolus is also characteristic. **B,** Dense collagen bundles are arranged in parallel layers.

hepatocellular atypia distinguishes FNH from FL-HCC. The presence of grossly detectable bile staining and a diameter greater than 5 cm strongly suggest FL-HCC. Diffuse lamellar fibrosis combined with oncocytic cellular features is not found in typical HCC. In metastatic carcinomas, the collagen is more haphazardly arranged and lacks the lamellar features characteristic of FL-HCC. The tumor cells in scirrhous HCC are smaller, do not display oncocytic features, and form glandular patterns.

PROGNOSIS AND THERAPY

FL-HCC is often resectable and thus associated with a better outcome than usual HCC. Hepatic transplantation may be considered for nonresectable tumors confined to the liver. The most common metastatic sites are abdominal lymph nodes, peritoneum, and lung.

HEPATOBLASTOMA

CLINICAL FEATURES

Hepatoblastoma (HB) is the most common primary hepatic tumor in children, accounting for about 50% of all primary pediatric hepatic malignancies; the majority occurs by 2 years of age. There is a male predominance (2:1). Patients generally present with an abdominal mass noticed by the parent, but some patients present with precocious puberty related to human chorionic gonadotropin production by the tumor. Roughly 5% of patients have an associated congenital abnormality. Familial adenomatous polyposis is associated with higher risk for HB. Although the etiologic factors of HB are unknown, an association with low birth weight is recognized, although it is not clear if an environmental cause is responsible. The serum AFP level is elevated in 90% of cases.

RADIOLOGIC FEATURES

HB is visualized as a solid or multifocal mass on CT, with calcification in more than half of cases. MRI shows decreased signal relative to the normal liver on T1-weighted images and increased signal on T2-weighted images.

PATHOLOGIC FEATURES

GROSS FINDINGS

HB is typically a solitary mass most often located in the right lobe. Tumors may be quite large, measuring up to 20 cm. Purely epithelial HB is a soft, fleshy, tan-white mass (Fig. 20-14); those with a prominent mesenchymal component are often firm and may be calcified. Cystic degeneration, necrosis, and hemorrhage may be seen.

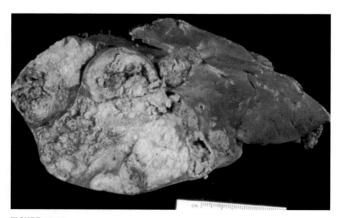

FIGURE 20-14
Hepatoblastoma (HB) is a single large mass; epithelial tumors are soft and fleshy.

MICROSCOPIC FINDINGS

HBs may be classified as either epithelial or mixed epithelial-mesenchymal and are subclassified into six patterns.

1. Fetal pattern (30%). In this pattern the hepatocytes are uniform and similar to normal hepatocytes, although they have a slightly higher N:C ratio. An alternating light and dark pattern is characteristic on low power (Fig. 20-15A). Mitoses are typically rare (less than 2 per 10 high-power fields). The tumor cells form cords two to three cells thick, separated by sinusoids, in a pattern reminiscent of normal liver. However, normal structures such as portal tracts, bile ducts, and bile ductules are absent.
2. Embryonal pattern (20%). The tumor cells in the embryonal pattern are less differentiated and cohesive compared with those of the fetal pattern and have a higher N:C ratio and coarser chromatin. The trabecular pattern is not well developed, and the tumor cells may form sheets. Mitoses and necrosis are more common than in the fetal pattern.
3. Macrotrabecular pattern (3%). This pattern is characterized by broad trabeculae 10 or more cells thick. Trabeculae may be composed of embryonal or fetal cells.
4. Small cell undifferentiated pattern (3%). This pattern is the least differentiated pattern and resembles other small blue cell tumors of childhood. The tumor is composed of loosely cohesive sheets of uniform small cells with scanty cytoplasm. The tumor cells are positive for CK.
5. Mixed epithelial and mesenchymal pattern (44%). This pattern is characterized by areas of both epithelial and mesenchymal differentiation. The primitive mesenchymal component may be primitive, with spindle or stellate cells with little cytoplasm, or display differentiation along chondroid and rhabdomyoblastic lines. Osteoid is the most frequent heterologous element and may be more prominent after chemotherapy (see Fig. 20-15B). The mesenchymal elements may be CK positive, suggesting sarcomatoid metaplasia of the epithelial component.
6. A subtype of mixed pattern tumors displays teratoid features and may contain elements of mature teratoma such as keratinized squamous epithelium, intestinal epithelium, and neuroectodermal structures.

ANCILLARY STUDIES

FINE-NEEDLE ASPIRATION BIOPSY

FNA biopsy yields highly cellular smears with cohesive nests and sheets of small atypical hepatocytes. The aspirate may contain a spindle cell or mesenchymal component.

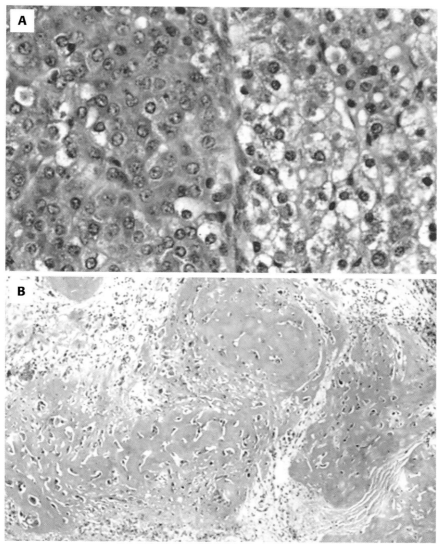

FIGURE 20-15

A, The fetal pattern of HB exhibits alternating areas of light- and dark-staining tumor cells showing hepatocellular differentiation.
B, Osteoid is the most common mesenchymal element and may be abundant following chemotherapy.

DIFFERENTIAL DIAGNOSIS

HB with a predominantly or exclusively small cell component may be difficult to distinguish from the small, round cell tumors such as neuroblastoma, lymphoma, and rhabdomyosarcoma. The presence of more differentiated areas of HB and the tumor cell immunophenotype (CK positive; leukocyte common antigen, neurofilament, and desmin negative) distinguish small cell HB from other neoplasms. The absence of a renal mass generally excludes Wilms' tumor. The macrotrabecular variant of HB closely resembles HCC; however, HCC is exceedingly rare in the age group affected by HB.

Other considerations include sarcomas, such as undifferentiated (embryonal) sarcoma, which are excluded by the lack of an epithelial component. Germ cell tumor must be considered in the differential diagnosis but is generally excluded by the focal nature of the teratoid areas in HB.

PROGNOSIS AND THERAPY

Outcome is dependent on tumor resectability. Most patients are treated with neoadjuvant multiagent chemotherapy, and currently the rate of resection is over 90%. More than 70% of patients have long-term survival. The most frequent metastatic sites are regional lymph nodes and lung. Liver transplantation may be considered in some cases in which tumor is limited to the liver but is unresectable.

HEPATOBLASTOMA—FACT SHEET

Definition

- Malignant liver tumor occurring in children, mimicking fetal or embryonal liver and often containing heterologous cell types

Incidence and Location

- Rare; annual incidence in United States is 0.2 per 100,000 children
- 47% of pediatric malignant liver tumors

Morbidity and Mortality

- Overall survival is 65% to 70%

Gender, Race, and Age Distribution

- Male predominance 2:1
- No racial predilection
- 90% occur within first 5 years of life

Clinical Features

- More common in low-birth-weight infants
- Presenting symptom is enlarging abdomen noted by parent
- Weight loss and anorexia are less common
- 5% of children with HB have congenital anomalies
- Human chorionic gonadotropin production may lead to presentation with precocious puberty

Radiologic Features

- Solid or multifocal mass on CT
- Calcification in greater than 50% of cases
- MRI shows decreased signal relative to normal liver on T1-weighted images, increased signal on T2-weighted images

Prognosis and Therapy

- Tumor stage is key prognostic factor
- Pure fetal type may have a better prognosis; small cell undifferentiated pattern has a worse prognosis
- Treatment is surgical excision when possible
- Preoperative chemotherapy allows many previously unresectable cases to be completely resected

HEPATOBLASTOMA—PATHOLOGIC FEATURES

Gross Findings

- Single well-circumscribed mass in 80% of cases
- Pure fetal tumors are soft, tan to brown, and coarsely lobulated
- Mixed epithelial and mesenchymal tumors have a variegated, heterogeneous cut surface

Microscopic Findings

- Six histologic subtypes
- Pure fetal epithelial pattern (approximately 30%) is composed of sheets of uniform cells resembling fetal hepatocytes
- Embryonal pattern consists of a mixture of fetal-type cells and smaller less differentiated cells with higher N:C ratio
- Macrotrabecular pattern: epithelial HB with trabeculae more than 10 cells thick
- Small cell undifferentiated pattern is composed of discohesive sheets of small cells indistinguishable from other small blue cell tumors of childhood
- Mixed epithelial and mesenchymal pattern contains fetal and embryonal epithelial cells and primitive mesenchyme with various mesenchymal tissues such as fibrous tissue, osteoid, and cartilage
- Teratoid pattern contains a variety of tissue types in addition to those found in the mixed pattern, such as skeletal muscle, bone, or squamous epithelium

Ultrastructural Findings

- Small cell tumors have relatively dense cytoplasm with tonofilaments, intercellular junctions, and microvilli
- Glycogen accumulation and bile canaliculi may be seen in epithelial components

Fine-Needle Aspiration Biopsy Findings

- Very cellular smears
- Cohesive nests and sheets of small, crowded, atypical hepatocytes
- High N:C ratio and vacuolated or granular cytoplasm
- May contain spindle cell or mesenchymal component
- Small cell type is indistinguishable from other small round blue cell tumors on smear

Genetics

- Associated with familial adenomatous polyposis (APC gene mutations)
- Trisomy 2, trisomy 20, 4q structural rearrangements are the most common chromosomal abnormalities
- Stabilizing mutations in β-catenin activate Wnt pathway

Immunohistochemistry

- Epithelial components are hepatocyte positive, AFP positive, epithelial membrane antigen positive
- Small cell pattern is CK positive
- Mesenchymal areas are vimentin positive

Differential Diagnosis

- HCC
- Other small blue cell tumors of childhood

Histologic pattern is generally not an independent predictor of prognosis, although the small cell undifferentiated pattern does appear to correlate with a poorer prognosis, and completely resected pure fetal tumors may have a more favorable outcome. Other unfavorable prognostic features are increased mitotic activity, vascular invasion, incomplete tumor resection, and AFP levels of less than 100 ng/mL at diagnosis.

BILIARY TUMORS

BILE DUCT HAMARTOMA

CLINICAL FEATURES

Bile duct hamartomas (BDHs), also known as von Meyenburg complexes, are small, incidental, clinically asymptomatic lesions, reported in up to 27% of all autopsies.

BDH is considered part of the spectrum of ductal plate malformation and may be related to autosomal dominant polycystic kidney disease, congenital hepatic fibrosis, or other genetic disorders, as well as being found on a sporadic basis.

PATHOLOGIC FEATURES

GROSS FINDINGS

BDHs appear as single or multiple subcapsular, gray-white, or occasionally green nodules less than 0.5 cm in diameter.

MICROSCOPIC FINDINGS

BDHs are found directly adjacent to portal tracts and consist of ectatic, branched bile ducts lined by a single layer of bland, low columnar to cuboidal biliary epithelium

(Fig. 20-16). The lumina may contain granular eosinophilic material or bile. The stroma is dense and hyalinized, with minimal inflammation.

DIFFERENTIAL DIAGNOSIS

A BDH is distinguished from a bile duct adenoma (BDA) by its dilated, rather than compact, biliary channels and the presence of intraluminal bile. It is distinguished from CC by its circumscribed nature and the lack of cellular atypia.

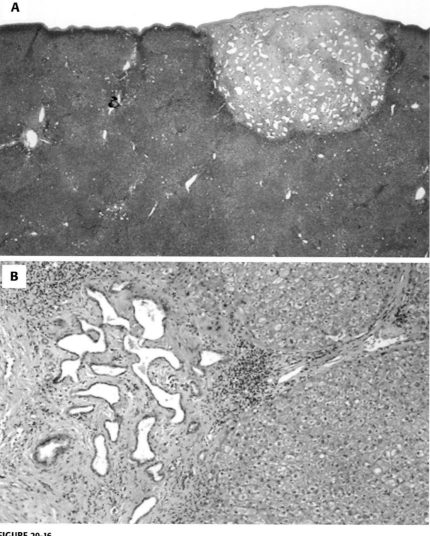

FIGURE 20-16

A, On low power, bile duct hamartomas (BDHs) are well circumscribed and frequently subcapsular. **B,** Dilated biliary channels at the periphery of a portal tract are characteristic.

BILE DUCT HAMARTOMA (VON MEYENBURG COMPLEX)—FACT SHEET

Definition

- Bile duct malformation at the level of the interlobular bile duct, caused by failure of involution of the embryonic ductal plate

Incidence and Location

- Common incidental finding at autopsy or surgery
- No geographic predilection

Morbidity and Mortality

- Sporadic lesions are innocuous; not associated with increased morbidity or mortality
- As part of the spectrum of ductal plate malformations, associated with increased risk for CC

Gender, Race, and Age Distribution

- Equal gender distribution
- No race predilection
- All ages, but more common in adults

Clinical Features

- Most commonly, sporadic asymptomatic incidental finding
- When multiple and numerous, may be part of the spectrum of ductal plate malformation and adult polycystic disease

Prognosis and Therapy

- Treatment is not indicated; lesion is excised for diagnostic purposes when identified during surgery
- Prognosis is excellent—innocuous finding

BILE DUCT HAMARTOMA (VON MEYENBURG COMPLEX)—PATHOLOGIC FEATURES

Gross Findings

- Small gray-white nodule, often subcapsular

Microscopic Findings

- Dilated biliary channels embedded in fibrous stroma
- Located at periphery of portal tract
- Channels may contain bile

Fine-Needle Aspiration Biopsy Findings

- Numerous groups of normal-appearing biliary epithelium

Differential Diagnosis

- BDA
- Metastatic adenocarcinoma or CC

PROGNOSIS AND THERAPY

BDHs are innocuous incidental findings. Rarely, CC has been reported in association with multiple BDHs, as with other ductal plate malformation disorders.

BILE DUCT ADENOMA

CLINICAL FEATURES

A BDA is an innocuous lesion, usually an incidental finding at autopsy or in the resected liver. It is not clear that a BDA is a true neoplasm, and it is regarded by some investigators as a hamartoma of peribiliary glands.

PATHOLOGIC FEATURES

GROSS FINDINGS

BDHs are solitary, well-circumscribed, firm, gray-white or tan, subcapsular nodules. Most measure 5 mm or less.

MICROSCOPIC FINDINGS

BDHs consist of a compact proliferation of simple tubular ducts embedded in a variable amount of fibrous stroma. The tubules have small lumina, unlike the dilated channels of a BDH, and do not contain intraluminal secretions or bile. The cuboidal/low columnar lining epithelium resembles that of interlobular bile ducts (Fig. 20-17). The cells of a BDA are uniform and lack nuclear pleomorphism and hyperchromasia. Mitoses and vascular or lymphatic invasion are not seen. The stromal inflammatory is variable.

DIFFERENTIAL DIAGNOSIS

A BDA is distinguished from a BDH by its lack of intraluminal bile and the compact nature of the proliferation. It is distinguished from CC by its circumscribed nature and the lack of cellular atypia.

PROGNOSIS AND THERAPY

A BDA is an innocuous incidental finding. However, some lesions, particularly larger BDAs, may carry a potential for malignant transformation.

SOLITARY BILIARY CYST

CLINICAL FEATURES

Solitary biliary cysts are found in up to 14% of autopsies but rarely come to clinical attention. They occur predominantly in women and are usually asymptomatic. Their origin is obscure, but many may develop from BDHs that become isolated from the biliary tree.

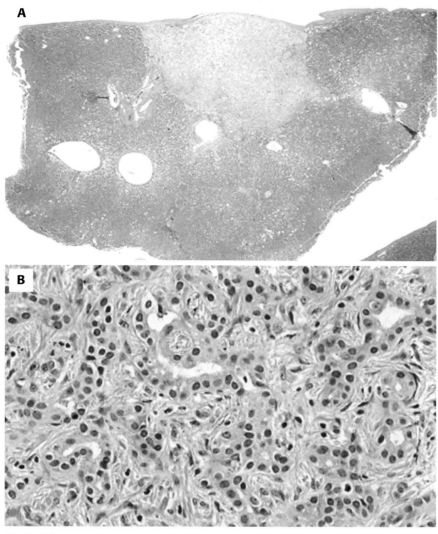

FIGURE 20-17

A, On low power, bile duct adenomas (BDAs) are well circumscribed, similar to BDHs. Most measure less than 2 cm. **B,** The BDA is composed of a tightly packed proliferation of bland biliary structures.

PATHOLOGIC FEATURES

GROSS FINDINGS

Most cysts are subcapsular (Fig. 20-18). Size is variable, from a few centimeters in incidental lesions to up to 40 cm. Biliary cysts usually contain thin clear yellow fluid, and the cyst lining is flat and glistening. Connection to the biliary tree is not demonstrated.

MICROSCOPIC FINDINGS

Biliary cysts are frequently lined by a single layer of cuboidal, flattened, or columnar biliary-type epithelium. The cyst wall is thin and fibrous and lacks the mesenchymal ovarian-type stroma of biliary cystadenomas. A ciliated lining and smooth muscle in the cyst wall are characteristic of ciliated hepatic foregut cyst.

BILE DUCT ADENOMA—FACT SHEET

Definition

- Small benign lesion composed of acini and tubules, regarded by some as a peribiliary gland hamartoma

Incidence and Location

- No geographic variation in incidence reported
- Considered rare, but found in approximately 25% of livers at autopsy when livers were closely examined

Morbidity and Mortality

- No increase in morbidity or mortality

Gender, Race, and Age Distribution

- Male predominance 3:2
- No race predilection
- Older adults (mean age 55 years), but all age ranges

Clinical Features

- Incidental finding at surgery or autopsy

Prognosis and Therapy

- Excellent prognosis
- Excised for diagnosis; no treatment indicated

SOLITARY BILIARY CYST—FACT SHEET

Definition

- Non-neoplastic unilocular cyst lined by single layer of cuboidal to columnar epithelium

Incidence and Location

- Up to 14% of autopsies
- No geographic variation in incidence reported

Morbidity and Mortality

- Low; often incidental finding

Gender, Race, and Age Distribution

- Female predominance 4:1
- No race predilection
- Rare in children; more common in 30- to 50-year-old age range

Clinical Features

- Smaller cysts are usually asymptomatic
- Usual symptoms are nonspecific: abdominal fullness, mass, nausea, rarely jaundice

Radiologic Features

- Circumscribed lesion with water density on CT

Prognosis and Therapy

- Surgical excision, laparoscopic fenestration, or aspiration with sclerotherapy are treatment options

BILE DUCT ADENOMA—PATHOLOGIC FEATURES

Gross Findings

- Usually solitary, subcapsular lesion
- One centimeter or less, well-demarcated gray-white mass

Microscopic Findings

- Densely packed tubules and acini lined by single layer of cuboidal to columnar cells
- Fibrous stroma with variable inflammatory infiltrate

Immunohistochemistry

- Immunophenotype is that of peribiliary glands: CK19+, D10+, 1F6+, CEA+, EMA+

Differential Diagnosis

- BDH (von Meyenburg complex)
- CC

SOLITARY BILIARY CYST—PATHOLOGIC FEATURES

Gross Findings

- More common in right lobe
- Round, with smooth lining
- Fluid is usually clear but may be bile stained, or purulent if secondarily infected

Microscopic Findings

- Single layer of biliary-type epithelium
- Cyst wall is fibrous tissue and lacks ovarian-type mesenchymal stroma

Fine-Needle Aspiration Biopsy Findings

- Cystic debris

Differential Diagnosis

- Biliary cystadenoma
- Polycystic liver disease

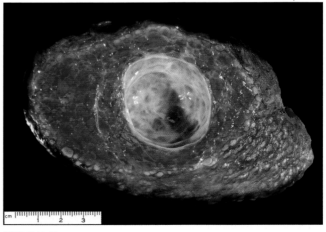

FIGURE 20-18

The biliary cyst is a unilocular, smooth-walled cyst, usually found just under the hepatic capsule. It is a common finding at autopsy.

PROGNOSIS AND THERAPY

Asymptomatic biliary cysts do not require treatment. Partial or complete surgical excision or cyst fenestration may be performed in symptomatic cases.

■ POLYCYSTIC LIVER DISEASE

CLINICAL FEATURES

Polycystic liver disease belongs to the family of fibrocystic disorders of the liver and represents one of the ductal plate malformation disorders, with the malformation occurring at the level of the interlobular bile duct. Patients with polycystic liver disease usually have autosomal dominant polycystic kidney disease. The liver cysts are not present at birth but develop over time as fluid accumulates in the dilated biliary spaces of BDHs (von Meyenburg complexes). Up to 30% of young adults have liver cysts; this prevalence increases to 90% in older patients.

PATHOLOGIC FEATURES

GROSS FINDINGS

Multiple unilocular cysts resembling simple biliary cysts and ranging in size from a few millimeters to over 10 cm in diameter are scattered diffusely throughout the liver or, more rarely, are limited to one lobe (Fig. 20-19).

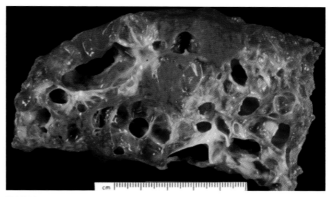

FIGURE 20-19
Polycystic liver disease. The liver is distorted by multiple cysts of varying sizes.

POLYCYSTIC LIVER DISEASE—FACT SHEET

Definition
- Multiple hepatic cysts, associated with autosomal dominant polycystic kidney disease

Incidence and Location
- Incidence of autosomal dominant polycystic kidney disease is 1 in 1000
- Numerous hepatic cysts are found in approximately 20% of patients with polycystic kidney disease
- More common in patients of Northern European descent

Morbidity and Mortality
- Morbidity is associated with infection of cysts and development of CC
- Mortality is usually due to renal disease, not hepatic involvement

Gender, Race, and Age Distribution
- Symptomatic hepatic cysts are more common in women, related to number of pregnancies
- More common in whites
- Average age for manifestation of liver cysts is approximately 53 years; number and size of cysts increases with age

Clinical Features
- Hepatomegaly and upper abdominal pain
- Jaundice and portal hypertension are rare
- Hepatic outflow obstruction may be seen
- Manifestations in other organs include colonic diverticula, cardiac valve abnormalities, and intracranial aneurysms

Radiologic Features
- Multiple circumscribed lesions with water density on CT

Prognosis and Therapy
- Excision or fenestration of cysts is rarely indicated
- Liver transplantation has been performed in selected patients
- Prognosis is related to underlying renal disease

POLYCYSTIC LIVER DISEASE—PATHOLOGIC FEATURES

Gross Findings
- Numerous cysts of various sizes, sometimes involving one lobe more than the other
- Cysts contain clear colorless or yellow fluid

Microscopic Findings
- Cysts are lined by columnar-to-flattened biliary epithelium
- Origin in von Meyenburg complex may be demonstrated for smaller cysts

Genetics
- Associated with autosomal dominant polycystic kidney disease
- Mutations in PKD1 and PKD2 have been implicated

Differential Diagnosis
- Solitary biliary cyst
- Biliary cystadenoma

MICROSCOPIC FINDINGS

Cysts in polycystic liver disease resembled solitary biliary cysts microscopically. Origin from BDHs may be demonstrated (Fig. 20-20).

PROGNOSIS AND THERAPY

The cysts usually do not compromise hepatic function but may produce hepatomegaly (sometimes massive) and abdominal discomfort. Women are more likely to be symptomatic from the cysts, and morbidity is related to number of pregnancies, use of oral contraceptives, and severity of renal involvement. Hepatic complications include secondary infection of cysts and development of CC. Treatments include resection of more severely affected areas of liver and in some cases liver transplantation.

BILIARY CYSTADENOMA AND CYSTADENOCARCINOMA

CLINICAL FEATURES

Biliary cystadenomas are analogous to mucinous cystadenomas of the pancreas. About 95% of cases develop in women, with the mean age at diagnosis 45 years. Patients may present with abdominal pain or an abdominal mass. Although most mucinous cystadenomas are intrahepatic, these tumors may also be found in the common bile duct, hepatic ducts, cystic duct, and gallbladder.

Biliary cystadenocarcinomas are rare hepatic malignancies; some arise in a preexisting cystadenoma. However, unlike cystadenomas, cystadenocarcinomas show no female predominance and usually arise in older patients.

PATHOLOGIC FEATURES

GROSS FINDINGS

Intrahepatic mucinous biliary cystadenomas are encapsulated and solitary multicystic lesions ranging from 2.5 to 28 cm in diameter. The cyst fluid is usually clear and mucinous. The cyst lining is smooth, with a few coarse trabeculations (Fig. 20-21A). Solid areas suggest possible malignant change (cystadenocarcinoma) (see Fig. 20-21B).

MICROSCOPIC FEATURES

The cysts of biliary cystadenomas are lined by tall columnar mucinous epithelium and resemble ovarian mucinous cystadenomas. Intestinal metaplasia is found in a minority of cases, and neuroendocrine cells can occasionally be identified. Roughly 10% of cases show dysplasia that in an ovarian mucinous neoplasm would be classified as borderline malignancy. A characteristic dense subepithelial mesenchymal spindle cell stroma resembling normal ovarian stroma is found in most cases from women and is not found in cystadenomas occurring in men (Fig. 20-22).

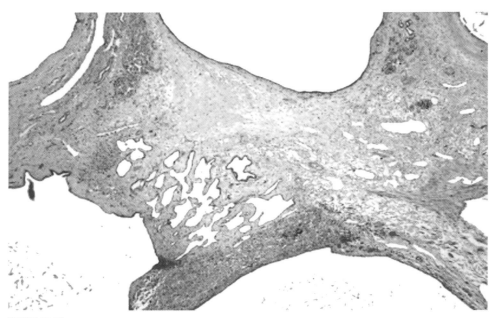

FIGURE 20-20

Polycystic liver disease. The cysts are lined by flattened or cuboidal biliary epithelium. Origin from bile duct hamartomas may be demonstrated.

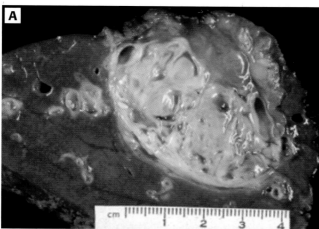

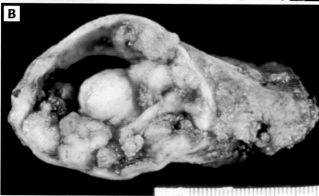

FIGURE 20-21

A, Most biliary cystadenomas are multilocular lesions arising in a normal liver. The cyst walls are smooth, without exophytic projections. **B,** The biliary cystadenocarcinoma often displays solid areas projecting into the cyst lumen.

Biliary cystadenocarcinomas most often grow in complex papillary fronds that project into the cysts (Fig. 20-23A); higher-grade lesions may have a solid growth pattern. Invasion of the underlying stroma is definitive evidence of cystadenocarcinoma (see Fig. 20-23B), although some pathologists diagnose malignancy when high-grade cytologic and architectural dysplastic changes are present.

ANCILLARY STUDIES

FINE-NEEDLE ASPIRATION BIOPSY

Occasional aggregates of bland, cuboidal-columnar epithelial cells, rarely arranged in papillary clusters, are reported on FNAs of biliary cystadenomas.

DIFFERENTIAL DIAGNOSIS

Biliary cystadenomas are distinguished from simple biliary cysts by their multilocular nature and tall columnar lining. The presence of mesenchymal ovarian-type stroma is a particularly helpful feature, particularly in frozen sections.

PROGNOSIS AND THERAPY

Some pathologists regard all hepatic mucinous cystic neoplasms to be of uncertain malignant potential. Complete excision of a cystadenoma is the treatment of

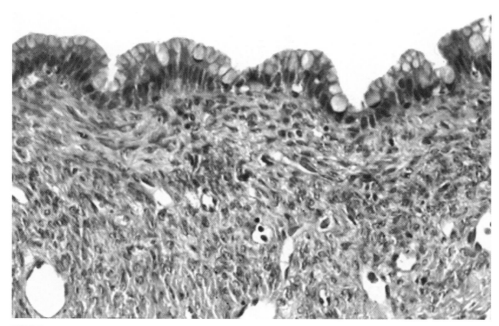

FIGURE 20-22

Biliary cystadenomas are lined by tall columnar to flattened mucinous epithelium. Note the mesenchymal ovarian-type stroma.

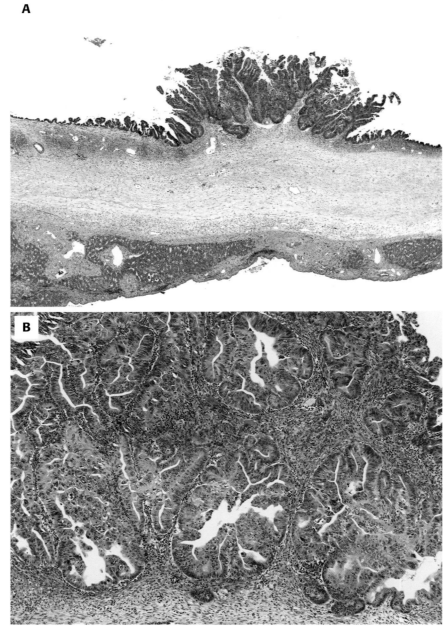

FIGURE 20-23

Biliary cystadenocarcinoma. **A,** Areas of complex papillary projections correspond to exophytic areas noted on gross examination. **B,** Stromal invasion is diagnostic of malignancy, but some pathologists require only complex architecture and severe cytologic atypia for diagnosis of cystadenocarcinoma.

BILIARY CYSTADENOMA AND CYSTADENOCARCINOMA—FACT SHEET

Definition
- Multilocular cystic neoplasm lined by mucinous biliary-type epithelium

Incidence and Location
- Rare tumors
- Geographic variation in incidence not reported

Morbidity and Mortality
- Survival is excellent for completely resected lesions
- Recurrence rate of approximately 13% for completely resected cystadenocarcinomas

Gender, Race, and Age Distribution
- Cystadenoma: Most patients (approximately 96%) are female; for cystadenocarcinoma, equal distribution between sexes
- More common in whites
- Mean age 45 years for cystadenoma, 59 years for cystadenocarcinoma

Clinical Features
- Present with upper abdominal discomfort or pain

Radiologic Features
- Solitary, multilocular cystic lesions
- Papillary areas, thickened internal septa, enhancing mural nodules suggest cystadenocarcinoma

Prognosis and Therapy
- Complete surgical excision is treatment of choice
- Prognosis is excellent for completely resected lesions

BILIARY CYSTADENOMA AND CYSTADENOCARCINOMA—PATHOLOGIC FEATURES

Gross Findings
- Multilocular cystic mass, 2.5 to 28 cm
- Cyst fluid is usually clear but may be blood tinged in cystadenocarcinoma
- Papillary or solid areas suggest cystadenocarcinoma

Microscopic Findings
- Lined by mucin-producing cuboidal to columnar epithelium
- Characteristic mesenchymal stroma is found only in females
- Foci of dysplasia are seen, with frank progression to cystadenocarcinoma
- Cystadenocarcinoma is distinguished by loss of polarity, densely packed glands, nuclear atypia, and stromal invasion

Fine-Needle Aspiration Biopsy Findings
- Occasional aggregates of bland, cuboidal-columnar epithelial cells
- Rare papillary clusters
- No significant atypia in cystadenoma; cytologic features of malignancy in cystadenocarcinoma

Immunohistochemistry
- Epithelium is CEA+, CA19-9+
- Stroma is vimentin positive, may be muscle-specific actin positive, desmin positive

Differential Diagnosis
- Simple biliary cyst
- Metastasis from mucinous cystic neoplasms of other organs (pancreas, ovary, appendix)

choice and is curative. Incomplete resection or cyst fenestration usually results in persistent disease. About 50% of patients with cystadenocarcinoma survive up to 4 years; prognosis may be worse for men.

CHOLANGIOCARCINOMA

CLINICAL FEATURES

Cholangiocarcinomas are generally subdivided into peripheral (intrahepatic) or hilar types. Peripheral CC is defined as CC arising in a segmental duct or a more peripheral duct. A third subtype of cholangiocarcinoma has also been described—the papillary (intraductal) cholangiocarcinoma—which may be biologically distinct from the other patterns.

The global incidence of intrahepatic CC, but not extrahepatic biliary malignancies, appears to be increasing. The etiology of CC is usually unknown. However, these tumors are associated with chronic inflammatory lesions of the bile ducts and conditions associated with bile stasis, including primary sclerosing cholangitis (PSC), parasitic infections with liver flukes such as *Clonorchis* and *Opisthorchis*, and recurrent bacterial cholangitis with hepatolithiasis. Intrahepatic CCs have also been reported in association with exposure to Thorotrast and are associated with all forms of fibropolycystic liver disease, including the presence of multiple BDHs.

Cholangiocarcinoma generally occurs in older adults, with most patients between 50 and 70 years of age. Intrahepatic CC is often clinically silent until late in the course; patients typically complain of fever, weight loss, anorexia, and vague abdominal pain. Patients with intrahepatic CC rarely present with jaundice, in contrast to those with hilar CC. However, the intraductal variant of intrahepatic CC may be associated with right upper quadrant pain, fever, and jaundice because of duct obstruction by tumor or tumor-related mucus production.

Elevated serum CA19-9 levels, if greatly elevated, may be of utility, although considerable overlap with PSC without cancer is seen. Serum CEA is elevated in about 40% of PSC patients with CC but is less sensitive and specific than CA19-9. The serum AFP level is not typically elevated.

CHOLANGIOCARCINOMA—FACT SHEET

Definition

- Malignant hepatic neoplasm demonstrating glandular (biliary) differentiation

Incidence and Location

- Approximately 46,000 cases worldwide per year; 19% of primary liver malignancies
- Incidence is rising
- Geographic variation, with higher incidence in Japan and East Asia, compared with United States

Morbidity and Mortality

- Most patients have unresectable tumors
- Patients undergoing resection have longer survival (23 months median survival vs. 6 months with unresectable tumors)

Gender, Race, and Age Distribution

- Male predominance 3:2
- More common in Asian population
- Affects older adults: mean age 62 years

Clinical Features

- Associated with inflammatory conditions involving the biliary tree (PSC, recurrent pyogenic cholangitis, parasitic liver diseases)
- Patients with intrahepatic cholangiocarcinoma present with nonspecific symptoms (upper abdominal pain, ascites, weight loss, anorexia)
- Patients with hilar cholangiocarcinoma present with obstructive jaundice

Radiologic Features

- Usual finding on CT is homogeneous low-attenuation mass
- Calcification is present in some cases
- On MRI, tumors are usually hypointense relative to liver on T1-weighted images and hyperintense on T2-weighted images

Prognosis and Therapy

- Poor prognosis, with median survival approximately 6 months in patients with unresectable tumors

Prognosis may be more favorable for papillary CCs

- Chemotherapy and radiation therapy are of little benefit
- Survival depends on tumor stage; tumor grade is of lesser prognostic impact

CHOLANGIOCARCINOMA—PATHOLOGIC FEATURES

Gross Findings

- Intrahepatic CCs may form large single tumor masses or infiltrate diffusely
- Tumors are firm, white to tan
- Satellite nodules are common
- Hilar CCs are associated with dense fibrous scar
- Papillary lesions with intraductal growth in papillary CCs

Microscopic Findings

- Most common pattern is adenocarcinoma
- Most are composed of small glands lined by cuboidal to columnar mucin-producing epithelium
- Dense fibrous stroma
- Perineural invasion is common
- Intraductal papillary architecture with pancreatobiliary, gastric foveolar, or intestinal-type epithelial lining with at least focal high-grade dysplasia in papillary CCs; invasive component may be present, most commonly of tubular or mucinous types

Fine-Needle Aspiration Biopsy Findings

- Irregular three-dimensional clusters of cells resembling biliary epithelium
- Prominent nucleoli but not as large as in HCC
- Features of adenocarcinoma, but not specific for CC

Genetic

- Mutations in *KRAS* and *TP53* are most common genetic abnormalities
- Overexpression of MET is common and correlated with tumor differentiation

Immunohistochemistry

- Most are CK7 positive
- Variable expression of CK20 (more common in hilar and papillary subtypes)
- Hep Par 1 negative
- CDX-2 negative (except in some cases of papillary CCs)

Differential Diagnosis

- Metastatic adenocarcinoma
- Hepatocellular carcinoma
- Benign lesions such as florid bile ductular proliferation and bile duct adenoma

PATHOLOGIC FEATURES

GROSS FINDINGS

On gross examination, intrahepatic CCs are generally gray-white to tan masses arising in a noncirrhotic liver (Fig. 20-24A); larger lesions may contain areas of central necrosis or, less commonly, hemorrhage. Central umbilication may be seen in subcapsular tumors. Most CCs are firm because of the prominent desmoplastic stroma, which may be gritty because of dystrophic calcifications. Satellite lesions resulting from intravascular or intraductal spread may be present. The margins may be infiltrative or deceptively well circumscribed on gross

RADIOLOGIC FEATURES

Cholangiocarcinomas are visualized on CT as a homogeneous low-attenuation mass, with calcification in some cases. On MRI, the tumors are usually hypointense relative to liver on T1-weighted images and hyperintense on T2-weighted images. Cholangiography is useful in visualizing biliary strictures in hilar CC, but distinction from benign lesions may be difficult.

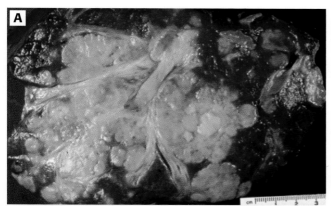

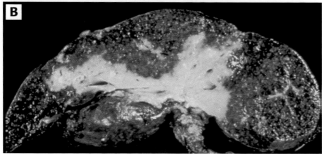

FIGURE 20-24

A, Peripheral or intrahepatic cholangiocarcinoma arises as a single firm mass, usually in a noncirrhotic liver. **B,** Hilar cholangiocarcinoma leads to biliary obstruction, resulting in severe bile staining, and may be indistinguishable from hilar scarring in primary sclerosing cholangitis.

examination. Rarely, involvement of portal or hepatic veins may be seen, and occasionally intraductal growth occurs. Intraductal CCs appear as papillary excrescences within dilated ducts. Hilar CCs appear as firm, tan or white, ill-defined lesions indistinguishable from scar in the hepatic hilum; the liver is frequently bile stained because of biliary obstruction (see Fig. 20-24B).

MICROSCOPIC FINDINGS

Most CCs are adenocarcinomas. The most common microscopic pattern is a well to moderately differentiated adenocarcinoma forming small tubular glands and duct-like structures (Fig. 20-25A). The tumor cells are low cuboidal to columnar, with clear to eosinophilic cytoplasm and round to oval nuclei. Intracellular mucin production may be scant but is usually demonstrable with special stains for mucin. A desmoplastic stroma is generally prominent. Perineural and lymphovascular invasion is common (see Fig. 20-25B), and CCs often involve portal tracts, either by spread within portal vein radicals or by spread within the intrahepatic biliary tree. Bile ducts in adjacent portal tracts may demonstrate varying degrees of epithelial dysplasia; however, it is usually not possible to identify a specific bile duct of origin.

Papillary CCs are distinct from peripheral and hilar CCs in many regards. Prominent intraductal papillary architecture is typical, and the epithelial lining may be of pancreatobiliary, gastric foveolar, or intestinal types, showing at least focal high-grade dysplasia. When an invasive component is present, it most commonly shows a tubular or mucinous (colloid) morphology. Some authors have suggested that papillary CCs represent the hepatic counterpart of pancreatic intraductal papillary mucinous neoplasms (IPMNs) due to their morphological and biological similarities. Other special variants of CCs include signet ring cell, squamous, adenosquamous, sarcomatoid (spindle cell), clear cell, and lymphoepithelioma-like variants.

ANCILLARY STUDIES

FINE-NEEDLE ASPIRATION BIOPSY

FNA biopsy of CC yields cells with features of adenocarcinoma, consisting of irregular three-dimensional clusters of cells resembling biliary epithelium (Fig. 20-26). Nucleoli are prominent, but not generally as large as in HCC.

IMMUNOHISTOCHEMISTRY

Cholangiocarcinomas are positive for CK7. Peripheral cholangiocarcinomas are usually negative for CK-20, whereas hilar and papillary CCs (especially intestinal-type papillary CCs) are commonly positive for this marker. CDX-2 is negative in peripheral and hilar cholangiocarcinoma but may be positive in some cases of papillary CCs. CCs show cytoplasmic reactivity for CEA and usually are negative for AFP HepPar-1.

DIFFERENTIAL DIAGNOSIS

The primary challenge in diagnosing most CCs is distinction from metastatic adenocarcinoma, particularly pancreas, gastrointestinal tract, breast, and occasionally lung. Immunohistochemical stains are of limited use in distinguishing CC from other primary tumors; distinction between CC and metastatic adenocarcinoma therefore depends heavily on the exclusion of a primary site elsewhere. Comparative immunohistochemical studies suggest that CK7 and CK20 may be useful in some cases in distinguishing peripheral CCs, which are generally CK7+/CK20−, from colorectal metastases, which are usually CK7−/CK20+. Non-papillary cholangiocarcinomas are also negative for CDX-2, distinguishing them from metastatic colorectal lesion. TTF-1 is positive in most cases of metastatic bronchogenic adenocarcinoma and negative in CCs.

The distinction between HCC and CC is usually more straightforward. HCCs display a trabecular architecture with scant fibrous stroma, a distinctly different morphology from the usual CC. Polyclonal (cross-reactive) CEA staining in CC will usually show a cytoplasmic staining pattern, without the canalicular pattern seen in HCC. CD-10 staining showing a canalicular pattern, likewise, indicates hepatocytic differentiation. Glypican-3 immunohistochemistry may also be useful in this setting,

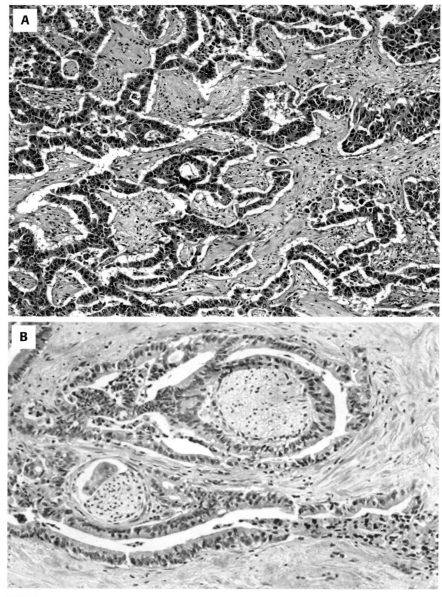

FIGURE 20-25

A, Most cholangiocarcinomas (CCs) are adenocarcinomas; dense fibrous stroma is common and helps distinguish CC from pseudoglandular hepatocellular carcinoma. **B,** Perineural invasion is an almost universal finding in CC.

especially in cases of poorly differentiated lesions. Glypican-3 is negative in CCs but positive in approximately 90% of poorly differentiated HCCs. Immunostain for AFP is negative in CC and positive in some HCCs.

Ultrastructural examination is seldom indicated, but electron microscopy of CC cells shows typical features of adenocarcinoma, such as microvilli and true lumen formation. Epithelioid hemangioendothelioma (EH) is easily distinguished from CC by its immunophenotype, with expression of factor VIII–related antigen, CD34, and other endothelial cell markers in EH.

PROGNOSIS AND THERAPY

Complete resection of the tumor appears to be an important factor in prognosis in CC. Median survival for resectable intrahepatic CC is as high as 30 months

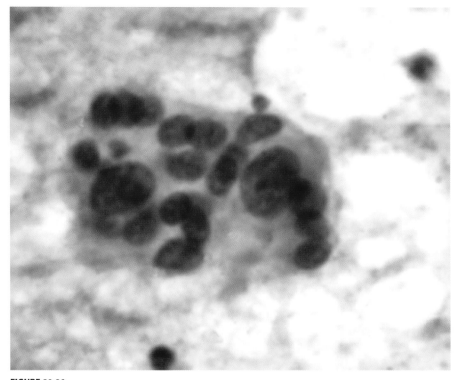

FIGURE 20-26

Cholangiocarcinomas may be difficult to diagnose by FNA because of low cellularity of the aspirate. Cells with cytologic features of adenocarcinoma are seen; CC cannot be differentiated from metastatic adenocarcinoma by FNA.

in some series, and the 5-year survival rate ranges between 35% and 45%. Median survival for unresectable intrahepatic tumors is only 6 to 7 months, even with adjuvant therapy. Papillary CCs, with or without an invasive component (usually tubular of mucinous), may have a significantly more favorable prognosis. At autopsy, 75% of patients have metastases, usually to porta hepatis lymph nodes, peritoneal surfaces, lung, bone, and adrenal gland. Tumor grade is significantly associated with outcome in some but not all series. Positive hilar lymph nodes are a poor prognostic sign.

■ MESENCHYMAL TUMORS

BENIGN

HEMANGIOMA

CLINICAL FEATURES

Cavernous hemangioma (CH), the most common primary hepatic tumor, is usually an incidental finding at autopsy. It is more frequent in adults; symptomatic CH is more common in women in most surgical series. The most common presenting symptom is abdominal pain. Most CHs are static over time, but the lesions can rapidly increase in size in pregnancy or with estrogen therapy. CHs may occur in conjunction with FNH.

PATHOLOGIC FEATURES

GROSS FINDINGS

Most CHs are small (<4 cm) solitary lesions in an otherwise normal liver. They are soft, spongy, and well circumscribed, and may be subcapsular or deep within the parenchyma. On sectioning, CH has an empty mesh-like appearance, due to escape of blood from the dilated vascular channels (Fig. 20-27).

MICROSCOPIC FINDINGS

Cavernous hemangiomas consist of large variably sized vascular spaces lined by bland, flattened endothelial cells (Fig. 20-28). The underlying stroma consists of fibrous tissue. Thrombi in various stages of organization are commonly found within the channels. As these thrombi undergo organization, the CH may undergo sclerosis that begins centrally but may sometimes spread to obscure the entire lesion, resulting in a fibrous nodule (sclerosed hemangioma).

HEMANGIOMA—FACT SHEET

Definition
- Benign vascular tumor of the liver

Incidence and Location
- Common; found in approximately 7% of autopsies
- No geographic variation

Morbidity and Mortality
- Usually incidental, innocuous finding
- Rarely, hemangiomas increase rapidly in size and rupture

Gender, Race, and Age Distribution
- More frequent in women
- More common in adults (mean age 46 years)
- No race predilection

Clinical Features
- Most patients (more than 85%) are asymptomatic
- Upper abdominal mass or pain is seen in approximately 50%
- Rupture may be spontaneous or related to trauma

Radiologic Features
- Mass isodense to large blood vessels on CT, with cloudlike peripheral enhancement

Prognosis and Therapy
- Excellent prognosis for incidental lesions
- Rarely, surgical excision is performed for symptomatic lesions

HEMANGIOMA—PATHOLOGIC FEATURES

Gross Findings
- Single or multiple
- Vary from less than 1 cm to greater than 30 cm
- Spongy honeycombed surface on sectioning

Microscopic Findings
- Blood-filled spaces lined by single layer of bland endothelium
- Extensive fibrosis may be seen
- Some vascular spaces may contain recent or organized thrombi

Fine-Needle Aspiration Biopsy Findings
- FNA is generally contraindicated because of risk for bleeding
- Bloody smear with scant fibrous tissue and benign endothelial cells

Differential Diagnosis
- Hepatic lymphangioma
- Peliosis hepatis

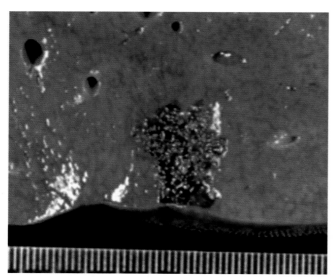

FIGURE 20-27

Hemangiomas are spongy red-brown lesions, usually incidentally discovered at autopsy.

DIFFERENTIAL DIAGNOSIS

Major differential diagnostic considerations include hereditary hemorrhagic telangiectasia, lymphangioma (extremely rare), and peliosis hepatis. In hereditary hemorrhagic telangiectasia (Rendu-Osler-Weber disease), hepatic involvement is rarely symptomatic. Telangiectatic lesions, composed of dilated veins and small capillaries, arise in relation to portal tracts and are frequently found in fibrous septa. In peliosis hepatis, the blood-filled cavities are not lined by endothelium. Sclerosed hemangioma may be confused with other hepatic lesions that may have prominent fibrosis; the relatively acellular nature of the fibrosis should prevent confusion with malignant processes.

PROGNOSIS AND THERAPY

Because most CHs are not associated with morbidity or increased mortality, asymptomatic CH is not treated. Symptomatic lesions greater than 10 cm are often treated by resection or enucleation.

INFANTILE HEMANGIOENDOTHELIOMA

CLINICAL FEATURES

Infantile hemangioendothelioma (IHE) is the most common mesenchymal tumor of the liver in childhood, accounting for about 20% of all primary pediatric hepatic tumors. The vast majority of patients are younger than 6 months of age at the time of diagnosis. Females are affected slightly more often than males. Typical presenting signs include an abdominal mass and high-output cardiac failure, although a significant number of cases are asymptomatic and are discovered incidentally at autopsy. Platelet sequestration within

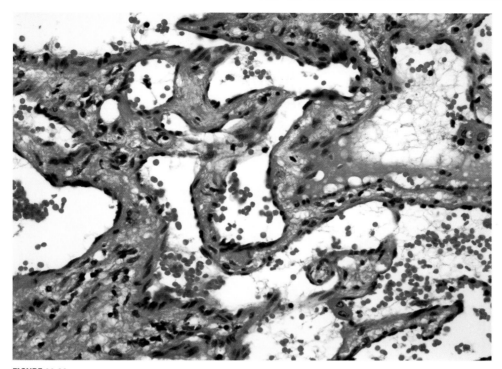

FIGURE 20-28
Hemangioma. Large, dilated blood-filled channels are lined by a single layer of bland endothelium.

the lesion may lead to severe thrombocytopenia and bleeding (Kasabach-Merritt syndrome). IHE is associated with hemangiomas of skin and other organs in up to 40 % of cases. The serum AFP level is usually normal.

PATHOLOGIC FEATURES

GROSS FINDINGS

IHE s may be solitary or multicentric. The tumor nodules are variable in size and are well circumscribed. Smaller lesions have a vascular appearance and are red to tan, soft, and spongy; larger nodules are variegated and have a gray-white, scarred central area with calcification.

MICROSCOPIC FINDINGS

IHE is composed of a proliferation of small, capillary-like, or dilated vascular spaces lined by bland endothelial cells (Fig. 20-29A and B). Occlusion of the lumen by the endothelial cells may be seen, but mitoses are rare. The vascular channels of IHE are separated by loose connective tissue. Extramedullary hematopoiesis is present in most cases. Portal tracts may be identified embedded within the lesion (see Fig. 20-29C). Areas indistinguishable from CH are often present in the center of the lesion. Degenerative changes such as thrombi, fibrosis, and stroma calcification are common in larger lesions.

ANCILLARY STUDIES

IMMUNOHISTOCHEMISTRY

The endothelial nature of the lining cells is easily demonstrated by immunohistochemical tests (factor VIII-related antigen, CD34, CD31).

DIFFERENTIAL DIAGNOSIS

IHE should be differentiated from angiosarcoma. An infiltrative margin can be found in IHE and is not a discriminating feature. Mitotic activity is more pronounced in angiosarcoma, and hypercellularity due to densely packed tumor cells and cytologic atypia suggests malignancy. Of note, pediatric patients with angiosarcoma are typically older than 1.5 years. The presence of extrahepatic tumors in patients with IHE is not indicative of metastatic spread. Myxoid stroma in IHE may be confused with mesenchymal hamartoma (MH), but the presence of calcification suggests the possibility of IHE. CH lacks the proliferation of numerous small blood vessels found in IHE.

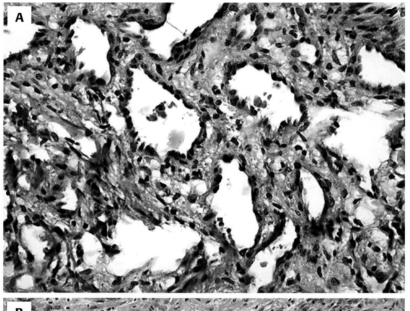

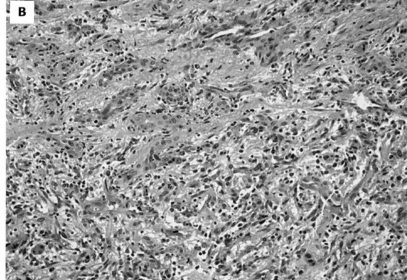

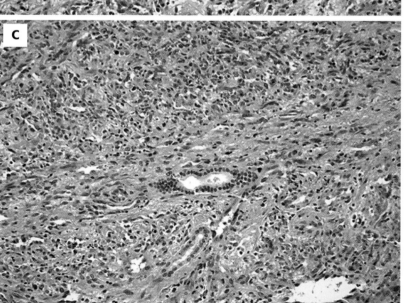

FIGURE 20-29

Infantile hemangioendothelioma. **A,** Irregular vascular channels are separated by loose edematous stroma. **B,** More densely cellular areas resemble granulation tissue. **C,** Entrapped portal structures may be identified.

INFANTILE HEMANGIOENDOTHELIOMA—FACT SHEET

Definition
- Low-grade vascular neoplasm occurring in first year of life

Incidence and Location
- Approximately 17% of all pediatric liver tumors
- 40% of benign liver tumors in first 21 years of life

Morbidity and Mortality
- Spontaneous regression in up to 10% of cases
- Overall survival is 70%
- Most deaths are associated with operative complications or congestive heart failure

Gender, Race, and Age Distribution
- Female predominance (63%)
- No racial predilection
- 90% are seen in first 6 months of life
- Almost all cases present by 2 years of age

Clinical Features
- Many patients are asymptomatic; symptoms are usually nonspecific (nausea, gastrointestinal bleeding, lethargy, liver failure)
- Most present with hepatomegaly and diffusely enlarged abdomen
- 15% present with congestive heart failure
- Associated with extrahepatic hemangiomas in approximately 10% of cases

Radiologic Features
- Hypoechoic or complex mass on ultrasonography
- Low-attenuation mass on nonenhanced CT
- Fine calcifications in 50% of cases
- MRI helpful in determining multifocality
- Enlarged tortuous feeding arteries on arteriography

Prognosis and Therapy
- Surgical resection is often curative for unifocal lesions
- Transplantation is used for large or multifocal lesions
- Hepatic artery embolization is also used for large lesions
- Jaundice and multiple tumor nodules are poor prognostic features

PROGNOSIS AND THERAPY

Roughly 70% of patients survive at least 7 years; most deaths occur within 1 month of diagnosis. Congestive heart failure and jaundice are the factors most often associated with death, but multiple nodules and the absence of cavernous differentiation are also adverse prognostic features. Solitary lesions may be resected. In some cases, corticosteroids have been used. Ablative therapies may be considered, and in some cases liver transplantation has been performed. Spontaneous regression may occur.

INFANTILE HEMANGIOENDOTHELIOMA—PATHOLOGIC FEATURES

Gross Findings
- Single tumor in 55%
- Spongy red-brown lesions; may have areas of hemorrhage, necrosis, calcification

Microscopic Findings
- Thin vascular channels lined by single layer of flattened-to-plump endothelial cells
- Myxoid to dense fibrous stroma
- Margins may be well demarcated or infiltrative
- Solid areas with atypical endothelial cells are considered angiosarcoma (type II lesions)

Genetics
- Most tumors are diploid; aneuploidy may be associated with poor outcome
- Balanced translocations reported

Immunohistochemistry
- Endothelial cells are positive for vascular markers: factor VIII–related antigen, CD31, CD34, exposure to *Ulex europaeus* (gorse shrub)
- Pericytes surrounding vessels are positive for α-smooth muscle actin

Differential Diagnosis
- Hemangioma
- MH

MESENCHYMAL HAMARTOMA

CLINICAL FEATURES

Mesenchymal hamartoma is the second most common benign pediatric tumor. Most patients are male, and three fourths of the patients show symptoms by 1 year of age. Serum AFP levels are usually normal but can be markedly elevated for age. The neoplastic nature of MH has not been conclusively established; alternative theories include aberrant development of primitive mesenchyme in portal tracts associated with ductal plate malformation and localized ischemia during development.

PATHOLOGIC FEATURES

GROSS FINDINGS

Mesenchymal hamartoma is solitary and well circumscribed, is usually large (up to 23 cm), and is more common in the right lobe. In most cases, multiple cysts are present, imparting a multilocular appearance (Fig. 20-30). The cysts contain clear or mucoid fluid and are separated by solid areas that become fibrotic with age.

MESENCHYMAL HAMARTOMA—FACT SHEET

Definition
- Benign lesion occurring in young children; composed of large fluid-filled cysts surrounded by mesenchymal stroma

Incidence and Location
- 8% of all pediatric liver tumors
- No geographic variation

Morbidity and Mortality
- 90% survival rate
- Mortality and morbidity are primarily related to surgical complications

Gender, Race, and Age Distribution
- Male predominance 2:1
- No race predilection
- Median age 10 months

Clinical Features
- Most common presentation is enlarging abdomen
- Physical examination reveals nontender mass

Radiologic Features
- Ultrasonography shows complex multicystic mass
- May be detected in utero
- CT shows variation in cyst size and septal thickness

Prognosis and Therapy
- Surgical excision is preferred therapy
- Rare examples of embryonal sarcoma arising in conjunction with MH are reported

MESENCHYMAL HAMARTOMA—PATHOLOGIC FEATURES

Gross Findings
- Involves right lobe in 75% of cases
- Pedunculated in up to 30% of cases
- Vary from a few centimeters to more than 30 cm
- Cysts in greater than 85% of cases; cysts are filled with clear amber fluid
- Hemorrhage and necrosis are rare and suggest undifferentiated sarcoma

Microscopic Findings
- Mixture of bile ducts, hepatocytes, loose mesenchyme, and cystic structures
- Cystic structures lack epithelial lining
- Loose edematous stroma with scattered bland stellate cells
- Dilated bile ducts at periphery of lesion may be surrounded by dense collar of fibrosis
- Extramedullary hematopoiesis is common

Ultrastructural Findings
- FNA biopsy findings
- Clusters of epithelial and mesenchymal cells
- Loose connective tissue
- Admixed normal hepatocytes and bile duct epithelium

Genetics
- Balanced translocation between chromosomes 11 and 19 has been reported

Differential Diagnosis
- Myxoid change in IHE
- Undifferentiated (embryonal) sarcoma

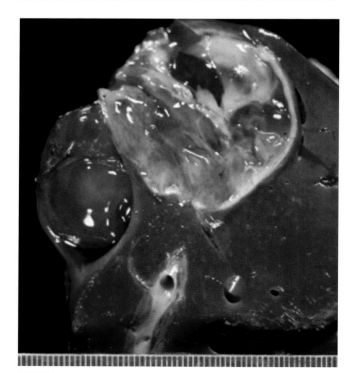

FIGURE 20-30

Mesenchymal hamartomas (MHs) are well circumscribed; cysts are variable in size and display a smooth lining.

MICROSCOPIC FINDINGS

Mesenchymal hamartoma is characterized by a mixture of different cell types. The cysts represent dilated bile ducts lined by attenuated biliary epithelium (Fig. 20-31A) or pools of fluid accumulated in the primitive mesenchyme. This stroma consists of bland stellate and spindle cells embedded in a myxoid matrix that may show variable fibrosis (see Fig. 20-31B). Extramedullary hematopoiesis is an almost universal finding. The bile ducts may show progressive dilatation and an aberrant architecture reminiscent of ductal plate malformation. The biliary epithelium is often flattened, with atrophic or degenerative changes, and a periductal neutrophilic infiltrate may be present.

ANCILLARY STUDIES

FINE-NEEDLE ASPIRATION BIOPSY

FNA biopsy cytologic findings include abundant myxoid stroma with scattered bland stromal cells arranged as individual cells or loose clusters. The chromatin pattern is evenly distributed, and nucleoli are inconspicuous.

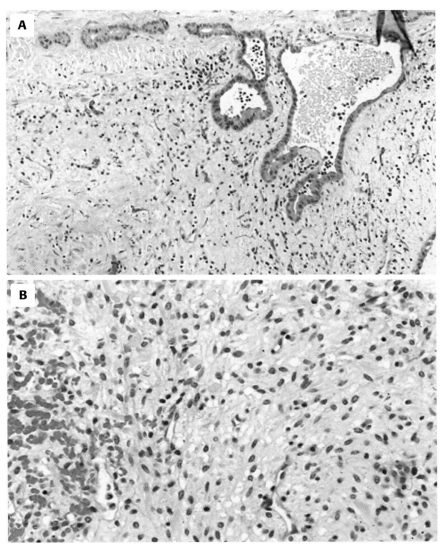

FIGURE 20-31

A, Bile ducts in MH may undergo progressive cystic dilatation. **B,** The abundant stroma is loose and edematous, with bland stellate stromal cells.

PROGNOSIS AND THERAPY

Treatment of choice is total excision, which is curative. Perioperative mortality is relatively high (up to 17%) and is related to technical difficulties with surgical resection. Recurrence of incompletely resected lesions has not been reported. MH has rarely been associated with undifferentiated (embryonal) sarcoma, raising the possibility of malignant transformation of MH.

ANGIOMYOLIPOMA

CLINICAL FEATURES

Hepatic angiomyolipomas (AML) are rare, benign tumors that affect adult patients, predominantly females. Although usually detected incidentally, large tumors

may cause abdominal discomfort. Tumor rupture with intraabdominal bleeding is an uncommon complication. Association of hepatic AML with tuberous sclerosis occurs in only 6% to 10% of cases, compared to 20% to 40% of cases of renal AML. Tumors with a low fat content are often mistaken for other benign or malignant lesions on imaging studies.

PATHOLOGIC FEATURES

GROSS FINDINGS

Hepatic angiomyolipomas are usually solitary, well-circumscribed, nonencapsulated lesions. Tumor size varies from a few millimeters to greater than 36 cm. The gross appearance is highly dependent on the tumor composition. The fatty component may be evident as soft,

ANGIOMYOLIPOMA—FACT SHEET

Definition

- Rare benign lesion composed of a combination of abnormal blood vessels, myoid cells, and fat cell

Incidence and Location

- Rare
- No known geographic variation

Morbidity and Mortality

- Generally benign
- Rare malignant examples reported

Gender, Race, and Age Distribution

- Female predominance 1.4:1 to 9:1
- No known race predilection
- Adult patients, no specific age group

Clinical Features

- Most lesions are asymptomatic and detected incidentally
- Large lesions may present with abdominal pain

Radiologic Features

- Heterogeneous, circumscribed, hyperechoic lesion on ultrasound
- Computed tomography shows a hypodense mass with marked early contrast enhancement, as well as delayed enhancement in the portal venous phase
- MRI is very sensitive for the detection of the fatty component on T1-weighted images (high-signal intensity)

Prognosis and Therapy

- Surgical excision usually indicated; non-surgical management may be an option for selected patients
- Excellent prognosis

ANGIOMYOLIPOMA—PATHOLOGIC FEATURES

Gross Findings

- Well-circumscribed lesion, variable size (0.1 to 36 cm)
- Gross appearance varies according to tumor composition—combination of hemorrhagic foci (vascular component), white-tan, solid, homogeneous areas (myomatous component), and soft, yellow areas (lipomatous component)
- Normal non-neoplastic liver

Microscopic Findings

- Angiomatous—abnormal, thick-walled vessels
- Myomatous—myoid cells, which may have a spindle cell, epithelioid, or intermediate morphology
- Myoid cells with epithelioid morphology are common in hepatic AMLs and may be misinterpreted as neoplastic hepatocytes, or epithelial malignancy
- Lipomatous component usually present but may be inconspicuous

Fine-Needle Aspiration Biopsy Findings

- Admixture of spindle or epithelioid smooth muscle cells and adipocytes
- Thick-walled blood vessels may be present

Genetics

- Most hepatic AMLs are monoclonal lesions, although no characteristic molecular abnormalities have been described
- Similar gene expression profile as activated stellate cells by cDNA microarray

Differential Diagnosis

- Benign and malignant hepatocellular tumors (myomatous variant)
- Metastatic carcinomas and melanoma (myomatous variant)
- Focal fatty change, steatotic hepatocellular tumors (lipomatous variant)
- Hemangioma, vascular malformations (angiomatous variant)

---

yellow regions, whereas the vascular component may appear as hemorrhagic foci (Fig. 20-32). Myomatous areas are soft, white-tan, and homogeneous. Necrosis is not commonly present.

MICROSCOPIC FINDINGS

Hepatic AMLs are composed of three basic histologic elements: blood vessels, myoid cells, and fat cells (Fig. 20-33A). Tumors have been classified as angiomatous, myomatous, lipomatous, or mixed, depending on the proportion of each element present in an individual lesion. Although a lipomatous component is usually present in hepatic AMLs, the fatty areas may be inconspicuous and may not be represented in core biopsies. Myoid cells may show different histologic appearances, including spindled, epithelioid, and intermediate morphology. Epithelioid myoid cells are commonly present in hepatic AMLs and may cause significant diagnostic difficulties. They are large, polygonal cells, with abundant clear to eosinophilic cytoplasm, and a round nucleus with a single, often

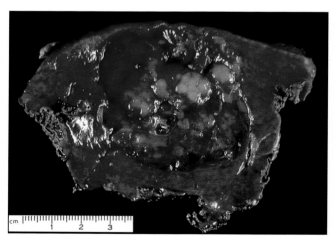

FIGURE 20-32

Hepatic angiomyolipoma with typical gross appearance: a well-circumscribed lesion with hemorrhagic areas and islands of fatty tissue in a background of normal liver parenchyma.

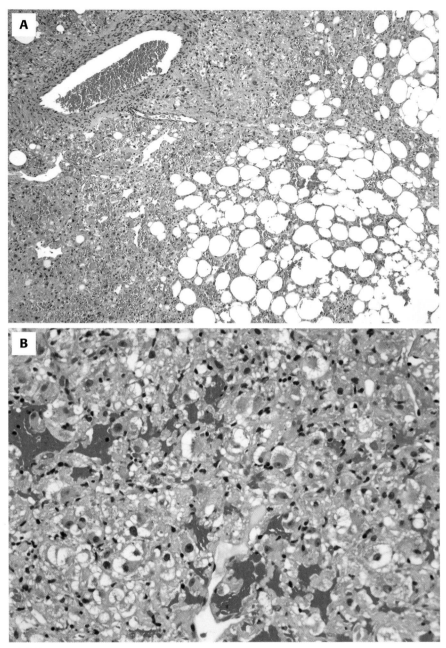

FIGURE 20-33

A, Low-power image showing the three elements found in angiomyolipomas: thick-walled vessels, myoid cells, and fatty tissue. **B,** Myoid cells in hepatic angiomyolipomas often have an epithelial morphology, as in this example.

prominent nucleolus (see Fig. 20-33B). Although mitoses are not numerous, the epithelioid myoid component may show considerable cytologic atypia. Hemosiderin and melanin pigment may be present. The vascular component is comprised of tortuous, thick-walled blood vessels. In addition, extramedullary hematopoiesis may also be present in hepatic AMLs—a feature not typically seen in renal AMLs. Infiltrating growth pattern with tumor invasion of portal tracts and liver parenchyma has been reported in AMLs that had a benign clinical course upon follow-up; these features, therefore, should not be regarded as an indication of malignant behavior. Malignant AMLs resulting in metastatic disease and/or death have only rarely been reported.

ANCILLARY STUDIES

IMMUNOHISTOCHEMISTRY

Hepatic AMLs are positive for HMB-45 (Fig. 20-34), Melan-A, and smooth muscle actin. Pancytokeratin and Hepar-1 are negative and may be used to differentiate AMLs from metastatic carcinomas and hepatocellular lesions.

DIFFERENTIAL DIAGNOSIS

Hepatic angiomyolipomas with one predominant component may pose diagnostic dilemmas. Angiomatous AMLs must be distinguished from hepatic hemangiomas and vascular malformations, whereas lipomatous AMLs may be confused with focal fatty change, and hepatocellular lesions with prominent steatosis. The differential diagnosis of myomatous AML is broader and includes hepatocellular lesions (liver cell adenoma and hepatocellular carcinoma), metastatic carcinomas from various sites, and metastatic melanomas. Recognition of the additional components of the lesions is the key for a correct diagnosis, which may be confirmed by HMB-45 and Melan-A immunohistochemistry. Metastatic carcinomas and hepatocellular lesions can be excluded with cytokeratins and hepatocytic immunohistochemical markers. The non-fatty components of hepatic AMLs

is S-100 negative, which is helpful in excluding metastatic melanomas.

PROGNOSIS AND THERAPY

Most cases of hepatic AML are managed surgically, although observation may be appropriate in selected cases. Hepatic AML are generally benign lesions and have an excellent prognosis. Only rare, anecdotal cases of malignant AMLs have been reported.

MALIGNANT

ANGIOSARCOMA

CLINICAL FEATURES

Although hepatic angiosarcoma (HAS) is the most common primary malignant mesenchymal tumor of the liver in adults, overall it is quite rare, with only about 200 cases of HAS diagnosed annually worldwide, for an estimated annual occurrence of 10 to 20 cases in the United States. HAS usually occurs in older men and has been associated with vinyl chloride exposure and Thorotrast administration. HAS due to environmental exposure is associated with a prolonged latency period. Patients present with abdominal pain, fatigue, weight loss, or an abdominal mass.

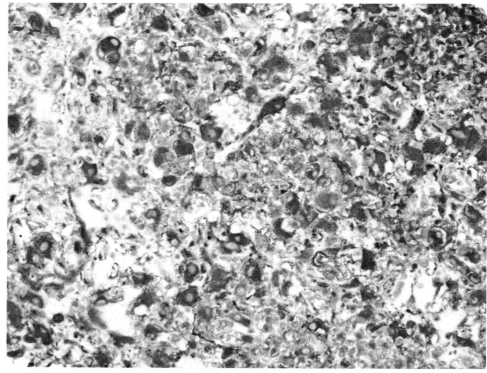

FIGURE 20-34

Angiomyolipoma. Strong HMB-45 reactivity is characteristic.

ANGIOSARCOMA—FACT SHEET

Definition
- High-grade malignant neoplasm of endothelial cells

Incidence and Location
- Most common primary hepatic sarcoma
- 200 cases diagnosed worldwide annually

Morbidity and Mortality
- Rapidly fatal tumor, with most patients dead within 6 months of liver failure or hemorrhage

Gender, Race, and Age Distribution
- Males predominance 3:1
- No race predilection
- Peak age incidence is in the seventh decade of life

Clinical Features
- Patients may present with symptoms of liver disease, hemoperitoneum due to tumor ruptures, splenomegaly, or symptoms related to metastasis
- Most important known etiologic factors are exposure to vinyl chloride, Thorotrast, or androgenic steroids

Radiologic Features
- Nonenhanced CT shows hypodense masses, becoming isodense on delayed postcontrast scans
- Abnormal vascular pattern on angiography

Prognosis and Therapy
- Prognosis is dismal
- Chemotherapy is ineffective
- Surgery and radiation have been used in rare cases

ANGIOSARCOMA—PATHOLOGIC FEATURES

Gross Findings
- Gray-white tumor tissue alternates with hemorrhagic areas
- Entire liver is usually involved

Microscopic Findings
- Tumor cells grow along sinusoids and other preformed vascular channels and replace normal endothelial cells
- Tumor cells are highly pleomorphic spindle cells and may grow as solid nodules
- Areas of infarct, atrophy, and fibrosis are frequent

Ultrastructural Findings
- Weibel-Palade bodies

Fine-Needle Aspiration Biopsy Findings
- Pleomorphic hyperchromatic spindle cells
- Tumor cells may be associated with benign hepatocytes in interdigitating growth pattern

Genetics
- *TP53* mutations in tumors associated with vinyl chloride exposure

Immunohistochemistry
- Tumor cells are positive for endothelial markers: factor VIII-related antigen, CD31, CD34, exposure to *Ulex europaeus* (gorse shrub)

Differential Diagnosis
- Other primary or metastatic sarcomas
- Hepatic metastases of angiosarcoma arising in other organs

PATHOLOGIC FEATURES

GROSS FINDINGS

Hepatic angiosarcoma is usually multicentric and involves both lobes. The spleen is often involved at the time of diagnosis. Individual tumor foci are infiltrative, variable in size, and heterogeneous, with solid areas alternating with large blood-filled spaces (Fig. 20-34).

MICROSCOPIC FINDINGS

Hepatic angiosarcoma is composed of highly atypical, large, plump, pleomorphic endothelial cells with hyperchromatic nuclei (Fig. 20-35). Solid areas resembling fibrosarcoma and bizarre tumor giant cells may be seen. Numerous mitotic figures are present. At the periphery of the lesion, tumor cells of HAS display a characteristic growth pattern of spread along pre existing sinusoids. Obliteration of sinusoids by tumor cells leads to hepatocyte atrophy. Tumor invasion of portal or hepatic vein branches is common.

ANCILLARY STUDIES

ELECTRON MICROSCOPY

Demonstration of Weibel-Palade bodies by electron microscopy may confirm the diagnosis, but ultrastructural examination is rarely necessary.

IMMUNOHISTOCHEMISTRY

Immunoreactivity for endothelial markers (CD34, CD31, factor VIII–related antigen, *Ulex europaeus*) confirms the vascular nature of the tumor. Roughly 10% of cases are CK positive.

DIFFERENTIAL DIAGNOSIS

Subtle foci, especially at the infiltrate edge of the lesion, may be mistaken for inflammatory or benign vascular disorders. The atypia of the sinusoidal lining cells distinguishes HAS from benign, however. The pattern of infiltration along sinusoids seen in HAS should not be confused with HCC, in which the hepatocytes, not the endothelial cells, are malignant. Kaposi's sarcoma may

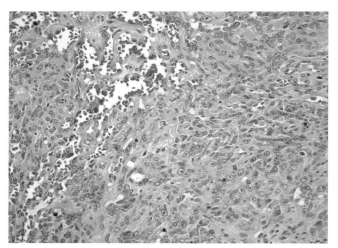

FIGURE 20-35
Angiosarcoma. Densely packed proliferation of highly atypical endothelial cells forming narrow vascular channels.

be confused with HAS; however, clinical history of acquired immunodeficiency syndrome (AIDS) facilitates diagnosis.

PROGNOSIS AND THERAPY

Prognosis for HAS is dismal, with most patients dying within months of diagnosis. Available therapies are ineffective. Hepatic failure and intra-abdominal bleeding are the most common causes of death. At autopsy, most patients have metastases, most frequently0 to the lung.

EPITHELIOID HEMANGIOENDOTHELIOMA

CLINICAL FEATURES

Epithelioid hemangioendothelioma (EH) is a malignant vascular neoplasm most commonly developing in middle-aged women. Common presenting symptoms are abdominal pain or weight loss, and, rarely, hepatic rupture or liver failure. Involvement of major hepatic vein branches or terminal hepatic venules may produce hepatic venous outflow obstruction. In about 40% of cases, EH may be an incidental finding. The etiology of EH is unknown, although OCS use has been suggested as an etiologic factor.

PATHOLOGIC FEATURES

GROSS FINDINGS

Grossly, EH lesions are usually multiple ill-defined tumor nodules of variable size, with involvement of both lobes. Tumor nodules are typically gray to white, firm, and sometimes gritty. Vascular channels are not appreciated on gross examination.

MICROSCOPIC FEATURES

EH often demonstrates a zonal pattern. At the periphery, portal tracts are spared and are surrounded by a sinusoidal proliferation of tumor cells (Fig. 20-36A), with residual intact hepatocytes and scanty myxoid stroma. Progressive obliteration of the sinusoids results in atrophic hepatocyte plates in the midzonal portion of the hepatic acinus. In zone 3, the tumor stroma becomes progressively sclerotic and central veins may be partially or totally obliterated by tumor cells.

The tumor cells are embedded in the matrix in cords, small nests, or as single cells and may be classified into two different cell types, dendritic and epithelioid (see Fig. 20-36B). Dendritic cells are spindle shaped or stellate. Epithelioid cells are rounded and display a greater amount of eosinophilic cytoplasm. A notable feature is the presence of one or more well-defined intracytoplasmic vacuoles of variable size (blister cells) that may contain erythrocytes.

ANCILLARY STUDIES

ELECTRON MICROSCOPY

Ultrastructural examination reveals Weibel-Palade bodies, characteristic of endothelial cells, and numerous intermediate filaments, which are responsible for the epithelioid histologic appearance.

IMMUNOHISTOCHEMISTRY

The tumor cells demonstrate immunoreactivity for CD34 (Fig. 20-37) and other endothelial markers but are negative for CEA. Nearly 15% of EHs are positive for CK.

DIFFERENTIAL DIAGNOSIS

The differential diagnosis includes other neoplasms such as metastatic adenocarcinoma (particularly the signet ring cell carcinoma), CC, and neuroendocrine neoplasms. These tumors can be distinguished from EH by their lack of zonal growth pattern, cytologic features, and negative staining for endothelial markers. While neuroendocrine tumors may contain dense sclerotic stroma, their trabecular growth pattern and other characteristic features make the diagnosis straightforward.

Non-neoplastic lesions such as sclerosed hemangioma, fibrous scarring, granulation tissue, and cirrhosis may also be confused with EH. Sclerosed hemangiomas are paucicellular and well circumscribed and do not invade veins. The distinction between primary hepatic EH and metastatic EH, usually from the lung, is not possible on morphologic grounds.

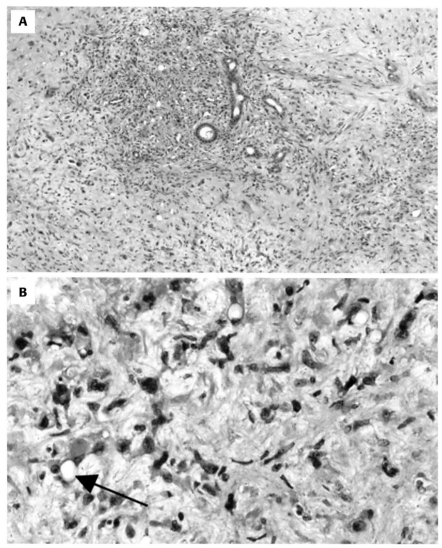

FIGURE 20-36

A, The tumor cells infiltrate around portal structures, leaving residual intact bile ducts. **B,** Neoplastic cells in epithelioid hemangioendothelioma (EH) are embedded in fibrotic stroma; note intracytoplasmic lumina (*arrow*) in some cells (blister cells).

PROGNOSIS AND THERAPY

The clinical course of EH is variable and unpredictable. Some patients die within months of initial diagnosis, whereas roughly 20% survive for at least 5 years. Resection is usually performed if possible, and hepatic transplantation has led to improved survival even in selected unresectable cases showing signs of extrahepatic disease. Prolonged survival with metastatic disease has been reported. Extrahepatic involvement (lung, omentum/mesentery, lymph nodes) is noted in 50% of cases and may reflect multicentricity rather than metastatic spread.

UNDIFFERENTIATED SARCOMA

CLINICAL FEATURES

Undifferentiated (embryonal) sarcoma (US) is a rare malignancy occurring almost exclusively in the pediatric population. Most patients with US are between 6 and 10 years of age, and more than 90% are 21 years or younger. There is no sexual preference. An abdominal mass or abdominal pain is the most common presentation.

EPITHELIOID HEMANGIOENDOTHELIOMA—FACT SHEET

Definition
- Low-grade malignant neoplasm of endothelial cells

Incidence and Location
- Rare tumor
- No reported geographic variation

Morbidity and Mortality
- Approximately 75% 5-year survival rate, independent of therapy
- Metastases in 25%, primarily to lung, abdominal lymph node, omentum, and peritoneum

Gender, Race, and Age Distribution
- Female predominance (62%)
- No race predilection
- Wide age range (12 to 86 years)

Clinical Features
- Incidental finding in many cases
- Presenting symptoms are nonspecific: weakness, anorexia, nausea, jaundice, hepatomegaly
- Two thirds have elevated alkaline phosphatase at presentation

Radiologic Features
- On CT, low-attenuation, peripheral tumor nodules
- Signal halo around nodules on MRI

Prognosis and Therapy
- Outcome is unpredictable
- Approximately 30% metastasize or involve other organ systems
- Treatment ranges from observation only, to chemotherapy and radiation, to liver transplantation

EPITHELIOID HEMANGIOENDOTHELIOMA—PATHOLOGIC FEATURES

Gross Findings
- Multiple white to tan firm nodules involving entire liver
- Margins of lesions appear hyperemic
- Nodules vary from a few millimeters to several centimeters

Microscopic Findings
- Ill-defined lesions involving multiple acini
- In early stages, tumor spares portal areas
- Tumor cells grow along sinusoids and cause atrophy of liver cell plates
- Tumor cells demonstrate epithelioid, dendritic spindle cell, or intermediate morphology
- Cytoplasmic vacuoles represent intracellular vascular lumina and may contain erythrocytes

Ultrastructural Findings
- Tumor cells have basal lamina, pinocytotic vesicles, and Weibel-Palade bodies
- Tumor cells contain large amounts of intermediate filaments compared with normal endothelial cells

Immunohistochemistry
- Tumor cells are positive for vascular markers such as factor VIII-related antigen, CD31, CD34

Differential Diagnosis
- Angiosarcoma
- CC
- Non-neoplastic diseases

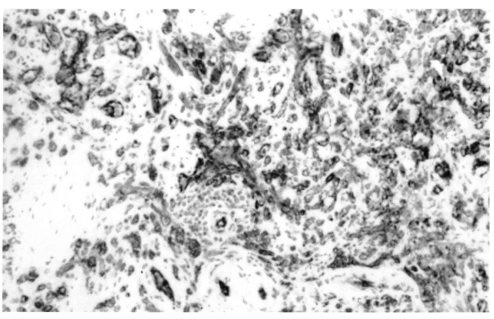

FIGURE 20-37
The cells of epithelioid hemangioendothelioma mark strongly with vascular markers, such as CD34, shown here.

UNDIFFERENTIATED SARCOMA—FACT SHEET

Definition
- Primitive primary sarcoma of liver, more common in children

Incidence and Location
- Approximately 6% of primary liver neoplasms in childhood

Morbidity and Mortality
- Prolonged survival and cure possible with multiagent chemotherapy followed by surgical resection
- Morbidity related to massive local tumor growth

Gender, Race, and Age Distribution
- Equal distribution between sexes
- No race predilection
- Most common between 6 and 10 years of age; rare in adults

Clinical Features
- Most patients present with abdominal swelling, with or without a palpable mass

Radiologic Features
- CT reveals a hypodense mass with solid and cystic areas
- Tumor is usually hypovascular

Prognosis and Therapy
- Multiagent chemotherapy followed by surgical resection
- Combined modality treatment has improved survival, previously reported as 15% 5-year survival rate

UNDIFFERENTIATED SARCOMA—PATHOLOGIC FEATURES

Gross Findings
- Most occur in the right lobe and measure up to 20 cm in diameter
- Cut surface is gray-white, variegated, and glistening with cystic areas

Microscopic Findings
- Tumor cells are stellate or spindle shaped and loosely arranged in myxoid stroma
- Tumor cells are often bizarre, with numerous mitotic figures
- Multiple eosinophilic PAS-positive cytoplasmic globules are a characteristic feature

Ultrastructural Findings
- Fibroblastic, smooth muscle, and skeletal muscle differentiation may be demonstrated

Fine-Needle Aspiration Biopsy Findings
- Large, markedly spindle anaplastic cells
- Tumor giant cells
- Tumor cells with PAS-positive, diastase-resistant cytoplasmic globules

Genetics
- No single characteristic abnormalities
- Multiple cytogenetic alterations reported

Immunohistochemistry
- Tumor cells may express CK
- Tumor cells are positive for vimentin and may express α_1-antitrypsin and α_1-chymotrypsin

Differential Diagnosis
- MH
- Mixed epithelial and mesenchymal HB
- Other hepatic sarcomas

RADIOLOGIC FEATURES

Undifferentiated sarcoma is usually hypodense on CT scan, with solid and cystic areas. The tumor is generally hypovascular.

PATHOLOGIC FEATURES

GROSS FINDINGS

US is usually a large, bulky solitary mass measuring up to 30 cm in diameter. On macroscopic examination, the tumor is a well-circumscribed, soft, gray, mass; degenerative changes are common and include necrosis, hemorrhage, and cystic degeneration.

MICROSCOPIC FINDINGS

US are composed predominantly of large, highly atypical spindle to stellate cells with ill-defined cell borders embedded in abundant myxoid stroma (Fig. 20-38A). Cell density may be quite variable. Multinucleation, cellular anaplasia, and numerous mitotic figures are usually found. Cytoplasmic hyaline globules that are PAS positive and diastase resistant are a characteristic finding and may represent α_1-antitrypsin uptake by tumor cells (Fig. 20-38B).

ANCILLARY STUDIES

ELECTRON MICROSCOPY

Ultrastructural features are consistent with mesenchymal differentiation.

FINE-NEEDLE ASPIRATION BIOPSY

Large, markedly anaplastic spindle or stellate cells are seen on smears. Tumor giant cells and PAS-positive, diastase-resistant cytoplasmic hyaline globules may be seen.

IMMUNOHISTOCHEMISTRY

Immunohistochemical studies have indicated variable immunoreactivity with antibodies to desmin, muscle-specific actin, and CK. US is negative for myoglobin. The consensus is that US is a primitive mesenchymal neoplasm, possibly derived from a primitive multipotential precursor cell, and may demonstrate areas of specific sarcomatous differentiation.

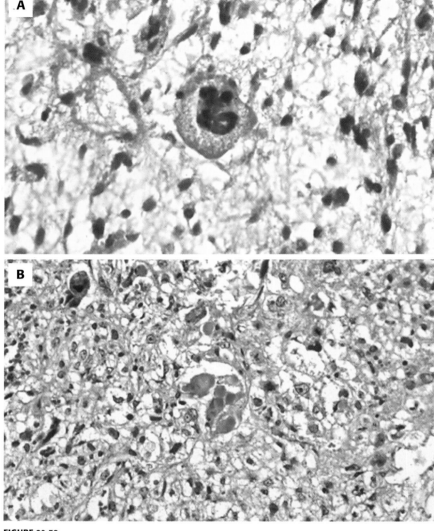

FIGURE 20-38

A, Large bizarre tumor cells in a variably cellular background of neoplastic spindle to stellate cells characterize undifferentiated sarcoma. **B,** Globular cytoplasmic inclusions are common and often represent α_1-antitrypsin uptake by tumor cells.

DIFFERENTIAL DIAGNOSIS

The sarcomatoid (spindle cell) variant of HCC is distinguished by identification of typical foci of HCC. HB should also demonstrate epithelial areas. MH is cytologically bland and paucicellular relative to US.

PROGNOSIS AND THERAPY

Survival in US has improved with modern therapy. Multiagent chemotherapy followed by complete resection has resulted in long-term disease-free survival (more than 10 years) in some cases. Lung, pleura, and peritoneum are the most common sites of metastasis.

PRIMARY HEPATIC LYMPHOMA

CLINICAL FEATURES

Primary hepatic lymphoma is rare and represents less than 0.5% of all extranodal non-Hodgkin's lymphomas. However, reported cases vary in lymph node, bone marrow, and splenic involvement, resulting in difficulties in comparing clinicopathologic features. In particular, the spleen is often involved at the time of detection.

PRIMARY HEPATIC LYMPHOMA—FACT SHEET

Definition
- Malignant neoplasm of lymphoid differentiation that arises in liver

Incidence and Location
- Rare; only approximately 0.4% of extranodal non-Hodgkin lymphomas
- No geographic predilection

Gender, Race, and Age Distribution
- Male predominance 2:1
- No racial predilection
- Usually occurs in adults (median age 53 years)

Clinical Features
- Reported in setting of chronic viral hepatitis (hepatitis B and hepatitis C) and AIDS
- Patients present with abdominal pain, distension, and hepatomegaly

Radiologic Features
- Lesions are hypoechoic on ultrasonography
- Low-attenuation lesions with variable enhancement on CT

Prognosis and Therapy
- Prognosis is poor for HIV-positive and cirrhotic patients
- Approximately 60% 2-year survival rate
- Combination chemotherapy is generally used

PRIMARY HEPATIC LYMPHOMA—PATHOLOGIC FEATURES

Gross Findings
- Large cell lymphomas produce bulky white to yellow masses
- A discrete mass may not be evident

Microscopic Findings
- Most are diffuse large cell B-cell lymphomas
- T-cell lymphomas are more likely to infiltrate sinusoids diffusely

Fine-Needle Aspiration Biopsy Findings
- Large cell type produces characteristic pattern of diffuse monomorphic population of atypical lymphocytes
- Smear contains discohesive single cells
- Scant cytoplasm, open nuclei with prominent nucleoli
- Lymphoglandular bodies in background

Immunohistochemistry
- Depend on type of lymphoma; most hepatic lymphomas are CD20+
- Sinusoidal T-cell lymphomas are CD3+, CD45RO+

Differential Diagnosis
- Chronic hepatitis is distinguished by the mixed nature of the infiltrate and characteristic pattern of tissue damage and inflammation
- Epstein-Barr virus hepatitis is best distinguished by clinical findings

A male predominance is seen among reported cases, which include a wide age range. Patients may present with abdominal pain with hepatomegaly; liver test results are variably abnormal. Human immunodeficiency virus (HIV), hepatitis B virus, hepatitis C virus, and autoimmune diseases have been implicated in some cases.

PATHOLOGIC FEATURES

GROSS FINDINGS

In most cases, a single large mass or multiple bulky deposits are present in the liver (Fig. 20-39). A diffusely infiltrative pattern may also be seen, depending on the type of lymphoma.

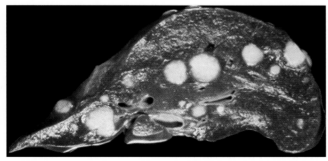

FIGURE 20-39
Hepatic lymphoma. Diffuse large cell B-cell lymphomas form nodular masses in the liver.

MICROSCOPIC FINDINGS

Most cases are of B-cell lineage, with the diffuse large cell type accounting for more than 75% of cases. However, reported cases include many of the lymphoma histologic subtypes, including primary hepatic follicular dendritic cell tumors. Some B-cell lymphomas are manifested primarily by the presence of a relatively monomorphic portal infiltrate (Fig. 20-40).

DIFFERENTIAL DIAGNOSIS

The presence of a lymphoid infiltrate that does not fit a recognized pattern of inflammatory disease in the liver should prompt consideration of hepatic lymphoma. Although immunohistochemical markers for various lymphoid markers may be helpful, gene rearrangement studies may be necessary. Lymphoma is not usually mistaken for carcinoma in the liver; immunostains for CKs and leukocyte common antigen are useful in making this distinction.

PROGNOSIS AND THERAPY

In general, prognosis depends on the specific type of lymphoma and the presence or absence of underlying liver disease. Treatment has included surgery, chemotherapy,

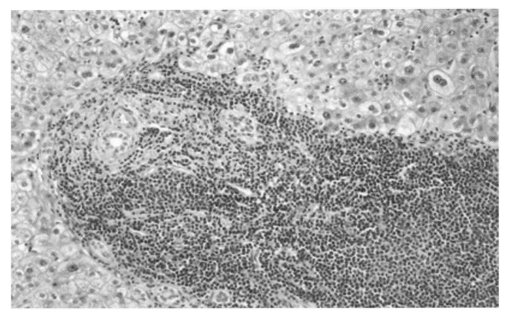

FIGURE 20-40
Low-grade B-cell hepatic lymphomas often result in monomorphic portal infiltrates of small lymphocytes, a pattern that can mimic chronic hepatitis.

and radiation therapy. Patients with HIV infection and those with cirrhosis have a poor prognosis.

METASTASES

Metastatic tumors account for the overwhelming majority of all hepatic malignancies in the noncirrhotic liver in developed Western countries. In the cirrhotic liver, however, primary hepatic malignancies are more common than metastatic tumors. Carcinomas of the lung, breast, colon, and pancreas are the most common primary sites in adults; neuroblastoma, Wilms' tumor, and rhabdomyosarcoma are the most common sites in children.

Clinical features range from asymptomatic to fulminant hepatic failure because of the diffuse replacement of the liver. Obstructive jaundice may occur secondary to tumor growth within large bile ducts or compression of extrahepatic biliary tree by involved perihilar lymph nodes.

PATHOLOGIC FEATURES

GROSS FINDINGS

In most cases, multiple tumor deposits of varying sizes are present (Fig. 20-41A), although in some cases the liver parenchyma is diffusely replaced and nodules are

not apparent on gross examination (see Fig. 20-41B). Large subcapsular nodules may demonstrate central necrosis and fibrosis, producing umbilication. Highly vascular tumors such as choriocarcinoma, angiosarcoma, or thyroid carcinoma appear hemorrhagic.

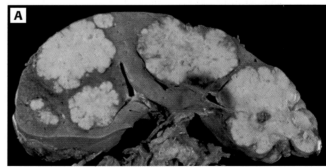

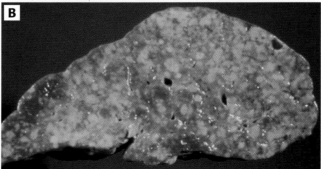

FIGURE 20-41
A, Multiple nodules of metastatic colon cancer with central necrosis and umbilication. **B,** Metastatic breast cancer producing diffuse involvement of the liver, without discrete nodule formation.

HEPATIC METASTASES—FACT SHEET

Definition

- Malignant tumor that secondarily involves the liver

Incidence and Location

- Most common malignant neoplasm involving liver
- 40% of patients dying from cancer have liver metastases
- No geographic variation

Morbidity and Mortality

- High morbidity, with many patients having signs of liver failure
- High mortality, with most patients dying within 2 years of diagnosis

Gender, Race, and Age Distribution

- Depends on primary site of cancer

Clinical Features

- Most common primary sites are lung, breast, colon, and pancreas
- Hepatomegaly, anorexia, and weight loss are common
- Jaundice may be seen when tumors near the hilum cause large duct obstruction
- Patients may present with acute liver failure from massive diffuse hepatic involvement

Radiologic Features

- Imaging studies show multiple hepatic lesions
- Solid, hypoechoic masses on ultrasonography
- CT appearance is variable, usually decreased attenuation
- MRI shows high lesion-to-liver contrast

Prognosis and Therapy

- Treatment is usually palliative: systemic or intrahepatic artery chemotherapy; chemoembolization or cryotherapy
- Resection of isolated hepatic metastases from colorectal cancer produces approximately 30% 5-year survival rate for carefully selected patients
- Prognosis is related to growth characteristics of tumor, extent of hepatic involvement, and comorbid conditions

HEPATIC METASTASES—PATHOLOGIC FEATURES

Gross Findings

- Usually multiple irregular nodules of varying sizes
- Central necrosis with retraction produces an umbilicated appearance
- Tumors are firm due to desmoplastic stromal response

Microscopic Findings

- Features are similar to primary tumors
- Metastatic adenocarcinoma may grow within bile ducts and simulate CC

Fine-Needle Aspiration Biopsy Findings

- Features are similar to primary tumors

Differential Diagnosis

- HCC
- CC
- Primary hepatic sarcomas
- Benign bile duct lesions

MICROSCOPIC FINDINGS

Metastases usually retain the histologic features of the primary tumor (Fig. 20-42). Intrasinusoidal growth should not be mistaken for a trabecular architecture or origin from hepatocytes. Vascular invasion of portal vein radicals may be noted. Colon carcinoma may involve large bile ducts, with an intrabiliary growth pattern that mimics CC.

DIFFERENTIAL DIAGNOSIS

Hepatocellular carcinoma displays a trabecular growth pattern and obvious hepatocellular differentiation, including bile production, in many cases. A panel of immunohistochemical markers including hepatocyte, CD10 or polyclonal CEA, and AFP distinguishes most HCCs from metastases. If metastatic neuroendocrine carcinoma is a consideration, positivity for chromogranin, synaptophysin, and neuron-specific enolase is generally diagnostic (see Fig. 20-43). CDX2 and TTF-1 immunohistochemistry may help distinguish metastatic gastrointestinal (especially midgut) carcinoids from metastatic pulmonary carcinoids. In general, metastatic adenocarcinoma from the pancreas, extrahepatic biliary tree, and gastrointestinal tract may be difficult to distinguish from primary ICC, although a panel of CK markers is sometimes helpful.

PROGNOSIS AND THERAPY

Most patients with hepatic metastases die within 1 year, and treatment is largely aimed at palliation. Exceptions include patients with metastatic neuroendocrine tumors; these patients may enjoy prolonged survival. Carefully selected patients with colorectal metastases with single or few tumor deposits and no extrahepatic spread are candidates for surgical resection; survival rates of approximately 30% are reported.

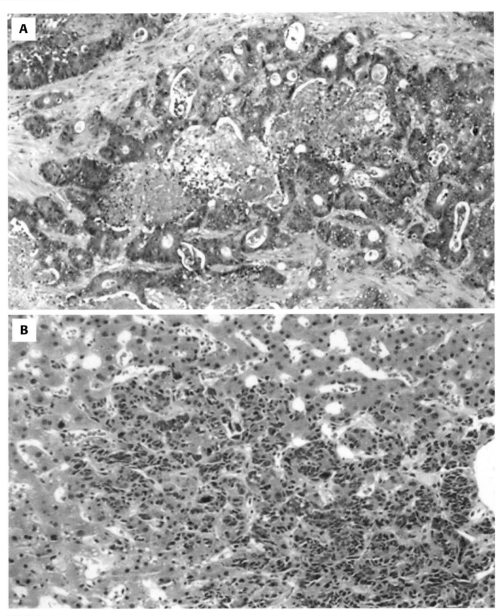

FIGURE 20-42

A, Metastatic colon cancer resembles the primary tumor; note central necrosis in neoplastic gland. **B,** Metastatic small cell carcinoma may infiltrate the liver diffusely in a sinusoidal pattern; this pattern of involvement may result in fulminant hepatic failure.

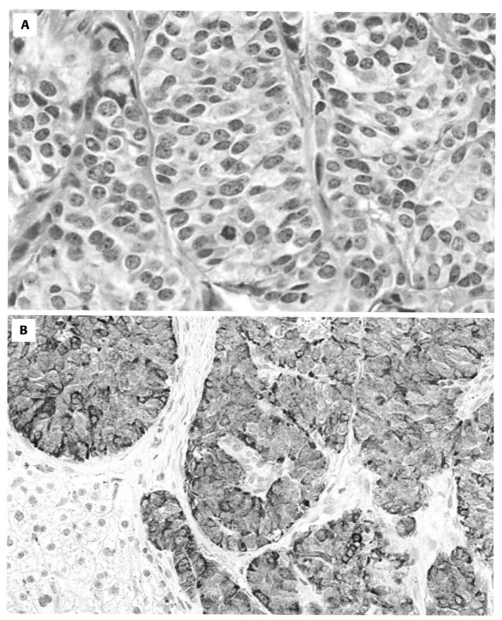

FIGURE 20-43

A, Metastatic low-grade neuroendocrine tumor grows in a trabecular pattern with tumor cell nests separated by delicate stroma. **B,** Chromogranin stain may be useful in distinguishing neuroendocrine tumor from hepatocellular carcinoma.

21

Gastrointestinal Lymphoma

■ **Shiyama Mudali, MD** ■ **H. Parry Dilworth, MD**
■ **Hubert H. Fenton, MD** ■ **Marc R. Lewin, MD**
■ **Christopher D. Gocke, MD**

The gastrointestinal tract is the most common site of extranodal non-Hodgkin lymphoma. Approximately 10% to 15% of all non-Hodgkin lymphoma primarily involves the gastrointestinal tract. Secondary GI tract involvement is also relatively common but typically incidental, both diagnostically and clinically. Hodgkin lymphoma of the GI tract is exceedingly rare and essentially always secondary. This chapter concentrates on the non-Hodgkin lymphomas that primarily involve the GI tract.

■ EXTRANODAL MARGINAL ZONE B-CELL LYMPHOMA

CLINICAL FEATURES

The gastrointestinal tract is the most common site of extranodal marginal zone B-cell lymphoma of mucosa-associated lymphoid tissue (MALT lymphoma). MALT lymphomas develop in sites of inflammation in response to either infectious conditions or autoimmune processes. Within the GI tract, approximately 85% of MALT lymphomas occur in the stomach. MALT lymphoma is also the most common primary lymphoma of the small intestine in Western countries. There is a unique form of MALT lymphoma seen in Mediterranean areas and the Middle East referred to as *immunoproliferative small intestinal disease* (IPSID), which encompasses a spectrum of diseases including alpha heavy chain disease (discussed separately in this chapter).

Most gastric MALT lymphomas are associated with *Helicobacter pylori* infection. The normal stomach has no significant lymphoid compartment. Infection by *H. pylori* leads to development of a reactive lymphocyte response with typical B-cell germinal centers (MALT). Gastric lymphoma is thought to arise from this acquired lymphoid tissue. However, as lymphoma evolves from chronic gastritis, the density of microorganisms and detectability of *H. pylori* infection decreases.

PATHOLOGIC FEATURES

GROSS FINDINGS

The endoscopic diagnosis of a MALT lymphoma is often difficult because of the various macroscopic patterns. Endoscopically, primary gastric lymphomas display a variety of morphologies: ulcerated (single, multiple, or diffuse), polypoid, granulonodular, erythematous, edematous, and infiltrated folds (Fig. 21-1). Most commonly, MALT lymphomas of the stomach are seen as an ulcerative lesion either alone or in combination with the other morphologies. MALT lymphomas are more commonly diffusely infiltrative than high-grade lymphoma. The differentiation between lymphomas and adenocarcinomas may not be easy; however, lymphomas tend to produce larger tumors than adenocarcinomas and may be multifocal as well. Gastric lymphomas more frequently involve the antrum and corpus. Rarely, the neoplasm may occupy the entire stomach.

MICROSCOPIC FINDINGS

MALT lymphomas are derived from marginal zone B-cells, which they resemble cytologically, phenotypically, and genotypically. MALT lymphomas comprise both reactive (B-cell follicles and plasma cells) and neoplastic (marginal zone B-cells) components. At low magnification, the lamina propria is expanded with small uniform cells that infiltrate the muscularis mucosa (Fig. 21-2A). These neoplastic cells invade the surrounding gastric gland epithelium to form "lymphoepithelial lesions" (see Fig. 21-2B). Lymphoepithelial lesions are the defining characteristics of MALT lymphomas but may not be seen in every case, particularly when the biopsy is small. They are clusters of B-cells within the epithelium, typically distorting or destroying the gland architecture. High-power assessment of the lymphoid infiltrate reveals cells similar to follicle-center centrocytes admixed with small lymphocytes referred to as *monocytoid* B-cells, which have eccentric small nuclei, abundant clear cytoplasm, and well-defined cell borders. Plasma cell differentiation

MALT LYMPHOMA—FACT SHEET

Definition

- Low-grade extranodal marginal zone B-cell lymphoma arising from mucosa-associated lymphoid tissue (MALT)

Incidence and Location

- Most common location is stomach (85%)
- Account for less than 5% of primary gastric neoplasms
- Associated with *Helicobacter pylori* gastritis in the stomach
- Most common primary small intestinal lymphoma in Western countries

Morbidity and Mortality

- Indolent behavior in low-grade lesions with excellent prognosis
- Minority of lesions show transformation to high-grade B-cell lymphomas

Gender, Age, and Race Distribution

- Slight female predominance in gastric MALT lymphoma
- Male predominance in small intestinal MALT lymphoma
- Presents in the fifth and sixth decades

Clinical Features

- Physical examination is normal in 55% to 60%
- Abdominal pain
- Bleeding
- Intestinal obstruction or perforation
- Weakness, night sweats, or fever
- Palpable abdominal mass
- Hematemesis or melena rare

Prognosis and Treatment

- Good prognosis associated with age < 65 years, low-grade histology, and/or initial complete remission
- 5-year survival rates for gastric MALT lymphoma: 50% to 90%
- 5-year survival rate for small intestinal MALT lymphoma: 50% to 80%
- Progression to diffuse large B-cell lymphoma may occur in 8% of MALT lymphomas
- Negative prognostic factors include nodal involvement, extension beyond the bowel wall, and high-grade histology

MALT LYMPHOMA—PATHOLOGIC FEATURES

Gross Findings

- Ulcerated, polypoid, granulonodular, or edematous and infiltrated mucosal folds
- Single or multiple masses
- Most commonly found in gastric body and prepyloric area

Microscopic Findings

- Monotonous infiltrate of monocytoid cells mixed with immunoblasts and plasmacytoid cells
- Lymphoepithelial lesions
- Infiltrate expands interfollicular space and effaces normal architecture
- Reactive follicles often present
- Presence of moderate nuclear atypia, Dutcher bodies, and prominent lymphoepithelial lesions are features highly suggestive of lymphoma

Immunohistochemistry

- CD20+, CD5−, CD10− and low Ki-67 proliferation index, CD43+ especially in gastric

Genetic Abnormalities

- Translocations t(11;18)(q21;q21)
- Trisomy of chromosomes 3, 12, and 18

Differential Diagnosis

- Reactive lymphoid hyperplasia
- Mantle cell lymphoma
- Follicular lymphoma
- Diffuse large B-cell lymphoma

may be seen, typically toward the luminal surface but also within the bulk of the tumor. Light chain restriction may be used to differentiate the clonal plasma cells from reactive plasma cells that are present as part of the inflammatory background. Often the background is scattered with larger transformed lymphoma cells, some of which have a "halo" around them. When these larger cells comprise greater than 5% of the cells, this may signify slightly worse prognosis. Sheets of large cells indicate high-grade transformation and should be diagnosed as large B-cell lymphoma.

ANCILLARY STUDIES

Immunohistochemistry can aid in establishing the diagnosis of MALT lymphoma (Fig. 21-3). The neoplastic B-cells, similar to marginal zone B-cells, are CD20-positive and negative for CD10, CD5, and CD23. CD43 is aberrantly expressed in approximately one half of gastric MALT lymphomas. In a gastric biopsy showing a dense, monotonous lymphocytic infiltrate, an initial immunophenotyping panel of CD3, CD20, and CD43 can be performed. If the infiltrate is composed predominantly of

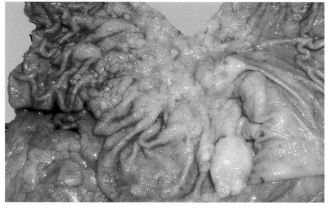

FIGURE 21-1

Gross appearance of mucosa-associated lymphoid tissue (MALT) lymphoma. In this example, prominent polypoid and nodular effacement of the gastric mucosa is seen.

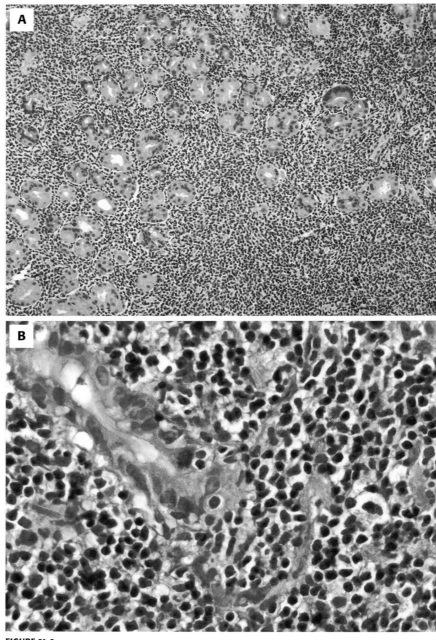

FIGURE 21-2

Mucosa-associated lymphoid tissue (MALT) lymphoma. **A,** At low magnification, the lamina propria is markedly expanded by small lymphocytes. Residual oxyntic glands are present within the neoplastic infiltrate. **B,** The infiltrate is composed of monomorphic, monocytoid lymphocytes with eccentric small nuclei, abundant clear cytoplasm, and well-defined cell borders. The lymphocytes invade the gastric glandular epithelium to form lymphoepithelial lesions.

CD20+ B-cells with coexpression of CD43, the diagnosis of MALT lymphoma can be rendered. Because admixed reactive T-cells and plasma cells are strongly positive for CD43, care must be taken in interpreting CD43 coexpression by the B-cells. Similarly, normal mantle zone B-cells and many T-cells are BCL2 positive, so only the putative tumor cell population should be interpreted. When there is high suspicion for a MALT lymphoma, but CD43 coexpression cannot be demonstrated, IgH rearrangement studies by PCR may be pursued. In the small intestine where normal B-cells can coexpress CD43, IgH rearrangement studies are often necessary to establish the diagnosis. When the lymphoid infiltrate is markedly nodular due to the presence of reactive follicles, follicular lymphoma should be excluded with CD10 and BCL6 immunohistochemical staining. Light chain stains are generally not useful because of low-density staining or high background.

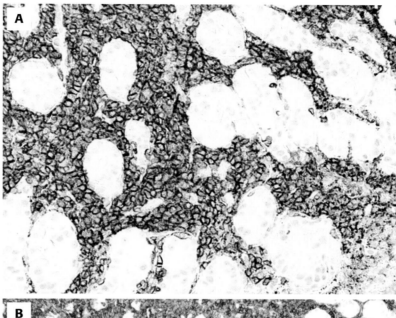

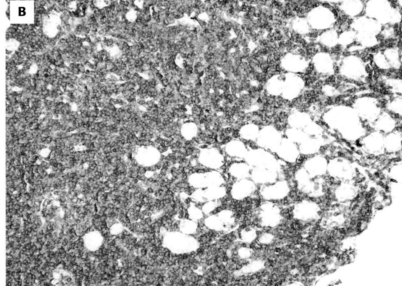

FIGURE 21-3

Immunohistochemical features of mucosa-associated lymphoid tissue (MALT) lymphoma. Immunohistochemical staining highlights a dense B-cell infiltrate highlighted by CD20 **(A)** with aberrant coexpression of CD43 **(B),** while CD3 highlights the scattered reactive T-cells in the background.

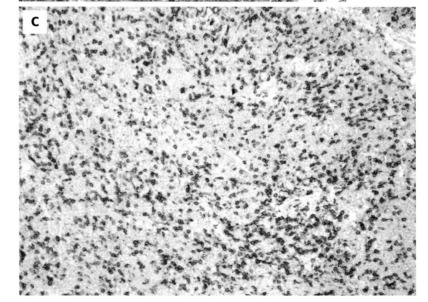

The presence or absence of *Helicobacter* organisms should be documented, for clinical management of the patient and further substantiation of the process leading to MALT development.

Four recurrent chromosomal translocations are recognized in MALT lymphomas: t(11;18)(q21;q21)/API2-MALT1, t(1;14)(p22;q32)/IgH-BCL10, t(14;18)(q34;q21)/IgH-MALT1, and t(3;14)(p14.1;q32). *H. pylori*-related gastric MALT lymphoma is most commonly associated with t(11;18) translocation. It is suspected that early low-grade forms of MALT carry trisomy of chromosomes 3, 12, and 18, leading to the subsequent emergence of a higher-grade B-cell clone.

DIFFERENTIAL DIAGNOSIS

The differential diagnosis of MALT lymphomas in the stomach includes a reactive lymphoid process and lymphocytic gastritis. Reactive lymphoid aggregates can be distinguished from MALT lymphomas by their normal cytologic features and normal immunophenotype, as described. In lymphocytic gastritis, despite a prominent inflammatory infiltrate, the absence of lymphoepithelial lesions and cytologic features of the infiltrate should reliably distinguish this lesion from lymphoma. Additionally, the infiltrate of lymphocytic gastritis is T-cell rich (CD3 and CD5 positive), unlike the B-cell infiltrate in MALT (CD20 positive). Gene rearrangement analysis may be needed to diagnose difficult cases.

PROGNOSIS AND THERAPY

Long-term remissions can be induced in low-grade MALT lymphomas in 70% to 80% of cases. The lymphomas that are most likely to respond to *H. pylori* eradication by antibiotics are those that are located superficially within the gastric mucosa. Certain genetic abnormalities, such as t(11;18) and BCL-10 mutation, may be associated with lack of response to this therapy. Recurrences of low-grade lymphoma are encountered in patients treated by *H. pylori* eradication, but these appear to be infrequent and may be self-limiting and regress spontaneously without further therapy. Transformation to diffuse large B-cell lymphoma may occur.

■ DIFFUSE LARGE B-CELL LYMPHOMA

CLINICAL FEATURES

Diffuse large B-cell lymphoma (DLBCL) of the GI tract is most frequent in the stomach. No good survey data are available on the incidence of DLBCL. Some cases show histologic evidence of coincident low-grade B-cell

---

DIFFUSE LARGE B-CELL LYMPHOMA—FACT SHEET

Definition
- High-grade B-cell neoplasm composed of large, pleomorphic B-cells with a diffuse growth pattern

Incidence and Location
- Most commonly involves the stomach but can be anywhere in the GI tract

Morbidity and Mortality
- Aggressive clinical behavior
- Mortality varies with extent of disease and other clinical parameters

Gender, Race, and Age Distribution
- Median age is in the sixth to seventh decade
- Slightly more common in males than in females

Clinical Features
- Presents with pain, dyspepsia, sometimes asymptomatic
- Rapidly enlarging mass may cause site-specific symptoms

Prognosis and Treatment
- Preliminary data suggest that gastric DLBCL may be effectively treated with antibiotics
- Aggressive but potentially curable with multiagent chemotherapy
- Overall survival is approximately 50%

DIFFUSE LARGE B-CELL LYMPHOMA—PATHOLOGIC FEATURES

Gross Findings
- Ulcerative or mass-forming lesion

Microscopic Findings
- Diffuse infiltration by large lymphoid cells
- Most commonly have oval to round vesicular nuclei with multiple nucleoli and scant to moderate cytoplasm
- Effacement of normal structures

Immunohistochemical
- CD20+ B-cells with a Ki-67 proliferation index greater than 40% to 50%
- Variable coexpression of CD10, BCL-6, BCL-2, and MUM-1

Differential Diagnosis
- Burkitt and Burkitt-like lymphoma
- Poorly differentiate carcinomas

---

lymphoma; the WHO classification indicates that the two should be diagnosed separately and discourages use of the term *high-grade MALT lymphoma*. One study reported that primary gastric lymphomas, including many DLBCL, were more often symptomatic than secondary lymphomas. However, low-grade and high-grade lymphomas do not differ significantly in the type of symptoms or clinical presentation. *Helicobacter* infection undoubtedly plays a role in DLBCL arising from indolent MALT lymphoma, but whether it is directly involved in the transformation process or whether *H. pylori* is involved in de novo gastric DLBCL is unclear.

PATHOLOGIC FEATURES

GROSS FINDINGS

Macroscopic findings in the stomach include gastric body and antrum locations and unifocal disease, particularly in patients with primary disease. The diffusely infiltrative pattern is relatively less common in DLBCL than in low-grade MALT lymphoma. Most cases present with polypoid or ulcerative lesions. Nongastric disease has a similar gross appearance. The majority of gastric DLBCL has spread to adjacent nodes by the time of diagnosis.

MICROSCOPIC FINDINGS

The definitional feature of DLBCL in the GI tract does not differ from disease in other sites (e.g., sheets of B-cell immunoblasts or centroblasts) (Fig. 21-4). The extent of the clusters of large cells varies, with some cases exhibiting only a few fields of large cell lymphoma and others showing massive infiltration and destruction of the bowel wall. There may or may not be lymphoepithelial lesions. Gastric DLBCL, in particular, may show coincident low-grade MALT lymphoma. In most cases examined, these two entities are clonally related, both by light chain restriction and at the DNA sequence level. As with systemic DLBCL, the immunologic profile may suggest either a follicle center origin (CD10 or BCL-6 positive) or a non-follicle center origin. The absence of CD5, CD10, and BCL-6 raises the possibility of origin from a MALT lymphoma.

ANCILLARY STUDIES

Gene rearrangement analysis, with or without microdissection, may reveal genetic identity of a DLBCL with an underlying MALT lymphoma. However, this is not clinically important because there is no difference in behavior of de novo DLBCL and large cell lymphoma transformed from MALT lymphoma. As with other low-grade lymphomas that transform, a minority of GI tract DLBCL carry mutations or loss of p53 and p16. Classic cytogenetics and array-based analysis suggest that there are at least two pathways to lymphomagenesis in the stomach, with t(11;18) (API2/MALT1) lymphomas remaining low grade and tumors with chromosomal instability and no t(11;18) having the potential to progress to DLBCL.

DIFFERENTIAL DIAGNOSIS

It is most important to distinguish primary DLBCL from secondary lymphoma. Immunohistochemistry can provide some assistance if the tumor cells have a follicle center phenotype, but this is primarily a clinical and radiographic distinction. The occasional case with a particularly cohesive appearance or an infiltrative pattern may raise the differential of carcinoma, but this is easily excluded by immunohistochemistry.

PROGNOSIS AND THERAPY

Standard therapy for GI tract DLBCL tracks the approach in nodal DLBCL: chemotherapy with rituximab and CHOP (cyclophosphamide, doxorubicin, vincristine, and prednisone). This may be followed by radiation therapy. Surgery—in the past a common therapeutic approach—has generally fallen out of favor except for rare cases with extensive hemorrhage or perforation. The role of antibiotic therapy in aggressive large cell lymphoma of the stomach has not been extensively studied, but several groups report lasting regression of DLBCL with MALT lymphoma after antibiotic therapy alone (albeit not as often as in pure MALT lymphoma).

■ IMMUNOPROLIFERATIVE SMALL INTESTINAL DISEASE

Immunoproliferative small intestinal disease (alpha heavy chain disease, Mediterranean lymphoma, and diffuse small intestinal lymphoma) is a special form of MALT lymphoma restricted to a limited geographic distribution, which is characterized by synthesis of a mutated alpha heavy chain immunoglobulin without corresponding light chains.

CLINICAL FEATURES

IPSID typically afflicts young adults and is slightly more common in males. It is seen almost exclusively in the Middle East and Mediterranean regions. Common risk factors include low socioeconomic status, endemic parasitic infestation, poor sanitation, and infantile infectious enteritis. *Campylobacter jejuni* has been proposed as an infectious trigger to IPSID, analogous to *Helicobacter* and gastric MALT, but there is not agreement on this. Some genetic factors have also been implicated. Presentation is typically severe malabsorption with chronic severe intermittent diarrhea and weight loss. Nearly half of patients experience peripheral edema, tetany, and clubbing of fingers. Alpha heavy chain paraproteinemia (α heavy chain without associated light chain) is present in up to 70% of IPSID cases, which are at their highest levels early in the course and may diminish with progression of disease.

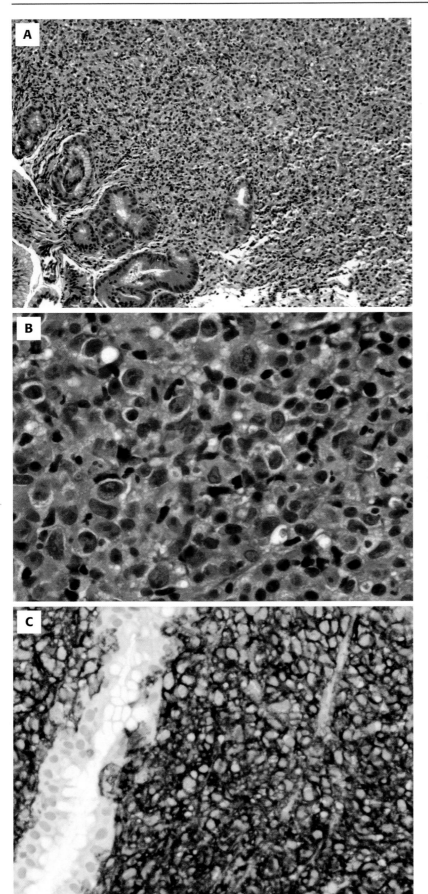

FIGURE 21-4

Diffuse large B-cell lymphoma. **A,** At low magnification, a dense lymphoid infiltrate with a pushing border is noted. **B,** The infiltrate is composed of sheets of pleomorphic large cells with prominent nucleoli and moderate amounts of cytoplasm. **C,** Immunohistochemical stain for CD20 shows a membranous staining pattern of the B-cells and emphasizes the pleomorphic nature of the cells.

PATHOLOGIC FEATURES

GROSS FINDINGS

IPSID is generally a diffuse infiltrating lesion; initially, the mucosa may appear normal and then develop a cobblestone appearance. Eventually, lymphomatous masses may form, leading to polyp formation. Mesenteric lymph node involvement happens early in the course. The primary site of involvement is the proximal small intestine, but IPSID may involve any part of or the entire small intestine. The stomach and colon can also be involved.

MICROSCOPIC FINDINGS

IPSID demonstrates a histologic spectrum ranging from low- to high-grade histology, divided into stages A through C. All stages exhibit at least some features typical of other MALT lymphomas, but they tend to have more marked plasma cell differentiation.

Stage A is characterized by a lymphoplasmacytic infiltrate with features of a typical MALT lymphoma (reactive follicles with parafollicular clusters of clear cells and lymphoepithelial lesions) that is confined to the mucosa and expands the lamina propria, causing broad villi (Fig. 21-5). Mesenteric lymph nodes may be involved. In stage B disease, the infiltrate becomes nodular and extends beyond the mucosa into the submucosa. The macroscopic appearance at this stage is typically abnormal, with thickened mucosal folds. Stage C is characterized by the presence of large masses and transformation to large cell lymphoma.

Lymph node involvement is initially seen as mature plasma cells that fill the sinuses and then progresses to infiltration of the marginal zone and colonization of follicle centers.

ANCILLARY STUDIES

The lymphoma cells are CD20+, CD5−, CD10−, and CD23−. Alpha immunoglobulin heavy chains can be demonstrated in the cytoplasm of the infiltrating plasma cells, centrocytes, and transformed large cells.

DIFFERENTIAL DIAGNOSIS

The differential considerations depend on the stage of IPSID. The early disease (stage A) may have a similar appearance to gluten sensitive enteropathy

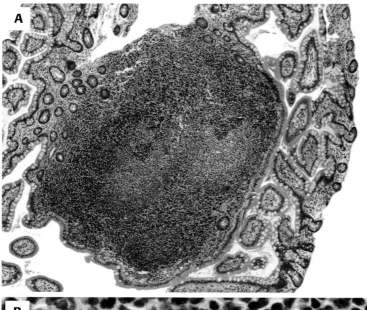

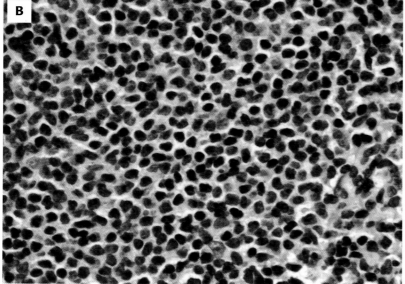

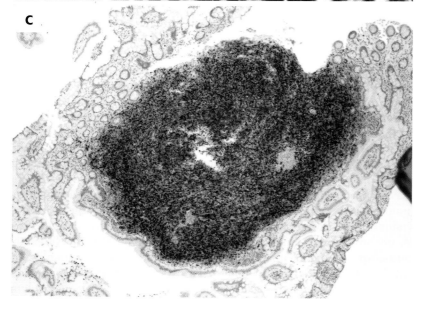

FIGURE 21-6

A, Mantle cell lymphoma often forms polypoid masses in the gastrointestinal tract (lymphomatous polyposis). **B,** At high magnification, the infiltrate is composed of a monomorphic population of small lymphocytes with minimally irregular nuclei. Note the absence of large lymphs. **C,** Immunohistochemical stain for cyclin D1 displays nuclear staining of the neoplastic cells with sparing of residual germinal centers seen in the middle of the infiltrate.

ANCILLARY STUDIES

The tumor cells are CD20+ B-cells that are CD5+, CD43+, BCL-2+, CD10− and CD23−. Nuclear cyclin D-1 (BCL-1) is virtually always present if properly performed (see Fig. 21-6C). Surface light chains are present (usually IgM or IgD) and are typically lambda restricted.

Chromosomal translocation t(11;14)(q13;q32) between the cyclin D1 gene and the IGH gene is the most sensitive and specific measure and can be demonstrated in almost all cases.

DIFFERENTIAL DIAGNOSIS

The main diagnostic considerations are other low-grade lymphomas, primarily follicular lymphoma (FL). Both MCL and FL can present as polypoid masses and appear histologically as nodular lesions. Although MCL cells have slightly irregular nuclear outlines, they lack the nuclear irregularities typical of FL (Fig. 21-7). Immunohistochemical stains are useful to distinguish MCL and FL: MCL is CD5+, cyclin D1+, and CD10− whereas FL is CD10+, CD5−, and cyclin D1−. Follicular lymphoma also may express BCL6 and BCL2. The mantle zone pattern and diffuse pattern are more easily recognized as MCL. Patients typically have systemic disease as well, so clinical history can be very helpful.

PROGNOSIS AND THERAPY

Although systemic chemotherapy is the treatment of choice, MCL is presently considered incurable, with a median survival of 3 to 5 years. Aggressive chemotherapy followed by autologous stem cell transplantation may benefit younger patients. Surgery has a relatively small role in the management of this disease but may be necessary to relieve bowel obstruction.

■ BURKITT LYMPHOMA

Burkitt lymphoma (BL) is a highly aggressive B-cell neoplasm that occurs in three major clinical forms: endemic, sporadic, and immunodeficiency associated. All three types present primarily in extranodal sites, including the GI tract.

CLINICAL FEATURES

Endemic BL is found primarily in Africa, where it is the most common childhood malignancy and has a male predominance (males to females, 2:1). It typically presents with jaw, orbit, or paraspinal lesions and is strongly associated with Epstein-Barr virus (EBV) infection. It is unusual for African endemic BL to affect the GI tract. However, in other endemic regions (particularly the Middle East), BL frequently presents with intestinal obstruction or intussusception due to ileocecal involvement.

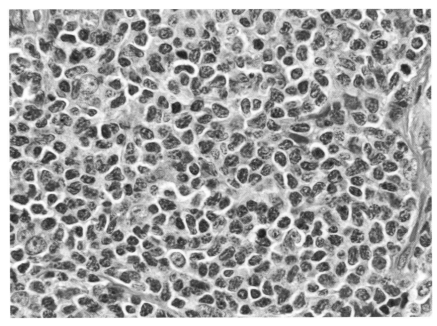

FIGURE 21-7

Follicular lymphoma. The neoplastic infiltrate is composed of mixture of small centrocytes with nuclear irregularities and no nucleoli and larger centroblasts with vesicular chromatin and prominent nucleoli.

BURKITT LYMPHOMA (BL)—FACT SHEET

Definition

- Highly aggressive B-cell neoplasm
- Occurs in three major clinical forms: endemic, sporadic, and immunodeficiency associated
- All three types may present in the GI tract

Incidence and Location

- Endemic
  - Primarily in Africa, but also seen in other areas rarely
  - Associated with EBV infection in nearly all cases
  - Most common childhood malignancy in endemic areas
- Sporadic
  - Seen throughout the industrialized societies
  - Associated with EBV infection <30% of cases
  - 1% to 2% of all lymphomas, 30% to 50% childhood lymphomas
- Immunodeficiency associated
  - Seen throughout the world—associated with HIV infection
  - Associated EBV infection in 25% to 40% of cases
  - BL can be seen in other non-HIV immunodeficiency states, but not as often

Gender, Race, and Age Distribution

- Endemic
  - Disease of childhood
  - Male predominance (males-to-females, 2:1)
- Sporadic
  - Wider age distribution, half of cases children, and remaining young adults
  - Male predominance (males-to-females, 2:1)
  - Immunodeficiency associated
  - Primarily seen in association with HIV infection, less often other immunodeficiency conditions

Clinical Features

- All subtypes—bulky disease and frequently widespread with bone marrow involvement and acute leukemia common
- Endemic
- Mass in the jaw, orbit, or paraspinal lesion; GI tract involvement less common, usually ileocecal
- Sporadic
  - Children: abdominal mass, typically in ileocecal region, causes abdominal pain and obstructive symptoms
  - Adults: tumors found in any part of GI tract, most common in the ileocecal region and the rectum

Prognosis and Treatment

- Highly aggressive tumor, but potentially curable in the majority of patients
- Prognosis depends on stage and is generally better in children
- Mainstay of treatment is intensive combination chemotherapy regimens
- Prognosis for HIV-associated Burkitt-like lymphomas is related more to HIV syndrome
- Surgical therapy has a role in treatment for obstruction/intussusception and debulking

BURKITT LYMPHOMA (BL)—PATHOLOGIC FEATURES

Gross Findings

- Predilection for the ileocecal region and less often rectum and stomach
- Bulky masses typically replace normal structures in areas of involvement
- Solid glistening white cut surface (fish flesh appearing) often associated with hemorrhage and necrosis
- Lymph nodes not usually involved but instead are surrounded by tumor

Microscopic Findings

- Round nuclei with finely clumped chromatin and contain three to four centrally located small basophilic nucleoli
- Scant cytoplasm
- Cytoplasmic vacuoles on touch and smear preparations
- Extremely high proliferation rate
- Tingle-body macrophages yielding a "starry sky" appearance

Immunohistochemistry

- CD20+, CD10+, CD5−, BCL-2− and TdT−
- Ki-67 labeling is seen in nearly 100% of cells

Differential Diagnosis

- Diffuse large cell lymphoma
- Lymphoblastic lymphoma

is at least 2:1, and about one third of cases are associated with EBV infection, particularly early in life. Sporadic BL frequently presents as an abdominal mass due to primary intestinal involvement (usually ileocecal), typically causing abdominal pain and obstructive symptoms. In adults, tumors can arise at any site in the GI system but are most common in the ileocecal region and rectum.

Immunodeficiency-associated BL is primarily seen with human immunodeficiency virus (HIV) infection, often as the first manifestation of AIDS. One quarter to one half of cases are associated with EBV infection. BL can be seen in other non-HIV immunodeficiency states, but not as often.

Small bowel contrast radiography or CT scan may suggest the diagnosis. However, laparotomy is often required for confirmation. In selected cases, colonoscopic retrograde intubation of the terminal ileum and biopsy may be diagnostic. Unlike for other lymphomas, CT-guided biopsy can be attempted because BL often forms bulky masses. The bone marrow is often involved; therefore, examination of the bone marrow and peripheral blood may be diagnostic and may obviate the need for laparotomy or other biopsy procedures.

PATHOLOGIC FEATURES

GROSS FINDINGS

GI tract BL of all clinical types has a predilection for the ileocecal region and less often the rectum and stomach. It is characterized by bulky tumor masses that typically

Sporadic BL is seen throughout the industrialized world, where it exhibits a wider age distribution. Half of the cases involve children, and the remaining cases occur in young adults. For endemic BL, the male-to-female ratio

replace areas of involvement. These masses have a solid glistening white cut surface ("fish flesh" appearing) that is often associated with hemorrhage and necrosis. Lymph nodes are often surprisingly uninvolved but are instead enveloped by tumor.

MICROSCOPIC FINDINGS

The tumor shows a monomorphous infiltrate of medium-sized lymphocytes with round nuclei, finely clumped chromatin, several small nucleoli, and scant cytoplasm. Numerous admixed macrophages with ingested apoptotic tumor cells, so-called tingible body macrophages, are present, leading to a "starry sky" appearance (Fig. 21-8A). On cytologic, smear and touch preparations, the cytoplasm is deeply basophilic with characteristic cytoplasmic lipid vacuoles. Some cases may be associated with a florid granulomatous reaction.

ANCILLARY STUDIES

The tumors cells are CD20+, CD10+, BCL6+, CD43+, CD5−, BCL-2−, and TdT−. A definitional feature, Ki-67 labeling is seen in nearly 100% of cells (see Fig. 21-8B). Tumor infiltrating CD3+ T-cells are typically less common than in diffuse large B-cell lymphoma.

Three MYC translocations characterize BL; they involve translocation of the MYC oncogene on chromosome 8q24 to the heavy chain gene on chromosome 14q32 (t8;14) or less commonly to one of the light chain genes on 2q11 t(2;8) or 22q11 t(8;22). MYC deregulation through the translocation is believed to play an important role in the tumorigenesis by accelerating cells through the cell cycle. The EBV genome can be demonstrated in nearly all endemic cases, 25% to 40% of immunodeficiency cases, and less than 30% of sporadic cases.

DIFFERENTIAL DIAGNOSIS

Other high-grade lymphomas need to be considered. Diffuse large B-cell lymphoma is significantly more pleomorphic than BL and will not have the 100% labeling with Ki-67 typical of BL. Lymphoblastic lymphoma lacks mature B-cell markers (e.g., CD20) and is TdT+. In the GI tract, MYC gene translocations are essentially restricted to cases of BL.

PROGNOSIS AND THERAPY

BL is a highly aggressive tumor but is potentially curable in the majority of patients. Prognosis depends on stage and is generally better in children. The mainstay of treatment is intensive combination chemotherapy regimens that result in a 90% cure rate in low-stage disease and a 60% to 80% cure rate in advanced-stage disease. The prognosis for HIV-associated Burkitt-like lymphomas is related more to the underlying HIV pathology than to the lymphoma itself. Even patients with Burkitt leukemia and those with central nervous system involvement can be cured. Surgical therapy has a role in treatment when debulking or decompression is required.

■ T-CELL LYMPHOMAS

Intestinal T-cell lymphomas are far less common than those of B-cell origin. The majority of T-cell primary GI lymphomas occurs in the setting of gluten-sensitive enteropathy (GSE) and is specifically referred to as enteropathy-associated T-cell lymphoma (EATL). Although other T-cell lymphomas only infrequently involve the GI tract, the liver is more commonly affected. Hepatosplenic T-cell lymphoma, in particular, frequently involves the liver and as the spleen.

ENTEROPATHY-ASSOCIATED T-CELL LYMPHOMA

CLINICAL FEATURES

EATL is rare (approximately 5% of all GI tract lymphomas) and is associated with a history of gluten-sensitive enteropathy (GSE) or celiac disease. Although it may present after a long-standing history of GSE, it is more commonly seen in adult celiac disease or in association with dermatitis herpetiformis. The mean age of patients with EATL is 60 years, with no gender predilection. The geographic distribution of EATL follows that of GSE, with the highest incidence in Northern Europe. Immunodeficiency states are not known to be associated with EATL. In 10% to 20% of cases, the lymphoma is composed of monomorphic medium-sized cells. This monomorphic variant, designated type II EATL, may occur sporadically without risk factors for GSE and has a broader geographic distribution.

The most common presentation of EATL is a several-month to several-year history of abdominal pain and weight loss. About 40% present acutely with bleeding, obstruction, or perforation. Clinical deterioration of celiac disease, despite compliance with a gluten-free diet, should raise the possibility of lymphoma. Many patients presenting with EATL appear to have subclinical GSE, and thus all patients with T-cell lymphoma of the gut likely should be tested for underlying, previously unrecognized celiac disease.

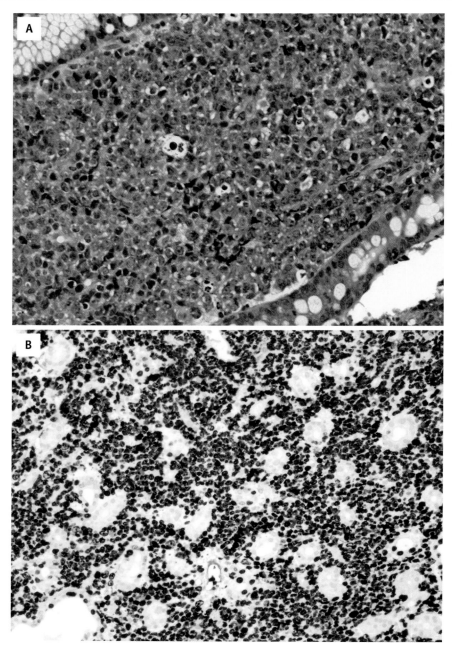

FIGURE 21-8

Burkitt lymphoma. **A,** The neoplastic infiltrate is composed of a highly monotonous, monomorphic population of medium-sized lymphocytes with round nuclei, finely clumped chromatin, several small nucleoli, and scant cytoplasm. Admixed tingible-body macrophages containing apoptotic debris lead to a "starry-sky" appearance within the dense infiltrate. **B,** An immunohistochemical stain for Ki-67 shows nuclear positivity in virtually all neoplastic cells, corresponding to a high proliferative index.

ENTEROPATHY-ASSOCIATED T-CELL LYMPHOMA—FACT SHEET

Definition
- An intestinal T-cell lymphoma associated with gluten-sensitive enteropathy, it carries a poor prognosis

Incidence and Location
- Rare, approximately 5% of all GI tract lymphomas
- Geographic distribution follows that of GSE, highest incidence in Northern Europe

Gender, Race, and Age Distribution
- Mean age 60 years
- No particular sex predilection

Clinical Features
- Typical presentation: several month to year history of abdominal pain and weight loss
- May present acutely with acute bleeding, obstruction, or perforation
- Deterioration of celiac disease may herald the presence of lymphoma
- GSE history typically of recent onset
- Subclinical GSE may be present
- Most have localized intestinal disease with or without contiguous lymph node involvement
- Disseminated disease has predilection for liver, spleen, lung, testes, and skin

Prognosis and Treatment
- Prognosis is poor (median survival 3 months; 5-year survival 10%)
- Patients suffer complications of peritonitis and malnutrition, and later from progressive disease

ENTEROPATHY-ASSOCIATED T-CELL LYMPHOMA—PATHOLOGIC FEATURES

Gross Findings
- Most common in jejunum, alone or in combination with other sites in the GI tract
- Affected bowel segment is often dilated and edematous
- Large circumferential ulcers, ulcerated plaques, and strictures with intervening areas of normal mucosa
- Bulky exophytic or infiltrating masses are not typical but can be seen
- Mesenteric lymph node involvement is common

Microscopic Findings
- Variable between individual cases and between different sites in the same patient
- Monotonous medium-sized to large cells with round or angulated vesicular nuclei, prominent nucleoli, and moderate to abundant pale-staining cytoplasm
- Less commonly, marked pleomorphism with multinucleated cells
- Inflammatory infiltrate of histiocytes and eosinophils
- Destruction of the overlying epithelium by the lymphoma cells
- Upper and intermediate villous regions are most affected
- Background mucosa shows changes of GSE (intraepithelial lymphocytosis, increased lamina propria lymphocytes and plasma cells, villous blunting, and crypt hyperplasia)
- Monomorphic form of EATL (type II EATL):
  - Medium-sized round, darkly staining nuclei with a rim of pale cytoplasm
  - Florid infiltration of intestinal crypt epithelium
  - Inflammatory background is usually absent

Immunohistochemistry
- Most cases are CD3+, CD4−, CD8−, CD7+, CD5−, and express cytotoxic granule associated protein TIA-1, often with granzyme B
- CD56 used to describe two variants: Type A CD56− and type B CD56+ (and CD8+)
- Both the medium to large pleomorphic and the anaplastic variants of ETL are usually type A (CD56−) often with CD30 positive, but are always ALK1 negative
- Most of the type B (CD56+) lymphomas are the small to medium-sized variant

Differential Diagnosis
- Celiac disease
- Diffuse large B-cell lymphoma
- Extranodal natural killer cell lymphoma
- Peripheral T-cell lymphoma, NOS
- Poorly differentiated malignancies (melanoma, carcinoma)

Most patients present with localized intestinal disease with or without contiguous lymph node involvement. Dissemination, when present, has a predilection for liver, spleen, lung, testes, and skin, but only rarely the bone marrow.

Endoscopy with biopsy is the diagnostic test of choice. When endoscopy is not feasible or nondiagnostic, laparotomy may be necessary to confirm the diagnosis.

PATHOLOGIC FEATURES

GROSS FINDINGS

EATL occurs most commonly in the jejunum, alone or in combination with other sites in the GI tract. The affected bowel segment is often dilated and edematous, with large circumferential ulcers, ulcerated plaques, and strictures with intervening areas of normal mucosa. Bulky, exophytic, or infiltrating masses are not typical but may be seen on occasion. Mesenteric lymph node involvement is common. Adhesion formation between loops of bowel can be present.

MICROSCOPIC FINDINGS

The histologic appearance of EATL is variable between individual cases and between different sites in the same patient. Most commonly, the tumor cells are relatively monotonous medium-sized to large cells with round or angulated vesicular nuclei, prominent nucleoli, and moderate to abundant pale-staining cytoplasm (Figs. 21-9 and 21-10). Less commonly, the tumor exhibits marked pleomorphism with multinucleated cells bearing a resemblance

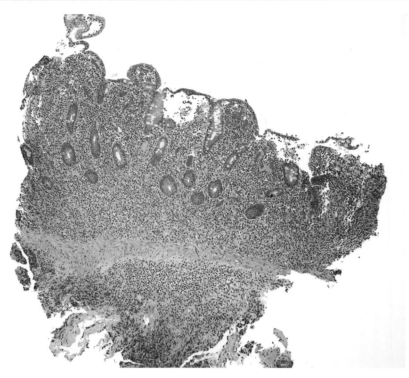

FIGURE 21-9

Enteropathy-associated T-cell lymphoma (EATL). The small intestine shows transmural involvement with marked architectural effacement by a diffuse proliferation of neoplastic T-cells.

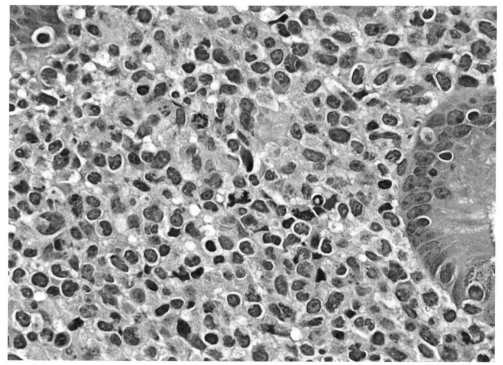

FIGURE 21-10

Enteropathy-associated T-cell lymphoma (EATL). At higher magnification, the infiltrate is composed of monotonous medium-sized to large cells with round or angulated vesicular nuclei, prominent nucleoli and moderate to abundant pale-staining cytoplasm. Numerous mitotic figures are present.

to anaplastic large cell lymphoma. An accompanying inflammatory infiltrate of histiocytes and eosinophils is usually seen. All the subtypes are associated with destruction of the overlying epithelium by the lymphoma cells. The areas of epithelium most affected are the upper and intermediate villous regions or, in the presence of villous atrophy, the upper aspect of the crypts. In the majority of cases, endoscopically normal background mucosa shows changes of GSE (intraepithelial lymphocytosis, increased lamina propria lymphocytes and plasma cells, villous blunting, and crypt hyperplasia) (Fig. 21-11).

In the monomorphic form of EATL (type II EATL), the neoplastic cells have medium-sized round, darkly staining nuclei with a rim of pale cytoplasm. There is usually florid infiltration of intestinal crypt epithelium, but the inflammatory background is absent.

In cases of refractory GSE or celiac disease where the intraepithelial lymphocytes show immunophenotypic features such as loss of CD8, monoclonal TCR rearrangements, or gains of chromosome 1q, the lesion is considered intraepithelial T-cell lymphoma or EATL in situ.

ANCILLARY STUDIES

Most cases are CD3+, CD5−, CD7+, CD4−, CD8−, CD103+, and CD56− and express cytotoxic granule–associated protein TIA-1, often with granzyme B. The monomorphic variant, in contrast, is CD3+, CD4−, CD8+, and CD56+. The immunohistochemical labeling pattern of EATL correlates to some extent with the histologic pattern. In almost all cases a varying proportion of the tumor cells are CD30+.

More than 90% of patients have HLA DQA1*0501 or DQB1*0201. Complex segmental amplifications of chromosome 9q31 or deletions of 16q12 are prevalent. The classic form of EATL displays gains of 1q and 5q, whereas the monomorphic variant is characterized by 8q24 (MYC) amplification.

DIFFERENTIAL DIAGNOSIS

Celiac disease also is a diffuse disease with prominent intraepithelial lymphocytes but lacks erosions and ulcerations and lacks aberrant T-cell antigen expression by immunohistochemistry and T-cell clonality by gene rearrangement studies. Diffuse large B-cell lymphoma usually forms masses and is clearly distinguished by immunohistochemistry. Extranodal natural killer cell lymphoma and peripheral T-cell lymphoma, not otherwise specified, are more difficult to distinguish; the absence of clinical features of GSE is helpful. Poorly differentiated malignancies (melanoma, carcinoma) can be sorted out by morphologic features and immunohistochemical stains.

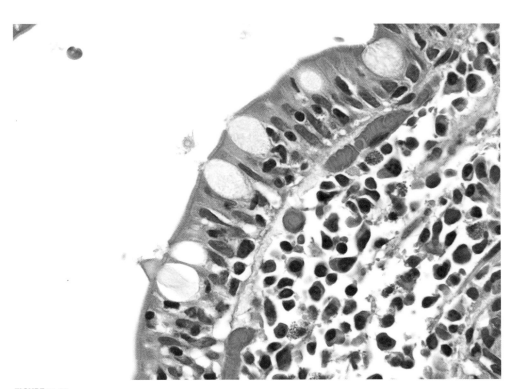

FIGURE 21-11

Intraepithelial lymphocytes in enteropathy-associated T-cell lymphoma (EATL). Microscopic evidence of epithelial infiltration by the neoplastic T-cells is seen in endoscopically normal areas adjacent to those involved by EATL.

PROGNOSIS AND THERAPY

The prognosis is dismal, with a median survival of only 3 months and 5-year survival rates of approximately 10%. Patients suffer complications of peritonitis and malnutrition initially and later from progressive disease. A significant number of patients cannot tolerate chemotherapy due to underlying malabsorption. Factors associated with long-term survival include absence of a previous diagnosis of GSE and tolerance of a complete course of chemotherapy.

HEPATOSPLENIC T-CELL LYMPHOMA

CLINICAL FEATURES

Hepatosplenic T-cell lymphoma (HSTL) is rare neoplasm that involves the sinusoids of the liver, spleen, and bone marrow. It occurs largely in adolescents and young adults with a male predilection. Approximately 10% to 20% of patients have a history of immunosuppression, including solid organ transplantation, Hodgkin lymphoma, acute myelogenous leukemia, inflammatory bowel disease treated with azathioprine or infliximab, and malaria infection.

Initial presentation includes splenomegaly, usually with concomitant hepatomegaly, marked thrombocytopenia, and systemic symptoms such as fever, abdominal pain, and weakness. Anemia may also be present. Slight elevations in liver function tests (AST, ALT, and alkaline phosphatase) and marked elevations in lactate dehydrogenase levels may be observed.

PATHOLOGIC FEATURES

GROSS AND MICROSCOPIC FINDINGS

Diffuse hepatic and splenic enlargement are noted with no discrete nodules. The lymphoma predominantly involves the red pulp of the spleen. The liver shows sinusoidal infiltration by tumor cells with relative sparing of portal triads (Fig. 21-12A). The infiltrate consists of a monotonous population of cells with medium-sized nuclei, small inconspicuous nucleoli, and a rim of pale cytoplasm (see Fig. 21-12B). Occasional mitotic figures and single-cell necrosis may be noted. Cytologic atypia with large cell changes may be seen, especially with disease progression.

ANCILLARY STUDIES

The commonly reported T-cell phenotype is CD2+, CD3+, CD4−, CD5−, CD7+/−, CD8−, with gamma-delta T-cell receptor expression (see Fig. 21-12C). CD7

HEPATOSPLENIC T-CELL LYMPHOMA—FACT SHEET

Definition
- Extranodal and systemic neoplasm of cytotoxic T-cells

Incidence and Location
- Up to 20% arise in the setting of chronic immune suppression
- Involves the spleen, liver, and bone marrow

Gender, Race, and Age Distribution
- Peak incidence in adolescents and young adults
- Male predominance
- Median age of 35 years

Clinical Features
- Marked splenomegaly usually with hepatomegaly
- No lymphadenopathy
- Thrombocytopenia often with anemia and leukopenia
- Systemic symptoms

Prognosis and Treatment
- Aggressive course
- Initial response to chemotherapy
- Median survival < 2 years

HEPATOSPLENIC T-CELL LYMPHOMA—PATHOLOGIC FEATURES

Gross Findings
- No gross lesions
- Diffuse enlargement of spleen and liver

Microscopic Findings
- Monotonous lymphocytes with medium-sized nuclei and a rim of pale cytoplasm
- Diffuse involvement of the cords and sinuses of the splenic red pulp
- Splenic white pulp atrophy
- Hepatic sinusoid involvement
- Cytologic atypia with large cell or blastic changes seen in disease progression

Immunohistochemistry
- Usually γδ T-cell receptor type, but a minority are αβ type
- CD3+, CD56+/−, CD4−, CD8-/+, and CD5−
- Express cytotoxic granule associated proteins, TIA1, and granzyme M
- Negative for granzyme B and perforin

Genetic Abnormalities
- Isochromosome 7q is present in most cases
- EBV is usually negative

Differential Diagnosis
- Extranodal natural killer cell lymphoma
- Peripheral T-cell lymphoma, NOS

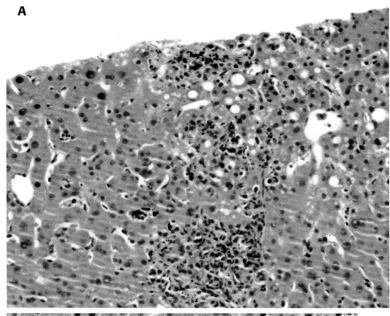

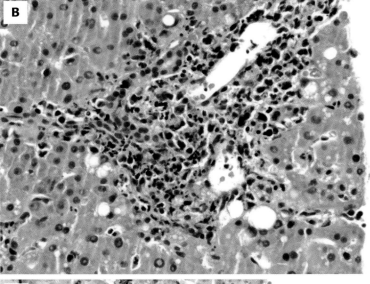

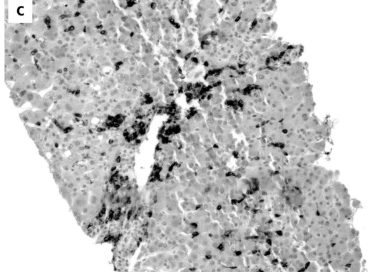

FIGURE 21-12

Hepatosplenic T-cell lymphoma. **A,** A core biopsy of the liver shows a lymphocytic infiltrate involving the sinusoids with relative sparing of the portal triads. **B,** At higher power, the infiltrate is composed of a monotonous population of cells with medium-sized nuclei, small inconspicuous nucleoli, and a rim of pale cytoplasm. Scattered single-cell necrosis with apoptotic bodies is also seen. **C,** An immunohistochemical stain for CD3 highlights the predominantly sinusoidal pattern of infiltration by the neoplastic T-lymphocytes.

expression may be lost during treatment. NK cell markers, CD56 and CD16, are often expressed, but CD57 is usually negative. The cells also express the cytotoxic granule-associated proteins, TIA1 and granzyme M. EBV is generally negative.

Although most cases are derived from T-cells in the gamma-delta T-cell receptor (TCR) class, a minority of cases in the alpha-beta TCR class have been reported. Isochromosome 7q is a recurrent chromosomal abnormality observed in most cases of HSTL. Trisomy 8 and loss of a sex chromosome have also been reported.

DIFFERENTIAL DIAGNOSIS

The differential diagnosis of hepatosplenic T-cell lymphoma includes aggressive NK leukemia/lymphoma. This disease also presents with marked hepatosplenomegaly and has an aggressive clinical course. The tumor cells in NK-cell lymphoproliferative disorders are immunophenotypically similar to HSTL, but they lack expression of a T-cell receptor and CD3. The tumor cells share many functional and phenotypic similarities with NK cells and NK-like cytotoxic T-cells, and therefore, clinical overlap among these malignancies is perhaps not surprising. Morphologic overlap is seen as well, although the exquisite localization of the HSTL tumor cells within sinusoids in spleen and bone marrow is a feature not seen in other large granular lymphocyte disorders.

PROGNOSIS AND THERAPY

The clinical course is aggressive with a dismal prognosis. Patients may initially respond to chemotherapy, but there is a high relapse rate and a short median survival of 8 months.

Index